OPTIMUM VITAMIN NUTRITION

for More Sustainable Ruminant Farming

OPTIMUM VITAMIN NUTRITION

for More Sustainable Ruminant Farming

S. Calsamiglia, E.O. Oviedo-Rondon, L. Tamassia, G. Litta
and J.M. Hernandez

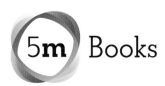

First published 2024

Copyright © dsm-firmenich 2024

Published by
5M Books Ltd
Lings, Great Easton
Essex CM6 2HH, UK
Tel: +44 (0)330 1333 580
www.5mbooks.com

Follow us on
X @5m_Books
Instagram 5m_books
Facebook @5mBooks
LinkedIn @5mbooks

A catalogue record for this book is available from the British Library

ISBN 9781789183566
eISBN 9781789183665
DOI 10.52517/9781789183566

Book layout by Cheshire Typesetting Ltd, Cuddington, Cheshire
Printed by Bell & Bain Ltd, Glasgow

This book is dedicated in memory of Prof. Sergio Calsamiglia (1964–2023)

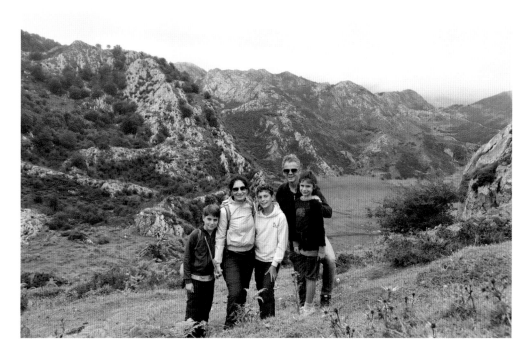

Sergio graduated in veterinary medicine at the UAB (Autonomous University of Barcelona, Spain) and followed his master and doctorate studies at the University of Minnesota (USA).

He was a member of the Animal Nutrition and Welfare Service (SNiBA) of the Autonomous University of Barcelona and his specialty was the nutrition and management of dairy cattle.

Sergio initiated his collaboration in the first version of this vitamin book in 2012 and, since then, participated in the different updates, with this current publication in 2024 unfortunately being the last one.

Sergio was not only an excellent and dedicated professional full of enthusiasm and joy, with always an extremely positive attitude. He was much more: a beloved husband, father, son, brother and friend of many people who will miss him deeply. Rest in peace, Sergio, you will be always in our hearts.

CONTENTS

Authors and acknowledgements

Sergio Calsamiglia
Department of Animal and Food Science, Autonomous University of Barcelona, Spain

Edgar O. Oviedo-Rondon
Prestage Department of Poultry Science, North Carolina State University

Luis Tamassia, Gilberto Litta and José Maria Hernandez
dsm-firmenich, Animal Nutrition and Health

The authors are grateful to the students of Dr. Lina Piedad Penuela Sierra at University of Tolima, and Thiago H. Yabuta from North Carolina State University who supported the work of Dr. Edgar O. Oviedo-Rondon.

Abbreviations

ABS	avidin-binding substances
ACP	acyl groups carrier protein
ADF	acid detergent fiber
ADP	adenosine diphosphate
AFM	afamin gene
AFS	automatic component feeding system
AI	adequate intake
ANOVA	analysis of variance
AOP	antioxidant potential
ARS	apparent ruminal synthesis
AST	aspartate aminotransferase
ATP	adenosine triphosphate
BCoV	bovine coronavirus vaccine
BGP	bone Gla protein
BHB	β-hydroxyl butyrate
BHMT	betaine homocysteine methyltransferase
BRSV	bovine respiratory syncytial virus
BW	body weight
CCN	cerebrocortical necrosis
CFA	coated folic acid
CNS	central nervous system
CoA	constituent of acetyl-coenzyme
CPK	creatinine phosphokinase
CRALBP	cellular retinaldehyde binding protein
CRF	coated riboflavin
CSF	cerebrospinal fluid
DBP	d binding protein
DBS	dried blood spots
DCAD	dietary cation-anion difference
DIM	days-in milk
DM	dry matter
DMI	dry matter intake
EC	ethyl cellulose-coated
ELISA	enzyme-linked immunosorbent assay
ETC	electron transport chain
ETKA	erythrocyte transketolase activity
FAD	flavin adenine dinucleotide
FBP	folate-binding proteins
FCR	feed conversion ratio
FMN	flavin mononucleotide

G6P	glucose 6-phosphate
GABA	γ-aminobutyric acid
GDH	glutamate dehydrogenase
GHG	greenhouse gas
GIT	gastrointestinal tract
GLO	gulono-γ-lactone oxidase
GPX	glutathione peroxidase
HC	haptocorrin
HDL	high-density lipoprotein
HF	high forage
HG	high grain
HPLC	high-performance liquid chromatography
HVA	high vitamin A
IGF	insulin-like growth factor
IgG	immunoglobulin G
IM	intramuscular
IMF	intramuscular fat
IU	international Unit
KGDH	α-ketoglutarate dehydrogenase
LCA	life cycle assessment
LATD	latissimus dorsi
LDA	left displaced abomasum
LDH	lactic dehydrogenase
LDL	low-density lipoproteins
LPS	lipopolysaccharides
LT	longissimus thoracis
LVA	low vitamin A
LW	liveweight
MCF	manual component feeding
MDH	malic dehydrogenase
ME	metabolizable energy
MG	mammary gland
MK	menaquinone
MMA	methylmalonic acid
MNB	menadione nicotinamide bisulfate
MoDC	monocyte-derived dendritic cells
MPB	menadione dimethylpyrimidinol bisulfite
MSB	menadione sodium bisulfite
MSBC	menadione sodium bisulfite complex
MSU	Michigan State University
MTHFR	methylenetetrahydrofolate reductase
NAD	nicotinamide adenine dinucleotide
NADH	nicotinamide adenine dinucleotide (reduced form)
NADP	nicotinamide adenine dinucleotide phosphate
NADPH	nicotinamide adenine dinucleotide phosphate (reduced form)
NASEM	National Academy of Science Engineering and Medicine
NDF	neutral-detergent fiber
NEFA	non-esterified fatty acid

NFC	non-fiber carbohydrates
NMD	nutritional muscular dystrophy
NRC	National Research Council
OG	orchard grass
OxBC	oxidized β-carotene
PABA	para-aminobenzoic acid
PAF	platelet-activating factor
PAG	pregnancy-associated glycoproteins
PARP	poly (ADP-ribose) polymerase
PCV	packed cell volume
PDH	pyruvate dehydrogenase
PEM	polioencephalomalacia
PGC	primordial germ cells
PL	post-larvae
PLP	pyridoxal-5'-phosphate
PM	pyridoxamine
PMP	pyridoxamine-5'-phosphate
PN	pyridoxol or pyridoxine PNP
PNG	pyridoxine-5'-β-D-glucoside
PNP	pyridoxine-5'-phosphate
PNS	peripheral nervous system
PPARG	peroxisome proliferator-activated receptor γ
PPP	pentose phosphate pathway
PRF	post-ruminal flow
PTH	parathyroid hormone
PUFA	polyunsaturated fatty acids
R5P	ribose 5-phosphate
RA	retinoic acid
RAR	retinoic acid receptor
RBP	retinol-binding protein
RE	retinol equivalents
RFM	retention of fetal membranes
RIA	radioimmunoassay
RNA	ribonucleic acid
RNI	reference nutrient intakes
ROS	reactive oxygen species
RP	rumen-protected
RPBC	rumen-protected blend of B vitamins and choline
RPC	rumen-protected choline
RPFA	rumen-protected folic acid
RPM	rumen-protected methionine
RUSITEC	rumen simulation technique
RXR	retinoid X receptor
S2-	sulfide
SAL	saline
SARA	subacute rumen acidosis
SCC	somatic cell counts
SGOT	serum glutamic-oxaloacetic transaminase

SM	sphingomyelin
SNP	single nucleotide polymorphism
SO3–2	sulfite
SO4–2	sulfate
SOD	superoxide dismutase
SRS	salmonid rickettsial syndrome
TC	transcobalamin
TCA	citric acid cycle
TCA	tricarboxylic acid
TDP	thiamine diphosphate
THF	tetrahydrofolate
THFA	tetrahydrofolic acid
TK	transketolase
TMP	thiamine monophosphate
TMR	total mixed ration
TPP	thiamine pyrophosphate
TPPK	thiamine pyrophosphokinase
TTP	thiamine triphosphate
TTPA	α-tocopherol transfer protein gene
UPLC	ultra-performance liquid chromatography
USMARC	United States Meat Animal Research Center
USP	United States Pharmacopeia
UV	ultraviolet
VAD	vitamin A deficient
VAS	vitamin A sufficient
VBP	vitamin D binding protein
VDR	vitamin D receptor
VERS	vitamin E regeneration system
VFA	volatile fatty acids
VLDL	very low-density lipoproteins
VPG	vitamin-producing genomes
WDGS	wet distillers grains plus solubles
WMD	white muscle disease

Chapter 1

Contribution of vitamin nutrition to a more sustainable ruminant farming

ADDRESSING THE CHALLENGES OF TODAY AND TOMORROW

Today, well into the 21st century, the crucial issues relating to food production are changing. Key concepts such as productivity and efficiency continue to be of vital importance. Increasingly, the emphasis is on the significance of terms such as sustainability, animal health and welfare, food quality, and decreased food waste.

Everything indicates that continuous development in the field of animal nutrition is becoming essential to meet current and future challenges such as:

- produce cost-effective animal protein production – for all
- provide high-quality food and feed – for a better life for all
- develop proper livelihoods – for the 30% of the world population working today in agriculture
- treat animals well until the end of their life – all of them
- eliminate the negative impact of food production – on us and the environment.

In parallel, it is important for the feed industry to lead by example, constantly seeking to reduce the carbon and environmental footprint of products and processes. That means closely managing absolute greenhouse gas (GHG) emissions and energy efficiency in all phases of the production, starting with the feed footprint. A growing number of companies are setting long-term goals, validated by the science-based targets initiative (SBTi) aligned with the 2015 Paris agreement on climate change to reach net-zero emissions before 2050.

These are ambitious and long-term challenges in which the optimal use of vitamins in animal nutrition should be part of the solution.

COMMITMENT TO SUSTAINABILITY

Providing the right levels of high-quality and sustainably produced vitamins to feed mills, integrators, and farmers help them improve animal health, well-being, and performance while also protecting the environment, succeeding in a dynamic and ever-changing global market, enhancing both profits and environmental sustainability.

Optimizing the performance and improving the sustainability of feed additives and premixes plays an important role in reducing the environmental challenges of animal protein production. Excipients such as rice hulls and calcium carbonate can make up to 50% of a premix composition, but little can be done to reduce their carbon footprint further. The critical products with the potential to contribute to carbon footprint and environmental impact reductions in premixes are the nutritional supplements like vitamins.

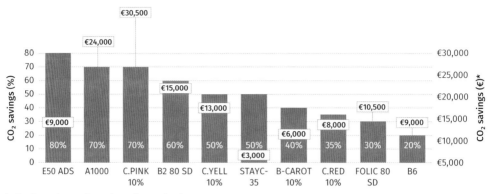

Figure 1.1 Carbon dioxide savings and potential value (carbon tax) per 10 t of feed additive: dsm-firmenich product versus the main alternative (source: dsm-firmenich Animal Nutrition and Health, unpublished)

Reducing the impact of vitamins and other feed additives operations might enable feed mills and farmers to become more sustainable, reduce their risk profile, and potentially benefit from the value created from future carbon tax savings. Some of the leading vitamin companies now share environmental impact information on their nutrient products, and their manufacturing processes and technology (including, when possible, comparisons to alternative products). This information is mainly based on life cycle assessment (LCA) standards. Figure 1.1 shows an example of potential carbon dioxide savings available to a premixer or feed producer when selecting specific vitamin sources.

Carbon pricing – whether implemented as a tax or cap and trade system – seeks to reduce GHG emissions by putting a direct financial liability on industries and activities that are large GHG emitters. It is a policy intervention to encourage the reduction of harmful activities. The sustainability of mainstream animal production is increasingly questioned as demand rises. International bodies agree that animal protein production is one of the activities that need to reduce carbon emissions if we want to solve the climate crisis. Reductions in the impact of agricultural and animal production processes can be supported by greater use of sustainably produced nutritional solutions.

Additionally, governments may seek to impose low-carbon product standards, further environmental regulation, or tax schemes on animal protein production or products as an incentive to reduce emissions and steer consumer consumption. The groundwork for these interventions is already being laid. In Germany, value-added tax increases on meat and dairy products are being proposed. The New Zealand government has agreed to include farm-level emissions in its Emissions Trading Scheme by 2025 (New Zealand legislation, 2019), and the Dutch government has committed to studying 'fair meat prices' ahead of fiscal reforms in 2022.

The agricultural and animal protein products supply chain prepares to minimize the risk posed by these changes or face severe financial penalties. The only way to do this is to significantly reduce animal production's impact on the climate and the environment. Equally, redesigning existing incentive systems (i.e., subsidies) and scaling up high-quality voluntary carbon credit systems to directly reward emissions reductions can significantly accelerate the transition.

This transition to a lower-carbon future for animal proteins can be facilitated by supplying nutritional ingredients such as vitamins with industry-leading performance to

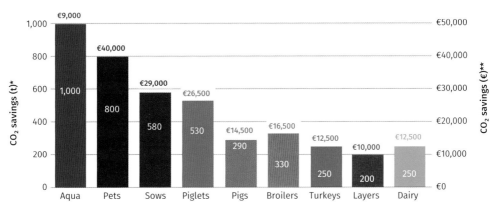

*Examples of CO_2 savings based on average vitamin levels used in 100k t feed
** Value of CO_2 saving assuming a carbon credit or tax of €50/ton CO_2

Figure 1.2 Carbon dioxide savings and potential value (carbon tax) of a more sustainable vitamin source for 100,000 t of feed produced (source: dsm-firmenich Animal Nutrition and Health, unpublished)

improve the efficiency of animal production systems while reducing the carbon footprint of these feed additives and those within which they are utilized. By considering the potential carbon dioxide savings when using certain sources of vitamins (as illustrated in Figure 1.1) and the average vitamin inclusion level in feed for different animal species, we can calculate the environmental benefits for those farmers interested in the sustainability of vitamins within their strategies to achieve more sustainable farming practices (Figure 1.2). Vitamins can contribute to at least 3 United Nations Sustainable Development Goals (SDGs): 2 (Zero hunger), 3 (Good health and well-being) and 13 (Climate action).

UPDATING THE NUTRITIONAL STANDARDS OF VITAMINS IN A CONSTANTLY EVOLVING WORLD

Vitamins play a decisive role in both human and animal nutrition. As organic catalysts present in small quantities in most foods, they are essential for the normal functioning of metabolic and physiological processes such as growth, development, health, and reproduction. The requirements for vitamins in animals are dynamic: they vary according to new genotypes, levels of yield, and production systems. Vitamin functions and requirements are becoming increasingly well known.

The concept of Optimum Vitamin Nutrition® (OVN™) for animals is essential today. Its objective is to develop a new standard for vitamin supplementation in feed to improve animal health status and resilience to diseases and environmental stress, which will translate into better animal productivity and homogeneity. Moreover, the quality of food produced by those animals can be enhanced, improving human health and reducing food waste. The latter is critical in a global society in which, unfortunately, many people still do not have access to the correct quantity and quality of food.

When we talk about optimum vitamin supplementation in the diet of animals, we refer to the provision of vitamin levels both over and above the established minimum requirements for avoiding deficiencies and adapted to the specific conditions of each animal species to achieve the objectives mentioned above.

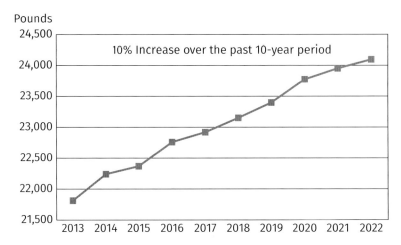

Figure 1.3 Production per cow, 2012–2021, in the United States (source: USDA, 2023)

Historically, the objective of the vitamin recommendations provided by various international scientific organs – such as the National Academy of Science Engineering and Medicine (NASEM, 2021) – was preventing nutritional shortages or deficiencies. Some of the studies on which they are based are sometimes 40 years old. We all know that the livestock industry today has little in common with the industry as it was at that time.

For example, Figure 1.3 shows that in the last 10 years yearly milk production per cow has increased 2.250 lb or 1.020 kg or roughly 1% per year.

Therefore, it is logical to infer that nutrition programs for farm animals must be adjusted, including vitamin supplementation, consistently with improved animal management techniques and genetic makeup.

Likewise, in recent times there have been important legislative changes in the world that are limiting or banning the use of compounds such as antibiotics, substances that were regular additives of animals' diets as well as of the diet of the animal trials where vitamins requirements were based on. At the same time, many countries are developing new rules on animal welfare which, in short to medium term, will entail less "intensiveness" in the livestock industry, aiming to improve the animals' health and well-being. Meanwhile, our farmers need to be competitive enough regarding livestock productivity (weight gain, milk yield, feed conversion ratio (FCR), the final weight of the animal, mortality, etc.) to survive strong international competition where free trade is a tangible reality.

From the nutritional point of view, in these fast-changing circumstances, so different from those we have become accustomed to in the last years, it is essential to re-evaluate the vitamin requirements of animals with the aim of safely and efficiently producing healthy and nourishing food that meets consumer expectations, always under sustainable farming practices.

VITAMINS: ESSENTIAL MICRONUTRIENTS IN THE ANIMAL ORGANISM

Vitamins are unique and crucial nutrients in the diet of people and animals. They are essential elements in the organism's vital functions: maintenance, growth, development, health, and reproduction. They also combine 2 characteristics.

- The daily requirement for each of the vitamins is very small, an aspect in which they differ from macronutrients such as carbohydrates, fats, and proteins.
- Vitamins are organic compounds, unlike other essential nutrients such as minerals (iron, iodine, zinc, etc.).

The discovery of vitamins and their function in preventing classical deficiency diseases are events that stand among the most important achievements of the last century. Vitamins are particularly important because they allow optimum metabolism of other nutrients in the animal diet. In general, humans and animals need to derive them from their diet as they cannot produce the appropriate quantities by themselves. Vitamins are present in many reactions of the cellular metabolism and play, particularly in combination, a critical role in biochemical pathways like the Krebs or citric acid cycle (Figure 1.4).

Vitamins may only represent less than 1% of the cost of animal feed, but they are present in 100% of metabolic functions. This fact gives them the status of micronutrients of macro importance. Vitamins are found in minimal quantities in most feedstuffs. Their absence from the diet gives rise to specific deficiency diseases because of their significance for the normal functioning of the metabolism. While the need to provide additional vitamins in feed is unquestioned, the levels of supplementation needed to achieve an optimum economic return in field conditions are open to debate. As a general rule, the optimum economic supplementation level is that which achieves the best index of growth, feed conversion, health status – including immunocompetence – and which, in addition, provides the reserves appropriate for the organism. Nutrition is optimal when an animal efficiently utilizes the nutrients provided in the feed for survival, health, growth, and reproduction. Although all the nutrients, including proteins,

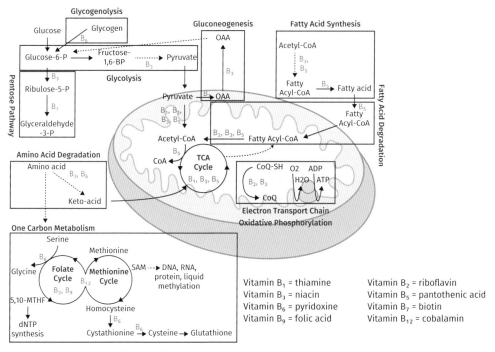

Figure 1.4 Metabolic functions and interactions of B vitamins (source: Godoy-Parejo et al., 2020)

fats, carbohydrates, minerals, and water, are essential for carrying out these vital functions, vitamins play a key role in basic functions such as an appropriate immune response in animals.

As mentioned already, several factors – e.g., increased productivity, intensive farming, and higher handling and higher susceptibility to diseases – give rise to a growing vulnerability to vitamin deficiencies and a yield below the maximal potential. A great majority of nutritionists and investigators recognize that the minimum vitamin requirements needed to prevent clinical deficiency symptoms may not be sufficient to achieve an optimum state of health and yield. In Chapter 4 we will review the multiple metabolic functions specific to each of the vitamins in greater depth.

VITAMIN LEVELS IN ANIMAL DIET: THE NUTRITIONIST'S GREAT UNKNOWN QUANTITY

Establishing the vitamin supplementation level is something all nutritionists should concern themselves with. Economic cost and benefit must be a fundamental reason for revising and determining vitamin supplements in feed. The cost of supplementing feed with essential vitamins must be assessed considering the risk of suffering losses from deficiency symptoms and productive yields below the optimum. The great challenge for nutritionists is choosing a particular level from the various recommended tables. There are currently various sets of recommendations for vitamin levels in feed available from industries in the animal feed sector, research institutes, and vitamin manufacturers themselves. In turn, fundamental differences can be seen in how the studies have been produced.

For example, latest NASEM recommendations (NASEM, 2021) for dairy cattle show that not all vitamins had an established requirement. Nevertheless, NASEM recommendations constitute reference sources of limited value from the viewpoint of commercial feed formulation as they are based on establishing vitamin levels necessary to prevent clinical deficiency symptoms in optimal trial conditions and therefore far removed from commercial conditions. For instance, they do not account for the stress factor, a frequent part of livestock rearing, which can drastically influence nutritional needs.

To make more efficient use of the NASEM's vitamin recommendations, it is advisable to consider the following aspects.

- The indicated levels have been established to prevent deficiencies in the animal.
- They do not include any kind of safety margin to prevent loss of vitamin activity stemming from usual feed processing or feed storage conditions. In other words, the recommended NASEM (2021) levels must be those present in the animal's feed and when it is eating it.
- They do not include safety margins for the eventuality that the animals are subjected to some sort of stress or subclinical disease.
- They do not consider possible adverse environmental conditions, such as high temperatures, or increased handling.
- In most cases, they are not specific to the new animal genotypes and improved farming practices.

Nutritionists usually consider stress and other economically important variables in their formulations. There is a great disparity between the levels of supplementation prescribed by the industry and those indicated by NASEM (2021). While the industry continues to adjust vitamin supplementation in feed to achieve an optimum yield and state of health in the animal, the NASEM (2021) has introduced only a few minor changes for most animal species in the last few decades. Logically, the vitamin needs established decades ago do not apply to today's animals. Most nutritionists agree on this aspect, and supplements of many vitamins are given in practice at levels 3 to 10 times higher than those recommended by the NASEM (2021).

BIOAVAILABILITY OF VITAMINS IN ANIMALS

Many feed materials used in animal nutrition contain variable quantities of vitamins. The amounts of vitamins available in the feedstuffs are limited by the nutritional requirements of these materials: hence, the vitamin levels in the diets tend to vary considerably. The overall content is low, and their presence in the feed does not guarantee their bioavailability or that the animal will indeed benefit from them.

It is well accepted that vitamin levels in feedstuffs vary significantly from one geographical region to another as well as depending on the time of harvesting and the climatic conditions at each harvest. Long storage periods and the use of preservatives, fungicides, etc., negatively affect the vitamin content. Some of the factors which most adversely affect the level of vitamins in the ingredients of feed are:

- origin of the harvest
- use of fertilizers
- genetic modifications which increase productive yield
- climate
- agricultural practices such as crop rotation
- harvesting conditions
- storage conditions and the use of preservatives
- vitamin form and consequently vitamin stability and bioavailability.

The real content of vitamins in feed is determined by complex chemical and microbiological analysis methods in authorized laboratories, which provide the real value at a given time for a certain sample or batch of the respective ingredient. But given the great number of factors that affect the stability of vitamins (temperature, humidity, light, etc.), it would be necessary to undertake costly systematic analyses of the principal feed materials to be able to use those values reliably in the formulation – at minimum cost – of the feed, with the constant adaptation of the values to avoid possible variations of the desired level.

In many cases, vitamins derived from the feedstuffs are present in compound forms that are not bioavailable, hence, not available to be absorbed and participate in the animal's physiological and metabolic processes. At the practical level only the content of the vitamin in its free form is considered when calculating the total vitamin content in feed.

The term bioavailability refers exclusively to the vitamin content of an ingredient that is available to be absorbed and participate in the animal's different physiological and metabolic processes.

In commercial vitamin preparations various substances protect vitamins from harm during feed production processes and from aggressive environmental agents during storage. Therefore, it is essential to consider the bioavailability of these substances when determining the vitamin content of any feed ingredient.

In contrast, in nature, both in vegetable and animal products, substances can effectively destroy the vitamin activity or limit their bioavailability. These antinutritional agents can also be released by certain types of bacteria or fungi – e.g., mycotoxins – as by-products of their metabolic activity, as well as being present in the normal environment of the production facilities.

Their most frequent mechanism of action consists of deactivating the free form of the vitamin or preventing its absorption. Among the most common scenarios are:

- deactivation of thiamine (B_1) by thiaminase
- formation of a compound with a metabolite, as in the case of the deactivation of biotin by avidin
- blocking the site of absorption or an independent chemical reaction, as in the case of dicumarol and vitamin K.

The addition of fats and oils as an energy source is common practice in the manufacture of feed. Attention should be paid to the total content of unsaturated fatty acids since they increase the likelihood that the oils and fats will become rancid. This would affect the absorption of fat-soluble vitamins such as A, E and D. Likewise, oxidation of the fats would also contribute to biotin deactivation.

STABILITY OF VITAMINS IN ANIMAL FEED

Diverse factors can affect the stability of substances as volatile as vitamins, whether in their pure commercial form, in vitamin-mineral premixes, or after the manufacture of compound feed and its subsequent storage. Some of these factors are connected with the catalytic activity of the molecules themselves, the handling of commercial forms and their premixes, the characteristics of the blend, the presence of various antagonistic substances, and the storage conditions. The vitamins present in primary materials are very susceptible to the adverse conditions mentioned above, and a heavy loss of vitamin activity is a common occurrence in these macroingredients. In contrast, the highest-quality commercial forms of vitamins are produced from industrial processes, which stabilize and protect the molecules of active substance during manufacture and storage, both in premixes and the feed.

Recent data from a European premix company shows large differences in vitamin A stability in pelleted feed at 90°C with 30, 60, or 120 seconds of holding time (up to 50%) when comparing 3 different vitamin A product forms (Figure 1.5).

However, it must again be emphasized that the stabilization of the vitamins must not compromise their bioavailability in the animal. Different methods are used for stabilizing vitamins.

- **Use of antioxidants** – Antioxidants are included in the formulation of commercial vitamin products to prevent fat-soluble vitamins' oxidation and prolong these compounds' shelf life. In general, those commercial forms with an appropriate quantity of antioxidant substances have a longer effective shelf life. This period, during which vitamin content is guaranteed, will depend to a great extent on storage conditions. The ban of ethoxyquin in the EU and some other countries has put additional pressure on vitamin, premix, and feed manufacturers to adapt their product formulation technologies and sources to guarantee the right content of the active substance in the products they market.
- **Mechanical methods** – The process, in this case, covers the active substance with a stabilizing coat. This covering protects the vitamin molecule inside it from the adverse effect of aggressive external agents such as the presence of oxygen, ultraviolet radiation, sunlight, humidity, different temperatures, etc. Figure 1.6 shows that all of the fat-soluble vitamins (A, D, E, K), vitamin B_1 and vitamin C are sensitive to oxidizing agents like inorganic minerals.

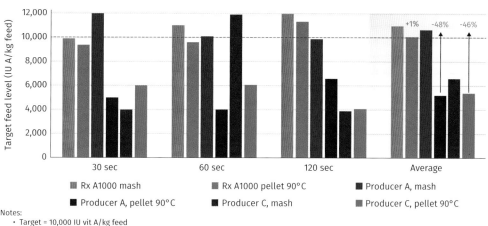

Notes:
 • Target = 10,000 IU vit A/kg feed
 • Premixes produced by large EU premixer with 3 different vitamin A products
 • Feed corn/wheat/soy produced by Kolding Tech. Institute, Denmark
 • Vitamin analyses carried out by LUFA Kiel lab, Germany (method REG(EC) 152/2009, IV, A)

Figure 1.5 Vitamin A stability in a 90°C pelleted feed at 30, 60, and 120 seconds holding time (source: elaboration by dsm-firmenich Animal Nutrition and Health based on data from a European premix company, 2020 unpublished)

Additive	Temperature	Oxygen	Humidity	Light
Vitamin A	++	++	+	++
Vitamin D	+	++	+	+
25OHD$_3$ (calcifediol)	++	++	+	+
Vitamin E	0	+	0	+
Vitamin K$_3$	+	+	++	0
Vitamin B$_1$	+	+	+	0
Vitamin B$_2$	0	0	+	+
Vitamin B$_6$	++	0	+	+
Pantothenic acid	+	0	+	0
Nicotinates	0	0	0	0
Biotin	+	0	0	0
Folic acid	++	0	+	++
Vitamin C	++	++	++	0

++ Marked effect

+ Moderate effect

0 No effect

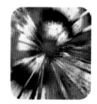

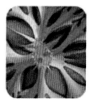

Figure 1.6 External factors influencing the stability of non-formulated vitamins (source: dsm-firmenich Animal Nutrition, dsm-firmenich Product Forms. Quality feed ingredients for more sustainable farming, 2022a)

On a practical level, this method has proved highly effective in protecting these substances and, depending on their characteristics, can be combined with a process of spray drying, which provides a large number of active particles (all with the active form of the vitamin) which facilitates a subsequent homogenous mixture in the animal's food. This is particularly relevant for vitamins like biotin or vitamin B$_{12}$ added into feed at very low levels (Figure 1.7).

Physical characteristics	ROVIMIX® Biotin 2% SD	ROVIMIX® Biotin HP 10% SD	Biotin 2% Triturate A
Soluble in water	yes	yes	no
Flowability (sec-100g)	medium	medium	low flow, tapping required
Average practical size (μm)	66	73	296
Mixability in feed, CV %	6%	5.7%	10.8%
Total particles per g product	>21 mio	>20 mio	>10 mio
Active particles per g product	100%	100%	2% (98% carrier)
Active Biotin particles per animal/day @ 0.2 mg biotin/Kg feed @ 10 g feed/day/chick	2000	400	20

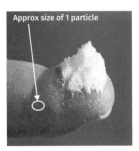

Approx size of 1 particle

*Biotin consumed by **1 sow** (or 20 birds, or 1 dog or 4 salmon) per year*

Figure 1.7 Confrontation of physical characteristics of biotin spray-dried form against biotin triturate (source: dsm-firmenich Animal Nutrition and Health, unpublished)

At all events, the factors mentioned above affect vitamins in different ways:

- Vitamins A, D, and carotenoids:
  - are prone to oxidation when exposed to air
  - are sensitive to oxidizing agents
  - isomerize in acid pH
  - are sensitive to prolonged heat
  - are sensitive to the catalytic effect of minerals.
- Vitamin E:
  - is prone to oxidation in the presence of air
  - is sensitive to alkaline mediums
  - the ester is relatively more stable.
- Vitamin K:
  - is sensitive to heat
  - is prone to oxidation in the presence of oxygen.
- Vitamin B_1 (thiamine):
  - is stable with low pH, loss of activity when pH of medium increases
  - is sensitive to the presence of oxygen and other oxidizing agents in neutral or alkaline
  - solutions
  - splits on reacting with sulfites, with immediate separation at pH 6
  - is sensitive to metallic ions such as copper
  - the thiaminases present in some animal and vegetable products are known antagonists of this vitamin.
- Vitamin B_2 (riboflavin):
  - is sensitive to light, especially in alkaline solutions
  - is stable in acid and neutral mediums
  - is unstable in alkaline solutions

- o   is sensitive to reducing agents.
- Vitamin B$_6$ (pyridoxine):
  - o   is sensitive to light
  - o   is relatively stable in acid solutions and dry mixes.
- Vitamin B$_{12}$ (cobalamin):
  - o   has little stability in alkaline or slightly acid mediums
  - o   is sensitive to oxidizing reactions and reducing agents
  - o   the metabolites of ascorbic acid, thiamine and nicotinamide accelerate this vitamin's decomposition
  - o   is sensitive to light in very dilute solutions.
- Niacin:
  - o   is relatively stable under practical conditions.
- Pantothenic acid:
  - o   has little stability in alkaline or acid mediums
  - o   is very hygroscopic, especially in its dl-calcium pantothenate form
  - o   decomposes through hydrolysis, especially at low and high pH values.
- Biotin:
  - o   is stable in air, acids and at neutral pH
  - o   is slightly unstable in alkaline solutions.
- Folic acid:
  - o   little stability in acid solutions below pH 5
  - o   is sensitive to oxidizing reactions and reducing agents
  - o   decomposes in sunlight
  - o   little stability in hygroscopic environments and in the presence of minerals.
- Ascorbic acid:
  - o   is sensitive to radiation
  - o   oxidizes rapidly in all types of solution
  - o   is catalyzed by metallic ions, such as copper and iron
  - o   degrades rapidly at high temperatures.

OPTIMUM VITAMIN NUTRITION® IN PRACTICE

The objective of OVN™ is to supplement the diet of animals with the amounts of each vitamin considered most appropriate (the optimum) to optimize the state of health and the productivity of farm animals while guaranteeing the efficiency (desired effect at minimum cost) of the recommended levels. As already outlined, the levels of supplementation required for OVN™ are generally higher than those necessary to prevent clinical deficiency symptoms. These optimum supplementation levels should likewise compensate for the stress factors affecting the animal and its diet, thus guaranteeing these factors do not limit the animal's yield and health.

   The following describes the concept of a cost-effective window for vitamin supplementation. This level must satisfy but not exceed the aim of achieving a state of optimum health and productivity. Below are some definitions of terms applicable to the OVN™ concept (Figure 1.8).

1   **Average animal response** refers to productivity results – FCR, growth rate, reproductive status, level of immunity, the animal's health status, etc. – because of the ingestion of vitamins.
2   **Total vitamin intake** describes the total level of vitamins in the diet, feedstuff's bioavailable quantity, and supplementation.

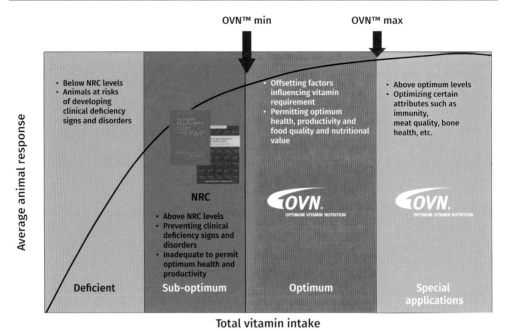

Figure 1.8 The OVN Optimum Vitamin Nutrition® concept (source: DSM Nutritional Products (2022b) OVN Optimum Vitamin Nutrition® guidelines)

3 **Deficient or minimum vitamin intake** refers to the vitamin level which puts the animal in danger of showing clinical deficiency symptoms and metabolic disorders and in which the level of vitamins falls short of the NRC supplementation level.

4 **A suboptimum intake** prevents the appearance of clinical deficiency symptoms. Its supplementation levels comply with or exceed the NRC's guidelines but are inadequate to permit an optimum state of health and productivity.

5 **An optimum intake** compensates for the negative factors which influence an animal's yield and therefore contributes to achieving an optimum state of well-being, health, and productivity.

6 **Special applications** are above optimum intake levels of vitamin supplementation for optimizing certain attributes such as immunity, meat quality, bone health, etc., or are directly used to produce vitamin-enriched animal-origin foods. There is a growing demand for food with a greater added value, such as vitamin-rich eggs, meat, or milk, the occasional consumption of which contributes to a balanced human diet. This would necessitate such a higher vitamin content in the feed. Concerning the safety of vitamins, only very large quantities (between 10 and 100 times the levels used in practice) of some vitamins such as A and D_3 in feed might occasionally cause some sort of disorder in animals. However, the suggested supplementation level for obtaining an enrichment of animal origin foods is not posing any risk of vitamin over supply.

There are various factors that affect an animal's vitamin requirements, and some may have an influence on the vitamin intake/supplement in the diet and its utilization. Among these factors are how we assess primary materials for their vitamin content, the process of harvesting these primary materials, as well as the processing and storage conditions of the ingredients in the feed, and the variability of the vitamins and their bioavailability.

Factors that influence vitamin requirements include the type and level of production, housing (especially whether or not animals are kept under cover), causes of stress, illnesses, other environmental conditions (for example, a warm environment or contamination by mycotoxins), vitamin antagonists, and the use of medicaments that may limit or even block the action of certain vitamins. Requirements will therefore vary depending on the severity of the above factors.

In summary, we can say that implementing a nutritional program with the most appropriate levels of all the vitamins in an animal's diet aims to offer the following benefits to the food chain:

1 **Optimum health and welfare of animals** are a prerequisite for producing safe and healthy meat.
2 **Optimum productivity**, given better sanitary conditions and greater efficiency in animal farming within parameters such as FCR, milk yield, final weight, weight gain, mortality, etc.
3 **Reduced food waste and optimum food quality** offered to consumers provides them with whole food with balanced nutrient content.

1. Optimizing animal's health and welfare
It is common knowledge that there is a close relationship between nutrition, health, and welfare. Improving the robustness of an animal nowadays constitutes a crucial aspect in the production of any food type of animal origin, so one essential objective regarding nutrition and management programs would be limiting the incidence of diseases and their debilitating effect on animals. Supplementing an animal's diet with optimum quantities of vitamins at times of greatest vulnerability to infection reduces the risk of contracting a disease.

Health and immunity
Vitamins, in sufficient quantities, play a fundamental role in the capacity of an animal's organism to develop an effective immune response to disease. Since the onset of an illness cannot be predicted, the immune system must be prepared to act before the disease attacks the organism.

Various studies have demonstrated a close relationship between low levels of vitamin E in the tissues and a decrease in immunocompetence (the immune system's response) long before any clinical signs of disease appear. Vitamins E and C are powerful antioxidants that protect cells from free radicals and other types of by-products harmful to an animal's metabolism.

Research shows that high levels of vitamin E have several benefits in ruminants' immune response by increasing bacteria killing and protecting neutrophils and prolonging their lifespan. When plasma level is below 3 mg/l the risk of mastitis is dramatically increased as shown by Weiss *et al.* (1990a) (Figure 1.9).

Welfare
As is well known, infections cause pain and suffering in animals. In general, farmers, rearing businesses, and other people involved in their care have the greatest interest in them and will assume responsibility for ensuring satisfactory standards of well-being.

In the food sector, too, there are ever more retailers, wholesale distributors, and even fast-food chains which have incorporated certain animal welfare standards in their best practices, aiming to give animals a healthy life that will contribute to guaranteeing more nutritious food to their consumers. Optimum vitamin supplementation in an animal's diet will contribute to improving its welfare because:

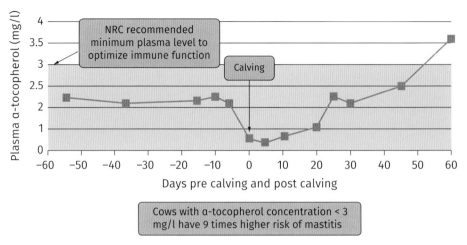

Figure 1.9 Changes in plasma α-tocopherol values during the dry period and early lactation in 270 cows. Points are averages of cows from 9 different herds (source: adapted from Weiss *et al.*, 1990a).

- optimum vitamin levels contribute to improving the metabolism, nutrition, and well-being of the animal
- improving immunity increases resistance to diseases
- some vitamins, such as biotin, contribute to reducing the incidence of digital dermatitis, thus preventing certain types of lameness, while others, such as vitamin C, alleviate the negative effects of stress on health and others like 25OHD$_3$, a more active D$_3$ metabolite, will improve bone health reducing lameness and other painful skeletal issues.

2. Optimizing productivity

In animals, advances have been achieved over decades through a process of natural genetic selection, accelerating growth rates and favoring certain genotypes to increase production of milk or meat. These have changed the nutritional requirements of cows because of improvements in the use of feed.

Recent data have demonstrated that animals grow faster under experimental and commercial conditions when the supplementation of vitamins in the diet is increased according to their requirements. From the economic viewpoint, the improvement in productive yield after optimizing the supply of vitamins in the feed gave rise to a significantly better cost–benefit ratio, in turn recompensing the farmer.

In commercial conditions, stress represents a serious threat to achieving optimum yield. It reduces feed intake, increasing vitamin concentration required to satisfy an animal's needs. Moreover, stress alters the animal's metabolic needs, turning a nutritionally balanced meal into a diet with possible nutritional deficiencies.

3. Increasing shelf life and optimizing the quality of food for the consumer

Meat is an essential source of protein in the human diet. A gradual and continuous increase in demand for processed meat products has been observed. This fact should be considered when defining the nutritional strategy that should be developed in animal diets. Lipid oxidation constitutes a problem for the conservation of meat since it can give rise to undesirable smells and flavors associated with rancidification, a fact of major relevance in processed meat particularly susceptible to this oxidation process.

Meat color is the main factor affecting meat product appearance at the time of consumer purchase. The quality of the color of meat is dependent on the chemical state of the muscle pigment myoglobin. Myoglobin can exist in a ferrous oxygenated form as cherry-red oxymyoglobin or in a ferric oxidized form as brownish red metmyoglobin (Faustman and Cassens, 1990). During storage and retail display, oxymyoglobin is oxidized to metmyoglobin; consumers consider the undesirable brown color less wholesome.

Feeding animals a diet rich in unsaturated vegetable fats can considerably increase levels of monounsaturated and polyunsaturated fatty acids in meat. There is a series of polyunsaturated fatty acids that react with molecular oxygen until they are finally degraded to undesirable compounds with short chains, which cause the meat's organoleptic characteristics to deteriorate and, consequently, reduce acceptance of the meat by the consumer. Animals fed on diets with high levels of vitamin E can counteract this effect and so improve the final quality of the meat:

- by protecting the meat's lipids from oxidation and reducing the formation of undesirable smells and flavors and preserving the reddish meat color
- by reducing the loss of exudates and improving the texture of the meat.

OPTIMUM VITAMIN NUTRITION: A DYNAMIC PROCESS IN CONSTANT EVOLUTION

Optimum vitamin supplementation in an animal's diet, over and above the established minimum needs and adapted to the specific conditions of each animal species, will permit an improvement in the state of health and welfare of the animal, thus optimizing its productive potential at the same time as facilitating the production of high-quality food that is nutritionally balanced.

These optimum levels are based on many studies carried out in university and industrial centers, on the requirements published by different associations and vitamin manufacturers, and on the continuous experience of the worldwide agricultural industry. These optimum levels guarantee farmers minimum impact of negative nutritional factors, such as variability in the natural content of feed ingredients, the existence of antinutritional factors and different levels of stress.

Although the vitamin recommendations for feed also attempt to compensate for the majority of the factors mentioned above, which influence an animal's vitamin needs, in extreme conditions where the processing of premix or feed is very aggressive (e.g., the inclusion of trace minerals or choline chloride, the use of feed expanders or extruded feed) supplementary quantities of some vitamins may be necessary. The negative effect on the stability of vitamins can be reduced by using high-quality commercial vitamin forms where their covering and the bioavailability of the active substance they contain are key elements to be considered. And all this is considering the environmental impact of how vitamins are manufactured.

Chapters 5 and 6 review the impact of vitamins in beef cattle and dairy cattle nutrition as reported in the international research literature. These studies have endeavored to emphasize the beneficial effects that optimum vitamin levels have on an animal, both on the level of health and welfare and concerning productivity. The chapters also identify aspects on which there is currently insufficient information available, intending to address these gaps in future research and editions of this book.

Given that animal farming is a dynamic process levels of vitamin supplementation need to be reassessed more frequently – this is a change demanded, in most cases, by society, for economic reasons related to the productivity of animals and by farming systems.

The concept of OVN™ always considers the costs of vitamin supplementation in an animal's diet (in many cases, less than 1% of the cost of feed, even less if we consider the impact on meat and milk production cost) against the risk of suffering losses through vitamin deficiencies and through working with yield indices below the optimum.

Nutritionists who follow the recommended guidelines based on the OVN™ concept ensure that vitamins will not constitute the limiting factor in developing an animal's genetic potential and contribute to a more sustainable animal farming.

Chapter 2

A brief history of vitamins

Vitamins were mostly discovered in the 20th century and were once regarded as "unknown growth factors" (Eggersdorfer *et al.*, 2012). The first phase of developing the concept of vitamins began many centuries ago and gradually led to the recognition that night blindness, xerophthalmia, scurvy, beriberi, and rickets are dietary diseases. These diseases had long plagued humankind and were mentioned in the earliest written records. Records of medical science from antiquity attest that researchers had already linked certain foods and diseases or infirmities, postulating that food constituents played a causal or a preventive role. These are considered the nebulous beginnings of essential nutrients (Eggersdorfer *et al.*, 2012).

Beriberi is probably the earliest documented deficiency disorder being recognized in China as early as 2697 BC. By 1500 BC, scurvy, night blindness, and xerophthalmia were described in Egyptian writings. Two books of the Bible contain accounts that point to vitamin A deficiency (McDowell, 2006). Jeremiah 14:6 states: "and the asses did stand in high places, their eyes did fail because there was no grass." In addition, the Bible mentions that fish bile was used to cure a blind man named Tobias.

In 400 BC, the Greek physician Hippocrates, known as the Father of Medicine, reported using raw ox liver dipped in honey to prevent night blindness. He also described soldiers afflicted with scurvy. Scurvy took a heavy toll on the Crusades of the Middles Ages because the soldiers traveled far from home, and their diet was deficient in vitamin C. During the long sea voyages between 1492 and 1600, scurvy posed a serious threat to the health of sailors and undermined world exploration. For example, while sailing worldwide, Magellan lost 80% of his crew to the disease. Vasco de Gama, another great explorer, lost 60% of his 160-man crew while mapping the coast of Africa. In 1536, during Jacques Cartier's expedition to Canada, 107 out of 110 men became sick with scurvy. However, the journey was saved when the Indians shared their knowledge of the curative value of pine needles and bark. In 1593, British Admiral Richard Hawkins wrote: "I have seen some 10,000 seamen die of scurvy; some sailors tried treating themselves by trimming the rotting, putrid black flesh from their gums and washing their teeth in urine."

In 1747, James Lind, a British naval surgeon, carried out the first controlled clinical experiment aboard a ship to find a cure for scurvy. Twelve patients with scurvy were divided into 6 treatment groups. Two sailors received a dietary supplement of oranges and lemons, while the other treatment groups were given nutmeg, garlic, vinegar, cider, and seawater, respectively. The 2 men who had received the citrus fruit were cured of scurvy. Where did Lind get the idea that scurvy was related to nutrition? He had been told a story of an English sailor with scurvy who was left to die on a lonely island with no food. Feeling hungry, the man nibbled a few blades of beach grass. The next day, he felt stronger and ate some more grass. After a few weeks on this "diet," he was completely well.

In the second half of the 19th century, there was another disease that killed thousands of sailors in the Japanese navy. In 1880, the Japanese navy recorded almost 5,000 deaths from beriberi in 3 years. Patients with beriberi became weak and eventually partially paralyzed, lost weight, and died. Doctors tried to find the germ that was causing beriberi. Finally, they listened to Japanese naval surgeon Kamekiro Takaki, who believed the sailors' diet was causing beriberi. Takaki noted a 60% incidence of beriberi on a ship returning from a 1-year voyage during which the sailors' diet had been mostly polished rice and some fish. He sent out a second ship under the same conditions but substituted barley, meat, milk, and fresh vegetables for some of the rice. The dietary change eliminated beriberi, but Takaki incorrectly concluded that the additional protein prevented the beriberi. Regardless, the Japanese knew they could avoid beriberi by not relying on polished rice as the only dietary staple.

Before the beginning of the 20th century, there was a growing body of evidence that nutritional factors, later known as vitamins, were implicated in certain diseases. Louis Pasteur was the chief opponent of the "vitamin theory," which held that certain illnesses resulted from a shortage of specific nutrients in foods. Pasteur believed there were only 3 classes of organic nutrients: carbohydrates, fats, and proteins. His research showed that microorganisms caused disease and made scientists with medical training reluctant to believe the vitamin theory. It has been said that the immensely successful "germ theory" of disease, coupled with toxin theory and the successful use of antisepsis and vaccination, convinced scientists of the day that only a positive agent could cause disease (Guggenheim, 1995). Until the mid-1930s, most US doctors still believed that pellagra was an infectious disease (McDowell, 2006).

VITAMIN THEORY TAKES SHAPE

Beginning in the mid-1850s, German scientists were recognized as leaders in the field of nutrition. In the late 1800s, Professor C. von Bunge, who worked at the German university in Dorpat, Estonia, and then at Basel, Switzerland, had some graduate students conduct experiments with purified diets for small animals (Wolf and Carpenter, 1997). In 1881, N. Lunin, a Russian student studying in von Bunge's laboratory, observed that some mice died after 16 to 36 days when fed a diet composed solely of purified fat, protein, carbohydrate, salts, and water. Lunin suggested that natural foods such as milk contain small quantities of "unknown substances essential to life."

Many great scientific advances have come about due to chance observations made by men and women of inspiration. In 1896, Dutch physician and bacteriologist Christiaan Eijkman made a historic finding concerning a cure for beriberi. Eijkman was researching in Indonesia to identify the causal pathogen of beriberi. He astutely observed that a polyneuritis condition in chickens produced clinical signs similar to those in humans with beriberi. This chance discovery was made when a new head cook at the hospital discontinued the supply of "military" rice (polished rice), and the chickens fed the wholegrain "civilian" rice recovered from the polyneuritis. After extensive experimentation, Eijkman proved that both polyneuritis and beriberi were caused by eating polished white rice. Both afflictions could be prevented or cured when the outer portions of the rice grain (e.g., rice bran) were consumed. Thus, Eijkman became the first to produce a vitamin deficiency disease in an experimental animal. He also noted that prisoners with beriberi eating polished rice tended to get well when fed a less milled product. In 1901, Grijns, one of Eijkman's colleagues in Indonesia, was the first to come up with a correct interpretation of the connection between the excessive consumption of polished rice and the etiology of beriberi. He concluded that rice contained "an essential nutrient" found in the grain's outer layers.

In 1902, a Norwegian scientist named Holst conducted some experiments on "ship-beriberi" (scurvy) using poultry, but the experiments failed. In 1907, Holst and Frolich produced experimental scurvy in guinea pigs. Later it was learned that poultry could synthesize vitamin C while guinea pigs could not.

In 1906, Frederick Hopkins, working with rats in England, reported that "no animal can live upon a mixture of pure protein, fat, and carbohydrate and even when the necessary inorganic material is supplied, the animal cannot flourish." Hopkins found that small amounts of milk added to purified diets allowed rats to live and thrive. He suggested that unknown nutrients were essential for animal life, calling them "accessory food factors." Hopkins' experiments were like those of Lunin; however, they were more in depth. He played an important role by recording his views in memorable terms that received wide recognition (McCollum, 1957). Hopkins also expressed that various disorders were caused by diets deficient in unidentified nutrients (e.g., scurvy and rickets). He was responsible for opening a new field of discovery that largely depended on experimental rats.

In 1907, Elmer McCollum (Figure 2.1) arrived in Wisconsin to work on a project to determine why cows fed wheat or oats (versus yellow corn) gave birth to blind or dead calves. The answer was found to be that wheat and oats lacked the vitamin A precursor carotene. Between 1913 and 1915, McCollum and Davis discovered 2 growth factors for rats, "fat-soluble A" and "water-soluble B." By 1922, McCollum had identified vitamin D as a substance independent of vitamin A. He bubbled oxygen through cod liver oil to destroy its vitamin A; the treated oil remained effective against rickets but not against xeropthalmia. Thus, "fat-soluble vitamin A" had to be 2 vitamins, not just one (DeLuca, 2014).

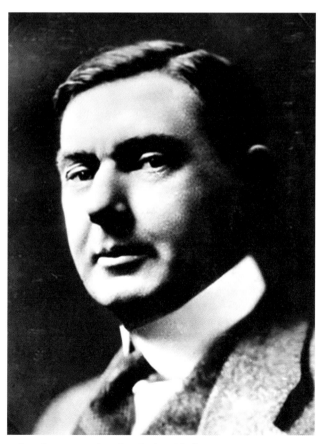

Figure 2.1 Elmer McCollum (source: Roche Historical Archive)

In 1912, Casimir Funk (Figure 2.2), a Polish biochemist working at the Lister Institute in London, proposed the "vitamin theory" (Funk and Dubin, 1922). He had reviewed the literature and made the important conclusion that beriberi could be prevented or cured by a protective factor present in natural food, which he successfully isolated from rice by-products. What he had isolated was named "beriberi vitamin" in 1912. This term "vitamin" denoted that the substance was vital to life and chemically an amine (vital + amine). In 1912, Funk proposed the theory that other "deficiency diseases" in addition to beriberi were caused by a lack of these essential substances, namely scurvy, rickets, sprue, and pellagra. He was the first to suggest that pellagra was a nutrient deficiency disease.

In 1923, Evans and Bishop discovered that vitamin E deficiency caused reproductive failure in rats. Steenbock (1924) showed that irradiation of foods as well as animals with ultraviolet light produced vitamin D. In 1928, Szent-Györgyi isolated hexuronic acid (later renamed "ascorbic acid") from foods such as orange juice. One year later, Moore proved that the animal body converts carotene to vitamin A. This experiment involved feeding 1 group of rats carotene and finding higher levels of vitamin A in their livers compared to controls. By 1928, Joseph Goldberger and Conrad Elvehjem had shown that vitamin B was more than one substance. After the "vitamin" was heated, it was no longer effective in preventing beriberi (B_1), but it was still good for rat growth (B_2). The 1930s and 1940s were the golden age of vitamin research.

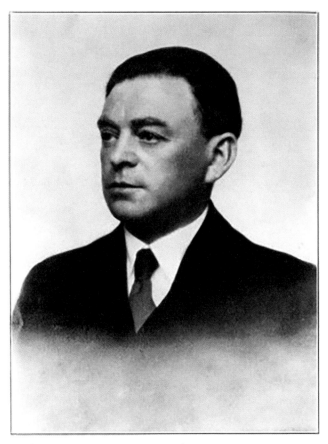

Figure 2.2 Casimir Funk (source: Roche Historical Archive)

During this period, the traditional approach was to (1) study the effects of a deficient diet, (2) find a food source that prevents the deficiency, and (3) gradually concentrate the nutrient (vitamin) in a food and test potency. Laboratory animals were used in these procedures.

Henrick Dam of Denmark discovered vitamin K in 1929 when he noted hemorrhages in chicks fed a fat-free diet. Ironically 1 year earlier, Herman Almquist, working in the United States, had discovered both forms of the vitamin (K_1 and K_2) in studies with chicks. Unfortunately, university administrators delayed the review of his paper, and when it was finally submitted to the journal *Science*, it was rejected. Therefore, only Henrick Dam received a Nobel prize for discovering vitamin K.

Vitamin B_{12} was the last traditional vitamin to be identified, in 1948. Shortly after that, it was discovered that cobalt was an essential component of the vitamin. Simple monogastric animals were found to require the vitamin, whereas ruminants and other species with large microbial populations (e.g., horses) require dietary cobalt rather than vitamin B_{12}.

Compared with the situation for night blindness, xeropthalmia, beriberi, scurvy, and rickets, there were no records from the ancient past of the disease of pellagra. The disease was caused by niacin deficiency in humans, a problem prevalent mainly in cultures where corn (maize) was a key dietary staple (Harris, 1919). Columbus took corn to Spain from America. Pellagra was not recognized until 1735, when Gaspar Casal, physician to King Philip V of Spain, identified it among peasants in northern Spain. The local people called it "mal de la rosa," and Casal associated the disease with poverty and spoiled corn. The popularity of corn spread eastward from Spain to southern France, Italy, Russia, and Egypt, and so did pellagra. James Woods Babcock of Columbia, South Carolina, who identified pellagra in the United States by establishing a link with the disease in Italy, studied the case records of the South Carolina State Hospital and concluded that the disease condition had occurred there as early as 1828. Most cases occurred in low-income groups, whose diet was limited to inexpensive foodstuffs. Diets characteristically associated with the disease were the 3 Ms, specifically meal (corn), meat (backfat), and molasses.

The word pellagra means rough skin, which relates to dermatitis. Other descriptive names for the condition were "mal de sol" (illness of the sun) and "corn bread fever." In the early 1900s in the United States, particularly in the South, it was common for 20,000 deaths to occur annually from pellagra. It was estimated that there were at least 35 cases of the disease for every death due to pellagra. Even as late as 1941, 5 years after the cause of pellagra was known, 2,000 deaths were still attributed to the disease. The clinical signs and mortality associated with pellagra are the 4 Ds: dermatitis (of areas exposed to the sun), diarrhea, dementia (mental problems), and death. Several mental institutions in the United States, Europe, and Egypt were primarily devoted to caring for pellagra sufferers or pellagrins.

In 1914, Joseph Goldberger, a bacteriologist with the US Public Health Service, was assigned to identify the cause of pellagra. His studies observed that the disease was associated with poor diet and poverty and that well-fed persons did not contract the disease (Carpenter, 1981). The therapeutic value of good diets was demonstrated in orphanages, prisons, and mental institutions in South Carolina, Georgia, and Mississippi. Goldberger, his wife, and 14 volunteers constituted a "filth squad" who ingested and injected various biological materials and excreta from pellagrins to prove that pellagra was not an infectious disease. These extreme measures did not result in pellagra, thus demonstrating the non-infectious nature of the disease. At the time, researchers and physicians did not want to believe that pellagra resulted from poor nutrition. They sought to link it to an infection in keeping with the popular "germ theory" of diseases (McDowell, 2006). An important step toward isolating the preventive factor for pellagra involved the discovery of a suitable laboratory animal for testing its potency in various concentrated preparations. It was found that a pellagra-like disease (black tongue) could be produced in dogs. Elvehjem and his colleagues (1974) isolated nicotinamide from the liver and identified it as the factor that could cure black tongue in dogs. Reports of niacin's dramatic therapeutic effects in human pellagra cases quickly followed from several clinics.

In 1824, James Scarth Combe first discovered fatal anemia (pernicious anemia) and suggested it was linked to a digestive disorder. George R. Minot and William Murphy reported in 1926 that large amounts of the raw liver would alleviate the symptoms of pernicious anemia. In 1948, E. L. Rickes and his colleagues in the United States and E. Lester Smith in England isolated vitamin B_{12} and identified it as the anti-pernicious anemia factor (McDowell, 2006). Much earlier, in 1929, W. B. Castle had shown that pernicious anemia resulted from the interaction between a dietary factor (extrinsic) and a mucoprotein substance produced by the stomach (intrinsic factor). Castle used an unusual but effective method to relieve the symptoms of pernicious anemia patients. He ate some beef, and after allowing enough time for the meat to mix with gastric juices, he regurgitated the food and mixed his vomit with the patients' food. With this treatment, the patients recovered because they received both the extrinsic (vitamin B_{12}) and intrinsic (a mucoprotein) factors from Castle's incompletely digested beef meal.

The importance of vitamins was well accepted in the first 3 decades of the 20th century. Table 2.1 provides an overview of the chronological evolution of the discovery, isolation, and assignment of the chemical structure and first production of the individual vitamins. The development of synthetic production of vitamins started in 1933 with ascorbic acid/vitamin C from Merck (Cebion®), which was isolated from plant leaves. However, the first industrial-scale chemical production of vitamin C was achieved by F. Hoffmann-La Roche in 1934 based on a combined fermentation and chemical process developed by Tadeus Reichstein. These scientific innovations were recognized with 12 Nobel Prizes and 20 laureates (Table 2.2). A complete description of the history of discovery, first syntheses, and current industrial processes used for producing each vitamin was described by Eggersdorfer et al. (2012) and McDowell (2013).

Table 2.1 Discovery, isolation, structural elucidation, and synthesis of vitamins (source: Eggersdorfer et al., 2012)

Vitamin	Discovery	Isolation	Structural elucidation	First synthesis
Vitamin A	1916	1931	1931	1947
Vitamin D	1918	1932	1936	1959
Vitamin E	1922	1936	1938	1938
Vitamin B_1	1912	1926	1936	1936
Vitamin B_2	1920	1933	1935	1935
Niacin	1936	1936	1937	1837/1940*
Pantothenic acid	1931	1938	1940	1940
Vitamin B_6	1934	1938	1938	1939
Biotin	1931	1935	1942	1943
Folic acid	1941	1941	1946	1946
Vitamin B_{12}	1926	1948	1956	1972
Vitamin C	1912	1928	1933	1933

Note: *1837: synthesis of niacin used in photography before discovering its nutritional function; 1940: nicotinamide.

Table 2.2 Nobel prizes for vitamin research (source: Eggersdorfer et al., 2012)

Year	Recipient	Field	Citation
1928	Adolf Windaus	Chemistry	Research into the constitution of steroids and connection with vitamins
1929	Christiaan Eijkman	Medicine, Physiology	Discovery of antineuritic vitamins
1929	Sir Frederick G. Hopkins	Medicine, Physiology	Discovery of growth-stimulating vitamin
1934	George R. Minot, William P. Murphy, George H. Whipple	Medicine, Physiology	Discoveries concerning liver therapy against anemias
1937	Sir Walter N. Haworth	Chemistry	Research into the constitution of carbohydrates and vitamin C
1937	Paul Karrer	Chemistry	Research into the constitution of carotenoids, flavins, and vitamins A and B_2
1937	Albert Szent-Györgyi	Medicine, Physiology	Discoveries in connection with biological combustion processes, with special reference to vitamin C and catalysis of fumaric acid
1938	Richard Kuhn	Chemistry	Work on carotenoids and vitamins
1943	Carl Peter Henrik Dam	Medicine, Physiology	Discovery of vitamin K
1943	Edward A. Doisy	Medicine, Physiology	Discovery of chemical nature of vitamin K
1953	Fritz A. Lipmann	Medicine, Physiology	Discovery of coenzyme A and its importance for intermediary metabolism
1964	Konrad E. Bloch, Feodor Lynen	Medicine, Physiology	Discoveries concerning mechanism and regulation of cholesterol and fatty acid metabolism
1964	Dorothy C. Hodgkin	Chemistry	Structural determination of vitamin B_{12}
1967	Ragnar A. Granit	Medicine, Physiology	Research which illuminated electrical properties of vision by studying wavelength discrimination by eye
1967	Halden K. Hartine	Medicine, Physiology	Research on mechanisms of sight
1967	George Wald	Medicine, Physiology	Research on chemical processes that allow pigments in the eye retina to convert light into vision

Vitamins became available in the following years through chemical synthesis, fermentation, or extraction from natural materials (Table 2.1). From 1930 to 1950, there was mainly small-scale production in several countries to reach local markets, but, as demand grew, larger plants became more common from 1950 to 1970. Still, it was not until 1987 that all the vitamins were accessible by industrial processes. Nowadays, chemical synthesis is still the dominant method of industrial production.

The large companies Hoffmann-La Roche (Figure 2.3) and BASF were market leaders, but numerous European and Japanese pharmaceutical companies produced and sold vitamins.

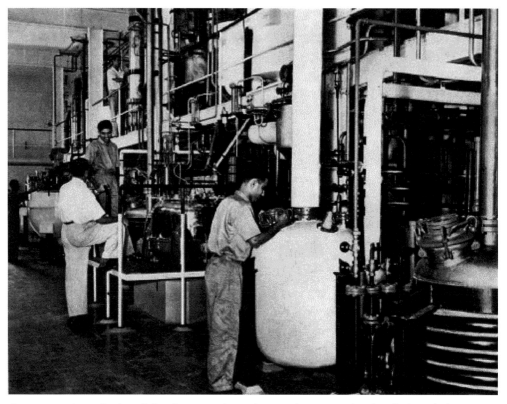

Figure 2.3 Early production of vitamin A at Roche Nutley, USA (source: Roche Historical Archive).

Between 1970 and 1990, production plants became even bigger and with global reach, and since 2000 China has become a larger producer. Fermentation technology started to gain importance, especially for vitamin B_{12} and B_2. New technologies have been emerging in the past 10 years, such as the overexpression of vitamins in plants by either using traditional breeding or genetically modified plants (Eggersdorfer *et al.*, 2012).

Chapter 3

Introduction to vitamins

VITAMIN DEFINITION AND CLASSIFICATION

A vitamin is an organic substance that is:

- a component of a natural compound but distinct from other nutrients such as carbohydrates, fats, proteins, minerals, and water
- present in most foods in a minute amount
- essential for normal metabolism in physiological functions such as growth, development, maintenance, and reproduction
- a cause of a specific deficiency disease or linked to a syndrome if absent from the diet or if improperly absorbed or utilized
- not (with very few exceptions) synthesized by the host in sufficient amounts to meet physiological demands and therefore must be obtained from the diet.

Vitamins are differentiated from trace elements, also present in the diet in small quantities, by their organic nature. Some vitamins deviate from the preceding definition in that they do not always need to be constituents of food (McDowell, 2000a; Combs and McClung, 2022). For example, companion animals and farm livestock can synthesize vitamin C (ascorbic acid) but not fish. Nevertheless, a deficiency has been reported in some species that synthesize vitamin C, and supplementation with this vitamin has been shown to have value for particular diseases or stress conditions (Cummins et al., 1992; Doğan, 2003; Doğan et al., 2021), toxicoses, restore productivity or maximize performance (Girard and Duplessis, 2022, 2023).

Likewise, for most species, niacin can be synthesized from the amino acid tryptophan, but not by the cat or the fish species studied to date, and choline from the amino acid methionine. Nevertheless, dietary supplementation with niacin and choline is necessary for animal farming. Finally, vitamin D can also be synthesized in the skin under UV-ray stimulation. Still, the diets of all farm animals are supplemented with this vitamin to provide the required quantity primarily for proper bone development, mineral mobilization during the prepartum and early lactation (Green et al., 1981; Kichura et al., 1982; Goff et al., 1991b; Horst et al., 1994; Eshaghian et al., 2013; Rodney et al., 2018; Poindexter et al., 2023a,b), improve mammary immunity (Poindexter et al., 2020) and general immunity among other functions (Hodnik et al., 2020; Ahmadi and Mohri, 2021; Eder and Grundmann, 2022).

The quantities of vitamins required are tiny, but they are essential for tissue integrity, normal development or physiological functions, and health maintenance. Their physiological and metabolic roles vary and are of great importance. They are involved in many biochemical reactions and participate in nutrient metabolism derived from the digestion of carbohydrates, lipids, and proteins (Wagner, 1995; Pinotti et al., 2002; Bindel et al., 2005; Alonso et al., 2023). In ruminants, vitamin dietary supplementation also affects the metabolism of ruminal microorganisms impacting nutrient digestion and production of other vitamins (Brusemeister and

Sudekum, 2006; Watanabe and Bito, 2018; Pan et al., 2018; McFadden et al., 2020). Rumen-protected vitamins have been used to have direct impact on the animal during critical life periods (Piepenbrink and Overton, 2003; Zahra et al., 2006; Benoit et al., 2010; Zom et al., 2010).

A single vitamin may have several different functions, and many interactions between them are known (McCay, 1985; Schelling et al., 1995; Zinn et al., 1996; Ashwin et al., 2018). Classically, vitamins have been divided into 2 groups based on their solubilities in fat solvents or water. Thus, fat-soluble vitamins include A, D, E, and K, while B complex vitamins C and choline are water-soluble. The list of the 13 recognized vitamins with main functions and deficiency symptoms are listed in Table 3.1.

Fat-soluble vitamins are found in feedstuffs in association with lipids. The fat-soluble vitamins are absorbed along with dietary fats, apparently by mechanisms like those involved in fat absorption (Blomhoff et al., 1991; Bierer et al., 1995; Goncalves et al., 2015).

Conditions favorable to fat absorption, such as adequate bile flow and good micelle formation, also favor the absorption of fat-soluble vitamins (Blomhoff et al.., 1991; Bramley et al., 2000; Harrison, 2012; Goncalves et al., 2015; Maurya and Aggarwal, 2017). Water-soluble vitamins are not associated with fats, and alterations in fat absorption do not affect their absorption. The fat-soluble vitamins A and D and, to a lesser extent, E are generally stored in appreciable amounts in the animal body. Water-soluble vitamins are not stored, and excesses are rapidly excreted, except for vitamin B_{12} and perhaps biotin (Said, 2011). Table 3.2 lists solubility characteristics of vitamins classified as either fat or water-soluble.

Vitamins can seldom be regarded as nutrients in isolation because they display various interactions with each other and other nutrients (Brusemeister and Sudekum, 2006; Calderón-Ospina and Nava-Mesa, 2020). For example, the fat-soluble vitamins compete for intestinal absorption, so an excess of one may cause deficiencies in the others (Goncalves et al., 2015; Stacchiotti et al., 2021). The vitamins of the B group are regulators of intermediary metabolism. Some metabolic processes are interdependent: for example, choline, B_{12}, and folic acid interact in the methyl groups' metabolism, so a lack of one increases the requirement for the others (Duplessis et al., 2015, 2017, 2022). The same happens between B_{12} and pantothenic acid (Rucker and Bauerly, 2013). It may also occur that an excess of one vitamin induces a deficiency of others. Thus, biotin status deteriorates if the diet is supplemented with high levels of choline and other vitamins of the B group (Bonjour, 1991). High choline levels may similarly affect other vitamins during feed storage.

Vitamins are also known to interact in diverse ways with other nutrients, such as amino acids (Benoit et al., 2010). Both methionine and choline can be a source of methyl groups, which are needed to synthesize both, and this relationship is of commercial importance because supplementation entails an economic cost (Davidson et al., 2008; Potts et al., 2020). Biotin, folic acid, and B_6 play a part in metabolic interconversions of amino acids, so their requirement increases if protein levels are high (Williams et al., 1998; Preynat et al., 2009). The same applies to those vitamins involved in the metabolism of carbohydrates (biotin, B_1), the requirements for which are higher with low-fat diets (Camporeale and Zempleni, 2006; Mock, 2013). Finally, there are also interactions between minerals and vitamins. The best-documented example is selenium and vitamin E (Bourne et al., 2008; Khan et al., 2022). All these aspects will be treated in more detail in Chapters 4, 5, and 6.

These interactions make it somewhat difficult to estimate the requirements for each vitamin precisely, and it is probably more appropriate to focus on the problem generally (NRC, 2016; NASEM, 2021). Chapters 5 and 6 provide a detailed explanation of the situation in beef cattle and dairy cows respectively. The classic evaluation of the dose-response curve, so widely used to estimate the requirements of other nutrients, is not an appropriate technique for vitamins, as their cost is generally low concerning the value of the response value and the potential consequences of inadequate levels. For these reasons, the usual practice is to define vitamin requirements by considering the maximum response obtained with the chosen evaluation criteria, traditionally milk production, weight gain or growth and FCR. However, both milk production and growth are not a specific response: they may be affected by other factors associated with the feed (palatability, particle size, levels of other nutrients, etc.). This issue may explain the variability in response levels between studies on a particular vitamin, even if they are almost concurrent. According to the extensive literature presented in this book, it would not be possible to establish precise mathematical relationships regarding vitamin requirements until all their interactions are known in detail, taking at the same time into account many factors like various diet types and changes in physical composition.

VITAMIN CONVERSION FACTOR

The recommended vitamin supplementation level is given in vitamin activity. Commercial products indicate the amount of vitamin activity: e.g., for vitamin A 1,000,000 international units (IU) per gram or for vitamin B_6 99% pyridoxine hydrochloride. In the latter case an additional correction must be applied: when supplementing 1 mg vitamin B_6 (pyridoxine) it is advised 1.215 mg pyridoxine hydrochloride is required. Table 3.3 provides the conversion factors, the product forms, and their content. In some countries regulatory authorities may have stated different rules for vitamin declaration in premixes and feeds. It could be, for example, the case for vitamin E: usually the declaration is in milligrams whereas in some countries the declaration could be required in IUs. However, as indicated in the table, the international standard is that 1 mg all-rac-α-tocopheryl acetate is equal to 1 IU.

VITAMINS IN FEEDSTUFFS

The vitamin content of feedstuffs is highly variable, and current values have not been wholly evaluated recently. There are severe limitations in relying on average tabular values of vitamins in feedstuffs. For example, the vitamin E content of 42 varieties of corn varied from 11.1 to 36.4 mg/ kg, a 3.3-fold difference (Chen *et al.*, 2019; Combs and McClung, 2022). As a reference, the average vitamin levels in some common forages are presented in Table 3.4 (Ballet *et al.*, 2000). However, the original sources of information still rely on data published in the 1980s or before.

Generally, these average values are based on a limited number of assays published more than 50 to 70 years ago and were not adjusted for bioavailability and variations of vitamin levels within ingredients. Therefore, they may not reflect the changes in genetic characteristics, handling, and storage of forages, cropping practices (Arizmendi-Maldonado *et al.*, 2003), and processing of feedstuffs over the years. Changing processing methods can significantly alter vitamin feed levels. For example, with changes in sugar technology, literature values for the pantothenic acid content of beet molasses have decreased from 50 to 110 mg/kg in the 1950s to about 1 to 4 mg/kg (Palagina *et al.*, 1990). Likewise, heat treatments in feed processing, like pelleting and extrusion, improve nutrient digestibility, reduce antinutritional factors, and eventually control *Salmonella* and other pathogens, resulting in more significant vitamin destruction (Gadient, 1986; Spasevski *et al.*, 2015). In addition, values for some vitamins were not determined by current, more precise assay procedures. Additional information on the limitations of using average values of vitamins in feedstuffs when formulating animal rations has been reported (Kurnick *et al.*, 1972; Chen *et al.*, 2019).

Table 3.1 Main Functions of Vitamins and Symptoms of Deficiency in Ruminants

Vitamin	Main functions	Deficiency symptoms
Vitamin A	• Essential for growth, health (immunity), reproduction (steroid synthesis), vision, development and integrity of skin, epithelia and mucosa	• Blindness or night-blindness (xeropthalmia) • Loss of appetite, poor absorption of nutrients, impaired growth and, in severe cases, death • Reproduction defects like failure of spermatogenesis and fetal resorption cr death • Increased risk of infections (respiratory and intestinal) • Keratinization of epithelial tissues
Vitamin D$_3$	• Homeostasis of calcium and phosphorus (intestine, bones and kidney) • Regulation of bones calcification • Modulation of the immune system • Muscular cell growth	• Rickets, osteomalacia and bone disorders • Lameness • Growth retardation • Muscular weakness and occasionally tetany
25OHD$_3$	• Major serum metabolite of vitamin D$_3$ • More efficient absorption in the intestine • Faster response for calcium homeostasis • More efficient modulation of the immune system and muscular cells than vitamin D$_3$	• Transition cow health (calcium homeostasis) • Colostrum quality • Calf health
Vitamin E	• Most powerful fat-soluble antioxidant • Immune system modulation • Tissue protection • Fertility • Meat quality	• Muscular dystrophy and myopathy • Reduced immune response • Increased mastitis incidence • Retained placenta • Fertility disorders • Meat quality/color case-life problems
Vitamin K$_3$	• Blood clotting and coagulation • Coenzyme in metabolic process related to bone mineralization (Ca binding proteins) and protein formation	• Increased clotting time • Haemorrhages • Anemia • Bone disorders
Vitamin B$_1$	• Coenzyme in several enzymatic reactions • Carbohydrate metabolism (conversion of glucose into energy) • Involved in ATP, DNA and RNA production • Synthesis of acetylcholine, essential in transmission of nervous impulses	• Loss of appetite up to anorexia • Growth retardation • Neuropathies and general muscle weakness • Poor leg coordination • Mucosal inflammation
Vitamin B$_2$	• Fat and protein metabolism • Flavin coenzyme (FMN and FAD) synthesis, essentials for energy production (respiratory chain) • Involved in synthesis of steroids, red blood cells and glycogen • Integrity of mucosa membranes and antioxidant system within cells	• Reduced feed intake and growth • Reduced absorption of zinc, iron and calcium • Inflammation of the mucous membranes (corner of the mouth) of the digestive tract • Rough hair coat, dermatitis and alopecia • More severe in young ruminants
Vitamin B$_6$	• Aminoacids, fats and carbohydrate metabolism • Essential for DNA and RNA synthesis • Involved in the synthesis of niacin from tryptophan	• Growth retardation, lesser feed intake and protein retention • Dermatitis, rough hair coat, scaly skin • Disorders of blood parameters • Muscular convulsions followed by paralysis

Vitamin	Functions	Deficiency symptoms
Vitamin B$_{12}$	• Synthesis of red blood cells and growth • Essential in utilization of propionic acid (and thus the production of glucose and lactose) • Involved in methionine metabolism • Coenzyme in nucleic acids (DNA and RNA) and protein metabolism • Metabolism of fats and carbohydrates	• Anaemia • Reduced milk yield in diets with low cobalt supply • Growth retardation and lower feed conversion • Reduced production of DNA and RNA • Leg weakness • Increased excitability
Niacin or Vitamin B$_3$	• Coenzyme (active forms NAD and NADP) in aminoacids, fats and carbohydrates metabolism • Required for optimum tissue integrity, particularly for the skin, the gastrointestinal tract and the nervous system	• Nervous system disorders • Skin and hair disorders • Inflammation and ulcers of mucous membranes • Ulcerative necrotic lesions of the large intestine • Reduced milk yield and feed efficiency • Increased risk of ketosis • Reduced reproductive performance
Biotin or Vitamin B$_7$	• Coenzyme in protein, fat and carbohydrates metabolism • Normal blood glucose level • Synthesis of fatty acids, nucleic acids (DNA and RNA) and proteins (keratin)	• Loss of appetite and growth retardation • Foot problems including brittle horns and cracks in hooves • Dermatitis • Fertility disorders
d-Pantothenic acid or Vitamin B$_5$	• Present in Coenzyme A (CoA) and Acyl Carrier Protein (ACP) involved in carbohydrate, fat and protein metabolism • Biosynthesis of long-chain fatty acids, phospholipids and steroid hormones	• Skin disorders • Fatty liver • Functional disorders of nervous system • Loss of appetite and poor feed utilization
Folic acid or Vitamin B$_9$	• Coenzyme in the synthesis of nucleic acids (DNA and RNA) and proteins (methyl groups) • Stimulates hematopoietic system • With vitamin B12 it converts homocysteine into methionine	• Megaloblastic (macrocytic) anaemia • Skin damages and hair loss • Fertility disorders • Loss of appetite and growth retardation
Vitamin C	• Intracellular (water-soluble) antioxidant • Immune system modulation (phagocytosis stimulation) • Collagen biosynthesis • Formation of connective tissues, cartilage and bones • Synthesis of corticosteroids and steroid metabolism • Conversion of vitamin D$_3$ to its active form 1,25(OH)2D$_3$	• Lower resistance to stress (e.g., low/high temperatures) • Weakness and fatigue • Reduced immune response • Haemorrhages of the skin, muscles and adipose tissues
Choline	• Membrane structural component (phosphatidylcholine) • Fat transport and metabolism in the liver • Support nervous system function (acetylcholine) • Source of methyl donors for methionine regeneration from homocysteine	• Fatty liver • Reduced milk yield, milk fat and protein • Ketosis • Growth retardation • Carcass characteristics
β-carotene	• Antioxidant • Source of vitamin A • Stimulation of progesterone synthesis • Reproductive tissue maintenance and function	• Poor reproduction: prolonged estrus, retarded follicle maturation and ovulation, cysts • Embryo losses and early abortion • Poor colostrum quality • Increased somatic cell counts in milk

Table 3.2 Vitamin solubility characteristics (source: dsm-firmenich Animal Nutrition and Health, unpublished)

	Molecular weight	Water	Glycerol	Alcohol	Propylene glycol	Ethyl acetate	Ethanol
Vitamin A (retinol)	286.44	Practically insoluble	Practically insoluble	Insoluble	Practically insoluble	Practically insoluble	Practically insoluble
Vitamin D$_3$	384.62	Practically insoluble	Practically insoluble	Practically insoluble	Practically insoluble	Practically insoluble	Practically insoluble
Vitamin E (tocopherol)	430.69	Practically insoluble	Practically insoluble	Insoluble	Practically insoluble	Practically insoluble	Practically insoluble
Vitamin K$_1$	450.68	Slightly soluble	Practically insoluble	Practically insoluble	Practically insoluble	Practically insoluble	Slightly soluble
Vitamin K$_2$	580.9	Insoluble	Practically insoluble	Practically insoluble	Practically insoluble	Practically insoluble	Slightly soluble
Vitamin K$_3$	17.21	Insoluble	Practically insoluble	Slightly soluble	Practically insoluble	Practically insoluble	Practically insoluble
Vitamin B$_1$ (thiamine)	337.28	Insoluble	Insoluble	Insoluble	Insoluble	Practically insoluble	Practically insoluble
Vitamin B$_2$ (riboflavin)	376.36	Insoluble	Practically insoluble	Practically insoluble	Practically insoluble	Practically insoluble	Practically insoluble
Niacin	123.11	Insoluble	Practically insoluble	Insoluble	Practically insoluble	Practically insoluble	Practically insoluble
Pantothenic acid (vitamin B$_5$)	219.23	Insoluble	Practically insoluble	Practically insoluble	Practically insoluble	Insoluble	Practically insoluble
Vitamin B$_6$ (pyridoxine hydrochloride)	205.64	Insoluble	Practically insoluble	Insoluble	Insoluble	Practically insoluble	Practically insoluble
Biotin (vitamin B$_7$)	244.31	Insoluble	Practically insoluble	Insoluble	Practically insoluble	Practically insoluble	Practically insoluble
Folic acid (vitamin B$_9$)	441.4	Slightly soluble	Practically insoluble	Practically insoluble	Practically insoluble	Practically insoluble	Practically insoluble
Vitamin B$_{12}$ (cyanocobalamin)	1355.42	Insoluble	Practically insoluble	Practically insoluble	Practically insoluble	Practically insoluble	Practically insoluble
Choline	121.18	Insoluble	Practically insoluble	Insoluble	Practically insoluble	Practically insoluble	Practically insoluble
Vitamin C (ascorbic acid)	176.12	Insoluble	Practically insoluble	Practically insoluble	Insoluble	Practically insoluble	Practically insoluble

Legend: Insoluble | Practically Insoluble | Slightly soluble

Methanol	Chloroform	Fats-oils	Organic solvents	Ether	Benzene	Acetone	Comments
Soluble	Soluble	Soluble					
			Soluble				
	Soluble	Soluble		Soluble		Soluble	
Soluble		Soluble		Soluble	Soluble	Soluble	
Soluble		Soluble		Soluble	Soluble	Soluble	
				Soluble			
				Soluble			
				Soluble			Freely soluble in dioxane and glacial acetic acid; moderately soluble in amyl alcohol
	Soluble	Soluble		Soluble		Soluble	
			Soluble				
Soluble	Soluble			Soluble	Soluble		Practically insoluble in butanol; Relatively soluble in acetic acid, phenol, pyridine, and solutions of alkali hydroxides and carbonates
	Soluble			Soluble	Soluble	Soluble	
				Soluble			
	Soluble	Soluble		Soluble	Soluble		

Soluble		Not mentioned

Table 3.3 Vitamin conversion factors (source: dsm-firmenich Animal Nutrition and Health, unpublished)

Vitamin (active substance)	Unit	Conversion factor active substance form to vitamin form	Product form
Vitamin A (retinol)	IU	1 IU Vitamin A = 0.344 µg Vitamin A acetate (retinyl acetate)	ROVIMIX® A 1000
			ROVIMIX® A 500 WS
			ROVIMIX® A Palmitate 1.6
			ROVIMIX® AD3 1000/200
Vitamin D$_3$ (cholecalciferol)	IU	1 IU Vitamin D$_3$ = 0.025 µg Vitamin D$_3$	ROVIMIX® D$_3$-500
			ROVIMIX® AD3 1000/200
25OHD$_3$ (25 hydroxy-cholecalciferol)	mg	1 µg 25OHD3 = 40 IU Vitamin D$_3$	ROVIMIX® Hy–D™ 1.25%
Vitamin E (tocopherol)	mg	1 mg Vitamin E = 1 IU Vitamin E = 1 mg all-rac-α-tocopheryl acetate	ROVIMIX® E-50 Adsorbate
			ROVIMIX® E 50 SD
Vitamin K$_3$ (menadione)	mg	1 mg of Vitamin K$_3$ = 2 mg of Menadione Sodium Bisulfite (MSB)	K$_3$ MSB
		1 mg of Vitamin K$_3$ = 2.3 mg of Menadione Nicotinamide Bisulfite (MNB)	ROVIMIX® K$_3$ MNB
Vitamin B$_1$ (thiamine)	mg	1 mg of Vitamin B$_1$ = 1.233 mg of Thiamine mononitrate	ROVIMIX® B$_1$
Vitamin B$_2$ (riboflavin)	mg		ROVIMIX® B2 80-SD
Vitamin B$_6$ (pyridoxine)	mg	1 mg Vitamin B$_6$ = 1.215 mg Pyridoxine hydrochloride	ROVIMIX® B$_6$
Vitamin B$_{12}$ (cyanocobalamin)	mg		Vitamin B$_{12}$ 1% Feed Grade
			ROVIMIX® B$_{12}$ 1% Feed Grade
Vitamin B$_3$ (Niacin; nicotinic acid and nicotinamide)	mg	1 mg Nicotinic acid = 1 mg Niacin	ROVIMIX® Niacin
		1 mg Nicotinamide (or Niacinamide) = 1 mg Niacin	ROVIMIX® Niacinamide
Vitamin B$_7$ (d-Biotin)	mg	1 mg of Biotin = 1 mg D-Biotin	ROVIMIX® Biotin ROVIMIX® Biotin HP
Vitamin B$_5$ (d-Pantothenic acid)	mg	1 mg d-Pantothenic acid = 1.087 mg Calcium d-pantothenate or 2.174 mg Calcium dl-pantothenate	ROVIMIX® Calpan
Vitamin B$_9$ (Folic acid)	mg		ROVIMIX® Folic 80 SD
Vitamin C	mg	1 mg Vitamin C = 1 mg L-Ascorbic acid	STAY-C® 35
			STAY-C® 50
			ROVIMIX® C-EC
			Ascorbic acid
β-Carotene	mg		ROVIMIX® β-Carotene 10%
			ROVIMIX® β-Carotene 10% P

* M: Mash; P: Pellet; EXP: Expansion; EXT: Extrusion; W: Water
For more information about further dsm-firmenich products and product forms please ask your local dsm-firmenich representative

Content (min.)	Formulation technology	Application*
1,000,000 IU/g	Beadlet	M, P, EXP, EXT
500,000 IU/g	Spray-dried powder, water dispersible	W/MR
1,600,000 IU/g	Oily liquid, may crystalize on storage	Oily solution
Vitamin A 1,000,000 IU/g Vitamin D₃ 200,000 IU/g	Beadlet	M, P, EXP, EXT
500,000 IU/g	Spray-dried powder, water dispersible	M, P, EXP, EXT, W/MR
Vitamin A 1,000,000 IU/g Vitamin D₃ 200,000 IU/g	Beadlet	M, P, EXP, EXT
1.25% 25OHD₃ (12.5 g/kg)	Spray-dried powder, water dispersible	M, P, EXP, EXT, W/MR
50% (500 g/kg)	Adsorbate on silicic acid	M, P, EXP, EXT
50% (500 g/kg)	Spray-dried powder, water dispersible	M, P, EXP, EXT, W/MR
Menadione: 51.5% (515 g/kg)	Fine crystalline powder	M, P, EXP, EXT, W/MR
Menadione: 43% (430 g/kg) Nicotinamide: 30.5% (305 g/kg)	Fine crystalline powder	M, P, EXP, EXT
98% (980 g/kg)	Fine crystalline powder	M, P, EXP, EXT
80% (800 g/kg)	Spray-dried powder	M, P, EXP, EXT, W/MR
99% (990 g/kg)	Fine crystalline powder	M, P, EXP, EXT, W/MR
1% (10 g/kg)	Fine powder	M, P, EXP, EXT
1% (10 g/kg)	Spray-dried powder	M, P, EXP, EXT
99.5% (995 g/kg)	Fine crystalline powder	M, P, EXP, EXT
99.5% (995 g/kg)	Fine crystalline powder	M, P, EXP, EXT, W/MR
2% (20 g/kg) 10% (100 g/kg)	Spray-dried powder, water dispersible	M, P, EXP, EXT, W/MR
98% Calcium d-pantothenate (980 g/kg) Calcium 8.2 – 8.6% (82 – 86 g/kg)	Spray-dried powder, water dispersible	M, P, EXP, EXT, W/MR
80% (800 g/kg)	Spray-dried powder, water dispersible	M, P, EXP, EXT, W/MR
35% of total phosphorylated ascorbic acid activity (350 g/kg)	Spray-dried powder	M, P, EXP, EXT
50% of total phosphorylated sodium salt ascorbic acid activity (500 g/kg)	Spray-dried powder	M, P, EXP, EXT, W/MR
97.5% (975 g/kg)	Ethyl-cellulose coated powder	M, P, W/MR
99 – 100% (990 – 1000 g/kg)	Crystalline powder	W/MR
10% (100 g/kg)	Encapsulated beadlet	M, P, EXP, EXT
10% (100 g/kg)	Cross linked beadlet	M, P, EXP, EXT

Vitamin levels from simple rations of feedstuff are generally lower than in complex rations. The currently used concentrated rations for beef cattle in feed lots and high-producing dairy cattle exclude or contain lower amounts of vitamin-rich ingredients. The vitamin fortification levels in these simpler diets should be increased to "fill in the gaps" resulting from the reduced amounts of vitamins supplied by feedstuffs or the higher requirements in some periods of life like prepartum and early lactation (Prom *et al.*, 2022; Poindexter *et al.*, 2023a; Duplessis *et al.*, 2023) or to enhance vitamin content or quality of meat (Yang *et al.*, 2002a; Descalzo *et al.*, 2005) and milk (Duplessis *et al.*, 2019; 2021). Since ingredient changes are frequent and unpredictable in computerized best-cost diet formulation, the low levels of vitamins likely to be supplied by feedstuffs should be disregarded, and adequate dietary vitamin fortification should be provided.

Vitamins, as pure substances, are almost all sensitive to various physical stress factors. Table 3.5 provides a simple qualitative overview of the sensitivity of each vitamin to these factors. This explains the importance, for industrial application, of properly formulating each vitamin to make it more stable and ensuring that the calculated amount per kg of feed reaches the animal.

FACTORS AFFECTING VITAMIN REQUIREMENTS AND UTILIZATION

1. Physiological makeup, genetics, and production function
Vitamin needs of animals and humans depend significantly on their physiological makeup related to the traits given by decades of genetic selection, age, health, and nutritional status and function, such as producing meat, milk, eggs, hair or wool, or carrying a fetus (Bourne *et al.*, 2007b; Zimmerly and Weiss, 2001; NASEM, 2021). For example, dairy cattle breeds with high milk yield have higher vitamin B requirements (Girard and Duplessis, 2023). Higher vitamins A, D$_3$, and E are needed in cows in the last gestation phase and early lactation than for drying cows (Enjalbert *et al.*, 2008; Zom *et al.*, 2010; Khan *et al.*, 2020a).

Table 3.4 Vitamin concentrations of feedstuffs [mean (standard deviation, SD), range] (source: adapted from Ballet *et al.*, 2000)

Forages	Vitamins, mg/kg DM [mean (standard deviation) range]				
	β-carotene	α-tocopherol	Vitamin D	Thiamine	Niacin
Green forages	196 (108) 15–606	161 (91) 9–400	365 (470) 31–1,800	4.6 (2.4) 1.9–8.3	37 (17) 13–56
Florakirk*	49.6	33.7	–	–	–
Florona*	47.7	29.9	–	–	–
Pensacola*	37.6	30.8	–	–	–
Tifton-85*	–	22.6	–	–	–
Dehydrated forages	159 (73) 66–271	125 (57) 28–238	176–617	4 (0.5) 3.8–4.5	53 (9) 39–64
Silages	81 (68) 2–276	0–310	440 (311) 80–866	0.1	1.1–3.4
Hays	36 (34) 1–162	61 (62) 10–211	1,156 (1,161) 90–5,560	2.7 (1.3) 0.2–4.5	28 (17) 6–52

Notes: Rows, excepting marked *, from Ballet et al. (2000) summarized information from Blaylock and Richardson (1950), Brown (1953), Keener (1954), Wallis et al. (1958), Albonico and Fabris (1958), Hjarde et al. (1963), Bunnel et al. (1968), Aitken and Hankin (1970), NRC (1989). *Arizmendi-Maldonado et al. (2003).

Table 3.5 Sensitivity of vitamins to physical stress factors (source: dsm-firmenich Animal Nutrition and Health, unpublished)

Additive	Temperature	Oxygen	Humidity	Light
Vitamin A	Marked	Marked	Marked	Marked
Vitamin D	Marked	Marked	Marked	Marked
25OHD$_3$ (calcifediol)	Marked	Marked	Marked	Marked
Vitamin E	No effect	Marked	No effect	Marked
Vitamin K$_3$	Marked	Marked	Marked	No effect
Vitamin B$_1$	Marked	Marked	Marked	No effect
Vitamin B$_2$	No effect	No effect	Marked	Marked
Vitamin B$_6$	Marked	No effect	Marked	Marked
Vitamin B$_{12}$	Marked	Marked	Marked	Marked
Pantothenic acid	Marked	No effect	Marked	No effect
Nicotinates	No effect	No effect	No effect	No effect
Biotin	Marked	No effect	Marked	No effect
Folic acid	Marked	No effect	Marked	Marked
Vitamin C	Marked	Marked	Marked	No effect
Carotenoids	Marked	Marked	Marked	Marked

Legend: **Marked effect** | **Moderate effect** | No effect

Higher levels of folacin and vitamin B$_{12}$ (Girard and Duplessis, 2023), ascorbic acid (Naresh *et al.*, 2002), and more available vitamin D (Guo *et al.*, 2018; Eder and Grundmann, 2022) could be necessary in the peripartum and early lactation to avoid mastitis, reproductive issues, and improve health.

The recent data discussed in Chapters 5 and 6, for beef cattle and dairy cows respectively, from diverse sources and industry applications in primary ruminant-producing countries indicates that current genetic potential has improved growth rate, FCR, and milk production. Consequently, vitamin requirements determined several decades ago might not apply to today's animals.

2. Confined production versus access to pasture
The complete confinement of dairy cattle in some regions has become more frequent: consequently, vitamin nutrition has played an essential role in the success of intensive dairy production (Nelson *et al.*, 2016a,b). In contrast, young, lush, green grasses or forages are good vitamin sources and could provide significant quantities of most vitamins. More available vitamins A and E are present in pastures and green forages, which contain ample amounts of β-carotene, α-tocopherol, and flavonoids, versus those found in grains, which are lower in bioavailability.

3. Antioxidants and immunological role of vitamins
Immunological response and disease conditions are intimately related to the requirements of specific vitamins (Bruns and Webb, 1990; Galyean *et al.*, 1999; Khan *et al.*, 2020c; Poindexter

et al., 2020; Doğan, 2023). Disease conditions influence the antioxidant vitamins like vitamins E, C, and β-carotene (Bendich, 1993; Ndiweni and Finch, 1996; Chawla and Kaur, 2004; Weiss *et al.*, 2004). These nutrients play essential roles in animal health by inactivating harmful free radicals from various stressors produced through regular cellular activity. Free radicals can damage biological systems (Celi, 2011; Abd Ellah, 2013). Free radicals, including hydroxy, hypochlorite, peroxyl, alkoxy, superoxide, hydrogen peroxide, and singlet oxygen, are generated by autoxidation, radiation, or some oxidases, dehydrogenases, and peroxidases. Also, phagocytic granulocytes undergo respiratory bursts to produce oxygen radicals to destroy pathogens. However, these oxidative products can, in turn, damage healthy cells if they are not eliminated. Antioxidants stabilize these highly reactive free radicals, maintaining cells' structural and functional integrity (McCay, 1985) and contributing to meat quality (Dikeman, 2007; Descalzo and Sancho, 2008).

Tissue defense mechanisms against free-radical damage generally include vitamin C, E, and β-carotene as significant vitamin antioxidant sources, but vitamin D can also play a role (Strickland *et al.*, 2021). In addition, several metalloenzymes, which include glutathione peroxidase (selenium), catalase (iron), superoxide dismutase (copper, zinc, and manganese), and even pyridoxine (Miller *et al.*, 1993; Xiao *et al.*, 2021; Khan *et al.*, 2022) are also critical in protecting the internal cellular constituents from oxidative damage. These nutrients' dietary and tissue balance protects tissues against free-radical damage (Combs and McClung, 2022).

A compromised immune system will reduce animal production efficiency through increased susceptibility to disease, leading to animal morbidity and mortality. Both *in vitro* and *in vivo* studies show that antioxidant vitamins enhance cellular and noncellular immunity. The antioxidant function of these vitamins could, at least in part, enhance immunity by maintaining the function and structural integrity of critical immune cells (Yue *et al.*, 2018; Khan *et al.*, 2020c).

Vitamin C is the most crucial antioxidant in extracellular fluids. It can protect biomembranes against lipid peroxidation damage by eliminating peroxyl radicals in the aqueous phase before the latter can initiate peroxidation (Ranjan *et al.*, 2012; Johnston *et al.*, 2013). Data from several animal species indicates that vitamin C is required for an adequate immune and antiviral response in limiting lung pathology after virus infection (Dwenger *et al.*, 1994). One of the protective effects of vitamin C may partly be mediated through its ability to reduce circulating glucocorticoids (Johnston *et al.*, 2013). In addition, ascorbate can regenerate the reduced form of α-tocopherol, perhaps accounting for the observed sparing effect of these vitamins (Ranjan *et al.*, 2005, 2012). In sparing fatty acid oxidation, tocopherol is oxidized to the tocopheryl free radical. Ascorbic acid can donate an electron to the tocopheryl free radical, regenerating the reduced antioxidant form of tocopherol (Roth and Kaeberle, 1985; Eicher-Pruett *et al.*, 1992).

Vitamin C and E supplementation resulted in a 78% decrease in the susceptibility of lipoproteins to mononuclear cell-mediated oxidation. Ascorbic acid, as an effective scavenger of reactive oxygen species, minimizes the oxidative stress associated with activated phagocytic leukocytes' respiratory burst, thereby controlling the inflammation and tissue damage associated with immune responses (Hidiroglou *et al.*, 1995). Ascorbic acid is very high in phagocytic cells, with these cells using free radicals and other highly reactive oxygen-containing molecules to help kill pathogens that invade the body. However, these reactive species may damage cells and tissues in the process. Ascorbic acid helps to protect these cells from oxidative damage (Combs and McClung, 2022).

Vitamin A strongly influences the immunological response, although it has less antioxidant potential than β-carotene. Animals deficient in vitamin A will show increased frequency and severity of bacterial, protozoal, and viral infections and other disease conditions (Jee *et al.*, 2013). As a function of vitamin A, part of the disease resistance is related to maintaining mucous membranes and normal adrenal gland functioning to produce corticosteroids needed to combat disease. An animal's ability to resist illness depends on a responsive immune system, and a vitamin A deficiency causes a reduced immune response (Combs and McClung, 2022).

Vitamin A deficiency affects several cells of the immune system. Vitamin A deficiency affects immune functions, particularly the antibody response to T-cell-dependent antigens (Ross and Harrison, 2013). The RAR-alpha mRNA expression and antigen-specific proliferative response of T-lymphocytes are influenced by vitamin A status *in vivo* and directly modulated by retinoic acid. Repletion with retinoic acid effectively re-establishes the number of circulating lymphocytes (Tjoelker *et al.*, 1988).

A diminished primary antibody response could also increase the severity and duration of an episode of infection. In contrast, a diminished secondary reaction could increase the risk of developing a second disease episode. Vitamin A deficiency causes decreases in phagocytic activity in macrophages and neutrophils. The secretory immunoglobulin A (IgA) system is an essential first line of defense against infections of mucosal surfaces.

An optimal vitamin A range enhances vitamin A responses because both deficient and excessive levels suppress immune function. In many experiments with laboratory and domestic animals, the effects of both clinical and subclinical deficiencies of vitamin A on the production of antibodies and the resistance of different tissues to microbial infection or parasitic infestation have frequently been demonstrated (Stephensen *et al.*, 1996; Twining *et al.*, 1997; Ahmed *et al.*, 1990).

Vitamin A and E supplementation improves the antioxidant capacity, immune status, intestinal cells, and growth performance of calves (Eicher *et al.*, 1994; Franklin *et al.*, 1998; Carter *et al.*, 2005). Supplementation of vitamin A can also inhibit the harmful action of lipopolysaccharides on the intestinal barrier function, contributing to maintaining gut health (He *et al.*, 2019). However, levels above 20,000 or 40,000 IU/kg of DM can decrease serum levels of vitamin E and inhibit vitamin K_2 synthesis, and liver metabolism.

Animal studies indicate that specific carotenoids like canthaxanthin, retinoic acid, and lycopene, with antioxidant capacities but without vitamin A activity, can enhance many aspects of immune functions and act directly as antimutagens and anticarcinogens (Chew and Park, 2004). They can protect against radiation damage and block photosensitizers' damaging effects. Also, carotenoids can directly affect gene expression, and this mechanism may enable carotenoids to modulate the interaction between B-cells and T-cells, thus regulating humoral and cell-mediated immunity (Wiedermann *et al.*, 1993; Zhao and Ross, 1995).

Vitamin E is perhaps the most studied nutrient related to the immune response (Meydani and Han, 2006). Evidence accumulated over the years and in many species indicates that vitamin E is an essential nutrient for the normal function of the immune system. Furthermore, studies suggest that the beneficial effects of certain nutrients, such as vitamin E, on reducing disease risk can affect the immune response. Deficiency in vitamin E impairs B- and T-cell-mediated immunity. Vitamin E partially reduces prostaglandin synthesis and prevents the oxidation of polyunsaturated fatty acids (PUFAs) in cell membranes (Shanker, 2006).

Considerable attention is being directed to vitamin E and selenium's role in protecting leukocytes and macrophages during phagocytosis, the mechanism whereby animals immunologically kill invading bacteria and viruses (Beck, 2007). Both vitamin E and selenium may help these cells survive the toxic products produced to effectively kill ingested bacteria (Badwey and Karnovsky, 1980). Most of the benefits of this combination depend on the excellent synergistic antioxidant effect of these 2 nutrients. Vitamin E and selenium can also improve immunoglobulin transfer in colostrum (Quigley and Bernard, 1995; Lacetera *et al.*, 1996; Debier *et al.*, 2005).

Since vitamin E acts as a tissue antioxidant and aids in quenching free radicals produced in the body, any infection or other stress factor may exacerbate the depletion of the limited vitamin E stores in various tissues. Regarding immunocompetency, dietary requirements may be adequate for average growth and production; however, higher levels have improved cellular and humoral immune status (Ndiweni and Finch, 1996; Azzi *et al.*, 2000). The former 2 responses are generally used as criteria for determining the requirements of a nutrient. There is an increase in glucocorticoids, epinephrine, eicosanoids, and phagocytic activity during stress and disease. Eicosanoid and corticoid synthesis and phagocytic respiratory bursts are prominent producers of free radicals that challenge the antioxidant systems. Vitamin E has been implicated in stimulating serum antibody synthesis, particularly IgG antibodies (Tengerdy, 1980). The productive effects of vitamin E on animal health may reduce immunosuppressive glucocorticoids (Golub and Gershwin, 1985). Vitamin E also likely has an immuno-enhancing impact by altering arachidonic acid metabolism and subsequent prostaglandin synthesis, thromboxanes, and leukotrienes. Under stress conditions, increased levels of these compounds by endogenous synthesis or exogenous entry may adversely affect immune cell function (Hadden, 1987). These results suggest that the criteria for establishing requirements based on overt deficiencies or growth do not consider optimal health.

4. Stress, disease, or adverse environmental conditions

Intensified production increases stress and subclinical disease-level conditions because of higher densities of animals in confined areas. Animal stress and disease conditions may increase the essential requirement for specific vitamins. Several studies indicated that nutrient levels adequate for growth, feed efficiency, gestation, and lactation might not be sufficient for normal immunity and maximizing the animal's resistance to disease (Cunha, 1985; Lee *et al.*, 1985; Nockels, 1988; Ndiweni and Finch, 1996; Zimbelman *et al.*, 2010).

The adverse effects of environmental stress, welfare, and performance cannot be overemphasized (Aréchiga *et al.*, 1998). Environmental stressors can cause an upsurge in stress hormone secretion, negatively affecting growth and leading to severe mortality. However, effective management techniques are crucial to raising healthy cattle and profit maximization in the ruminant industry. To enhance cattle adaptability under stress conditions, it is essential to understand the functions of different vitamins and the appropriate dosage in ruminant diets to alleviate stress. The synergistic effects of various vitamins and minerals could promote growth performance and reduce environmental stress in ruminants (Maldonado *et al.*, 2017; Khan *et al.*, 2018; Kirdeci *et al.*, 2021; Ahmadi *et al.*, 2022).

Diseases or parasites affecting the gastrointestinal tract will reduce the intestinal absorption of vitamins from dietary sources and those synthesized by microorganisms. If they cause diarrhea, they decrease intestinal absorption and increase vitamin needs. Vitamin A deficiency is often seen in heavily parasitized animals that supposedly receive adequate vitamins (Bruns and Webb, 1990; Esteban-Pretel *et al.*, 2010).

Any disease that includes bleeding of the intestinal wall increases both vitamin loss and vitamin requirements for tissue regeneration. Likewise, a condition that causes a loss in appetite and feed intake increases the need for vitamins per unit of feed consumed to meet daily body needs. Diseases that adversely affect the integrity of the intestinal wall may interfere with vitamin A conversion from carotene and increase the animal's vitamin A needs. Eder and

Grundmann (2022) suggested that the transformation of vitamin D to its functional forms in the liver and kidney would be affected by diseases of these organs.

Mycotoxins are known to cause digestive disturbance, such as vomiting, diarrhea, and internal bleeding, and interfere with the absorption of dietary vitamins A, D, E, and K (Surai and Dvorska, 2005). Moldy corn containing mycotoxins has been associated with deficiencies of vitamin D (rickets) and vitamin E, even though these vitamins were supplemented at levels regarded as satisfactory. Vitamin C has been found to promote vitamin D metabolism and is also known to counter the effects of multiple stresses (DeLuca, 2014; Eder and Grundmann, 2022).

Several research reports have confirmed that almost all vitamins may directly improve ruminal function, especially in dairy cows consuming high levels of concentrate and during the peripartum period (Hannah and Stern, 1985; Abdouli and Schaefer, 1986; Chiquette *et al.*, 1993; Brisson *et al.*, 2022). Vitamins can improve intestinal mucosa, enhance gut antioxidant status, modulate gut microbial communities, improve nutrient digestibility, and stimulate mucosa development and intestinal barrier functions in cows (Ragaller *et al.*, 2011; Pan *et al.*, 2016; Ren *et al.*, 2023).

5. Vitamin antagonists

Vitamin antagonists (antimetabolites) interfere with the activity of various vitamins, and Oldfield (1987) summarized the action of antagonists, which:

- could cleave the vitamin molecule and render it inactive, as occurs with thiaminase, found in raw fish and some feedstuffs, and thiamine. Pyrithiamine is another thiamine antagonist
- could bind with the metabolite, with similar results, as happens between avidin, found in raw egg white, and streptavidin, from *Streptomyces* mold and biotin
- could, because of structural similarity, occupy reaction sites and deny them to the vitamin, as with dicumarol, found in certain plants, and vitamin K.
- inactivate, through rancid fats, biotin and destroy vitamins A, D, E, and possibly others.

These effects were also reviewed by Woolley (2012).

Vitamin antagonists in animal and human diets should be considered when adjusting vitamin allowances, as most vitamins have antagonists that reduce their utilization. Mycotoxins are antagonists in the feed that can substantially decrease antioxidant nutrient assimilation and increase their requirements to prevent the damaging effects of free radicals and toxic products. It is now increasingly recognized that at least 25% of the world's grains are contaminated with mycotoxins (Surai and Dvorska, 2005). Mycotoxins cause digestive disturbances such as vomiting, diarrhea, and internal bleeding and interfere with the absorption of dietary vitamins A and vitamins D, E, and K (McDowell, 2006). On the other hand, vitamin C can reduce the toxicity of specific mycotoxins (Su *et al.*, 2018).

Toxic minerals may be antagonists and will likewise increase vitamin requirements. Vitamin E protects against the toxicity of certain heavy metals (e.g., cadmium, mercury, and lead), which increases the need for the vitamin (McDowell, 2000a).

Specific vitamins can likewise be antagonistic to other vitamins. Excess vitamin A, but largely above the upper safe level of 66,000 IU/kg diet, can affect the metabolism (e.g., absorption) of other fat-soluble vitamins. Large excesses of vitamin E have been shown to result in hemorrhages in some species, apparently by reducing vitamin K absorption. The problem can be eliminated with additional dietary vitamin K.

6. Levels of other nutrients in the diet

The fat level in the diet may affect the absorption of the fat-soluble vitamins A, D, E, and K and the requirements for vitamin E and possibly other vitamins. Fat-soluble vitamins may fail to be absorbed if fat digestion is impaired by liver damage or when the enterohepatic recirculation of bile acids is interrupted. Type (e.g., animal fats, vegetable oils, and blends) and quality (e.g., cis versus trans, saturated versus PUFAs, and oxidized sources) of fats can influence individual vitamin allowances (Charmley and Nicholson, 1994; Bindel et al., 2000; Drouillard et al., 1998; Pottier et al., 2006), and ruminal B vitamin synthesis (Castagnino et al., 2017).

For example, a precise vitamin E:PUFA ratio may not apply to all diet and health status types. Therefore, there has been no consensus on the exact vitamin E:PUFA ratio to determine the vitamin requirement. However, the published human data for a diet with an average concentration of PUFA and mainly linoleic acid indicates that the additional vitamin E requirement ranges from 0.4 to 0.6 mg RRR-α-tocopherol/g of PUFA in the diet. A ratio of 0.5 mg RRR-α-tocopherol/g of linoleic acid was used in the diet, and considered the degree of unsaturation of the dietary fatty acids to evaluate the required vitamin E. Thus, using the proposed equation, humans' estimated requirement for vitamin E varied from 12 to 20 mg/day for a typical range of dietary PUFA intake. Calculations in animal diets indicate that high dietary PUFA increases the vitamin E requirement by 3 mg/g of PUFA (Luciano et al., 2011). Many interrelationships of vitamins with other nutrients exist and affect requirements. For example, prominent interrelationships exist for vitamin E with selenium (Hogan et al., 1993), vitamin D with calcium and phosphorus (Montgomery et al., 2002; Hodnik et al., 2020), choline with methionine (Emanuele et al., 2007; Benoit et al., 2010; Potts et al., 2020), and niacin with tryptophan (Khan et al., 2018; Mishra et al., 2018).

7. Body vitamin reserves

The fat-soluble vitamins A, D, and E are more inclined to remain in the body. This is especially true of vitamin A and carotene, which may be stored by an animal in its liver and fatty tissue in sufficient quantities to meet its requirements for varying periods. Tissue accumulation of vitamin A and α-tocopherol is important for meat stability during storage (Hill et al., 1995; Hoppe et al., 1996; Yang et al., 2002b). Body storage of B group vitamins, except for vitamin B_{12}, is irrelevant (Schwab and Shaver, 2005; Santschi et al., 2005a). Overall, a daily supplementation at the proper levels typical of each species and growth stage is generally recommended in animal husbandry in industrial conditions.

Chapter 4

Vitamin description

FAT-SOLUBLE VITAMINS

Vitamin A
Chemical structure and properties

Vitamin A is a generic term for all the non-carotenoid β-ionone derivatives possessing the biological activity of all-*trans*-retinol (Combs and McClung, 2022). Retinol is the alcohol form of vitamin A. Replacement of the alcohol group (-OH) by an aldehyde group (-CHO) yields retinal, and replacement by an acid group (-COOH) gives retinoic acid (Ross and Harrison, 2013). Vitamin A products for feed use include retinyl acetate, propionate, and palmitate esters (Figure 4.1). Other vitamin A compounds in the body include retinoyl β-glucuronide in bile and retinyl phosphate, an intermediate in glycoprotein synthesis.

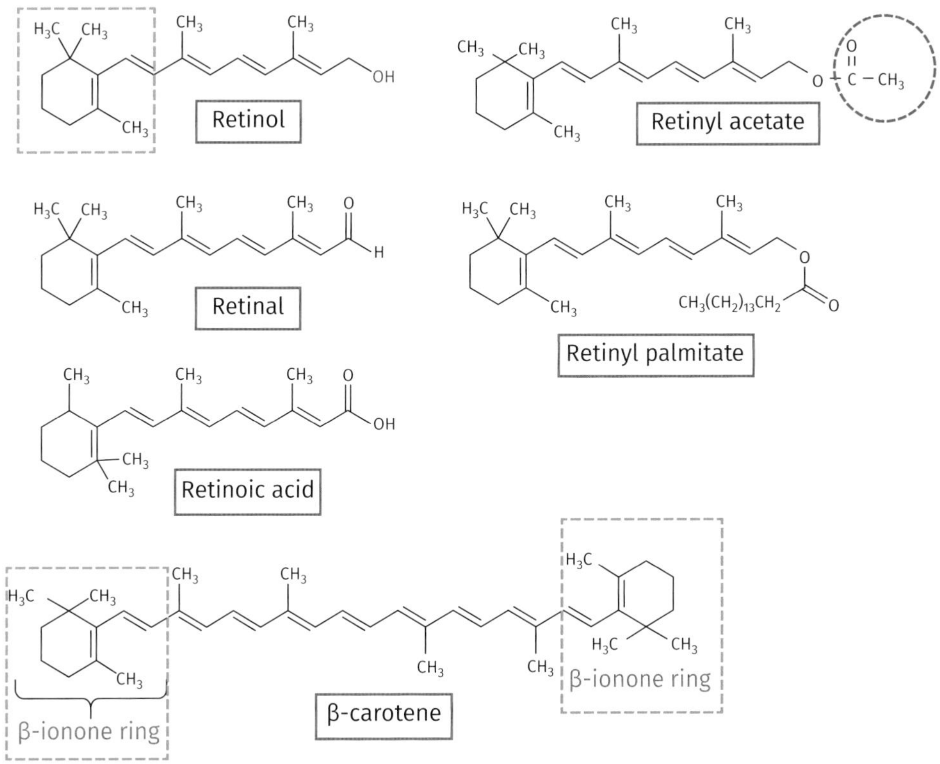

Figure 4.1 Vitamin A, natural and synthetic forms, and β-carotene chemical structures

Chemically, retinol consists of a substituted cyclohexene ring with an aliphatic side chain marked by a series of conjugated double bonds. This unique structure allows retinol and its derivatives to function as both a visual pigment and a regulator of cellular growth and differentiation (Olson, 1984; Ross and Harrison, 2013).

Vitamin A alcohol (retinol) is a nearly colorless, fat-soluble, long-chain, unsaturated compound with 5 bonds. Since it contains double bonds, vitamin A can exist in different isomeric forms. Oxygen, heat, light, and acids rapidly destroy vitamin A and its precursors, carotenoids. Carotenoids are usually found in nature in the all-*trans*-form; however, they are easily isomerized to form *cis* isomers following exposure to heat and light (Lindshield and Erdman, 2006). Moisture and trace minerals reduce vitamin A activity in feeds (Olson, 1984).

The combined potency in a feed, represented by its vitamin A and carotene content, is its vitamin A value. In animal tissues, they exist predominantly as retinal, retinol, retinaldehyde, retinoic, and retinyl esters (Ross and Harrison, 2013).

Vegetables contain a variety of carotenoids. Over 600 forms of carotenoids have been isolated; they differ in molecular structure and biological function (Goodwin, 1984; Ross and Harrison, 2013). Carotenoids are long hydrocarbons divided into carotenes (without oxygen), xanthophylls (with oxygen). Only 80 carotenoids have provitamin A activity. The carotenes are orange-yellow pigments, mainly in green leaves and, to a lesser extent, in corn grain. Six carotenoids are the focus of nutritional research: α-carotene, lutein, lycopene, β-carotene (the most active provitamin A carotenoid), γ-carotene, and β-cryptoxanthin, one of the main carotenoids of corn, possessing the β-ionone ring (C15=C15), are critical because of their provitamin A activity. In corn and corn by-products, β-carotene, β-zeacarotene, and β-cryptoxanthin are present in a ratio of 25:25:50.

Lycopene is an essential carotenoid for its antioxidant function but does not possess the β-ionone ring structure. It is not considered a precursor of vitamin A and is frequently listed as a food colorant (Johnson *et al.*, 1997). However, recently, it has been observed that ruminants are sensitive to lycopene. Positive effects of lycopene have been observed in the cellular and humoral immune responses of pregnant ewes and newborn lambs (Kiani, 2017; Fallah *et al.*, 2021). Lycopene (100 mg/day) increased lymphocyte cells in pregnant ewes, blood circulating IgG concentrations in ewes, and colostrum (6 hours) and lamb blood (24 hours) postpartum.

Lycopene also affected ruminal fermentation parameters, improved microbial protein production, and increased the feed intake of fattening lambs (Aminifard and Kiani, 2023). Lycopene can be considered a potent antioxidant that could be administered to ruminant animals during stressful periods such as the transition into lactation. Aminifard *et al.* (2022) determined that only 70% of dietary lycopene bypassed the rumen and observed that the de-oiled tomato pomace has good lycopene nutritional content for ruminants.

Vitamin A activity of β-carotene is substantially greater than that of other carotenoids (Ross and Harrison, 2013). For example, both α-carotene and cryptoxanthin have about one-half the conversion rate of β-carotene (Tanumihardjo and Howe, 2005). Theoretically, 2 molecules of vitamin A could be formed from 1 molecule of β-carotene. However, biological tests have consistently shown that pure vitamin A has twice the potency of β-carotene on a weight-to-weight basis, indicating a maximum conversion efficiency of 50%.

Natural sources

Vitamin A (retinol) does not occur *per se* in plants, but its precursors, the carotenes with provitamin A activity, occur in several forms. The vitamin A requirements of ruminants can potentially be met by carotenes in feedstuffs. Green plants contain almost 100 molecules with provitamin A activity. ß-carotene is the most abundant and active precursor of vitamin A. However, the content varies significantly in feedstuffs according to the species, state of maturity, preservation, etc. The content in ß-carotene in most feedstuffs is variable and subject to significant losses under less-than-ideal harvest and storage conditions. Vitamin A and the precursor carotenoids are rapidly destroyed by oxygen, heat, light, and the presence of acids. The presence of moisture and trace minerals accelerates the destruction of vitamin A activity in feeds (Olson, 1984; Nozière *et al.*, 2006; NASEM, 2021). The potency of the other carotenoids ranges from 0 to 57% of ß-carotene (Bauernfeind, 1981).

Carotenes are chemically unstable, so many stored feedstuffs are deficient in provitamin A activity. All green parts of growing plants are rich in carotene and, therefore, have a high vitamin A value. The degree of green color in roughage is a good index of its carotene content. Although the yellow color of carotenoids is masked by chlorophyll, all green parts of growing plants are rich in carotene and thus have a high vitamin A value. Good pasture always provides a liberal supply, and the type of pasture, plant (whether grass or legume), appears to be of minor importance. At maturity, however, leaves contain much more than stems, and thus, legume hay is richer in vitamin A content than grass hay (Maynard *et al.*, 1979). With all hays and other forage, vitamin A value decreases after the bloom stage. Plants at maturity can have 50% or less of the maximum carotenoid value of immature plants.

There is a negative correlation between the length of storage and concentration of β-carotenes in forages (Mora *et al.*, 1999; Chauveau-Duriot *et al.*, 2005). Williams *et al.* (1998) estimated that the average values of β-carotenes in forages are 196, 159, and 81 mg/kg DM for artificially dehydrated hay, silage, and sun-dried hay, respectively. Variables influencing carotene digestibility include the month of forage harvest and seasonality, type of forage (fresh or not), plant species and varieties, as tropical or temperate grass, plant DM content, and harvest, conservation methods and storage conditions (hay, silage, green chop, or pasture). Generally, carotene digestibility was above average during warmer months and below average during winter. Wing (1969) reported that the apparent digestibility of carotene in various forages fed to dairy cattle averaged about 78%.

Patel *et al.* (1966) studied carotenes in alfalfa harvested by different methods. Initial losses were most significant in alfalfa that wilted for 2 days after cutting and least in alfalfa that was dried under a shed to protect it from sunlight. Once harvested, the loss of carotene through the first 100 days of storage ranges from 44 to 74%. The alfalfa with the highest initial carotene value (the most negligible loss of activity during harvest) had the most considerable loss of carotene in storage. The highest carotene content was observed 100 days after harvest in alfalfa wilted for 1 day and then dried and stored under a protective shed. Under typical harvest and storage conditions in North America, carotene losses in forage crops would be significant.

Both carotene and vitamin A are destroyed by oxidation. This process is accelerated at high temperatures, but heat without oxygen has a minor effect. Much of the carotene content is destroyed by oxidation in the process of field curing. Many years ago, Russell (1929) already found that there may be a loss of more than 80% of the carotene in alfalfa during the first 24 hours of the curing process. This loss occurs chiefly during daylight hours, partly because of the photochemical activation of the destructive process. Much of the carotene content is destroyed not only by oxidation but also by plant enzymes during the process of field curing. In alfalfa leaves, sunlight-sensitized destruction is 7–8% of the total pigment, while enzymatic destruction amounts to 27 to 28% (Rousseau *et al.*, 1954; Bauernfeind, 1981). Enzymatic destruction requires oxygen, is most significant at high temperatures, and ceases after complete dehydration.

Hay crops cut in the bloom stage or earlier and are cured without exposure to rain or too much sun retain a significant portion of their carotene content. In contrast, those cut in the seed stage and exposed to rain and sun for extended periods lose most of their carotene activity. Green hay curing in the swath may lose one-half of its vitamin A activity in 1 day of exposure to sunlight. Thus, hay usually has only a tiny proportion of the carotene content of fresh grass. Under similar harvest and curing conditions, alfalfa and other legume hay can have less carotene content than grass hay of a good grade (Maynard *et al.*, 1979).

The carotene content of dried or sun-cured forages decreases in storage with the rate of destruction depending on factors such as temperature, exposure to air and sunlight, and length of storage. Concerning light, β-carotene has been shown to protect against photo-oxidation as it absorbs a significant portion of light below 500 nm, reducing reactions with photosensitizers (Airado-Rodriguez *et al.*, 2011). Under average conditions, the carotene content of hay can be expected to decrease by about 6–7% per month. In the artificial curing of hay with a "hay drier," there is only a slight loss of carotene because of the rapidity of the process and protection against exposure to oxygen, with the final product having 2 to 10 times the value of field-cured hay. Severe heating of hay in the mow or stack reduces vitamin content, and there is a gradual loss in storage, so old hay is poorer than new. All-trans-carotene is the predominant isomer in feeds; thermal processing can substantially increase the proportions of cis isomers (9-C and 13-C); β-carotene is the more bioavailable isomer (Deming *et al.*, 2002). It would likely seem that the isomers of β-carotene would increase in the silage fermentation process, resulting in a lower bioavailable β-carotene.

Aside from yellow corn and its by-products, practically all concentrates used in livestock feed are devoid or nearly devoid of vitamin A activity. In addition, yellow corn contains a high proportion of non-β-carotenoids (i.e., cryptoxanthin, lutein, and zeacarotene) that have much less or no provitamin A value than β-carotene. However, they are absorbed and deposited in body tissues (Yang *et al.*, 1992).

The provitamin A activity of yellow corn grain is only one-eighth that of good roughage. There is evidence that yellow corn loses carotene rapidly during storage. For example, a hybrid corn high in carotene lost 50% of its carotene content during 8 months of storage at 25°C and 75% in 3 years at same temperature. Carotene loss was reduced if corn grain was stored at 7°C (Quackenbush, 1963). Maize and its derivatives contain significant quantities of pigmenting carotenoids with much lower provitamin activity (cryptoxanthin) or do not possess provitamin activity like lutein and zeaxanthin. The potency of yellow corn is only about one-eighth that of good roughage. The bioavailability of natural β-carotene was less than that of chemically synthesized forms (White *et al.*, 1993; van Het Hof *et al.*, 2000). Aside from yellow corn and its by-products, practically all concentrates used in feeding animals lack vitamin A value, or nearly so.

The prime factor determining the bioavailability of a vitamin from a feedstuff is its stability. Prolonged storage of the vitamin in premixes or in the final product, vitamin premixes containing minerals, raised temperature, and humidity, pelleting, processing in blocks or by extrusion, or the presence of rancid fats in the ration all reduce the stability of vitamin A (Spasevski *et al.*, 2015). The bioavailability of vitamin A and β-carotenes in the animal depends on the degree of ruminal degradability, the absorption efficiency in the intestine, and the efficiency of conversion of β-carotenes to vitamin A. This process takes place in the intestinal mucosal cells. Dairy cattle can absorb and store a significant proportion of the β-carotenes in a ration. Vitamin A can be stored sufficiently in ruminants' liver and fatty tissue to cover their requirements for up to 6 months or more (McDowell, 2006). In calves, a small enhancing effect of mild heat treatment of carrots on serum and tissue accumulation of carotenoids has been reported (Poor *et al.*, 1993).

A marked discrepancy exists between the carotene content of corn silage, and the vitamin A status of ruminants fed corn silage. On average, corn silage-carotenes were only two-thirds as effective as β-carotene in maintaining liver vitamin A levels in rats (Miller *et al.*, 1969; Rumsey, 1975). Martin *et al.* (1971) reported 5-fold less carotene in corn silage harvested in October and November than in corn silage harvested in September. The more mature corn silage could not sustain liver vitamin A stores in beef steers, mainly if the silage were finely chopped. Diets high in corn silage harvested after a killing frost would be marginal in vitamins A and E. After a killing frost, 4 Florida types of grass showed dramatically reduced β-carotene and α-tocopherol concentrations (Arizmendi-Maldonado *et al.*, 2003). Miller *et al.* (1969) reported that ethanol, an occasional by-product of corn silage fermentation, may reduce liver vitamin A. Fungal mycotoxins occur in corn silage and may increase the vitamin A requirement.

Wing (1969) reported that carotene digestibility in plants is increased during the warmer months. Variations were found in the digestibility of carotenes in plants according to year, plant species, DM content, and form of forage: carotene digestibility was somewhat lower in silages than in pastures or hay. Average published values of carotene content can serve only as approximate guides in feeding practice because many factors affect the potency of individual samples as fed (NRC, 1982).

Naturally occurring sources of vitamin A (retinyl esters) include fish oils, liver, milk fat, egg yolk, and liver, although these are not typically significant contributors to ruminant diets. Animal by-product proteins may contribute some vitamin A activity, primarily to dairy cattle diets. Their contribution would depend on losses of vitamin A during rendering.

Vitamin A value can be decreased by exposure to light (Whited *et al.*, 2002). Light exposure can detrimentally affect fluid milk products' nutritional value and flavor quality. Previous reports have detailed light-induced chemical reactions that result in vitamin A degradation and light-oxidized flavor defects. The presence of milk fat appears to protect against vitamin A degradation in fluid products but adversely affects the flavor quality of milk after exposure to light (Whited *et al.*, 2002). Vitamin A loss was directly influenced by the length and intensity of light exposure and inversely influenced by the fat content of the milk. To illustrate, after 16 hours, vitamin A content was reduced by 29% in reduced-fat milk and 49% in nonfat milk.

Commercial forms

Chemical synthesis of vitamin A was introduced in 1949, and the synthetic form has become the major commercial source of vitamin A. The primary sources of supplemental vitamin A used in ruminant diets are all-trans-retinyl acetate and all-trans-retinyl palmitate (Donoghue *et al.*, 1983). Major vitamin A manufacturers all produce acetate, propionate, and palmitate esters. Propionate and palmitate esters are used in liquid feeds and human foods. The propionate ester is much less common (McGinnis, 1988). Vitamin A is esterified in these forms for stability. These are available in hardened or gelatin beadlet product forms for protection against oxidative destruction in premixes, mash, and pelleted and extruded feeds. Carbohydrates, gelatin, and antioxidants are generally included inside the beadlet to stabilize vitamin A to provide physical and chemical protection against factors either ordinarily present in the feed or due to feeding treatment and storage that are destructive to vitamin A. Unprotected vitamin A oxidizes rapidly in feedstuffs when moisture levels exceed 12%. The reaction between gelatin and sugar makes the beadlet insoluble in water, giving it a more resistant coating that can sustain higher pressure, friction, temperature, and humidity (Frye, 1994). Beadlets are usually formulated to produce a flowable product that will mix easily with minimal dust.

The most frequently used vitamin A acetate in ruminant feeds contains 500,000 to 1,000,000 international units (IU) or United States Pharmacopeia Units (USP) per gram of product. (Note that IU and USP units are equal in value, and one unit equals the activity of 0.3 μg of all-trans-retinol or 0.344 μg of all-transretinyl acetate.) Beadlet technology is also used to produce combination products containing, for example, 500,000 IU vitamin A and 100,000 IU vitamin D_3 per gram, or 1,000,000 IU vitamin A and 200,000 IU vitamin D_3 per gram of product. Similarly, stabilized, dispersible, flowable liquid vitamin concentrates are produced by significant vitamin manufacturers for use in liquid feeds for livestock. Major vitamin A manufacturers also produce water-dispersible dry vitamin A products for milk replacers.

Several factors influence the digestibility of carotene and vitamin A in ruminants. Working with lambs, Donoghue *et al.* (1983) reported that dietary vitamin A levels, ranging from mildly deficient to toxic, affect digestion and uptake. Percentage absorption from supplemental levels of 0, 100, and 12,000 μg retinol (0, 333, and 40,000 IU) per kg diet were 91, 58, and 14%, respectively. Enteric disease states, such as *Cryptosporidium* infection, reduce vitamin A absorption in calves (Holland *et al.*, 1992).

Several factors can influence the loss of vitamin A from feedstuffs during storage. The trace minerals in feeds and supplements, particularly copper, are detrimental to vitamin A stability (Yang *et al.*, 2021a). Dash and Mitchell (1976) reported the vitamin A content of 1,293 commercial feeds over 3 years, and the loss of vitamin A was over 50% in 1 year. Vitamin A loss in commercial feeds was evident even if the commercial feeds contained stabilized vitamin A supplements. It is, therefore, essential to carefully assess the quality of the commercial product.

Vitamin A supplements should not be stored for prolonged periods before feeding. Chen (1990) measured the stability of 3 commercial cross-linked vitamin A beadlets in trace mineral premixes and feeds on the market. After 3 months of storage at high temperatures and humidity, vitamin A retention varied from 30 to 80%, depending on the antioxidants present in the beadlet.

Vitamin A (and carotene) destruction also occurs from processing feed with steam and pressure. Pelleting effects of vitamin A in the feed are determined by die thickness and hole size, which produce frictional heat and a shearing effect that can break supplemental vitamin A beadlets and expose the vitamin. In addition, steam application exposes feed to heat and moisture. In a 30% concentrate pelleted at 93°C after 3 months of storage at high temperature and humidity, retention varied from 57 to 62%. Running fines back through the pellet mill exposes vitamin A to the same factors a second time.

Metabolism
Rumen Metabolism of Vitamin A
Several studies indicate that appreciable amounts of vitamin A are degraded in the rumen. Studies with various diets have reported pre-intestinal vitamin A disappearance values ranging from 40 to 70% (Ullrey, 1972). Warner *et al.* (1970) indicated that ruminal destruction of vitamin A was 55% in rations containing 50–75% forage and increased to 65% when the percentage of forage was reduced from 40 to 20% of the ration. The ruminal degradability of β-carotenes is lower than vitamin A and varies between 0 and 30% (Potanski *et al.*, 1974; Mora *et al.*, 1999). The concentration in a diet is one factor associated with ruminal destruction. Rode *et al.* (1990) compared microbial degradation of vitamin A (retinyl acetate) in steers fed concentrate, hay, or straw diets. The estimated effective rumen degradation of biologically active vitamin A was approximately 80% in animals fed with rations containing 30% forage, 67% for cattle fed high-concentrate diets, and 16% and 19% for animals fed hay and straw diets, respectively.

Weiss *et al.* (1995) reported 72% *in vitro* rumen degradation of retinyl esters with a 50% concentrate ration and 16 to 20% degradation when diets greater than 75% forage were fed.

On the other hand, β-carotene degradation was 23% in sheep, *in vivo*, across a wide range of dietary starch levels. Weiss (1998) interpreted these data to mean that in ruminants fed rations with 50% or more concentrate, retinyl esters would be only 50% as available on a weight basis compared to β-carotene. However, preformed vitamin A (e.g., retinyl acetate) has approximately 8 times the vitamin A activity per mg compared to β-carotene in cattle (3,000 IU/mg vs. 400 IU/mg), which must be considered in any comparison.

Interestingly, workers in Florida, USA reported that milk production significantly increased in 3 experiments where cows were fed 400 mg of β-carotene per head daily despite being supplemented with 200,000 to 250,000 IU of vitamin A per day (Aréchiga *et al.*, 1998). The 2 different rations averaged 28.8 and 28% forage on a DM basis, although fibrous by-product feeds comprised a significant portion. Ruminal destruction of vitamin A may have been a factor in this study. The results suggest that β-carotene supplementation in dairy cows may be warranted under certain dietary or climatic conditions.

These results suggest that, in rations containing 50% or more concentrate, the ruminal degradability of vitamin A is considerably greater than in those rations based on forage. Consequently, it seems reasonable to consider the possibility of using sources of protected vitamin A in rations rich in concentrate. Thus, for example, Alosilla *et al.* (2007) evaluated the bioavailability of 5 commercial sources of vitamin A (80,000 IU/day) using a concentrate-rich diet in beef cattle. They observed differences in the hepatic concentration of retinol – considered the best indicator for evaluating the status of vitamin A in the animal – between the different vitamin sources used. These differences were attributed to ruminal degradability and intestinal digestibility.

Stacchiotti *et al.* (2021) concluded, in a literature review, that fat-soluble vitamins, in general, directly or indirectly modify the microbial composition involving, for example, immune system-mediated and metabolic mechanisms of bacterial growth or inhibition in humans. The gut microbiota influences the synthesis, metabolism, and transport of fat-soluble vitamins at different levels, including their bioactive metabolites that are either introduced with the diet or released in the gut via entero-hepatic circulation. Understanding these interactions in ruminants and their impact on ruminal intestinal and metabolic homeostasis will be pivotal to designing new, more efficient disease prevention strategies.

Absorption and transport
The absorption and transport of vitamin A have been reviewed in more detail elsewhere (Bierer *et al.*, 1995; Solomons, 2006; Ross and Harrison, 2013; Álvarez *et al.*, 2015). Dietary carotenoids and retinyl esters (e.g., acetate) are released by pepsin in the stomach. Vitamin A and β-carotene become dispersed in micelles before absorption from the intestine (O'Byrne and Blaner, 2013). These molecules are hydrolyzed to retinol in the intestine (duodenum) by pancreatic retinyl ester hydrolase, absorbed as free alcohol retinol, and then re-esterified in the mucosa, primarily to palmitate. β-carotene in feed is cleaved in the intestinal mucosa by the enzyme 15,15' dioxygenase to retinaldehyde, which is then reduced to retinol (vitamin A), as described by Harrison (2012). Normal processes of fat digestion and absorption and adequate dietary fat content are required for the absorption and subsequent conversion of β-carotene to retinol. Consequently, pancreatic, liver, and biliary functions are required to absorb vitamin A and its precursors (Figure 4.2).

There is not much data on vitamin A absorption in the small intestine of ruminants. Data collected from humans and rats indicate that intestinal absorption varies between 20 and

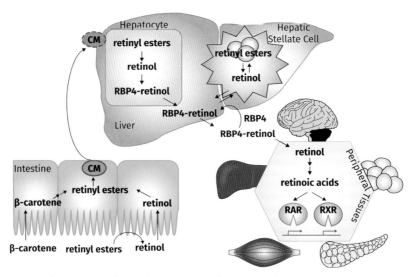

Figure 4.2 Schematic representation of intestinal vitamin A absorption, transport to, and storage in the liver and redistribution to peripheral tissues (source: Saeed *et al.*, 2018)

60% (Blomhoff *et al.*, 1991; Álvarez *et al.*, 2015). However, early reports have indicated that the absorption is lower in ruminants. Wing (1969) calculated that intestinal digestibility was 78%. However, Cohen-Fernandez *et al.* (1976) recovered 90% of marked β-carotene administered to lambs in their feces, suggesting a much lower absorption level. Another study carried out on sheep evaluated the digestion and absorption of carotenoids from red clover (Cardinault *et al.*, 2006) and observed that apparent digestibility increased (>53%). However, it varied according to the type of carotenoid considered. For β-carotenes, the values were over 100% in some cases, suggesting that the ruminal microorganisms can synthesize them.

The efficiency of absorption of β-carotenes and retinol depends on the quantity of fat and vitamins supplied in the diet (Blomhoff, 1994; Yeum *et al.*, 2000). Yeum *et al.* (2000) indicated that in the presence of α-tocopherol, β-carotene is converted exclusively into retinol, while if α-tocopherol is absent, it splits into apocarotenoids and retinol. In dairy cows, supplemental fat elevates plasma levels of β-carotene (Weiss *et al.*, 1994). Compared to goats, cattle have a low enzyme activity for converting β-carotene to retinol (Mora *et al.*, 2000). Lower enzyme levels of duodenal and jejunal 15 and 15-dioxygenase in cattle compared with goats may explain the more excellent pigmentation of adipose tissue in cattle.

The accepted conversion standard in dairy cattle is that 1 mg of all-trans β-carotene will provide 400 IU of vitamin A activity for a 12% conversion efficiency (Bauernfeind, 1981; NRC, 1989). Jersey and Guernsey's breeds absorb a more significant proportion of carotene intact from the intestine than Holstein cows, leading to the orange-yellow color of their body and milk fat. Still, they can convert carotene to retinol in the liver, lung, and other tissues (McGinnis, 1988). Cattle reportedly can convert β-carotene to retinol in the ovary (Sklan, 1983; Schweigert *et al.*, 1988), where β-carotene may act as a local supply of retinol.

Donoghue *et al.* (1983) observed that vitamin A absorption in lambs supplemented with 0, 100, and 12,000 µg of retinol/kg live weight was 91, 58 and 14%, respectively, suggesting an inverse relationship between intestinal concentration and vitamin A absorption. The leading site of vitamin A and carotenoid absorption is the mucosa of the proximal jejunum. These micelles are composed of mixtures of bile salts, monoglycerides, and long-chain fatty acids, together with vitamins D, E, and K, all of which influence the transfer of vitamin A and β-carotene to the intestinal cell (Bierer *et al.*, 1995).

An enzyme converts carotene present in feed to retinal in the intestinal mucosa. The retinal is then reduced to retinol (vitamin A). However, extensive evidence exists also for random (excentric) cleavage, resulting in retinoic acid and retinal, with a preponderance of apocarotenals formed as intermediates (Wolf, 1995). Carotenoids are typically converted to retinol in the intestinal mucosa. They may also be converted into the liver and other organs (McGinnis, 1988).

The absorption of vitamin A in the intestine is believed to be 80 to 90%, while that of β-carotene is about 50 to 60% (Olson, 1984; Bierer *et al.*, 1995). Many factors may modify it, either in a positive way, such as the inclusion of fats in the diet, the addition of antioxidants, and the use of moderate levels of vitamin E or other synthetic antioxidants (Baldi, 2005; Calderón *et al.*, 2007) or in a negative way, such as high levels of vitamin E, the presence of aflatoxins (Surai and Dvorska, 2005; Rodrigues, 2014) or enteric infections. The efficiency of vitamin A absorption decreases somewhat with very high doses. Thus, intestinal diseases reduce their levels of plasma and hepatic reserves, which increases the requirements of vitamin A because of poor absorption and oxidation induced by the cellular immune response. Vitamin A deficiencies reduce resistance to intestinal challenges.

Several factors affect the absorption of carotenoids and vitamin A. These include genetics, carotenoid form, fat sources, and antioxidant and protein levels. There are differences among mammalian species and breeds in a species. In the case of cattle, there is a substantial breed difference in the absorption of carotene. The Holstein is an efficient converter, having white adipose tissue and milk fat. However, the Guernsey and Jersey breeds readily absorb carotene, producing yellow adipose fat and butterfat.

Cis-trans-isomerism of the carotenoids is important in determining their absorbability, with the *trans*-forms being more efficiently absorbed (Stahl *et al.*, 1995). Dietary fat is important in absorption (Fichter and Mitchell, 1997). Dietary antioxidants (e.g., vitamin E) also affect the utilization and absorption of carotenoids. It is uncertain whether the antioxidants contribute directly to the efficient absorption or whether they protect both carotene and vitamin A from oxidative breakdown. Interactions between different fat-soluble compounds competing for the exact absorption mechanism have been described. Protein deficiency reduces the absorption of carotene from the intestine. Once the retinoids are transferred into the cell, they are quickly bound by specific binding proteins in the cytosol. The intracellular retinoid-binding proteins bind retinol, retinal, and retinoic acid to protect against decomposition, solubilize them in an aqueous medium, render them nontoxic, and transport them within cells to their site of action.

In most mammals, the product ultimately absorbed from the intestinal tract due to feeding carotenoids is mainly vitamin A. Pre-ruminant calves (Bierer *et al.*, 1995) readily absorb carotenoid compounds, especially β-carotene, which contributes to liver vitamin A stores (Hoppe *et al.*, 1996). Animals' conversion of carotene to retinol is inversely related to vitamin A status (McDowell, 1992). Conversion of carotene to retinol decreases with increasing intake of carotene or vitamin A and vitamin A concentrations in the liver (van Vliet *et al.*, 1996).

The retinyl esters, triglycerides, phospholipids, and cholesteryl esters are transported mainly in association with lymph chylomicrons to the liver (Blomhoff *et al.*, 1991; Bierer *et al.*, 1995; Stahl *et al.*, 1995). Chylomicrons, through exocytosis, pass from enterocytes into the lymph and eventually enter the general blood circulation.

There are notable species differences in the transport of carotenoids by plasma lipoprotein fractions. Sheep, goats, and cattle differ in the proportion of carotenoids associated with plasma's very low-density lipoproteins (VLDL), low-density lipoproteins (LDL), and high-density

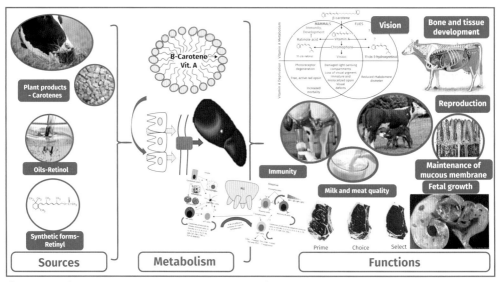

Figure 4.3 Main sources and types of the precursors of vitamin A. Schematic illustration of the absorption, the purpose of the metabolites, and the main functions developed

lipoproteins (HDL) fractions (Yang *et al.*, 1992). Compared to sheep and goats, cattle have ten-fold higher concentrations of β-carotene in the liver, 7 versus 0.7 µg/g of tissue (Yang *et al.*, 1992). Retinol is readily transferred to the egg in birds, but the transfer of retinol across the placenta is marginal, and mammals are born with meager liver stores of vitamin A.

Hydrolysis of the ester storage form mobilizes vitamin A from the liver as free retinol. Retinol is released from the hepatocyte as a complex with retinol-binding protein (RBP) and transported to peripheral tissues (Figure 4.2 and Figure 4.3). The liver takes up the majority of dietary vitamin A that is absorbed into the body within 4 to 6 hours. In lipocytes, which represent only 7% of total liver cells, the storage form of vitamin A represents a lipoglycoprotein complex consisting of 96% retinyl esters and 4% unesterified retinol (O'Byrne and Blaner, 2013). Small amounts of retinyl palmitate are absorbed directly into the portal blood and are adsorbed to plasma lipoproteins. In vitamin A toxicity, plasma retinyl palmitate concentrations are elevated while retinol concentrations remain normal.

Retinol, associated with RBP, circulates in peripheral tissues complex to a thyroxine-binding protein, transthyretin (Chew *et al.*, 1984; Blomhoff *et al.*, 1991; Ross and Harrison, 2013). Therefore, there is a metabolic interdependence between vitamin A and thyroid function. Iodine deficiency impairs vitamin A metabolism, and vitamin A deficiency impairs thyroid function (Olson, 1984). Goitrogenic feedstuffs in the diet may increase the vitamin A requirement or potentiate cattle responses to supplemental carotene.

In most species, 90% of serum RBP is saturated with retinol. The half-life of the *holo*-RBP-transthyretin complex in plasma is approximately 11 to 16 hours. Unbound *holo*-RBP and *apo*-RBP are turned over in about 4 hours.

The retinol-transthyretin complex is transported to target tissues, where the complex binds to a cell-surface receptor. The receptor was found in all tissues that require retinol, particularly the pigment epithelium of the eye (Wolf, 2007). Once the retinoids are transferred into the cell, they are quickly bound by specific RBP in the cytosol. These intracellular RBPs show high specificity and affinity for particular retinoids and seem to control retinoid metabolism both qualitatively and quantitatively. They protect retinoids from nonspecific interactions, and on the quantitative side, they have been stated to "chaperone" access of metabolic enzymes to retinoids. (Solomons, 2006). The intracellular RBP binds retinol, retinal, and retinoic acid to protect against decomposition, solubilize them in an aqueous medium, render them nontoxic, and transport them within cells to their site of action (Ross and Harrison, 2013). These intracellular RBP also present the retinoids to the appropriate enzymes for metabolism (Wolf, 1991; 1993).

In target cells, retinol can be either reconverted to retinyl esters or oxidized to retinal and, in a second step, to retinoic acid. The presence of specific cytoplasmic RBP influences the pathway selected. Conversion of retinol to retinyl esters occurs by lecithin: retinol acyltransferase and acyl-CoA: retinol acyltransferase. The nicotinamide adenine dinucleotide (NADH) retinol dehydrogenase mediates the oxidation of retinol to retinoic acid. Retinoic acid is formed from the irreversible oxidation of the retina (O'Byrne and Blaner, 2013).

The cells' final key mediators of vitamin A function are the all-*trans*-retinoic acid and 11-cis retinal. The all-*trans*-retinoic acid is a regulator of gene transcription for all biological roles in cell growth, differentiation, organogenesis, immunity, bone development, etc. In contrast, 11-*cis* retinal acts as a chromophore for visual functions (Figure 4.2 and Figure 4.3).

Some of the principal forms of intracellular or cytoplasmic RBP are cellular retinol-binding proteins (CRBP I and CRBP II), cellular retinoic acid-binding proteins (CRABP I and CRABP II), cellular retinaldehyde binding protein (CRALBP), and 6 nuclear retinoic receptors (RAR) and retinoid "x" receptors (RXR) (with α, β and γ forms). There are 2 classes of nuclear receptors with all-*trans*-retinoic acid as the ligand for RAR; 9-cis-retinoic acid is the ligand for RXR (Kastner *et al.*, 1994; Kliewer *et al.*, 1994). Vitamin A also contributes to maintaining lysozyme stability inside the cells.

Storage and excretion

The liver typically contains about 90% of the body's vitamin A. The remainder is stored in the kidneys, lungs, adrenals, and blood, with small amounts found in other organs and tissues. Serum retinol is not always sensitive to vitamin A status (Debier and Larondelle, 2005). In contrast to gastrointestinal tract absorption, some tissues, like eyes, prefer *cis* isomers of carotenoids (O'Byrne and Blaner, 2013).

Carotenoid interactions can affect uptake from the gastrointestinal tract and tissues, leading to differences in tissue storage levels. Non-provitamin A carotenoids such as lutein, lycopene, and xanthophylls can reduce β-carotene cleavage to retinal through competitive inhibition of β-carotene-15–15'-dioxygenase (O'Byrne and Blaner, 2013).

Among ruminants, only bovines accumulate high concentrations of carotenoids, mainly β-carotene, possibly due to lower vitamin A synthesis efficiencies in enterocytes (Nozière *et al.*, 2006). Carotenoid flows in plasma and tissues in dairy cows remain to be investigated, especially the ability of adipose tissue to release β-carotene in depleted or underfed animals. Carotenoids in cows' milk mainly consist of all-*trans*-β-carotene and lutein to a lesser extent (Nozière *et al.*, 2006). Milk concentration of β-carotene depends on its dietary supply (Nozière *et al.*, 2006). In milk, concentration is more variable for β-carotene than for retinol, for which the plasma concentration is well regulated.

Both animal and feeding factors that affect milk yield (i.e., breed, parity, physiological stage, level of intake) generally also control milk β-carotene concentration by concentration/dilution mechanisms and by the efficiency of extraction from plasma (Nozière *et al.*, 2006). The β-carotene concentration in cheese is highly linked to milk concentration, whereas high losses of retinol occur during cheese-making. The color of dairy products highly depends on their carotenoid concentration, suggesting that color may be a promising rapid measurement tool for the traceability of feeding conditions. Feeding management of dairy cows allows efficient control of carotenoid concentration and color in dairy products (Nozière et al., 2006).

Since ruminant animals are born with meager reserves of vitamin A, calves must receive adequate colostrum, which contains high levels of vitamin A activity and other vitamins (Table 4.1), within a few hours after birth. Colostrum deprivation during the first 24 hours of life impairs the overall absorption of vitamins A, D, and E through 7 days of age (Waldner and Uehlinger, 2016). Adequate fat intake is required for fat-soluble vitamin absorption in calves (Rajaraman et al., 1997) and is a consideration in the formulation of milk replacers. Low vitamin A intake by the cow during pregnancy increases the likelihood of vitamin A deficiency in the calf. This is because the cow's body reserves will be low, and thus, colostrum will have a subnormal vitamin A content (Miller et al., 1969). Deficiencies of dietary protein, phosphorus, zinc, and iodine during gestation can also impair vitamin A metabolism in the cow and reduce colostral vitamin A supply to the calf. Adding 200 g/day of extra fat to the diet of dry dairy cows increased plasma-carotene (as well as vitamin E) concentrations in the peripartum period (Weiss et al., 1994).

Changes in carotene and vitamin A and E status occur during the dairy cow's transition from the nonlactating to the lactating state. The regulatory role of the liver in maintaining retinol concentrations in plasma appears to be compromised in cows with fatty liver (Rosendo et al., 2010). In ordinary cows, the lower liver carotene and greater plasma retinol found at calving suggest that stored retinol in the liver first forces available carotene stores to be converted into retinol, thus decreasing liver carotene but not retinol. However, less β-carotene was mobilized at calving for cows with fatty liver. Cows that develop fatty liver during the transition have a higher risk for retained placenta, metritis, and mastitis, all associated with lower retinol, α-tocopherol, or β-carotene status (LeBlanc et al., 2002; 2004; Bobe et al., 2004).

The main excretory pathway for vitamin A is as glucuronide conjugates in the bile before fecal excretion, but it can also occur in the urine. Oxidized, polar metabolites of retinol, retinal,

Table 4.1 Concentrations of vitamins present in bovine colostrum and mature milk (source: Playford and Weiser, 2021)

Vitamins	Colostrum	Mature milk
Thiamine (B$_1$) (µg/ml)	0.58–0.90	0.4–0.5
Riboflavin (B$_2$) (µg/ml)	4.55–4.83	1.5–1.7
Niacin (B$_3$) (µg/ml)	0.34–0.96	0.8–0.9
Cobalamin (B$_{12}$) (µg/ml)	0.05–0.60[a]	0.004–0.006[a]
Pantothenic acid (µg/ml)	1.73[b]	3.82[b]
Biotin (µg/100 ml)	1–2.7[c]	8–9[d]
Folic acid (ng/ml)	440.3±18.8[e]	42–56[f]; 78.4±2.6[e]
Vitamin A (µg/100 ml)	25	34
Vitamin D (IU/g fat)	0.89–1.81	0.41
Tocopherol (E) (µg/g)	2.92–5.63[g]	0.06

Sources: [a]Marca et al. (1996) 10 µg/ml in colostrum and early milk. Concentrations declined after that to 50% or less by 21 days of lactation; [b]Foley and Otterby (1978); [b,c]Midla et al. (1998); [d]Fitzgerald et al. (2000); [e]Duplessis et al. (2015); [f]Girard and Matte (1989); [g]Hidiroglou (1989) reported a mean value of 1.9 µg/g, declining to 0.3 µg/g at 30 days postpartum.

and retinoic acid that retain intact chains in their structures are converted into β-glucuronides, which pass into bile. Once in the bile, these glucuronides can be lost in the feces or recycled in the enterohepatic circulation. Oxidized, chain-shortened metabolites of retinoic acid display little or no biological activity and are predominantly excreted in the urine. Esterification of retinol in tissues also represents a recycling mechanism and, together with enterohepatic recycling, influences the vitamin A status. The conversion of retinol to a retinyl-phosphomannose metabolite relates to vitamin A role in cell communication and differentiation. The regulation of vitamin A metabolism and expression of RBP depends on vitamin status or all-*trans*-retinoic acid production (O'Byrne and Blaner, 2013).

Biochemical functions

Vitamin A is necessary to support all major animal species' growth, immunity, health, reproduction, and life (Debier and Larondelle, 2005; Kadek *et al.*, 2021). Without vitamin A, animals will cease to grow and eventually die. Vitamin A and its derivatives, the retinoids, profoundly influence organ development, cell proliferation, and cell differentiation, and their deficiency originates or predisposes several disabilities (McDowell, 2000a; Esteban-Pretel *et al.*, 2010). During embryogenesis, retinoic acid has been shown to influence processes governing the patterning of neural tissue and craniofacial, eye, and olfactory system development; retinoic acid affects the outcome, regeneration, and well-being of neurons (Debier and Larondelle, 2005; Asson-Batres *et al.*, 2009).

Vitamin A is vital in forming rhodopsin in the retina, which is critical for vision, influences bone growth and maturation, and affects reproduction and epithelial tissues.

Recent discoveries have revealed that most, if not all, actions of vitamin A in development, differentiation, and metabolism are mediated by nuclear receptor proteins that bind retinoic acid, the active form of vitamin A (Iskakova *et al.*, 2015). A group of retinoic acid-binding proteins (receptors) function in the nucleus by attaching to promoter regions in several specific genes to stimulate their transcription and thus affect growth, development, and differentiation. Retinoic acid receptors in cell nuclei are structurally homologous and functionally analogous to the known receptors for steroid hormones, thyroid hormone (triiodothyronine), and vitamin D 1,25(OH)$_2$D$_3$. Very early, it was recognized that vitamin A sources affected the ergocalciferol requirement (Maurya and Aggarwal, 2017). Thus, retinoic acid is now recognized as a hormone regulating the transcription activity of many genes (Ross, 1993). Vitamin A can also inhibit the adverse action of lipopolysaccharides (LPS) on the intestinal epithelial barrier function and tight junction proteins (Zebeli and Ametaj, 2009; He *et al.*, 2019).

Vision

Retinol is utilized in the aldehyde form (all-*trans*-retinaldehyde) and transformed to 11-*cis*-retinaldehyde in the eye's retina. It forms part of the prosthetic group (opsin) in rhodopsin for dim light vision (rods) and as the prosthetic group in iodopsin for bright light and color vision (cones). When light falls on the retina, rhodopsin breaks down into opsin and all-*cis*-retinaldehyde, which reverts to all-*trans*-retinaldehyde, initiating an action potential that travels up the optic nerve. In the dark, the all-*trans*-retinaldehyde is isomerized back to all-*cis*-retinaldehyde, and the latter recombines with opsin to regenerate rhodopsin, resensitizing the retina to light. The mammalian visual cycle is represented in Figure 4.4. Retinoic acid has been found to support growth and tissue differentiation but not vision or all aspects of reproduction (McDowell, 2000a; Solomons, 2006; O'Byrne and Blaner, 2013).

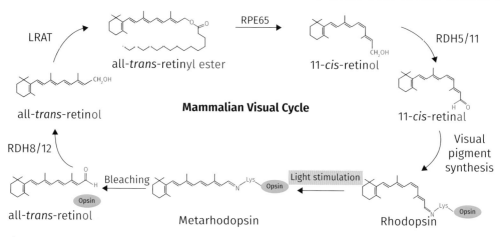

Figure 4.4 The mammalian visual cycle (source: Dewett *et al.*, 2021)

Tissue differentiation

Retinoic acid regulates the differentiation of epithelial, connective, adipose, and hematopoietic tissues (Safonova *et al.*, 1994; O'Byrne and Blaner, 2013). The nature of the growth and differentiation response elicited by retinoic acid depends upon cell type. Retinoic acid can inhibit many cell types, reducing adipose tissues in meat-producing animals (Kastner *et al.*, 1994; Pyatt and Berger, 2005; Gorocica-Buenfil *et al.*, 2007a,b,c; O'Byrne and Blaner, 2013). Proliferation and cellular aggregation are critical features for the survival and self-renewal of primordial germ cells (PGCs).

The activities of retinoic acid are crucial in early embryonic development (Kin Ting Kam *et al.*, 2012). Retinoic acid signaling regionalizes all 3 germ layers along the anteroposterior axis during gastrulation, especially in the mesoderm. Vitamin A-deficient rats fed retinoic acid were healthy in every respect, with normal estrus and conception, but failed to give birth and resorbed their fetuses (Chew *et al.*, 1984; Chew, 1993). When retinol was given even at a late stage in pregnancy, fetuses were saved, which can be related to proteins in uterine secretions induced by progesterone that are affected by retinol (Bindas *et al.*, 1984a, b; Tharnish and Larson, 1992; Arikan and Rodway, 2000; Kaewlamun *et al.*, 2011).

Keratinization of epithelial tissues results in loss of function in the alimentary, genital, reproductive, respiratory, and urinary tracts. Such altered characteristics increase the susceptibility of the affected tissue to infection. Abortions, increased prevalence of retained fetal membranes, and increased calf morbidity and mortality are indicators of vitamin A deficiency in gestating cows. Thus, diarrhea and pneumonia are typical secondary effects of vitamin A deficiency. The skin and hair coat are also affected.

Immunity

Adequate dietary vitamin A is necessary to help maintain resilience to stress and disease (Wiedermann *et al.*, 1993; Zhao and Ross, 1995; Chew and Park, 2004) and wound healing (Polcz and Barbul, 2019). Disease resistance is a function of vitamin A, which is the vitamin needed to maintain mucous membranes and the normal function of the adrenal gland (Nabi *et al.*, 2020). Vitamin A deficiency can impair the regeneration of normal mucosal epithelium damaged by infection or inflammation (Ahmed *et al.*, 1990; Stephensen *et al.*, 1996) and thus could increase the severity of an infectious episode and prolong recovery from that episode. An animal's ability to resist infectious disease depends on a responsive immune system, with a vitamin A deficiency causing a reduced immune response. In many experiments with laboratory and domestic animals, the effects of both clinical and subclinical deficiencies of vitamin A on the production of antibodies, the number of lymphocytes, and the resistance of different tissues against microbial infection or parasitic infestation have frequently been demonstrated (Tomkins and Hussey, 1989; Ahmed *et al.*, 1990; Stephensen *et al.*, 1996; Vlasova *et al.*, 2013; McGill *et al.*, 2019).

Several studies indicated that specific carotenoids without vitamin A activity have antioxidant capacities and can enhance many aspects of immune functions, act directly as antimutagens and anticarcinogens, protect against radiation damage, and block the damaging effects of photosensitizers (Chew and Johnston, 1985; Chew, 1995; Lindshield and Erdman, Jr., 2006). β-carotene can function as a chain-breaking antioxidant and aid in healing after injuries (Polcz and Barbul, 2019). It deactivates reactive chemical species, such as singlet oxygen, triplet photochemical sensitizers, and free radicals, that would otherwise induce potentially harmful processes like lipid peroxidation (McDowell, 2004; Nabi *et al.*, 2020). Vitamin A can also protect against the toxic effects of LPS in the gut (Zebeli and Ametaj, 2009; He *et al.*, 2019).

Neutrophil function is impaired by vitamin A deficiency (Twining *et al.*, 1997). Neutrophils and alveolar macrophages from young calves respond to increasing vitamin A concentrations *in vitro* (Eicher *et al.*, 1994). Vitamin A also affects the integrity of blood vessels, as evidenced by edema observed in the legs and brisket of deficient cattle.

McGill *et al.* (2019) working with newborn calves show that vitamin A-deficient calves are not able to respond to the vaccine, have no protection against respiratory disease challenges, and have significant abnormalities in the inflammatory response in the infected lung.

Bone development

Vitamin A plays a role in normal bone development by controlling the activity of osteoclasts of the epithelial cartilage, the cells responsible for bone resorption (Tanumihardjo, 2013). In vitamin A deficiency, the activity of osteoclasts is reduced with excessive deposition of periosteal bone due to stimulation of osteoblasts (depositing bone cells) and joint irritation. However, hypervitaminosis A also causes bone lesions.

Reproduction

The functions of vitamin A in reproduction have not been sufficiently clarified, but there is enough evidence of its influence on reproductive success (Debier and Larondelle, 2005; Kumar *et al.*, 2010). Vitamin A functions in the embryo begin soon after conception and continue throughout the life of all vertebrates (Ross *et al.*, 2000). Research findings have indicated that vitamin A increased ribonucleic acid (RNA) synthesis by polymerase II in rat testes, and the induced change in transcription was partly due to altered chromatin structure (Porter *et al.*, 1986). A hormonal effect is suggested for retinoic acid. Its actions are mediated by specific nuclear receptor proteins that control gene expression by binding to specific deoxyribonucleic acid (DNA) sequences in regulatory regions of target genes (Franceschi, 1992). The biological effect of retinoic acid is through nuclear RAR and RXR receptors. This allows binding to target DNA sequences of responsive genes to activate or repress gene transcription, thus regulating many biological processes (Ross, 2003).

Still, they could be related to the intracellular transport of vitamin A and its passage to the embryo, where it is probably needed to regulate cellular differentiation and proliferation, steroid production (Ikeda *et al.*, 2005), immune response (Thomas *et al.*, 1947; Meyer *et al.*, 2005), transcription of specific genes, etc.

Kolb and Seehawer (1997) reviewed the significance of carotenes and vitamin A for the reproduction of cattle, horses, and pigs. It was found that retinoic acid is necessary for the function of the germ cell epithelial, Sertoli cells, and interstitial cells. They promoted the synthesis of proteins, estrogens, and progesterone, which was included in the actions credited to cis- and all-*trans*-retinoic acid. During embryogenesis, retinoic acid has been shown to influence processes governing the patterning of neural tissue and craniofacial, eye, and olfactory system development. Retinoic acid influences neurons' development, regeneration, and well-being (Asson-Batres *et al.*, 2009). Retinoic acid also regulates the differentiation of epithelial, connective, and hematopoietic tissues (Safonova *et al.*, 1994). The nature of the growth and differentiation response elicited by retinoic acid depends upon cell type. Retinoic acid can inhibit many cell types, potentially reducing adipose tissues in meat-producing animals (Mora *et al.*, 2000; Pickworth *et al.*, 2012a).

At birth, ruminants have meager liver reserves of vitamin A, reflected by the low concentration of vitamin A in the blood (Swanson *et al.*, 2000; Zanker *et al.*, 2000). To prevent vitamin A deficiency, the newborn must ingest high amounts of vitamin A supplied by colostrum immediately after birth (Table 4.1). Because it is clear that nuclear receptors play a vital role in the expression of many essential enzymes, it is likely that feeding vitamin A would significantly affect the metabolism, health status, and growth performance of young ruminants. Krüger *et al.* (2005) fed high vitamin A levels to cows. The result was that calves fed the colostrum from supplemented cows were now more able to metabolize and eliminate foreign substances from external and internal sources. This further emphasizes the importance of vitamin A-rich colostrum and has great significance for other species that depend on colostrum for the health of their offspring (e.g., humans).

β-carotene and reproduction in dairy cattle
Since 1978, several studies have suggested that β-carotene has a function independent of vitamin A in bovine reproduction (Lotthammer, 1979; Larson *et al.*, 1983; Sklan, 1983; Rakes *et al.*, 1985; Ascarelli *et al.*, 1985; Bonsembiante *et al.*, 1986; Schweigert *et al.*, 1988; Graves-Hoagland *et al.*, 1988; Kolb and Seehawer, 1997; Aréchiga *et al.*, 1998; De Ondarza *et al.*, 2009; Kumar *et al.*, 2010). Cows fed supplemental β-carotene have exhibited a reduced interval to first estrus, increased conception rates, and reduced frequency of follicular cysts compared to animals receiving only vitamin A.

Aréchiga *et al.* (1998) reported an improvement in pregnancy rate, but only under heat stress conditions and only when β-carotene had been fed for 90 days or more. In this study, high levels of dietary vitamin A (200,000–250,000 IU/day) were fed to all cows, and β-carotene elicited a consistent increase in milk production across all 3 trials. Cystic ovarian degeneration is correlated with plasma-carotene reduction (Lopez-Diaz and Bosu, 1992). A study in Québec, Canada, reported a weak inverse correlation between plasma-carotene concentration and reproductive performance (Block and Farmer, 1987). However, other studies have found no significant effect (Folman *et al.*, 1979; Wang *et al.*, 1982, 1988b; Bindas *et al.*, 1984a; Marcek *et al.*, 1985; Greenberg *et al.*, 1986; Akordor *et al.*, 1986) or adverse effects (Folman *et al.*, 1987) of β-carotene supplementation on the fertility of cattle.

In some of these studies, there have been trends for improved reproduction whereas in others, there were no effects. The cow's corpus luteum and follicular fluid have a high concentration of β-carotene (Chew *et al.*, 1984; Arikan *et al.*, 2002; Haliloglu *et al.*, 2002). It has been suggested that carotene has a specific effect on reproduction and has a role as a precursor of vitamin A. The corpus luteum and the follicle possess the 15,15'-dioxygenase activity and convert β-carotene to retinol within the granulosa tissue (Sklan, 1983; Schweigert and

Zucker, 1988; Schweigert et al., 1988; Rapoport et al., 1998; Arikan and Rodway, 2000; Arellano-Rodriguez et al., 2009).

Uptake and conversion of β-carotene to retinol have been demonstrated in human and mouse fibroblasts, rabbit corneal epithelia, and rat liver cells maintained in cell culture (Wei et al., 1998). Graves-Hoagland et al. (1988, 1989) reported a positive relationship between postpartum progesterone production and plasma concentrations of β-carotene in dairy cows. Block and Farmer (1987) reported a modest positive correlation (0.23) between reproductive performance and plasma retinol and plasma-carotene in a survey of commercial farms in Québec. A Swedish survey reported no relationship between blood-carotene or vitamin A and reproduction (Jukola et al., 1996). Other surveys reported seasonal variability in plasma-carotene content, with significantly lower levels observed during winter and higher levels during spring and early summer, especially when green forages were fed. Jackson et al. (1981) reported that cows with low carotene levels during winter months exhibited irregular cycles of plasma reproductive hormones.

The results of several studies are summarized in Table 4.2. Five trials with 168 Holstein cows and 20 heifers (Tharnish and Larson, 1992) found no benefit of feeding very high levels of vitamin A (1 to 2 million IU versus 100,000 IU per day) on plasma progesterone concentration or measures of reproductive efficiency.

One potential interaction initially explored by Lotthammer et al. (1976) was that of β-carotene and thyroid function. The diets fed in these initial studies contained goitrogenic Brassica feedstuffs such as kale, forage rape, and turnips. β-carotene affected serum thyroxine (T_4) levels in these studies. Serum-carotene and T_4 were inversely related. β-carotene has been reported to increase the conversion of T_4 to T_3 in dairy cows (Pethes et al., 1985). This may have, in turn, mediated some of the reproductive responses observed in response to β-carotene supplementation in these studies. The rats (Coya et al., 1997) and chickens (Bhat and Cama, 1978) demonstrated an interdependency between vitamin A and carotene status and thyroid function. Seasonal variance in plasma carotenes (Block and Farmer, 1987; Cetinkaya and Ozcan, 1991) may also be partly related to seasonal changes in thyroid function in cattle. Interrelationships of vitamin nutrition, stress load, endocrine and immune function have been reported (Jackson et al., 1981; Miller et al., 1993; Aréchiga et al., 1998; Franklin et al., 1998; Chew and Park, 2004; Muri et al., 2005; McGill et al., 2019) and should prove to be a productive area of research in the future.

Milk production in dairy cattle, vitamin A, β-carotene, and mammary gland immune function

A sufficiently long dry period before parturition is well known to be a prerequisite for mammary gland (MG) regeneration and high milk yields during the subsequent lactation. During the dry period, the MG epithelium involutes, and regenerates (Capuco et al., 2003). Because milk production depends on the number of mammary secretory cells and their synthetic and secretory capacities, regulating the mammary epithelial cell population during the dry period has important consequences for milk production and lactation persistency (Capuco et al., 2003).

Milk production is dependent on vitamin A. In vitro studies show meaningful interactions among vitamin A, lactoferrin, and insulin-like growth factor (IGF) binding proteins (Muri et al., 2005; Puvogel et al., 2005; Schottstedt et al., 2005). Consequently, vitamin A is essential for MG epithelial cell proliferation and apoptosis during the dry period, and potential milk yield can be affected (Cheli et al., 2003; Puvogel et al., 2005). The β-carotene is related to the color of milk and all dairy products. β-Carotene has the highest binding affinity to κ-casein

Table 4.2 Studies of supplemental Vitamin A and/or β-carotene in cattle

Age, weight, or physiological state	Administration				Effect	Reference
	Amount	Form	Duration	Route		
Dairy cows from 4 weeks before to 23 weeks after parturition	β-carotene	N/A	190 days	Oral	Positive association with reproduction	Scharns et al. (1978)
Israel-Friesian heifers 7–17 months of age	free diet 8,3 mg β-carotene/kg BW	β-carotene	300 days	Oral	Some positive effects on reproduction	Folman et al. (1979)
Blood from Holstein cows lactating during four 2 week periods	Plasma concentrate of vitamin A and β-carotene	Vitamin A, β-carotene	56 days	N/A	Positive association with udder health	Chew et al. (1982)
Holstein heifers 12–16 months of age	300 mg/animal/day	β-carotene	56 days	Oral	No effect on reproduction	Wang et al. (1982)
Holstein cow from day 30–90 postpartum	600 mg/cow/day	β-carotene	60 days	Oral	No effect on reproduction	Bindas et al. (1984a)
Holstein cows seven days postpartum and on alternate weeks through the week of lactation	Plasma concentrate of vitamin A and β-carotene	Vitamin A, β-carotene	77 days	N/A	Positive association with udder health	Johnston and Chew (1984)
Dry and lactating dairy cows	500 mg/cow/day in dry period & 750 mg/cow/day during lactation; 60 mg/cow/day in dry period & 90 mg/cow/day during lactation	β-carotene	330 days	Oral	Positive effect on reproduction in winter	Ascarelli et al. (1985)
Postpartum (10–120 days) Holstein cows	300 mg/cow/day	Retinol	100 days	Oral	No effect on reproduction	Marcek et al. (1985)
Holstein cows at calving	300 mg/cow/day β-carotene + 3,919 IU vitamin A/kg of ration DM	β-carotene	100 days	Oral	Positive effect on reproduction and udder health	Rakes et al. (1985)
Holstein cows from day 10 postpartum until pregnant	400 mg/cow/day of β-carotene; 160,000 IU vitamin A/cow/day	Vitamin A, β-carotene	90 days	N/A	Some positive effects on reproduction	Akordor et al. (1986)

Subject	Amount	Compound/Form	Duration	Route	Effect	Reference
Pregnant, crossbred beef heifers	0 or 675 mg/day of β-carotene	Concentrate	Ten months	Oral	No effect on reproduction	Greenberg et al. (1986)
Holstein cows near parturition	Records of 20 years	β-carotene, Vitamin A	N/A	N/A	Positive association with reproduction	Inaba et al. (1986)
Lactation Holstein cows	10 ml jugular blood samples	Determination of β-carotene, Vitamin A	Once a month, by the way, Jan, & Mar	N/A	Positive association with reproduction	Block and Farmer (1987)
Holstein cows, 8 weeks before calving to new conception	69 mg retinyl acetate/cow/day before & 96 mg retinyl acetate after calving; 500 mg β-carotene before & 700 mg after calving	β-carotene, retinyl acetate	200 days	Oral	Negative effect on reproduction	Folman et al. (1987)
5-month-old Holstein heifers	105 mg β-carotene/heifer/day	β-carotene	Ten months	Oral	Positive effect on reproduction	Tekpetey et al. (1987a)
Holstein cow 4 years old	32-62 mg/kg DM of β-carotene in winter diet; 23-228 mg/kg DM of β-carotene in summer diet	Hay and fava bean silage, fresh pasture, grass haylage & alfalfa pellets	12 months	N/A	Positive association with reproduction	Tekpetey et al. (1987b)
Corpora lutea from non-pregnant Holstein cows and blood	52 corpora lutea	β-carotene, Vitamin A	N/A	N/A	Positive association with reproduction in winter	Graves-Hoagland et al. (1988)
Third-lactation cows from 6 weeks before dry-off to 2 weeks after	53,000 IU vitamin A/cow/day; 213,000 IU vitamin A/cow/day + 400 μg β-carotene/cow/day	Vitamin A palmitate, β-carotene	56 days	Oral	Positive effect on udder health and immunity	Tjoelcker et al. (1988)
Ovariectomized lactating Holstein cows at week 20 of a 28 week period	600 mg/cow/day	β-carotene	28 weeks	Oral	No effect on reproduction	Wang et al. (1988a)
Lactation Holstein cows from day 3–98 postpartum	300 mg/cow/day	β-carotene	96 days	Oral	No effect on reproductive performance	Wang et al. (1988b)

Table 4.2 (continued)

Age, weight, or physiological state	Administration				Effect	Reference
	Amount	Form	Duration	Route		
Postpartum Holstein & Jersey cows	100 µg GnRH; plasma β-carotene 53,000 IU vitamin A/cow/day; 53,000 IU vitamin A/cow/day + 400 µg β-carotene/cow/day	N/A vitamin A palmitate, β-carotene	N/A	IM	Positive association with reproduction	Graves-Hoagland et al. i(1989)
			56 days	Oral	positive effect on immunity	Tjoelker et al. (1990)
Blood from ~4,-1,o,1, and 4 weeks postpartum Holstein cows	10^{-9} and 10^{-8} M	β-carotene	72 hours	N/A	positive effect on immunity	Daniel et al. (1991)
	10^{-9} and 10^{-8} M	Retinol	72 hours	N/A	no effect immunity	
	10^{-9} and 10^{-8} M	Retinoic Acid	72 hours	N/A		
Holstein dairy cows	50,000 IU vitamin A; 170,000 IU vitamin A; 50,000 IU vitamin A + 400 µg β-carotene	Vitamin A	16 weeks	Oral	No effect on udder health	Oldham et al. (1991)
Commercial dairy herds: Finland	Plasma β-carotene	Observational study	N/A	N/A	No association with fertility	Jukola et al. (1996)
Holstein cows: 2 farms, 3 experiments	0 or 400 mg-day	β-carotene	60–90 days	Oral	Positive effect on reproduction in heat stress. Positive effect on milk, and all experiments	Aréchiga et al. (1998)
Holstein cow, postpartum 60–90 days	400 mg /cow/day	β-carotene	90 days	Oral	Positive effect on reproduction. Positive effect on milk production	Aréchiga et al. (1998)
Holstein cows, postpartum 120 days	425 mg /cow/day	β-carotene	120 days	Oral	Positive effect on reproduction. Positive effect on milk production	De Ondarza et al. (2009)

among casein fractions and its presence changes the conformation of caseins (Allahdad et al., 2018).

Feeding vitamin A to calves influenced concentrations of vitamin A, hemoglobin, and triglycerides and tended to affect the insulin growth factor (IGF)-binding proteins (Muri et al., 2005). Circulating vitamin A (retinol) and lactoferrin levels are low in calves at birth. Bovine colostrum contains relatively high amounts of vitamin A (Table 4.1) and lactoferrin, and neonatal calves intestinally absorb both substances. Ingestion of colostrum in the neonatal calf is followed by changes in the development and functions of the gastrointestinal tract, causing metabolic and endocrine changes (Blum and Baumrucker, 2002) and influencing the immune systems of the gastrointestinal tract (David et al., 2003; Norman et al., 2003).

Vitamin A and lactoferrin supplementation influenced the growth of the ileum and colon in neonatal calves. Interactions were observed between vitamin A and lactoferrin on epithelial cell maturation, villus growth, and size of follicles in intestinal immune tissues (Peyer's patches) (Schottstedt et al., 2005). The finding that supplemental β-carotene increased milk production in 3 experiments in Florida, USA, when fed to high-producing cows on low-forage rations with high levels of supplemental vitamin A suggests that β-carotene may complement preformed vitamin A in the diet under certain conditions (Aréchiga et al., 1998). In the latter study, rations were based on corn silage as the primary forage, and cows were intensively managed with milking and bovine somatotropin 3 times per day (Aréchiga et al., 1998).

Disease resistance is a crucial function of vitamin A, which is required for the development and function of immune cells, the maintenance of mucous membranes and epithelial linings of the respiratory, mammary, digestive, urinary, and reproductive tracts, and the normal functioning of the adrenal gland and thyroid glands. An animal's ability to resist infectious disease depends on a responsive immune system, and vitamin A deficiency reduces the immune response. In many experiments with laboratory and domestic animals, the effects of both clinical and subclinical deficiencies of vitamin A on the production of antibodies and the resistance of different tissues to microbial infection or parasitic infestation have been demonstrated (Tompkins and Hussey, 1989; Olson, 1984). Vitamin A has been used as an adjunct in treating ringworm (Trichophyton verrucosum) infestations in cattle. Cryptosporidia infection reduces vitamin A absorption (Holland et al., 1992).

Vitamin A and β-carotene are essential in disease resistance, including bovine mastitis (Bendich, 1993; Chew, 1993; NRC, 2001; LeBlanc et al., 2004). The immune cells involved in the MG, their functions, and the cytokines produced are described in Figure 4.5. Rezamand et al. (2007) reported that dairy cows with greater tissue energy stores prepartum and reduced plasma proteins, β-carotene, and α-tocopherol had a greater risk for developing a new intramammary infection during the periparturient period. In the last week's prepartum, a 100 ng/ml increase in serum retinol was associated with a 60% decrease in the risk of early lactation clinical mastitis (LeBlanc et al., 2004). There are reports of improved mammary health in dairy cows supplemented with β-carotene and vitamin A during the dry period (Dahlquist and Chew, 1985) and lactation (Chew and Johnston, 1985).

Dairy cows supplemented with 53,000 IU of vitamin A per head daily plus 300 mg of β-carotene starting 30 days prepartum had significantly lower milk somatic cell counts during lactation than unsupplemented animals (Chew et al., 1984). Additionally, cows fed 173,000 IU of vitamin A per head daily showed a reduction in somatic cell count compared to controls but not as large a response as the cows fed both vitamin A and β-carotene (Chew and Johnston, 1985; Chew, 1993; Chew and Park, 2004). Carotene improved calf neutrophil function in vitro (Eicher et al., 1994).

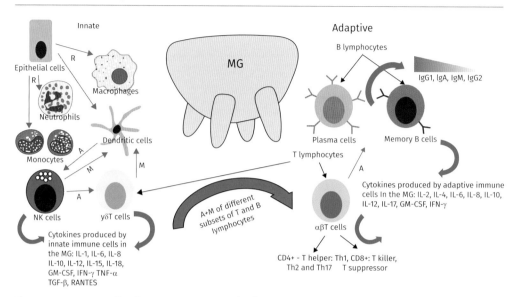

Figure 4.5 Immune cells of the mammary gland (MG), their functions, and cytokines produced. (source: Vlasova and Saif, 2021)

In addition to a reproductive effect, carotenoids have been shown to have other biological actions independent of vitamin A (Chew, 1995; De Ondarza *et al.*, 2009). Recent animal studies (Álvarez *et al.*, 2015) indicated that specific carotenoids with antioxidant capacities but without vitamin A activity can enhance many aspects of immune functions (Paul and Dey, 2015; El-Masry *et al.*, 2020), act directly as antimutagens and anticarcinogens, protect against radiation damage, and block the damaging effects of photosensitizers. Also, carotenoids can directly affect gene expression, and this mechanism may enable carotenoids to modulate the interaction between B-cells and T-cells, thus regulating humoral and cell-mediated immunity (Chew and Park, 2004; Ross and Harrison, 2013). Oxidized β-carotene (OxBC), a phytochemical that occurs naturally in plants, including fruits and vegetables, is formed by the spontaneous reaction of β-carotene with ambient oxygen. Synthetic OxBC, obtained by the full oxidation of β-carotene with air, is predominantly composed of β-carotene–oxygen copolymers that have beneficial immune-modulating effects. These compounds have shown considerable promise as a feed additive, added in parts per million, that enhances health and performance in poultry, swine, and ruminant species (Riley *et al.*, 2023).

In animal models, β-carotene and canthaxanthin have protected against UV-induced skin cancer and some chemically induced tumors. In some of these models, an enhancement of tumor immunity has been suggested as a possible mechanism of action of these carotenoids (Bendich, 1989). β-carotene can function as a chain-breaking antioxidant. It deactivates reactive chemical species such as singlet oxygen, triplet photochemical sensitizers, and free radicals, which would otherwise induce potentially harmful processes (e.g., lipid peroxidation; McDowell, 2004). Lymphocyte function, phagocytosis, and *in vitro* intracellular killing by blood neutrophils against *Staphylococcus aureus* were enhanced with increasing dietary α-tocopherol, retinol, and β-carotene in dairy cows (Erskine *et al.*, 1997).

Polymorphonuclear neutrophils (PMNs) are the primary line of defense against bacteria in the MG. β-carotene supplementation stabilizes PMNs and lymphocyte function during the early dry period (Tjoelker *et al.*, 1990). Daniel *et al.* (1991a,b) reported that β-carotene enhanced the bactericidal activity of blood and milk PMNs against *S. aureus* but did not affect phagocytosis. Vitamin A either had no effect or suppressed bactericidal activity and phagocytosis. Control of free radicals is essential for bactericidal activity but not for phagocytosis. β-carotene has significant antioxidant properties and effectively quenches singlet oxygen free radicals (Di Mascio *et al.*, 1991; Zamora *et al.*, 1991), which may explain its effects on immune cell function. In this role, β-carotene may complement the antioxidant activity of vitamin E.

The role of β-carotene in mammary disease resistance is unclear. While the above studies, conducted primarily in the northwestern United States, have found specific effects of β-carotene on immune cell function and beneficial effects of β-carotene supplementation on udder health in dairy cows, others have reported no effect of β-carotene on the incidence of mastitis or somatic cell count (Oldham *et al.*, 1991). Batra *et al.* (1992) reported that mastitic cows had lower plasma concentrations of vitamin A and β-carotene than healthy cows. Chew and Johnston (1985) reported a positive association between plasma-carotene postpartum and somatic cell count. Some studies aimed at assessing reproductive effects reported that β-carotene supplementation reduced somatic cell count (Rakes *et al.*, 1985) and reduced treatments required for clinical mastitis (Wang *et al.*, 1988b).

Meat quality
Vitamin A has also been associated with specific characteristics related to meat quality, such as intramuscular fat content in steers (Krone *et al.*, 2015; Harris *et al.*, 2018; Maciel *et al.*, 2022) or the percentage of specific fatty acids deposited in different tissues, thanks to the possible action of vitamin A in controlling the differentiation of adipocytes (Gregoire *et al.*, 1998; Siebert *et al.*, 2003; O'Byrne and Blaner, 2013) and in the activity of certain desaturating enzymes. However, the responses vary among genetic lines, age, length, and level of vitamin A supplementation (Siebert *et al.*, 2003).

In most cases, the mechanism of vitamin A action is similar to that of steroid hormones. It is carried out by binding to specific receptors in the target tissues' cellular cytoplasm. When the active form (retinoic acid) is bound to the receptor, the receptor translocates to the nucleus, where it attaches to chromatin acceptors and causes the production of a messenger RNA and, consequently, of a specific cytoplasmic protein (Shin and McGrane, 1997).

Nutritional assessment

Retinol and its fatty acid esters are the compounds relevant for determining vitamin A status. Serum or plasma retinol concentration is not always sensitive to vitamin A status because of its tight homeostatic regulation. Liver reserves are the gold standard because the liver contains most total body vitamin A stores unless the overall status is deficient. The liver store of vitamin A can be measured at slaughter or by biopsy (Figure 4.6).

In blood and tissues, retinol can be determined using reversed-phase high-performance liquid chromatography (HPLC). Retinol can be measured using dried blood spots (DBS), allowing the collection of small blood samples under field conditions with limited infrastructure. Stability issues have limited the widespread practical application. Still, some improvements have been made, indicating its validity for assessing, as said, a low retinol (or a high) status and not a broader evaluation of its nutritional status (Gannon *et al.*, 2020). The provitamin A carotenoids and primarily β-carotene could be used as an indirect measurement of vitamin A status by considering, as discussed in previous paragraphs, that the biological activity of these compounds relative to retinol is estimated to be in the order of 50% for β-carotene and 25% for carotenoids with only one β-ionone end group. Carotenoids are mainly assessed

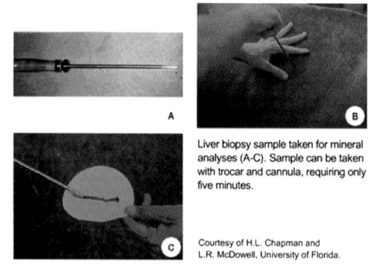

Liver biopsy sample taken for mineral
analyses (A-C). Sample can be taken
with trocar and cannula, requiring only
five minutes.

Courtesy of H.L. Chapman and
L.R. McDowell, University of Florida.

Figure 4.6 A liver Biopsy sample was taken for vitamin A analysis (A-C) (source: courtesy of Chapman, H.L. and McDowell, L.R., University of Florida)

from plasma using HPLC coupled with visible spectrophotometry. The feed industry has used spectrophotometric and chemical (Carr–Price) methods to determine the biopotency of vitamin A, but accuracy, sensitivity, and specificity have been variable, limiting their use. These methods have been replaced mainly by growth, microbiological, or analytical assays with assay variations for vitamin A and β-carotene ranging from 10 to 25% and 5 to 20%, respectively.

Deficiency signs
Vitamin A is required for normal visual function, healthy maintenance of epithelial tissues and mucous membranes, normal bone development, and functional immunity in animals. Vitamin A deficiency signs observed in ruminants vary, but most relate to degenerative changes in these tissues. Numerous studies have demonstrated increased frequency and severity of infection in vitamin A-deficient animals. Low vitamin A status reduces antibody production and impairs cell-mediated immune response against pathogens (Tompkins and Hussey, 1989). Vitamin A is required for the production of leukocytes and other cells of the immune system. Clinical signs of vitamin A deficiency may be specific or nonspecific. General signs observed include loss of appetite, loss of weight, unhealthy appearance, thick nasal discharge, and reduced fertility. The normal epithelia of the body are progressively replaced by stratified, keratinized tissue. This effect has been noted in the respiratory, alimentary, reproductive, and genitourinary tracts and the eye. Keratinization reduces the effectiveness of the epithelial tissues as a barrier to the entrance of infectious organisms. Thus, respiratory, and upper respiratory diseases are more severe in animals with vitamin A deficiency.

Signs of vitamin A deficiency:
In cattle, signs of vitamin A deficiency include reduced feed intake and growth rate; rough hair coat (Figure 4.7); edema of the joints and brisket (Figure 4.8); diarrhea; lacrimation; xeroph-thalmia; night blindness; blindness from corneal opacity (Figure 4.9); convulsive seizures,

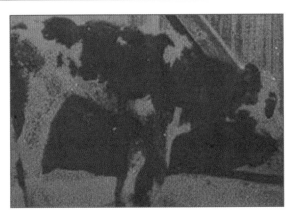

Figure 4.7 Vitamin A deficiency in cattle: unhealthy appearance. (source: courtesy of G. Patterson and Pfizer, Inc.)

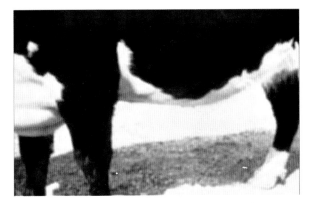

Figure 4.8 Vitamin A deficiency in cattle: edema of brisket. (source: USDA)

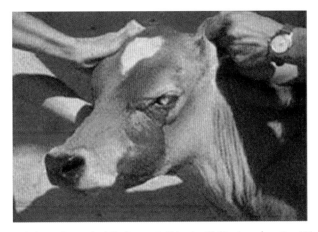

Figure 4.9 Vitamin A deficiency in cattle: blindness. Calf in the Philippines (south of Manila) showing vitamin A deficiency characterized by copious lacrimation and blindness; the 6-month-old animal had been fed reconstituted milk powder and poor-quality bleached hay (practically devoid of carotene). (source: courtesy of J.K. Loosli, University of Florida)

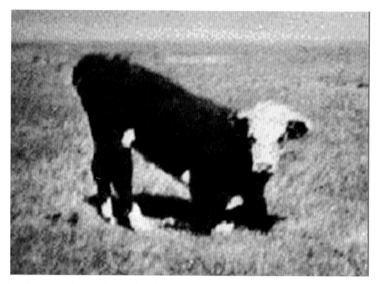

Figure 4.10 Vitamin A-deficient calf, showing incoordination and weakness.

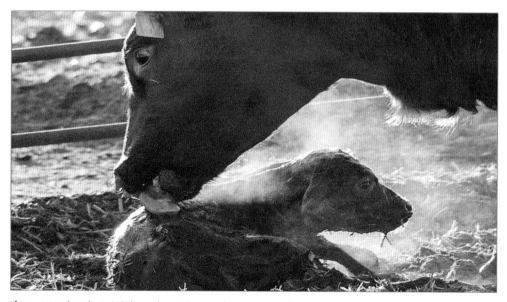

Figure 4.11 Vitamin A deficiency in cattle: Impaired reproduction.

incoordination and weakness (Figure 4.10); abnormal bone growth; impaired reproduction with low conception rates (Figure 4.11); abortion; stillbirths; weak, blind or stillborn calves; abnormal sperm and reduced libido in bulls; and increased susceptibility to respiratory and other infections (NRC, 1996; McDowell, 2000a). Cattle with marginal vitamin A status may be more susceptible to pinkeye or other diseases affecting the mucous membranes. Animals in advanced stages of deficiency may exhibit a staggering gait, convulsive seizures ("fainting" in feedlot cattle), and papilledema of the eye resulting from elevated cerebrospinal fluid pressure (Figure 4.12).

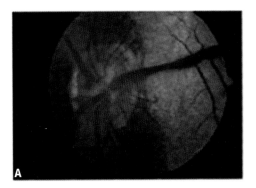

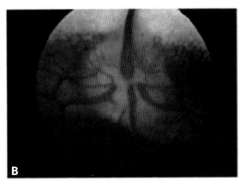

Fundus of the eye with point of entry of optic nerve and surrounding tissue of a healthy calf.

Papilledema of the optic disc—a diagnosis of vitamin A deficiency in the calf.

Figure 4.12 Vitamin A deficiency in cattle: Impaired vision.

Wellmann *et al.* (2020) studied the vitamin A depletion in castrated crossbred angus steers and animals not supplemented with vitamin A reduced the feed intake with no benefit on gain to feed ratio.

Defects in reproduction
Vitamin A is critical for successful reproduction. Vitamin A deficiency lowers reproductive efficiency in both males and females. Reduced libido and sterility in bulls with seminiferous tubular degeneration have been reported (Larkin and Yates, 1964). Spermatozoa decrease in number and motility, and the numbers of abnormal sperm increase markedly. In cows, key indications of deficiency are reduced conception rate (Table 4.3), shortened pregnancies, increased incidence of abortions, high incidence of retained placenta, and the birth of dead, weak, uncoordinated, or blind calves. Blindness in newborn calves is caused by malformation and closure of the optic foramen, constricting the optic nerve (Miller *et al.*, 1989; Van der Lugt and Prozesky, 1989). If born alive, calves have trouble gaining balance and lack the instinct to nurse. Vitamin A-deficient newborn calves may show very severe, often fatal diarrhea. In young calves, signs of vitamin A deficiency also include watery eyes, nasal discharge, muscular incoordination, staggering gait, and convulsive seizures (McDowell, 2000b). Elevated cerebrospinal fluid (CSF) pressure is the earliest change specific to vitamin A deficiency in the calf and is a precursor to most of the severe neurologic symptoms described.

In addition, some studies have shown that β-carotene has a favorable effect on the fertility of heifers and lactating cows (Lotthammer, 1979; Bonsembiante *et al.*, 1986; Aréchiga *et al.*, 1998), while others (Oldham *et al.*, 1991; Akordor *et al.*, 1986) have shown no effect of β-carotene on reproductive performance or incidence mastitis. Additional studies are needed to clarify the physiologic role of β-carotene as differences in results may relate to variations in body stores of β-carotene and (or) vitamin A in experimental animals.

Defects in vision
The classic sign of vitamin A deficiency in ruminants is night blindness due to the loss of activity of the rod cells in the retina, which are active in dim light. As vitamin A deficiency develops, the adaptation to dim light and darkness is reduced, eventually resulting in night blindness.

Table 4.3 Influence of Vitamin A on conception rate (source: modified from Bradfield and Behrens, 1968)

Age group	Control group		Vitamin A supplemented group	
	No. of animals	Pregnant (%)	No. of animals	Pregnant (%)
Mature cows	582	70.1	1.097	85.5
First-calf heifers	129	74.9	241	83.0
Replacement heifers	107	64.5	251	79.3

This condition is readily detected when animals encounter obstacles in dim light. Night blindness and blindness may be the first noticeable signs of vitamin A deficiency in rapidly growing cattle fed high-concentrate rations. In severe vitamin A deficiency, characteristic changes occur in the eye, including excessive lacrimation (tearing), keratitis, softening and clouding of the cornea, and the development of xerophthalmia, characterized by drying of the conjunctiva. In cattle, copious lacrimation (rather than xerophthalmia) is the most prominent clinical sign of vitamin A deficiency (Maynard *et al.*, 1979). The degenerative changes in the eye in vitamin A deficiency are shown in Figure 4.9. Blindness can result from either epithelial degeneration or secondary eye infections caused by the deficiency.

Defects in growth and bone development
Generalized edema can occur in finishing cattle, with signs of lameness in the hock and knee joints and swelling in the brisket area (NRC, 1996). Booth *et al.* (1987) reported feedlot cattle with low serum vitamin A concentration, apparent blindness, fixed dilated pupils, severe ataxia, and poor weight gains. Feedlot cattle with mild vitamin A deficiency exhibit reduced feed intake and weight gain. Reduced feed intake may result in deficiencies of other nutrients, mainly when the diet is marginal in those nutrients. Because vitamin A is involved in normal bone development, the long bones of deficient animals are altered in shape during growth.

Teeth are also affected. Failure of the spine and other bones to develop typically causes increased pressure on and degeneration of the nerves. For example, blindness in calves results from constriction of the optic nerve caused by a narrowing of the bone canal through which it passes, the optic foramen (Maynard *et al.*, 1979). Bone abnormalities in the spine and pelvis may be responsible for muscular incoordination and other neurologic symptoms exhibited by vitamin A-deficient cattle.

Impairment of the immune function and resistance to diseases
Vitamin A is required for normal immune system development, maintenance, and function. As part of the significant role of maintaining a healthy epithelium, vitamin A and β-carotene are vital in reducing the incidence and severity of mastitis in dairy cows (Chew, 1987). Feeding rations with low vitamin A activity has increased the incidence and severity of bovine mastitis (Chew, 1987, 1993). Adequate vitamin A and β-carotene intake is necessary for protection against mastitis. Vitamin A helps maintain epithelial integrity and normal immune cell function. At the same time, the antioxidant activity of β-carotene increases the bactericidal activity of blood and milk PMNs against *S. aureus* (Daniel *et al.*, 1991a, b).

Van Merris *et al.* (2004) confirmed the decrease in serum retinol during the peripartum period of dairy cows. They noted that profound changes in vitamin A metabolism occurred during the acute-phase reaction of coliform mastitis in heifers. All-trans-retinoic acid was found to be the most abundant circulating acid isomer during mastitis, indicating a possible key role of all-*trans*-retinoic acid in modulating the immune response.

Impairment of detoxifying systems

In the 1950s, it was discovered that cattle developed signs of vitamin A deficiency, initially referred to as X-disease (hyperkeratosis), from consuming feeds that contained chlorinated naphthalene found in lubricating oil. The depressed vitamin A levels in blood plasma led investigators to conclude that the toxic substance interfered with converting carotene to vitamin A (Maynard *et al.*, 1979). Removal of naphthalenes from oils eliminated X-disease. Studies have shown that vitamin A-deficient cattle lack heat tolerance. Deficient cattle stand panting and daily feed consumption are reduced (Perry, 1980).

Vitamin A-supplemented cattle show improved hot weather tolerance and spend more time ruminating. Vitamin A deficiency signs can result indirectly from deficiencies of zinc, iodine, phosphorus (P), protein, or vitamin E because these nutrients are required for the average utilization and metabolism of vitamin A. Zinc deficiency interferes with the synthesis in the liver of RBP which carries vitamin A (retinol) in plasma. Thus, decreased liver RBP levels in zinc deficiency may cause low plasma vitamin A concentrations. Zinc-deficient goats have been observed to have low serum vitamin A despite adequate dietary vitamin A (Chhabra *et al.*, 1980). In calves, serum vitamin A was significantly higher for animals supplemented with 50 mg per kg of zinc (Chhabra and Arora, 1987). Cattle from tropical Northern Australia showed a 12% annual mortality rate, partly because of a slow release of liver vitamin A (McDowell, 1985).

High calcium (Ca) and low zinc concentrations in native forages contributed to this slow liver vitamin A release. Since tropical forages have often been shown to be low in zinc (McDowell *et al.*, 1984), conditioned vitamin A deficiencies may result even though liver vitamin A values indicate adequate concentrations of this vitamin. This points out the importance of balanced vitamin-mineral nutrition for grazing livestock. Deficiencies of P, iodine, protein, or vitamin E reduce vitamin A utilization and may cause vitamin A deficiency signs. Retinyl phosphate is an intermediary in retinol metabolism. Transthyretin, a thyroid hormone-binding protein, forms a complex with RBP in plasma (Olson, 1984). Therefore, iodine status and thyroid activity can influence retinol transport and uptake. Protein deficiency can limit the synthesis of RBP, and vitamin E enhances vitamin A stability and utilization.

Vitamin A deficiency in sheep

Clinical signs of vitamin A deficiency in sheep (Figures 4.13 and 4.14) are similar to those of cattle. Night blindness is the common means of determining the deficiency, although severe vitamin A deficiency in feedlot lambs may progress to total blindness (NRC, 1985). Vitamin A deficiency results in keratinization of the respiratory, alimentary, reproductive, urinary, and ocular epithelia. Keratinization of these tissues reduces their resistance to infection (Weber, 1983).

Bruns and Webb (1990) found that vitamin A-deficient lambs had depressed humoral immune responses to ovalbumin. Adrenal function is compromised by vitamin A deficiency (Webb *et al.*, 1968). Additional clinical deficiency signs include growth retardation, bone malformation, degeneration of the reproductive organs, and elevated pressure in cerebrospinal fluid. A deficiency interferes with the normal development of bone, which may contribute to muscular incoordination and nervous signs (Figure 4.13). Also, a vitamin deficiency can result in lambs being born weak, malformed, or dead (Figure 4.14). Retained placenta also occurs in vitamin A-deficient ewes.

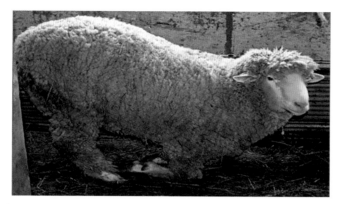

Figure 4.13 Vitamin A deficiency in sheep: Weakness, swayed back, followed by inability to stand. (source: T.J. Cunha and Washington State University, 1985)

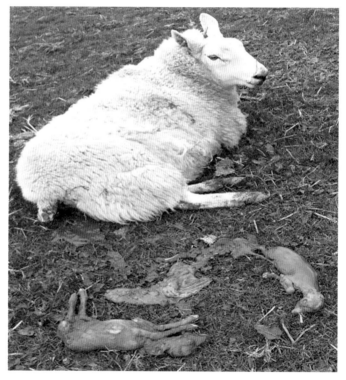

Figure 4.14 Vitamin A deficiency in sheep: Reproductive failure. Ewe fed low carotene ration during gestation. One lamb was born dead, and the other died 6 hours after birth. (source: CA AG. Experiment Station, NRC, 1985)

Vitamin A deficiency has resulted in low semen quality in rams (Lindley *et al.*, 1949). Vitamin A deficiency has detrimental effects on wool production and characteristics, including shortened wool fibers and decreases in fiber thickness, strength, and elongation (Guirgis *et al.*, 1982).

Vitamin A deficiency in Goats
Vitamin A deficiency in goats may first appear as a nonspecific rough, dull hair coat. Goats deficient in vitamin A exhibit keratinization of the epithelium of the respiratory, alimentary, reproductive, and urinary tracts and the eye (NRC, 1981). Signs include increased susceptibility to multiple infections, especially respiratory infections, poor bone development, the birth of abnormal offspring, and visual impairment. Night blindness is a classic deficiency sign. Experimentally produced signs of vitamin A deficiency in goats include loss of appetite, loss of weight, unhealthy appearance, night blindness, and a thick nasal discharge (Schmidt, 1941). In India, limited work with goats suggested that vitamin A deficiency leads to the development of urinary calculi (Majumdar and Gupta, 1960). Vitamin A deficiency impairs fertility, either temporarily or permanently. Metritis may be caused by damage to the integrity of the uterine mucosa (Guss, 1977). In adult goats, reduced fertility is a common clinical sign. Doe goats show poor conception rates and shortened or delayed estrus, and bucks exhibit reduced semen quality.

Safety
In general, the possibility of vitamin A toxicity in ruminants is remote because it has a wide margin of safety. However, vitamin A offers the greatest risk of accidental toxicity of all vitamins. Presumed upper safe levels are 4–10 times the nutritional requirements for monogastric animals, including birds and fish, and about 30 times the requirements for ruminants (NRC, 1987). The higher vitamin A tolerance of ruminants may be partly due to microbial degradation of vitamin A in the rumen (Rode *et al.*, 1990; Weiss, 1998).

Most harmful effects have been obtained by feeding over 100 times the daily requirements for an extended period. Thus, moderate excesses of vitamin A administered for short periods should not produce harmful effects. Recommended upper safe levels for adult cattle are 66,000 IU per kg, and for goats and sheep, 45,000 IU per kg. In a short-term study, steers were fed 2.56 million IU per head per day, with no gross evidence of toxicity (Hale *et al.*, 1961). Tharnish and Larson (1992) fed dairy cows 1.0 to 2.0 million IU daily for several months in 5 experiments. No outright toxicity symptoms of depression in performance were noted.

The most characteristic signs of hypervitaminosis A are skeletal malformation, spontaneous fractures, and internal hemorrhage (NRC, 1987). Other signs include loss of appetite, reduced growth or weight loss, skin thickening (hyperkeratosis), increased blood-clotting time, reduced erythrocyte count (hematocrit), enteritis, congenital abnormalities, and conjunctivitis. Degenerative atrophy, fatty infiltration, and reduced function of the liver and kidneys are also typical. For ruminants fed toxic levels of the vitamin, the most common clinical signs were osteoporosis, reduced feed intake, and decreased spinal fluid pressure (NRC, 1987).

The dietary level at which damage occurs in cattle varies among affected tissues; skeletal changes were observed with 132,000 IU vitamin A per 100 kg of body weight (BW) per day, or about 30 times the requirement (Hazzard *et al.*, 1964). In contrast, weight gains were depressed at 880,000 IU of vitamin A per kg of BW (Hazzard *et al.*, 1964). High excess intake of vitamin A impairs the absorption and metabolism of other fat-soluble vitamins.

Therefore, excess vitamin A in diets containing marginal levels of vitamins D, E, and K may impair animal performance by inducing a marginal deficiency of one or more fat-soluble vitamins (Schelling *et al.*, 1995). In the dairy cow, 675,000 IU of vitamin A acetate per head per day is required to depress vitamin E utilization significantly. This is approximately 10-fold greater than the highest levels currently fed to dairy or beef cattle and, therefore, should not cause a practical problem. In particular, caution should be observed in the formulation of milk replacers for veal calves and replacement calves in accelerated-growth schemes to avoid potential problems with excessive vitamin A intake (NRC, 2001).

Animals receiving direct exposure to sunlight will be protected to varying degrees from an induced vitamin D deficiency. Vitamin K is generally synthesized by rumen flora, but its absorption could be impaired by excess vitamin A. Vitamin E would be the most significant concern under practical conditions. The efficiency of conversion of β-carotene to vitamin A (retinol) declines progressively with increasing intakes of either carotenes or preformed vitamin A. This appears to be a natural homeostatic control mechanism that protects grazing livestock from any potentially harmful effects of the carotenes abundant in high-quality green forages.

Similarly, animals exhibit relatively rapid catabolism and excretion of excess vitamin A. The conversion of retinol to retinoic acid is irreversible in animal tissues and provides a metabolic outlet for retinol and retinaldehyde. Retinoic acid derivatives are formed by conjugation to glucuronic acid in the liver and excreted in the urine. Excess vitamin A is far more likely to produce toxicity than carotene. However, vitamin A toxicity is typically not a practical problem for ruminant livestock, except when unreasonably high levels are accidentally administered or fed for extended periods (NRC, 1987).

Vitamin D
Chemical structure and properties
The term vitamin D covers a group of closely related compounds possessing antirachitic activity. This includes ergosterol, ergocalciferol, and cholecalciferol. Provitamin D_2 ergosterol is a sterol found in green plants, fungi, and yeasts that undergoes a photochemical reaction caused by ultraviolet (UV) radiation from sunlight to form vitamin D_2 or ergocalciferol.

Vitamin D_3 or cholecalciferol is produced only in animals via UV radiation of provitamin D_3 or 7-dehydrocholesterol present in the skin. The provitamin 7-dehydrocholesterol, derived from cholesterol or squalene, is synthesized in the body and present in large amounts in the skin, the intestinal wall, and other tissues. (DeLuca, 2014; Combs and McClung, 2022). Sterols with vitamin D activity have a common steroid nucleus and differ like the lateral chain attached to carbon 17 (Figure 4.15). Vitamin D precursors have no antirachitic activity.

In its pure form, vitamin D is colorless crystals that are insoluble in water but readily soluble in alcohol and other organic solvents. Vitamin D can be destroyed by over-treatment with UV light and by peroxidation in the presence of rancidifying polyunsaturated fatty acids

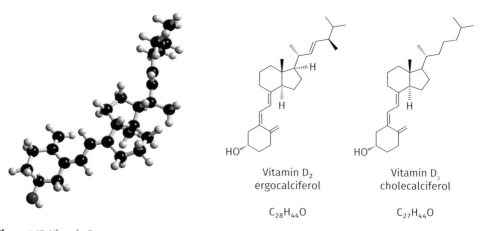

Vitamin D_2
ergocalciferol

$C_{28}H_{44}O$

Vitamin D_3
cholecalciferol

$C_{27}H_{44}O$

Figure 4.15 Vitamin D structure

(PUFA). Like vitamins A and E, it is destroyed by oxidation unless vitamin D_3 is stabilized. Its oxidative destruction is increased by heat, moisture, and trace minerals. There is less destruction of vitamin D_3 in freeze-dried fish meals during drying, possibly because of decreased atmospheric oxygen. There is negligible loss of crystalline cholecalciferol during storage for one year or crystalline ergocalciferol for 9 months in amber-evacuated capsules at refrigerator temperatures.

Natural sources

In most tables comprising the nutritional value of feedstuffs, the vitamin D content is calculated based on the equivalent bioactivity of vitamin D_2 plus D_3 (ergocalciferol and cholecalciferol). Vitamin D_2 and D_3 distribution in nature is limited, although their precursors, ergosterol in plants and 7-dehydrocholesterol in animals, occur widely. Grains, roots, and oilseeds, and their numerous by-products used in livestock feeds, contain insignificant amounts of vitamin D. Ergocalciferol occurs naturally in some mushrooms, and cholecalciferol occurs naturally in fish (Johnson and Kimlin, 2006).

The principal source of vitamin D in ruminant diets is vitamin D_2 (ergocalciferol), produced by the action of UV light on the ergosterol in forages. Green, uncured forages are poor sources of vitamin D, but vitamin D_2 is formed by UV radiation during the field curing of hay or silage. Potency depends on local climatic conditions. Hay or silage produced under cloudy conditions will have less vitamin D activity than when cured under bright sunlight. Artificially dried forages removed directly after harvest to drying facilities will have less vitamin D content than field-cured forage (Abrams, 1952). Even hay dried in the dark immediately after cutting has vitamin D activity because the dead or injured leaves on the growing plant are responsive to UV irradiation even though the living tissues are not. This phenomenon is also primarily responsible for the vitamin D activity found in corn silage (Maynard et al., 1979). Legume hay adequately cured to preserve most of its leaves and green color contains considerable vitamin D activity. Alfalfa, for example, will range from 650 to 2,200 IU per kg (Maynard et al., 1979).

Poor handling of hay, which can otherwise be an essential source of vitamin D for cattle, sheep, and goats, can lead to extensive shatter and leaf loss. Leaves are richer in vitamin D than the stem. Animals fed forages harvested or stored under poor conditions are susceptible to vitamin D deficiency if there is no vitamin D supplementation in the diet (Abrams, 1978).

The naturally occurring vitamin D activity in concentrate feeds is derived from animal products. Saltwater fish and their oils are wealthy sources of vitamin D. Milk fat contains a variable amount of vitamin D activity (5 to 40 IU in cow's milk per quart), depending on fat content. Still, neither cow's nor human milk contains sufficient vitamin D to protect the nursing young against rickets without sunlight (Maynard et al., 1979). Vitamin D in colostrum provides some reserve (Table 4.1). Cow's milk is reportedly higher in vitamin D when produced in the summer than in the winter (Zheng and Teegarden, 2013; Combs and McClung, 2022).

Commercial forms

Most vitamin D_3 used for fortifying animal feeds is a spray-dried formulation containing 500,000 IU/g. A combination of vitamin A and D_3, usually in a 5:1 ratio – i.e., vitamin A 1,000,000 IU/g and vitamin D_3 200,000 IU/g is also used in feed fortification.

Three commercial metabolites of vitamin D are used for animal feed supplementation: 25-hydroxy-cholecalciferol ($25OHD_3$ or calcidiol or calcifediol), 1-α-hydroxycholecalciferol, and 1,25-dihydroxy-cholecalciferol [$1,25(OH)_2D_3$ or calcitriol]. For over 25 years, the first metabolite, $25OHD_3$, has been largely used as a feed additive (tradename Rovimix® HyD) in spray-dried form.

Alfacalcidol, or 1-α-hydroxycholecalciferol or 1-α-hydroxyvitamin D$_3$, is a non-endogenous analog of vitamin D. Alfacalcidol is activated by the enzyme 25-hydroxylase in the liver to mediate its effects in the body, or most importantly, the kidneys and bones.

A form of calcitriol as 1,25(OH)$_2$D$_3$ – glycoside is also available as feed material. This metabolite is extracted from *Solanum glaucophyllum* (Bachman *et al.*, 2013).

Synthetic D$_2$, D$_3$, and metabolites are stable when stored at room temperature. In complete feeds and mineral-vitamin premixes, Schneider (1986) reported 10–30% activity losses after 4 or 6 months of storage at 22°C. However, pure vitamin D$_3$ crystals or vitamin D$_3$ resin are susceptible to degradation upon exposure to heat or contact with mineral elements. The resin is stored under refrigeration with nitrogen gas. Dry, stabilized supplements retain potency much longer and can be used in high-mineral supplements. It has been shown that vitamin D$_3$ is much more stable than D$_2$ in feeds containing minerals.

Studies with ruminants (Sommerfeldt *et al.*, 1981) suggest that vitamin D$_3$ is the preferred substrate for producing 1,25(OH)$_2$D$_3$. Sommerfeldt *et al.* (1983) reported that the concentration of 1,25(OH)$_2$D$_3$ in the plasma of ergocalciferol (D$_2$)-treated dairy calves was one-half to one-fourth the level in cholecalciferol (D$_3$)-treated calves. Discrimination against vitamin D$_2$ in ruminants may be partly a result of either its preferential degradation by rumen microbes or less efficient intestinal absorption. However, Sommerfeldt *et al.* (1983) also determined that vitamin D$_3$ (cholecalciferol) is more biologically active than vitamin D$_2$ (ergocalciferol) in dairy calves. Hymøller and Jensen (2011) report that vitamin D$_2$ impairs the utilization of vitamin D$_3$ in high-yielding dairy cows. Vitamin D$_3$ after D$_2$ was less efficient at increasing the plasma status of 25OHD$_3$ than D$_3$ given without previous D$_2$ administration.

Stabilization of the vitamin can be achieved by (a) rapid compression of the mixed feed, for example, into pellets so that air is excluded; (b) storing feed under cool, dry, dark conditions; (c) preventing close contact between the vitamin and potent metallic oxidation catalysts (e.g., manganese); (d) including natural or synthetic antioxidants in the mix. The vitamin can also be protected by enclosing it in durable gelatin beadlets.

The stability of dry vitamin D supplements is affected most by high-temperature, high-moisture content, and contact with trace minerals such as ferrous sulfate, manganese oxide, etc. Hirsch (1982) reports the results of a "conventional" or non-stabilized vitamin D$_3$ product being mixed into a trace mineral premix or animal feed and stored at ambient room temperature (20–25°C) for up to 12 weeks. The feed had lost 31% of its vitamin D activity after 12 weeks, and the trace mineral premix had lost 66% of its activity after only 6 weeks in storage.

Metabolism

Absorption, conversion to active forms, and transport

Vitamin D requirements can be covered in 2 ways: by ingestion and endogenous synthesis of vitamin D$_3$ from cholesterol. This process requires the animals to be exposed to sunlight (Eshaghian *et al.*, 2013; DeLuca, 2014).

Four important variables selectively determine the amount of vitamin D$_3$ that will be photochemically produced by skin exposure to sunlight (Norman and Henry, 2007). The 2 principal determinants are the quantity and intensity of ultraviolet light (UV) and the appropriate wavelength of UV light (290 and 315 nm). The third important variable determining skin vitamin D synthesis is the concentration of 7-dehydrocholesterol in the skin. The fourth determinant of vitamin D$_3$ production is the concentration of melanin in the skin (skin color). The darker the skin, the longer the time required to convert 7-dehydrocholesterol to vitamin D$_3$ (Zheng and Teegarden, 2013; Combs and McClung, 2022).

On average, only 50% of an oral dose of vitamin D is absorbed. However, considering sufficient vitamin D is usually produced by daily exposure to sunlight, it is unsurprising that the body has not evolved a more efficient mechanism for dietary vitamin D absorption (Horst et al., 1982; Norman and Henry, 2007).

The presence of the provitamin 7-dehydrocholesterol in the skin's epidermis and sebaceous secretions is well recognized, and vitamin D is synthesized in the skin of many herbivores and omnivores. The cholecalciferol formed by the UV irradiation of 7-dehydrocholesterol is removed from the skin into the circulatory system by the blood transport protein for vitamin D, the vitamin D binding protein (VBP or DBP) primarily bound to γ-globulin and becomes immediately available for further metabolism (Imawari et al., 1976). This mechanism is of little significance when animals are indoors, so vitamin D_3 must be provided in the feed. Some of the vitamin D_3 formed in and on the skin ends up in the digestive tract, as many ruminant animals consume it as they lick their skin and hair.

Vitamin D undergoes multiple transformations and multi-site interactions in the living system (DeLuca, 1992, 2008; Dittmer and Thompson, 2011). Vitamin D metabolism in ruminants begins before absorption because rumen microbes can degrade vitamin D to inactive metabolites (Sommerfeldt et al., 1983), which may explain the higher vitamin D requirements in ruminants. However, Hymøller and Jensen (2010b) showed no degradation of vitamin D in the rumen of high-producing dairy cows. Both ergocalciferol and cholecalciferol were added to the rumen contents through a rumen fistula. Later, both forms of vitamin D were found at constant levels, indicating no degradation in the rumen.

Dietary vitamin D is absorbed by passive diffusion from the ileal portion of the intestinal tract in association with fats, as are all the fat-soluble vitamins. Like the others, it requires the presence of bile salts for absorption (Braun, 1986) and is absorbed with other neutral lipids via chylomicron into the lymphatic system (Norman and Henry, 2007; Zheng and Teegarden, 2013; DeLuca, 2014; Maurya and Aggarwal, 2017; Combs and McClung, 2022; Eder and Grundmann, 2022).

Dietary $25OHD_3$ is absorbed virtually independently from fats due to its higher polarity and therefore makes it much less influenced by gut disorders impairing fat absorption.

Following its absorption, vitamin D and its metabolites circulate in the plasma, like other steroids, bound to the DBP. Regardless of their origin (conversion in the skin or absorption), the blood carries the vitamins to the liver to start an activation process. Vitamin D cholecalciferol is biologically inactive and must be converted to the active form through 2 hydroxy methylations. Over 30 vitamin D metabolites can be formed, among which $1,25(OH)_2D_3$ is the main active form.

In the liver, cholecalciferol is converted to $25OHD_3$. This first hydroxylation is catalyzed by the hepatic microsomal enzyme of the cytochrome P450 (CYP) family 25-hydroxylase (CYP2R1) with the transformation of cholecalciferol to $25OHD_3$ which is the circulating and storage form of vitamin D. This conversion step is not metabolically regulated. The concentration of $25OHD_3$ in the circulation is considered a good indicator of vitamin D status in general, able to indicate adequacy, deficiency, or toxicity of vitamin D (McDowell, 2000a; DeLuca, 2014).

By providing $25OHD_3$ through the diet allows to skip the first of the 2 hydroxylations hence providing the substrate for the second which converts $25OHD_3$ into the active, hormonal form $1,25(OH)_2D_3$.

$25OHD_3$ is then transported to the kidney, on the VBP, where it can be converted, in the proximal convoluted cells, to a variety of compounds, of which the most important is $1,25(OH)_2D_3$ by the action of 1α-hydroxylase (CYP27B1) (DeLuca, 2008; DeLuca, 2014).

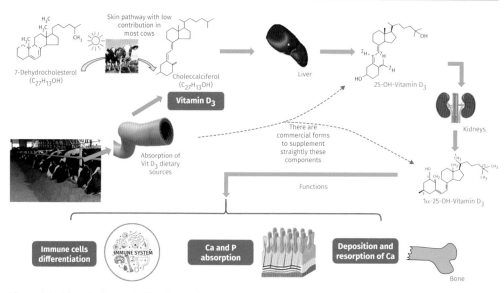

Figure 4.16 Vitamin D metabolism in ruminants

Vitamin C is involved in this stage. The parathyroid hormone regulates this second hydroxylation according to the concentrations of Ca and P. The $1,25(OH)_2D_3$ is more active but has a shorter half-life than $25OHD_3$. Other renal metabolites are of less practical interest, such as $24,25(OH)_2D_3$ or $1,24,25(OH)_3D_3$.

Subsequently, $1,25(OH)_2D_3$ is transported to the intestine, the bones, or another part of the kidney, which participates in Ca and P metabolism (Figure 4.16). VBP has the greatest affinity for $25OHD_3$, the main circulating form, then for cholecalciferol, and finally for $1,25(OH)_2D_3$. Another important enzyme is the renal 24-hydroxylase (CYP24A1), catalyzing the first step of its inactivation from $25OHD_3$ to $24,25(OH)_2D_3$. The physiological role of this metabolite is less clear: it is considered one of the primary metabolites destined for excretion. However, some research (Hove *et al.*, 1983) has identified a potential role in bone mineralization.

Although the kidney is the leading site of 1-α-hydroxylation, other cells and organs like intestinal cells, immune cells, endothelial cells, brain, mammary glands, pancreatic islets, parathyroid glands, placenta, prostate, and skin express active 1α-hydroxylase (Johnson and Kimlin 2006; DeLuca, 2008; Eder and Grundmann, 2022).

$1,25(OH)_2D_3$ acts metabolically as a hormone. Under conditions of Ca stress, parathyroid hormone (PTH) activates renal mitochondrial 1α-hydroxylase, which converts $25OHD_3$ to $1,25(OH)_2D_3$, and inactivates renal and extrarenal 24- and 23-hydroxylases (Goff *et al.*, 1991b).

In contrast, under conditions of low-Ca stress (when little PTH is secreted), the 1-α-hydroxylase can also be directly stimulated by low blood Ca or P concentration. High plasma $1,25(OH)_2D_3$ concentration has an inhibitory effect on renal 1-α-hydroxylase and a stimulatory effect on tissue 24- and 23-hydroxylases, which convert the $25OHD_3$ [and any $1,25(OH)_2D_3$ formed] to inactive metabolites (Eder and Grundmann, 2022). Thus, the production and catabolism of the hormone $1,25(OH)_2D_3$ are tightly regulated. It is now known that the most critical point of regulation of the vitamin D endocrine system occurs through stringent renal 1-a-hydroxylase activity control. In this way, the production of the hormone $1,25(OH)_2D_3$ can be modulated according to the Ca needs of the organism (Zheng and Teegarden, 2013; DeLuca, 2014).

Storage and excretion

For most mammals, vitamin D_3, 25OHD$_3$, and possibly 24,25(OH)$_2$D$_3$ and 1,25(OH)$_2$D$_3$ are all transported on the same protein, called transcalciferin, DBP. This protein is essential in maintaining the organism's adequate vitamin D level. VBP has a greater affinity for 25OHD$_3$, the main circulating form, then for cholecalciferol, and finally for 1,25(OH)$_2$D$_3$.

In contrast to aquatic species, which store significant amounts of vitamin D in the liver, land animals do not store appreciable amounts of the vitamin. The body can store vitamin D, although to a much lesser extent than vitamin A. Principal stores of vitamin D occur in fat, blood (as 25OHD$_3$), and the liver. It is also found in the lungs, kidneys, and elsewhere.

For mammals, 1,25(OH)$_2$D$_3$ is critical in maintaining sufficient maternal Ca to transport the fetus. It may play a role in the normal skeletal development of the neonate (Lester, 1986). A liberal vitamin D intake during gestation provides sufficient storage in newborns to help prevent early rickets. For example, newborn lambs can be provided enough to meet their needs for 6 weeks. During times of deprivation, vitamin D is released slowly, especially in the skin and adipose, thus meeting the vitamin D needs of the animal over a more extended period (Norman and Henry, 2007).

The excretion of absorbed vitamin D and its metabolites occurs primarily in feces with the aid of bile salts (Zheng and Teegarden, 2013; DeLuca, 2014). In addition to regulating 1,25(OH)$_2$D$_3$ synthesis, degradation of this potent hormone is also regulated by apparently separate but highly specific cytochrome P-450 enzymes. In degradation, 1,25(OH)$_2$D$_3$ is hydroxylated in the target tissue (bone and intestine) and the liver and kidney to an inert, water-soluble calcitroic. Both 25OHD$_3$ and 1,25(OH)$_2$D$_3$ undergo a 24-hydroxylation to form 24,25-dihydroxyvitamin D$_3$ (24,25(OH)$_2$D$_3$) and 1,24,25-trihydroxyvitamin D$_3$, respectively. The 24-hydroxylated derivatives are considered to be inert, first-step products of biodegradation. However, some observations imply possible, undefined roles for 24,25(OH)$_2$D$_3$ in bone formation, fracture healing, and embryonic development.

Biochemical functions

Classical functions

The classical function of vitamin D is to regulate the absorption, transport, deposition, and mobilization of Ca and P. The active form is 1,25(OH)$_2$D$_3$, which acts together with PTH, calcitonin, and fibroblast growth factor 23 (FGF23), similarly to steroid hormones. PTH, calcitonin, and FGF23 function in a delicate relationship with 1,25(OH)$_2$D$_3$ to control blood Ca and P levels (Nelson and Merriman, 2014; Eder and Grundmann, 2022). The production rate of 1,25(OH)$_2$D$_3$ is under physiological control. When blood Ca is below the normal range, PTH upregulates the production of calcitriol, elevating plasma Ca and stimulating specific ion pump mechanisms in the intestine, bone, and kidney (Deluca, 2014). FGF23 responds similarly in relationship to P level and interacts with the mechanism regulating Ca level.

These 3 sources of Ca and P provide reservoirs that enable vitamin D to elevate Ca and P in blood to levels necessary for normal bone mineralization and other functions ascribed to Ca. Contrary to the other 2, calcitonin regulates high serum Ca levels by depressing gut absorption, halting bone demineralization, and depressing reabsorption in the kidney.

McGrath *et al.* (2013), studying Ca and P retention in 18 steers fed a pelleted low-quality roughage diet containing an adequate Ca concentration (0.68%) with or without 25OHD$_3$ found a significant retention of Ca (8.1 g/day versus 4.1 g/day control) and P (8 g/day versus 4.9 g/day control).

The hormone enters the cell in the target tissue and binds to a cytosolic receptor or a nuclear receptor. $1,25(OH)_2D_3$ regulates gene expression by binding to tissue-specific receptors and subsequent interaction between the bound receptor and the DNA (Norman, 2006). The receptor-hormone complex moves to the nucleus. It attaches to the chromatin and stimulates the transcription of particular genes to produce specific mRNAs, which code for synthesizing particular proteins. Evidence for transcription regulation of a specific gene typically includes $1,25(OH)_2D_3$-induced modulation in mRNA levels.

Additionally, evidence may consist of measurements of transcription and a vitamin D-responsive element within the promoter region of the gene (Hannah and Norman, 1994). Several studies (Kliewer et al., 1992; Whitfield et al., 1995) have identified a heterodimer of the vitamin D receptor (VDR) and a vitamin A receptor (RXR) within the nucleus of the cell as the active complex for mediating positive transcriptional effects of $1,25(OH)_2D_3$. This classical function is driven by the effects of vitamin D at intestinal, bone, and kidney levels (Yang and Ma, 2021). The 2 receptors (vitamins D and A) selectively interact with specific hormone response elements composed of direct repeats of specific nucleotides in regulated gene promoters. The complex that binds to these elements consists of 3 distinct elements: the $1,25(OH)_2D_3$ hormonal ligand, the VDR, and one of the vitamins A (retinoid) X receptors (RXR) (Kliewer et al., 1992; Whitfield et al., 1995).

Intestinal effects

Vitamin D stimulates the active transport of Ca and P across the intestinal epithelium. This stimulation does not involve PTH directly but affects the active form of vitamin D (Zheng and Teegarden, 2013). PTH indirectly stimulates intestinal Ca absorption by stimulating the production of $1,25(OH)_2D_3$ under conditions of hypocalcemia.

Vitamin D promotes Ca and P absorption, but the mechanism is still not completely understood. Current evidence (Wasserman, 1981; Zheng and Teegarden, 2013; Combs and McClung, 2022) indicates that $1,25(OH)_2D_3$ is transferred to the nucleus of the intestinal cell, where it interacts with the chromatin material. In response to the $1,25(OH)_2D_3$, specific RNAs are elaborated by the nucleus. When these are translated into particular proteins by ribosomes, the events leading to Ca and P absorption enhancement occur (Hibbs and Conrad, 1983; Montgomery et al., 2004). In the intestine, calcitriol promotes the synthesis of calbindin (Ca-binding protein, CaBP) and other proteins and stimulates Ca and P absorption. Vitamin D has also been reported to influence magnesium (Mg) absorption and Ca and P balance.

Initially, it was felt that vitamin D did not regulate P absorption and transport. In 1963, through an in vitro inverted sac technique, it was demonstrated that vitamin D plays such a role (Harrison and Harrison, 1963). A more recently discovered phosphaturic hormone, FGF23, primarily produced in osteoblast and osteocyte cells, is responsible for P homeostasis through a pathway that involves feedback regulation between FGF23, vitamin D, P, and Ca (Sitara et al., 2006; David et al., 2013).

Bone effects

Vitamin D_3 plays an essential role in the metabolism and development of the skeleton in ruminants, maintaining complex balances with Ca and P. Increasing the dosage of vitamin D_3 increases the plasma concentration of ionized and total Ca and reduces the concentration of P and sodium. It also improves P absorption and retention, and utilization of phytic P (Ward et al., 1972; Wasserman, 1981; Liesegang et al., 2000; Eder and Grundmann, 2022) and intervenes in the differentiation and maturation of chondrocytes.

It must be noticed that other vitamins (B_6, folic acid, C, and K) and mineral trace elements (Cu, Zn, Mn, B, F, and Al) are also involved in the ossification process. Minerals are deposited on the protein matrix (Zheng and Teegarden, 2013; Combs and McClung, 2022). This is accompanied by an invasion of blood vessels that gives rise to trabecular bone. This process causes bones to elongate. This organic matrix fails to mineralize during a vitamin D deficiency, causing rickets in the young and osteomalacia in adults. The active metabolite calcitriol brings about the mineralization of the bone matrix.

Vitamin D has another function in bone: mobilizing Ca from bone to the extracellular fluid compartment. PTH shares this function. It requires metabolic energy and presumably transports Ca and P across the bone membrane by acting on osteocytes and osteoclasts. Rapid, acute plasma Ca regulation is due to the interaction of plasma Ca with Ca-binding sites in bone material as blood comes in contact with bone. Changes in plasma Ca are brought about by a difference in the proportion of high- and low-affinity Ca-binding sites, access to which is regulated by osteoclasts and osteoblasts, respectively (Bronner and Stein, 1995; Liesegang *et al.*, 2000). Another role of vitamin D is in bone collagen biosynthesis in preparation for mineralization (Rodney *et al.*, 2018; Combs and McClung, 2022; Eder and Grundmann, 2022). $25OHD_3$ is more potent than vitamin D_3 (2.5–4 times more) in improving Ca and P metabolism.

Kidney effects

There is evidence that vitamin D functions in the distal renal tubules to improve Ca reabsorption and is mediated by the Ca-binding protein calbindin (Bronner and Stein, 1995). It is known that 99% of renal-filtered Ca is reabsorbed without vitamin D and PTH. Although it is unknown whether they work in concert, the remaining 1% is controlled by these 2 hormonal agents. It has been shown that $1,25(OH)_2D_3$ improves renal Ca reabsorption (Sutton and Dirks, 1978).

Non-classical functions (beyond bone mineralization)

Other functions that we can call non-classical are connected with the discovery of the presence of 1α-hydroxylase and the receptor of the active metabolite in several tissues like the pancreas, bone marrow, cells of the ovary, cells of the brain, breast, and epithelial cells, suggesting a role in many other aspects like immune system modulation, muscle cells differentiation and reproduction (Machlin and Sauberlich, 1994; Deluca, 2014; Nelson and Merriman, 2014; Yang and Ma, 2021). More than 50 genes have been reported to be transcriptionally regulated by $1,25(OH)_2D_3$ (Hannah and Norman, 1994; Zheng and Teegarden, 2013; Combs and McClung, 2022). Yao *et al.* (2018) concluded that the diverse expression patterns of vitamin D receptors and vitamin D-metabolizing enzymes in the ram reproductive tract at different developmental stages and spermatozoa suggest it plays a potential role in spermatogenesis.

Immune system modulation

The actions of $1,25(OH)_2D_3$ are recognized as being involved in regulating the growth and differentiation of various cell types, including those of the hematopoietic and immune systems (Reinhardt and Hustmyer, 1987; Lemire, 1992; Yang and Ma, 2021). Recent studies have suggested $1,25(OH)_2D_3$ as an immunoregulatory hormone, and $25OHD_3$ appears more efficient than vitamin D in modulating immune response (Reinhardt and Hustmyer, 1987; Yue *et al.*, 2018; Poindexter *et al.*, 2020).

Elevated $1,25(OH)_2D_3$ was also associated with a significant 70% enhancement of lymphocyte proliferation in cells treated with pokeweed mitogen (Hustmyer *et al.*, 1994). Calcitriol or its metabolites have also been credited with functions regulating the cells of the immune system (Reinhardt and Hustmyer, 1987; Yue *et al.*, 2018; Poindexter *et al.*, 2020).

Feeding additional vitamin D in the last 3 weeks of gestation changed the profile of blood leukocytes and attenuated granulocyte phagocytosis during the transition period, whereas supplementing Ca prepartum increased mRNA expression of genes involved in immune cell function, including genes related to pathogen recognition and antimicrobial effects of leukocytes (Vieira-Neto *et al..*, 2021b).

Muscle cell differentiation and meat tenderization

It has been shown that feeding $25OHD_3$ affects ruminant vitamin D status and could stimulate satellite cell-mediated muscle hypertrophy response (Hines *et al.*, 2013; Półtorak *et al.*, 2017). Satellite cells are muscle stem cells giving rise, when activated, to a skeletal muscle cell precursors pool, able to differentiate and fuse to increase the nuclei accretion into existing muscle fibers or to form new fibers. These adult stem cells are involved in average skeletal muscle growth and regeneration following injury or disease.

Martins *et al.* (2020) studying supplementation of $25OHD_3$ in genes expression related to anabolism and catabolism of feedlot cattle concluded that the supplementation increased expression of genes correlated to muscular growth and protein synthesis, being a viable technology for beef cattle finished in feedlot systems. Feeding HyD® increased IGF 2 and tended to increase IGF 1 and mTOR gene expression These genes are related to protein synthesis, which may contribute to hypertrophy of muscular fibers and mass. $25OHD_3$ also enhanced expression of MSTN, a gene that controls muscular growth and protein turnover. No statistical difference ($P > 0.05$) was observed in gene expression of SOD 1 (antioxidant marker) and on genes related do muscular catabolism (FOXO 1, MURF 1, Atrogin 1).

Reproduction

One question that is still unanswered is whether the hormone form $1,25(OH)_2D_3$ acts alone or if there is some response from a second vitamin D metabolite or hormone (e.g., $24,25(OH)_2D_3$) (Feldman *et al.*, 2003; Nelson and Merriman, 2014). However, this question was probably answered in a study where the 24-position of $25(OH)D_3$ was blocked with fluoro groups to prevent 24-hydroxylation (DeLuca, 2008). All systems were normal for 2 generations, indicating a need for only $1,25(OH)_2D_3$. Therefore, research suggests that $1,25(OH)_2D_3$ appears to be the only functional form of vitamin D in biology (DeLuca, 2008; Yang and Ma, 2021).

For mammals, $1,25(OH)_2D_3$ is critical in maintaining sufficient maternal Ca to transport the fetus. It may play a role in the normal skeletal development of the neonate (Lester, 1986). A liberal vitamin D intake during gestation provides sufficient storage in newborns to help prevent early rickets. For example, newborn lambs can be provided enough to meet their needs for 6 weeks.

Nutritional assessment

As previously discussed, vitamin D undergoes, in the body, through successive metabolic hydroxylation into $25OHD_3$ and $1,25(OH)_2D_3$ in the liver and kidney, respectively. The first hydroxylation product $25OHD_3$ is recognized as the best status marker for humans and other mammals (Höller *et al.*, 2018). Very briefly, vitamin D cannot be used as a reliable marker as it undergoes quickly through 25-hydroxylation. In the case of $1,25(OH)_2D_3$, its production is regulated according to Ca and P plasma levels and therefore its quantification (in the order of pg/ml, hence thousand times smaller compared to $25OHD_3$) does not provide a reliable measurement of vitamin D nutritional status.

Since the body does not store 25OHD$_3$, the concentration in circulation (plasma or serum) can be used for vitamin D status determination and its monitoring is important for a proper diagnosis of adequate, marginal, or insufficient levels.

Both competitive chemiluminescence immunoassays and HPLC coupled with tandem mass spectrometry (HPLC-MS/MS) assays are used in clinical practice. The pros and cons of both technologies have been reviewed in depth (Van den Ouweland, 2016).

HPLC-MS/MS has been referred to as the "gold standard." Still, as happens for several delicate analyses, the result can also be erroneous as this technique requires the skills of an experienced analyst (Atef, 2018). Vitamin D is stable at room temperature on dry blood spots and was one of the first vitamins analyzed with this sampling method (Eyles *et al.*, 2009).

The varying selectivity of the antibodies for 25OHD$_3$ (and 25OHD$_2$) and the potential for cross-reactivity with related metabolites such as 24,25(OH)$_2$D$_3$ impact the repeatability between different immune-based assays. This aspect is highly critical when using immune assays with animal plasma. Most commercial immune kits are based on human antibodies, and few are "optimized" for use in different animal species.

Experts still debate about the adequate 25OHD$_3$ plasma level of humans for which a 75 nmol/l or 30 ng/ml (conversion factor 2,5) is considered a cut-off between adequate and inadequate vitamin D nutritional status (Holick, 2007). However, some authors and health bodies have placed this threshold at 20 ng/ml or 50 nmol/l (Cashman, 2018), while others consider such values low-end of adequacy (Heaney and Holick, 2011). Levels above 150 nmol/l or 60 ng/ml are considered excessive in humans, although these figures are debatable. One point of discussion is that vitamin D nutritional status is typically assessed using Ca and P metabolism and bone status (endocrine function) as an endpoint. Research has progressively indicated that vitamin D has broader autocrine and paracrine functions besides the endocrine function, like immune system modulation and muscle cell development. These functionalities seem to require higher 25OHD$_3$ circulating levels to be activated.

A direct transposition of human data to animals is impossible, and the establishment of clinical ranges upon which to adjust dietary supplementation is underway. Finally, the dietary administration of 25OHD$_3$ has been shown in different studies carried out in humans and animal species to increase more efficiently than vitamin D$_3$ in the 25OHD$_3$ plasma level (Wertz *et al.*, 2004; Guo *et al.*, 2018; Poindexter *et al.*, 2020).

The recommended 25OHD$_3$ serum level in beef and dairy cattle is around 100 ng/ml (Nelson *et al.*, 2018) to support, besides Ca and P metabolism, performance improvement (milk yield in dairy cows and muscle growth in beef cattle) and the modulation of the immune system. López-Constantino *et al.* (2022) assessed the 25OHD$_3$ plasma levels of Holstein-Friesian cows with a history of positive *M. bovis* culture. Tuberculin-negative cattle had a higher serum concentration of 25OHD$_3$ (87.12 ng/ml) when compared to tuberculin-positive cattle (45.86 ng/ml).

Serum levels between 30–100 ng/ml can be observed when providing through the diet vitamin D$_3$ (and D$_2$) to beef and dairy cattle. In case of animals spending part of the year on pasture there is also the contribution of the endogenous synthesis thanks to UV rays. However this contribution is influenced by the hours spent under sunlight and by the seasonality. Therefore, to obtain the above mentioned higher 25OHD$_3$ plasma levels (around 100 ng/ml) supporting immunity and muscle growth require the administration of 25OHD$_3$ in the diet.

Plasma levels between 10 and 20 ng/ml 25OHD$_3$ are definitely inadequate for Ca and P homeostasis and with levels <10 ng/ml 25OHD$_3$ there is a high probability of impaired Ca and P metabolism with consequences primarily on bone health.

Nelson *et al.* (2016a) did a survey checking the 25OHD$_3$ blood status in 702 dairy cows from 12 dairy herds receiving 30,000–50,000 IU of vitamin D$_3$ per head day and a vast majority of cows were below 100 ng/ml of 25OHD$_3$ and indeed for beef cattle, the majority of plasma samples of fattening cattle in the Northern and Southern regions of the USA were below 100 ng/ml of 25OHD$_3$.

Deficiency signs

Rickets, the primary vitamin D deficiency disease, is a skeletal disorder of young, growing animals generally characterized by decreased Ca and P concentrations in the organic matrixes of cartilage and bone. Vitamin D deficiency results in clinical signs similar to Ca and (or) P deficiency because all 3 nutrients are required for proper bone formation. In adult animals, osteomalacia is the counterpart of rickets. Cartilage growth in the adult has ceased, and thus, this condition is characterized by a decreased concentration of Ca and P in the bone matrix by demineralization (Uhl, 2018).

Symptoms of rickets include the following skeletal changes, varying somewhat with species depending on anatomy and severity: (1) weakened long bones, resulting in curvature and deformation; (2) enlarged, painful hock and knee joints; (3) general stiffness of gait, arched back and a tendency to drag hind legs; and (4) beaded ribs and deformed thorax. With osteomalacia in adults, the progressive demineralization of bones eventually results in fractures and breaks. The disturbance of Ca and P metabolism produces other symptoms, such as reduced performance, hypocalcemia, and reproductive failure (Dittmer and Thompson, 2011).

Although there appear to be differences among species in the susceptibility of different bones to degenerative changes, as well as differences that probably reflect body conformation (e.g., pigs compared with sheep), there is nevertheless an apparent typical pattern in vitamin D deficiency (Maynard *et al.*, 1979, Uhl, 2018). The spongy and cartilaginous parts of individual bones (mainly the bone ends or epiphysis) and bones relatively rich in this tissue, such as the ribcage, are generally the first and most severely affected. As in simple Ca deficiency, the vertebrae and the skull have the most significant degree of demineralization, followed by the scapula, sternum, and ribs. The most resistant bones are the metatarsals and shafts of long bones, which would have obvious survival value to the animal.

Other clinical signs of vitamin D deficiency in ruminants are decreased appetite and growth rate, digestive disturbances, stiffness of gait, labored breathing, irritability, weakness, and occasionally tetany and convulsions. These symptoms may precede the skeletal symptoms like enlargement of joints, slight arching of the back, and bowing of legs, with the erosion of joint surface causing difficulty in locomotion (NRC, 2000; Dittmer and Thompson, 2011; Uhl, 2018). There can be an increase in the birth of dead, weak, or deformed calves and lambs.

Grazing animals with regular exposure to direct sunlight are usually protected from vitamin D deficiency. However, under most conditions of commercial livestock production, where animals have limited exposure to direct sunlight and where growth or milk production rates are high, dietary supplementation with vitamin D is prudent and recommended.

Vitamin D deficiency in cattle

Vitamin D should be supplied to growing and lactating cattle housed in confinement or with limited sun exposure. In more northern latitudes during winter, the photochemical conversion of provitamin D to its active compound (cholecalciferol) in the skin can be limited because of insufficient ultraviolet radiation (Uhl, 2018).

Hidiroglou *et al.* (1979) reported that 25OHD$_3$ was higher in cattle plasma during summer than in winter. Richter *et al.* (1990) found higher concentrations of 25OHD$_3$ in blood plasma when bulls were outdoors compared to indoors: 21.1 versus 14.3 ng/ml, respectively. Therefore, even the bulls exposed to direct sunlight in this experiment appeared to have marginal vitamin D status.

Similar relationships have been observed in human populations (Romagnoli *et al.*, 1999), where plasma 25OHD$_3$ was significantly higher in summer than in winter. During winter, 15% of young adults, 32% of postmenopausal women, and 71–82% of hospital inpatients exhibited vitamin D deficiency based on plasma levels of 25OHD$_3$.

Clinical signs of vitamin D deficiency in calves involving the skeleton begin with thickening and swelling of the metacarpal or metatarsal bones (Figures 4.17 and 4.18). As the disease progresses, the forelegs bend forward or sideways. In severe or prolonged vitamin D deficiency, the force exerted by average muscle tension results in the bending and twisting of long bones and the characteristic bone deformity. There is an enlargement of bone ends (epiphyses) from the deposition of excess cartilage, giving the characteristic "beading" effect along the sternum at the point of attachment of the ribs (NRC, 1996; 2001).

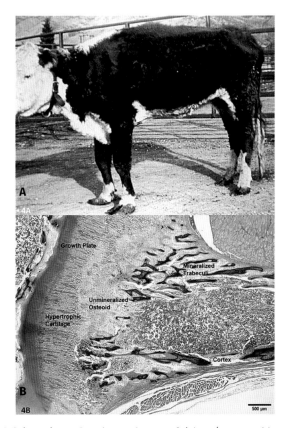

Figure 4.17 Vitamin D deficiency in cattle, advanced stage of rickets (source: Uhl, 2018). A cow with hypophosphatemic rickets is shown in the top panel; note the generalized poor condition and bowed front legs (photo courtesy of Dr. J. Carroll Woodard). Unlike osteoporosis, distortions of the bones are apparent in the living animal. In addition, affected cattle are often observed eating bones. The photomicrograph is of a long bone epiphysis from an opossum with rickets. The bones were so soft that they were not decalcified before processing, and the mineralized bone, which appears as dark spicules, is reduced in the cortex and trabeculi. The hypertrophic cartilage of the growth plate is expanded, and there are irregular aggregates of unmineralized, newly formed bone matrix (osteoid) at the distal edge of the growth plate (H&E, 20X).

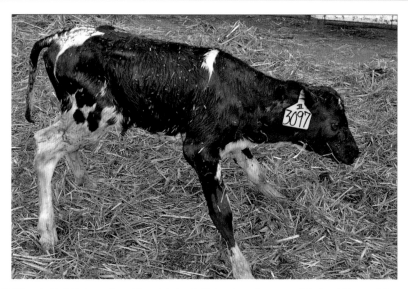

Figure 4.18 Vitamin D deficiency in cattle, rickets. Calf developed severe rickets while receiving ration deficient in vitamin D and without sunlight (source: Michigan Agriculture Experiment Station)

The mandible becomes thick and soft in calves, and in the worst cases, calves have difficulty eating. In calves so affected, there can be slobbering, inability to close the mouth, and tongue protrusion. Joints (particularly the knee and hock) become swollen and stiff, the pastern straight and the back arched. In severe cases, synovial fluid accumulates in the joints (NRC, 2001; Dittmer and Thompson, 2011; Uhl, 2018). Posterior paralysis may also occur as a result of fractured vertebrae. The structural weakness of the bones appears to be related to poor mineralization. The advanced stages of the disease are marked by stiffness of gait, dragging of the hind legs, irritability, tetany, labored and rapid breathing, weakness, anorexia, and cessation of growth. Calves born to vitamin D-deficient dams may be dead, weak, or deformed (Rupel *et al.*, 1933).

In older animals with vitamin D deficiency (osteomalacia), bones become weak and fracture easily, and posterior paralysis may accompany vertebral fractures. For dairy cattle, milk production may be decreased, and estrus may be inhibited by inadequate vitamin D (NRC, 2001). Cows fed a vitamin D-deficient diet and kept out of direct sunlight showed definite signs of vitamin D deficiency within 6–10 months (Wallis, 1946). Functions that deplete vitamin D are high milk production and advancing pregnancy, especially during the last few months before calving.

The visible signs of vitamin D deficiency in dairy cows are similar to those of rickets in calves. The animal begins to show stiffness in their limbs and joints, which makes it difficult to walk, lie down, and get up. The knees, hocks, and other joints become swollen, tender, and stiff. The knees often spring forward, the posterior joints straighten, and the animal is tilted forward on her toes. The hair coat becomes coarse and rough, with an overall unhealthy appearance (Wallis, 1946). The spine and back often become stiff, arched, and humped as the deficiency advances. Calving rates are lower in deficient herds; calves can be born dead or weak. Hypocalcemia, either milk fever (parturient hypocalcemia) or unexplained lactational hypocalcemia and paresis, may also be observed due to chronic vitamin D deficiency in dairy cattle. These signs are also produced by Ca, P, or electrolyte deficiency or imbalances and are not specific to vitamin D deficiency.

Milk fever in dairy cattle (parturient paresis)

Milk fever is a metabolic disease characterized by hypocalcemia at or near parturition in dairy cows. Goff et al. (1991b) and Horst et al. (1994) discussed milk fever and Ca metabolism of dairy cattle in detail. In essence, milk fever is a failure of Ca homeostasis due to increased metabolic demand for Ca. Causative and risk factors are partly, but not wholly, understood (Enevoldsen, 1993; Horst et al., 1994; Liesegang et al., 1998). Milk fever is related to factors such as (a) previous Ca and P intakes, (b) previous vitamin D intake, (c) previous intakes and dietary ratios of potassium, chloride, magnesium, sulfur, and sodium, and (d) age and breed of cow. Cows that develop milk fever cannot meet the sudden demand for Ca brought about by the initiation of lactation. Milk fever usually occurs within 72 hours after parturition and is manifested by circulatory collapse, generalized paresis, depression, and eventually coma and death.

The most obvious and consistent clinical sign is acute hypocalcemia, where serum Ca decreases from 8–10 mg to 3–7 mg (average 5 mg). Initially, a cow may exhibit some unsteadiness of gait. More commonly, the cow is observed lying on her sternum with her head turned sharply toward her flank in a characteristic posture. The eyes are dull and staring, and the pupils are fixed and dilated. If treatment is delayed, paresis will progress into a coma, which becomes progressively more profound, leading to death. Treatment with intravenous Ca boro-gluconate is a highly effective treatment. Some cows will relapse, sometimes with multiple episodes of paresis that indicate a severe failure of the Ca regulatory system or, in some cases, severe depletion of body Ca stores.

Oral Ca pastes and gels are also prophylactic and an adjunct to intravenous Ca treatment. Aged cows are at the most significant risk of developing milk fever. Heifers rarely develop milk fever, borne out by their superior Ca status at parturition (Shappell et al., 1987). Jersey cattle are generally more susceptible than Holsteins. Older animals have a decreased response to dietary Ca stress due to decreased production of $1,25(OH)_2D_3$ and a decreased responsiveness to the $1,25(OH)_2D_3$. In older cows, fewer osteoclasts exist to respond to hormonal stimulation, which delays the bone contribution of Ca to the plasma Ca pool (Goff et al., 1989, 1991b).

The aging process is also associated with a reduced renal 1-α-hydroxylase response to hypocalcemia, therefore reducing the amount of $1,25(OH)_2D_3$ produced from $25OHD_3$ (Goff et al., 1991b; Horst et al., 1994). Panda et al. (2001) demonstrated all adverse effects of low 1-α-hydroxylase activity with a mouse model. Mouse deficient in 1-α-hydroxylase were developed by targeted ablation of the hormone-binding and heme-binding domains of the 1-α-hydroxylase gene. Altered non-collagenous matrix protein expression and reduced numbers of osteoclasts were also observed in bone. Female mutant mice were infertile and exhibited uterine hypoplasia and absent corpora lutea. Furthermore, histologically enlarged lymph nodes in the vicinity of the thyroid gland and a reduction in CD4- and CD8-positive peripheral T-lymphocytes were observed. Reduced renal 1-α-hydroxylase negatively affected mineral and skeletal homeostasis, female reproduction, and immune function.

Other defects of vitamin D metabolism can occur, such as low activity of vitamin D receptors. Tissue receptors for $1,25(OH)_2D_3$ decline at parturition in cows (Goff and Horst, 1997), although there was no significant difference between paretic and nonparetic cows. Osteoblast activity also appears to be decreased during late pregnancy and around parturition (Naito et al., 1990). This may be related to reduced plasma calcitonin concentrations around parturition, especially in hypocalcemic, aged cows (Shappell et al., 1987). Low magnesium status is also a risk factor for parturient hypocalcemia and hypomagnesemia (Van de Braak et al., 1987; Van Mosel et al., 1991). Infection with the common brown stomach worm (*Ostertagia*) has been strongly implicated as a causative agent of milk fever and displaced abomasum in dairy cows (Axelsson, 1991), apparently due to an anaphylactic reaction at parturition.

Parturient paresis can be prevented effectively by feeding a low-Ca and adequate-P diet for the last weeks prepartum, followed by a high-Ca diet after calving (Horst *et al.*, 1994). Feeding low-Ca diets prepartum is associated with increased plasma PTH and $1,25(OH)_2D_3$ concentrations during the peripartum period (Kichura *et al.*, 1982; Green *et al.*, 1981). Green *et al.* (1981) suggested that the increased PTH and $1,25(OH)_2D_3$ concentrations resulted in "prepared" and effective intestinal absorption and bone resorption of Ca at parturition that prevents parturient paresis. P deficiency did not affect plasma concentrations of vitamin D_3 or its $25OHD_3$ or $1,25(OH)_2D_3$ active metabolites. Still, it did elevate plasma Ca and appeared to increase $1,25(OH)_2D_3$ receptor binding in the duodenum of P-depleted lactating goats (Schroder *et al.*, 1990).

Prepartal dietary cation-anion balance (DCAD) influences the degree and incidence of milk fever (Ender *et al.*, 1971; Block, 1984; Gaynor *et al.*, 1989; Oetzel *et al.*, 1988; Enevoldsen, 1993). Dietary excess of cations, especially sodium and potassium, relative to anions, primarily chloride and sulfur, tends to induce milk fever, while anionic diets can prevent milk fever. The cation-anion balance of the diet affects the acid-base status of the animal, with cationic diets producing a more alkaline state and anionic diets a more acidic state of metabolism. Mild metabolic acidosis, in turn, promotes Ca mobilization and excretion (Lomba *et al.*, 1978; Fredeen *et al.*, 1988; Won *et al.*, 1996). Anionic diets increase the amount of $1,25(OH)_2D_3$ produced per unit increase in parathyroid hormone (Goff *et al.*, 1991a). Debate remains regarding the mechanisms of action and the relative importance of individual mineral ions (Enevoldsen, 1993; Horst *et al.*, 1994).

Used correctly, anionic diets prepare the cow's metabolism for a sudden demand for Ca at calving and reduce the incidence of subclinical hypocalcemia and paresis (Horst *et al.*, 1994). Because most legumes and grasses are high in potassium, typical dry cow rations are alkaline. Adding anions, usually as anionic salts, to the diet for 2 to 4 weeks prepartum has been used successfully to reduce the incidence of milk fever. Goff *et al.* (1991a) concluded that low-Ca diets, anionic diets, and PTH administration increase renal 1-α hydroxylase activity, increasing production of $1,25(OH)_2D_3$ and milk fever prevention. Increased plasma $1,25(OH)_2D_3$ concentration in response to feeding acidified diets prepartum was reported by Phillippo *et al.* (1994).

Supplemental vitamin D has been used to prevent parturient paresis in dairy cows for several years (Hibbs and Conrad, 1976, 1983; Horst and Littledike, 1982). Feeding or injecting massive doses of vitamin D has effectively prevented milk fever, but toxicity symptoms and death have also occurred. In some cows, milk fever has been induced by the treatment. Due to the toxicity of vitamin D_3 in pregnant cows and the low margin of safety between vitamin D_3 doses that prevent milk fever and those that induce milk fever, Littledike and Horst (1982) concluded that injecting vitamin D_3 prepartum is not a practical solution to milk fever. However, more recent reports from the same laboratory have provided data suggesting that injection of $24-F_1,25(OH)_2D$ (fluoridation at the 24 positions) delivered at 7-day intervals before parturition can effectively reduce the incidence of parturient paresis (Goff, 1988).

Feeding high doses of vitamin D has been more successful than parental administration in preventing milk fever without inducing toxicity (Hibbs and Conrad, 1976). Feeding 20 to 30 million IU of vitamin D_2 for 3 to 8 days prepartum prevented 80% of expected milk fever cases in aged Jersey cows (Hibbs and Conrad, 1976). However, prolonging the treatment to 20 days prepartum has resulted in toxicity. The same authors fed cows 100,000 to 580,000 IU of vitamin D_2 per day continuously, year-roundly. They reported a reduction in milk fever in cows with a history of the disease but not in cows without a history of milk fever. The most practical approach to controlling milk fever appears to be optimizing macro-mineral levels with anionic diets and providing continuous supplementation with vitamin D at normal levels.

Subclinical hypocalcemia is still a concern with cows after postpartum as it affects the lactation and the health of dairy cows. Thus, the single oral Ca treatment approach gradually has shifted to a multi-treatment approach of subclinical hypocalcemia. Supplementing 25OHD$_3$ could solve the problem of vitamin D$_3$ insufficient synthesis and the limited conversion to 25OHD$_3$ in transition cows. Xu *et al.* (2021) feeding 25OHD$_3$ combined with oral Ca to transition cows improved serum 25OHD$_3$ status, Ca homeostasis and also improved the lactation performance and the health status during the transition period.

Vitamin D deficiency in sheep and goats

Clinical signs of vitamin D deficiency in sheep and goats are similar to those of cattle, including rickets in young animals and osteomalacia in adults (NRC, 1981; 1985) (Figure 4.19). An early report of rickets in Scotland referred to the condition as "bent leg," which occurred in ram lambs 7 to 12 months of age (Elliot and Crichton, 1926). The condition was prevented by administering small amounts of vitamin D in cod liver oil. Newborn lambs can receive enough vitamin D from their dams to prevent early rickets if the ewes have adequate vitamin D status (Church and Pond, 1974). Newborn kids develop rickets if the doe is fed a diet deficient in vitamin D during pregnancy (NRC, 1981).

Kohler *et al.* (2013) concluded that sheep and goats can produce vitamin D in the skin, but sheep depend more on vitamin D intake from feedstuffs, whereas goats rely more on cutaneous vitamin D production. However, genetic defects can also cause rickets that is not always associated with vitamin D deficiency. Dittmer *et al.* (2009) reported a new form of inherited rickets that causes skeletal disease in Corriedale sheep. This genetic defect may differ from other inherited rickets forms described in man and animals.

Vitamin D deficiency has been observed in young lambs or goat kids kept in complete confinement without access to sun-cured roughage, raised at high latitudes, during periods of

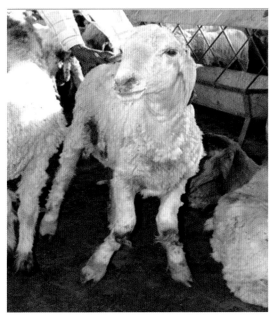

Figure 4.19 Vitamin D deficiency in sheep, rickets. Bilateral bent leg in yearling Rambouillet ram. Condition due to vitamin D deficiency. (source: Utah Agricultural Experiment Station)

decreased sunshine and forage low in P (Dittmer and Thompson, 2011; Kohler *et al.*, 2013). Hidiroglou *et al.* (1978) reported the clinical history of a flock of sheep kept in total confinement that showed a high incidence (8%) of an osteodystrophy condition, which was vitamin D-responsive. A form of osteodystrophy has also been produced experimentally in goats (NRC, 1981). Parturient paresis occurs in ewes. It is a disturbance of Ca metabolism in pregnant and lactating ewes and is characterized by acute hypocalcemia and the rapid development of hyperexcitability, ataxia, paresis, coma, and death. The disease occurs from 5 weeks before to 10 weeks after lambing, principally in over-conditioned, older ewes at pasture. The onset is often triggered by abrupt changes in diet, sudden weather changes, or periods of stress and fasting imposed by circumstances such as shearing or transportation. The extent of involvement of vitamin D in Ca metabolism in paretic ewes is unclear. Maternal Ca homeostasis is stressful in pregnant ewes (Paulson and Langman, 1990). Sheep differ from all other species studied thus far in that pregnancy does not increase circulating levels of $1,25(OH)_2D_3$ (Paulson and Langman, 1990). The signs (e.g., hyperexcitability) and conditions under which this disorder occurs (lush pasture, stressful events) suggest that hypomagnesemia is also involved.

Safety

After vitamin A, vitamin D is the next most likely to be consumed in concentrations toxic to animals (Fraser, 2021). Although vitamin D is toxic at high concentrations, short-term administration of as much as 100 times the required level may be tolerated. For cattle and sheep, the upper safe dietary level for short-term exposure is 25,000 IU per kg of diet, and for over 60 days, it is 2,200 IU per kg of diet (NRC, 1987).

Studies in several species, including ruminants, indicate that vitamin D_3 is 10 to 20 times more toxic than vitamin D_2 when provided in excess amounts (NRC, 1987). Excessive intake of vitamin D produces a variety of effects associated with hypercalcemia. Serum Ca concentration is elevated due to increased bone resorption and intestinal absorption of Ca. The main pathological effect of vitamin D toxicity is the widespread calcification of soft tissues. Pathological changes in these tissues include inflammation, cellular degeneration, and progressive calcification. Diffuse calcification affects joints, synovial membranes, kidneys, myocardium, pulmonary alveoli, parathyroid glands, pancreas, lymph nodes, arteries, conjunctivae, and cornea. In advanced cases, cartilage growth is disrupted. As a result, the skeletal system undergoes demineralization, losing bone mass and strength.

Other everyday observations of vitamin D toxicity are anorexia, extensive weight loss, bradycardia, reduced rumination, depression, polyuria, muscular weakness, joint pain and stiffness, elevated blood Ca, and lowered blood phosphate concentrations. Vitamin D toxicity in neonatal lambs may be characterized by clinical signs consisting solely of unhealthiness and weakness or an inability to stand (Roberson *et al.*, 2000). Cows receiving 30 million IU of vitamin D_2 orally for 11 days developed anorexia, reduced rumination, depression, premature ventricular systoles, and bradycardia (NRC, 1987). Littledike and Horst (1982) reported that moderate toxicity was characterized by delayed shedding of the winter hair coat; rough, dry hair coat; poor appetite and milk production; muscle and joint stiffness; excessive thirst; and air pockets under the skin of the neck and back with crepitation (crackling) of these areas. The same authors reported that severe toxicity resulted in pasty ocular discharge, flaccid udder, labored breathing, rapid, pounding pulse, fever, ketosis, severe anorexia, and death. Adipose tissue may provide some buffering effect against vitamin D toxicity. Brouwer *et al.* (1998) reported that in rats given large oral doses of vitamin D_3, adipose tissue accumulates and slowly releases vitamin D_3, thus mitigating the increase in plasma $25OHD_3$ and Ca.

Vitamin D toxicity is enhanced by increased dietary Ca and P supplies and is reduced when the diet is low in Ca. The route of administration also influences toxicity. Parenteral administration of 15 million IU of vitamin D_3 in a single dose caused toxicity and death in 71% of pregnant dairy cows (Littledike and Horst, 1982). On the other hand, oral administration of 20–30 million IU of vitamin D_2 daily for 7 days resulted in little or no toxicity in pregnant dairy cows (Hibbs and Pounden, 1955). Rumen microbes can metabolize vitamin D to the inactive 10-keto-19-nor vitamin D. This may partially explain the difference in toxicity between oral and parenteral vitamin D. The toxic dose of vitamin D is variable, with an essential factor being the duration of intake since this is cumulative toxicity. Pregnant cows are more susceptible to vitamin D toxicity than nonpregnant cows, possibly due to placental production of $1,25(OH)_2D_3$ (Littledike and Horst, 1982; DeLuca, 1992).

Although it is usually assumed that living plants do not contain vitamin D_2, certain plants contain compounds with vitamin D activity, predominantly $1,25(OH)_2D_3$ in glycoside form. Grazing animals in several parts of the world develop calcinosis, a disease characterized by the deposition of Ca salts in soft tissues (Carrillo, 1973; Morris, 1982). Ingestion of *Solanum malacoxylon* leaves by grazing animals causes enzootic calcinosis in Argentina and Brazil, where the disease is referred to as "enteque seco" and "espichamento," respectively. Consumption of as few as 50 fresh leaves per day (200 g of fresh leaves per week) over eight to 20 weeks will produce this toxicity disease in cows (Figure 4.20) (Okada *et al.*, 1977). The calcinogenic factor in *S. malacoxylon* is a water-soluble glycoside of $1,25(OH)_2D$ (Wasserman, 1975). The sterol is released during digestion, which results in a massive increase in dietary Ca and P absorption such that normal physiological processes cannot compensate, and soft tissue calcification results. Other plants that cause calcinosis in grazing animals are also reported in New Guinea, Florida, Hawaii, Australia, Jamaica and in the alpine regions in Europe (McDowell, 2000a).

During the development of plant-induced calcinosis diseases, the destruction of connective tissues precedes tissue mineralization in which Ca, P, and Mg are involved. Clinical signs of the disease are a stiff and painful gait and progressive weight loss. If animals are removed in the early stages from the affected areas, they recover quickly, but mortality is high after prolonged exposure. In advanced cases, joints cannot be extended completely, and animals tend to walk with an arched back, carrying their weight on the forepart of the hooves.

The calcinogenic plants are economically important due to losses in meat and milk production (Morris, 1982). In some fields in Argentina, between 10% and 30% of cattle show signs of "enteque seco," and *S. malacoxylon* is now regarded as one of the most important poisonous plants in that country. Other than these examples, most natural feedstuffs do not contain high

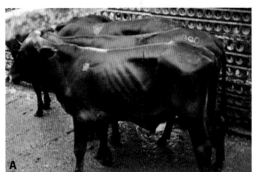 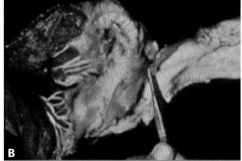

Figure 4.20 Vitamin D toxicity in cattle. "Enteque seco" in Argentina. Left: Cow that consumed shrub *Solanum malacoxylon*. Right: Ca deposits in soft tissue. (source: courtesy of Bernardo Jorge Carillo)

enough levels of vitamin D to cause toxicity. Marine fish oils are a rich source of vitamin D, but the amounts in livestock diets are not high enough to be of concern. In practice, vitamin D toxicity is unlikely.

Vitamin E
Chemical structure and properties
Vitamin E includes all tocopherol and tocotrienol derivatives that qualitatively have α-tocopherol activity (Bramley *et al.*, 2000), the most potent and standard plant form. This definition was given by the International Union of Pure and Applied Chemistry-International Union of Biochemistry (IUPAC-IUB, 1973) Commission on Biochemical Nomenclature. The tocopherols and the tocotrienols consist of a hydroquinone nucleus or chromanol ring and an isoprenoid side chain (4 carbon atoms in a straight chain and a side chain of a single carbon). Tocopherols have a saturated side chain, whereas tocotrienols have an unsaturated side chain containing 3 double bonds (Brigelius-Flohé, 2021).

There are 4 principal compounds of each of these 2 sources of vitamin E activity (α, β, γ and δ), differentiated by the presence of methyl (-CH3) groups at positions 5, 7, or 8 of the chroman ring (Figure 4.21). α-tocopherol, the most biologically active of these compounds, is the predominant vitamin E active compound in feedstuffs and the form used commercially to supplement animal diets. The biological activity of the other tocopherols is limited, but other functions have been found for non-α-tocopherol forms of vitamin E (Schaffer *et al.*, 2005; Freiser and Jiang, 2009; Traber, 2013). The differences between the different forms are due to the position and number of methyl groups in the chromanol ring. The other position of the methyl groups gives rise to the different racemic forms of tocopherols and tocotrienols. If the methyl groups are located on the same plane, they are called R forms, but if they are located on different planes, they are called S forms.

The tocopherol molecule has 3 asymmetric carbon atoms (methyl groups) at the 2', 4' and 8' positions. These 3 asymmetric carbon atoms generate 8 possible forms or stereoisomers: RRR-, RSR-, RRS-, RSS-, SRR-, SSR-, SRS-, and SSS-α-tocopherol. The d-form of α-tocopherol (d-α-tocopherol) has all of the methyl groups in these positions facing in one direction and is referred to as the RRR-form, which is the form found in plants and is considered the natural product. The all-*rac* (all racemic), or chemically synthesized form of DL-α-tocopherol, has an equal mixture of the R and S configurations at each of the 3 positions and contains the racemic mixture of all 8 stereoisomers (Traber, 2013).

Approximately 99% of what is found in tissues consists of R isomers in position 2, probably because of differences in the affinity of the α-tocopherol transporting hepatic protein. Of the total tocopherol retained in the tissues, the RRR-form predominates (more than 30%), followed by the RRS and RSR (around 27%) and the RSS (around 17%). The 4 isomers, SSS, SRR, SSR, and SRS, comprise less than 1%, even if the animals have a high supplementation of all-*rac*-α-tocopherol.

D-α-tocopherol is a yellow oil insoluble in water but in organic solvents, resistant to heat, but readily oxidized. Natural and synthetic forms of vitamin E are degraded by oxidation and accelerated by heat, moisture, rancid fat, copper, and iron. Inserting an acetate or succinate moiety on carbon 6 of the chromanol ring of either the natural or synthetic source stabilizes the compound. When acetate is inserted, the commercial names dl-α-tocopheryl acetate (all-*rac*-α-tocopheryl acetate) and d-α-tocopheryl acetate, more commonly known as RRR-α-tocopheryl acetate, are for the synthetic and naturally derived vitamin E products, respectively. The succinate form is less biologically active than the acetate form. D-α-tocopherol is an excellent natural antioxidant that protects carotene and other oxidizable materials in

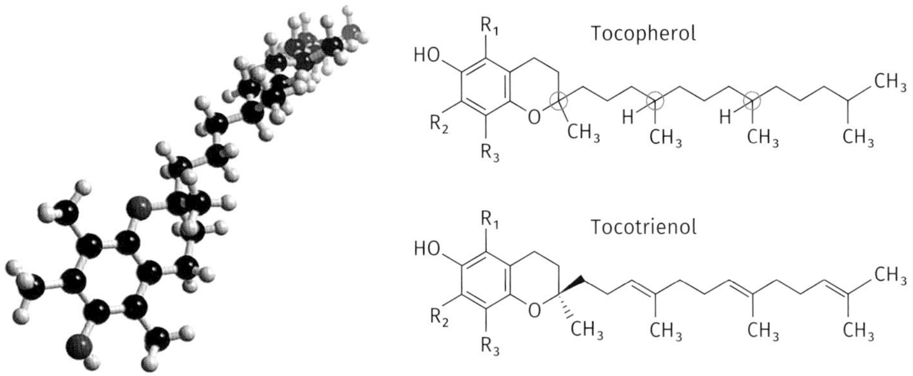

Figure 4.21 Vitamin E structure

feed and the body. In animal tissues, the most biologically active form of the vitamin is RRR-α-tocopherol, as it represents approximately 90% of the total (Bramley *et al.*, 2000). However, in the process of acting as an antioxidant, it is destroyed. The relative biological activity of vitamin E is expressed in international units (IU), 1 IU corresponding to the activity of 1 mg of (all-*rac*)-α-tocopheryl acetate.

Natural sources

Vitamin E is widespread. In nature, the synthesis of vitamin E is a function of plants; thus, their products are the principal sources. Published values of vitamin E analyses of feeds are based on various analytical techniques. As a result, there is a lack of characterization of individual tocopherols in most analyses. Total tocopherol analysis of a food or feed is of limited value in providing a reliable estimate of the natural vitamin E content in IU equivalents due to the inclusion of β-, γ- and δ-tocopherols.

In most cases, natural-derived vitamin E is esterified to acetate, forming the more stable dl-α-tocopheryl acetate ester, which has slightly lower biological activity than d-α-tocopherol. The richest sources are vegetable oils, cereal products containing these oils, eggs, liver, legumes, and green plants, especially leaves and buds. Tender grass contains around 200 mg/kg.

It is abundant in whole cereal grains (10–40 mg/kg), particularly in germ, and thus in by-products containing the germ (McDowell, 2000a; Traber, 2013). Rice bran, wheat germ, and some by-products of corn usually have larger quantities (50–70 mg/kg), although these are very variable depending on the technological treatment applied. Feed table averages are often of little value in predicting the individual content of feedstuffs or the bioavailability of vitamins. Barley (35–40 mg/kg) and oats (20–25 mg/kg) are the cereals that contain the most significant quantity. There is wide variation in the vitamin content of feeds, with many feeds having a three- to ten-fold range in reported α-tocopherol values. The vitamin E content of 42 varieties of corn varied from 11.1 to 36.4 IU per kg, a 3.3-fold difference.

Legumes generally have a moderate α-tocopherol content (around 10 mg/kg). Oleaginous feeds have very variable values depending on whether or not the oil has been extracted and the extraction procedure itself. For example, the α-tocopherol content of whole soy seed is around 50 mg/kg. The cake obtained by mechanical extraction contains approximately 7–10 mg/kg, and the cake obtained from solvent extraction has a value of around 3 mg/kg. In general, products of animal origin have insufficient quantities because, in live animals, the concentration rarely exceeds 2–4 mg/kg of tissue. The processing methods are usually very aggressive to tocopherols.

Naturally occurring vitamin E activity of feedstuffs cannot be accurately estimated from earlier published vitamin E or tocopherol values. α-tocopherol is exceptionally high in wheat germ oil and sunflower oil. Corn and soybean oil contain predominantly γ-tocopherol and some tocotrienols (McDowell, 2000a; Traber, 2013). Cottonseed oil contains both α- and γ-tocopherols in equal proportions. In practice, supplements are added in the more stable form of dl-α-tocopherol acetate.

The stability of all naturally occurring tocopherols is poor. Substantial losses (up to 90%) of vitamin E activity occur in feedstuffs in a few days or weeks when processed (drying, dehydration) and stored and in manufacturing (milling) and storage of finished feeds (Gadient, 1986; McDowell et al., 1996). For this reason, the vitamin E content of products like dried alfalfa can vary considerably depending on the production process (from 30 mg/kg or even less up to a value of around 180 mg/kg). Vitamin E sources in these ingredients are unstable under conditions that promote oxidation of feedstuffs – heat, oxygen, moisture, oxidizing fats, and trace minerals. Vegetable oils that are usually excellent sources of vitamin E can be deficient in vitamin E if oxidation has been promoted. Oxidized oil has little or no vitamin E, destroying the vitamin E in other feed ingredients and depleting animal tissue stores of vitamin E. The longer that mowed forages are exposed to sunlight (i.e., hay vs. wilted silage), the lower the concentration of α-tocopherol becomes. The concentration of vitamin E in feedstuffs is highly variable: coefficients of variation often were >50% for fresh and stored forages. Fresh green forages contain substantial amounts of alfa tocopherol (80 to 200 IU/kg), but vitamin E concentration in hay and silage are 20 to 80% lower (Weiss, 1998).

Oxidation of vitamin E increases after grinding, mixing with minerals, adding fat, and pelleting for balanced feed. When feeds are pelleted, the destruction of vitamins E and A may occur if the diet does not contain sufficient antioxidants to prevent accelerated oxidation under moisture and high-temperature conditions.

Iron salts (i.e., ferric chloride) can destroy vitamin E. They concluded that the oxidation rate of natural tocopherols is increased in diets containing increased levels of copper, iron, zinc, or manganese. The authors also indicated that corn-soybean meal diets containing high levels of copper might require α-tocopheryl acetate to maintain recommended vitamin E diets during storage, especially when unsaturated fat is added.

Artificial drying of corn results in a much lower vitamin E content. Studies testing vitamin E stability reported that artificial corn drying for 40 minutes at 87°C produced an average 10% loss of α-tocopherol and 12% loss of other tocopherols (Adams, 1973; Adams et al., 1975). When corn was dried for 54 minutes at 93°C, the α-tocopherol loss averaged 41%. Young et al. (1975) reported a concentration of 9.3 or 20 mg α-tocopherol per kg of artificially dried corn versus undried, respectively. The damage is not due to moisture alone but to the combined propionic acid/moisture effect.

Further decomposition of α-tocopherol occurs over an extended time until the grain eventually has α-tocopherol levels of less than 1 mg per kg, commonly found in propionic acid-treated barley. In alfalfa stored at 33°C for 12 weeks, 54–73% of vitamin E losses have been observed, and 5–33% losses have been obtained with commercial dehydration of alfalfa. The damage is not due to moisture alone but to the combined propionic acid/moisture effect (McMurray et al., 1980).

Vitamin E status is reduced in cows fed stored forages for extended periods, while pasture improves vitamin E status (Schingoethe et al., 1982; Lynch, 1983; Beeckman et al., 2010). A more available form of vitamin E is present in pastures and green forages, containing ample quantities of α-tocopherol versus the less bioavailable forms in grains (McDowell, 2004). Serum vitamin E levels are higher in summer and fall than in the winter and spring seasons (Miller *et al.*, 1995), which likely reflects the vitamin E level of forages consumed in the months before sampling. Besides seasonal effects, herd and time since parturition affected serum vitamin E and selenium concentrations (Miller *et al.*, 1995).

There can be a 5-fold seasonal variation in the α-tocopherol content of cow's milk. Colostrum is the primary source of vitamin E for the neonate (Table 4.1), whose tissue vitamin E levels at birth are low (Van Saun *et al.*, 1989; Njeru *et al.*, 1994a; Hidiroglou *et al.*, 1995). Colostrum from dairy cows has been reported to have a mean value of 1.9 µg α-tocopherol per gram, declining to 0.3 µg/g at 30 days postpartum (Hidiroglou, 1999). In this study, milk tocopherol was increased from 0.3 µg/g to 1.6 µg/g 12 hours after an intraperitoneal injection of dl-α-tocopheryl acetate. Four experiments conducted at Ohio State University (Weiss *et al.*, 1990b, 1992, 1994, 1997) reported higher overall values for colostral vitamin E. The mean α-tocopherol concentration in colostrum from unsupplemented cows was 4.7 µg/g with a range between 2.92 and 5.63 µg/g (Table 4.1). In contrast, colostrum from vitamin E-supplemented cows (fed 900 to 1,000 IU daily during the dry period) averaged 6.7 µg/g α-tocopherol. In one study, cows were injected twice with 3,000 IU supplemental vitamin E at 5 and 10 days prepartum. Injectable vitamin E also elevated colostral vitamin E to 8.9 µg/g in cows not fed supplemental vitamin E and to 11.6 µg/g in cows fed 1,000 IU supplemental vitamin E. Using a colostrum with a vitamin E content of 6.7 µg/g and an intake of 3.63 kg colostrum per calf per day, newborn calves would receive approximately 24 mg (24 IU) α-tocopherol per day while fed colostrum. Most commercial milk replacers supply a minimum of 40 IU of vitamin E per kg of milk powder. Higher levels have been shown to impact health benefits to calves, as will be discussed in later sections.

Green forage and good quality leaf meals, such as alfalfa meal, are good sources. The concentration of tocopherols per unit of DM in fresh herbage is 5 to 10 times as great as that in most cereals or their by-products (Hardy and Frape, 1983). Cattle grazed on green-lush pastures commonly had 4 to 6 µg α-tocopherol per g muscle compared with 1– 2 µg α-tocopherol per gram of muscle for standard grain-fed feedlot cattle (Yang *et al.*, 2002a). It was reported that variability in forage vitamin E content is so significant between and within farms that ongoing vitamin E analysis of forages and feeds must be conducted to ensure proper vitamin E fortification levels. These authors conclude that previously published forage vitamin E concentrations are unsuitable for feed formulation.

Preservation of grain by ensiling causes an almost complete loss of vitamin E activity. Corn stores as acid-treated (propionic or acetic-propionic mixture) high-moisture corn contains approximately 1 mg per kg of DM α-tocopherol, while artificially dried corn contains approximately 5.7 mg per kg of α-tocopherol. Destruction of tocopherol under these conditions is apparently due to the combination of moisture and acid (McMurray *et al.*, 1980). Tocopherol concentration of acid-treated, high-moisture grain continues to decline during storage to levels less than 1 mg/kg DM.

Drying or processing of forages can reduce tocopherol content. For example, in one study, 80% of the vitamin E was lost in haymaking (McDowell, 1985). Ensiled or rapidly dehydrated forages retain a more significant proportion of tocopherol content. Vitamin E content in forage is affected by the stage of maturity at harvest and by drying time. Frost dramatically reduced α-tocopherol and β-carotene concentrations in 4 tropical grasses (Arizmendi-Maldonado *et al.*, 2003). Losses during field drying can amount to as much as 60% within 4 days. Storage losses can reach 50% in one month. Vitamin E losses of 54–73% have been observed in alfalfa stored at 33°C for 12 weeks, and 5–33% losses have been obtained within commercial dehydration of alfalfa.

Commercial forms

Vitamin E is usually incorporated into feeds as all-rac or dl-α-tocopherol acetate (Chen *et al.*, 2019). Other vitamin E esters, like propionate or succinate, are produced, but the acetate form provides the best bioavailability. All-*rac*-α-tocopheryl acetate is manufactured by condensing trimethyl hydroquinone and isophytol and conducting ultra-vacuum molecular distillation, producing a highly purified form of α-tocopherol. This material may then be acetylated. As previously stated, all-*rac*-α-tocopherol is a mixture of α-tocopheryl acetate's 8 stereoisomers (4 enantiomeric pairs). The enantiomeric pairs, racemates, are in equimolar amounts (Cohen *et al.*, 1981). This finding indicates that the manufacturing processes lead to all-*rac*-α-tocopheryl acetate with similar proportions to all 8 stereoisomers (Weiser and Vecchi, 1982).

Vitamin E acetate product form, primarily used in animal feeding, is an adsorbate that provides good storage stability and physical treatments applied in feed manufacturing, like pelleting or extrusion with temperature and steam. Vitamin E acetate is also available in the spray-dried, water-soluble form for application in drinking water or milk replacers. The spray-dried formulation is also indicated when stability may be critical, like aggressive premixes with very high pH or canned pet food.

Commercially, not truly "natural" tocopherol products are available since the d-form, or RRR-form of α-tocopherol commercial products, are obtained from the original raw material (e.g., soybean oil) only after several chemical processing steps. Hence, it should be referred to as "natural-derived" and not "natural." In addition, the international unit (IU) is the standard of vitamin E activity: consequently, it is the same regardless of the source or the manufacturing process.

However, some studies in several species comparing the naturally derived RRR to the synthetic all-*rac*-α-tocopheryl acetate have shown the former to be more effective in elevating plasma and tissue concentrations when administered on an equal IU basis (Jensen *et al.*, 2006). Research in humans, poultry, sheep, pigs, guinea pigs, fish, and horses, in which the elevation of plasma concentrations was measured, indicated that the biopotency of RRR-α-tocopherol compared to all-*rac*-α-tocopherol can vary from the "official" figure of 1.36:1 up to closer to 2:1 (Traber, 2013), with differences among species. Considering the 1.36:1 ratio, 1 mg of all-*rac*-α-tocopheryl acetate can be replaced by 0.74 mg RRR-α-tocopheryl acetate. In Figure 4.22, the vitamin E activity of different forms is reported relative to DL-α-tocopheryl acetate or all-*rac*-tocopheryl acetate set at 1. In nutritional supplements, the α-tocopheryl succinate and α-tocopheryl acetate are the primary esterified forms of vitamin E. The esterified form of vitamin E is more stable, with a monthly loss of less than 1%. When it is subjected to extrusion, losses increase to 6% per month (Coelho, 1991).

However, some studies in several species, including cattle and sheep, show the naturally derived d-α-tocopheryl acetate, compared to the synthetic dl-α-tocopheryl acetate, is more effective in elevating milk, colostrum, plasma, and α-tocopherol concentrations when administered on an equal IU basis. Cattle and sheep discriminate between RRR and all-rac vitamin E with a preference for RRR-α-tocopheryl acetate. Thus, the official bioequivalence ratio of 1.36:1 RRR-α-tocopheryl acetate to all-*rac*-α-tocopheryl acetate is underestimated (Hidiroglou and McDowell, 1987; Hidiroglou *et al.*, 1988a, b; Meglia *et al.*, 2006; Waller *et al.*, 2007; Dersjant *et al.*, 2009; Weiss *et al.*, 2009).

Feeding a higher dietary level of dl-α-tocopheryl acetate could circumvent the lower bioavailability of the dl-form. It is not just naturally derived versus synthetic that is important for vitamin E biopotency, but also the ester and carrier used. In sheep, Hidiroglou and Singh (1991) reported that with equivalent IU dosage, the natural form of d-α-tocopheryl succinate had only one-third the biopotency of the synthetic dl-α-tocopheryl acetate, indicating that the

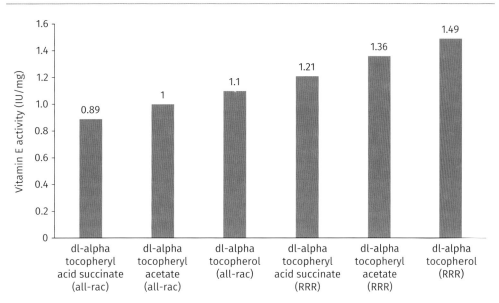

Figure 4.22 Vitamin E Activity of different chemical forms (IU/mg) relative to dl-α-tocopheryl acetate or all-*rac*-tocopheryl acetate set at 1 (source: United States Pharmacopeia, 1980)

ester succinate has less value than the acetate. Hidiroglou *et al.* (1992) also found acetate to be a better form of vitamin E than succinate.

As indicated previously, the acetate forms of α-tocopherol are commercially available from 2 primary sources: (1) D-α-tocopherol vegetable oil refining by-products, molecular distillation to obtain the a-form, and then acetylation to form the acetate ester; and (2) DL-α-tocopheryl acetate is made by complete chemical synthesis, producing a racemic mixture of equal proportions of 8 stereoisomers. Feeding a higher dietary level of dl-α-tocopheryl acetate could circumvent its lower bioavailability. The requirements of an animal and the level in the feed can be found expressed in IU of vitamin E (1 IU is equivalent to 1 mg dl-α-tocopherol acetate) or are expressed in mg of α-tocopherol equivalents (α-TE), which corresponds to the activity of d-α-tocopherol, the most active form (1 mg α-TE = 1 mg d-α-tocopherol =1.49 mg dl-α-tocopherol acetate).

Huang *et al.* (1995) evaluated the effectiveness of individual tocopherols and mixtures of these tocopherols in inhibiting the formation and decomposition of hydroperoxides in bulk corn oil, which had been stripped of natural tocopherols. Based on hydroperoxide formation, the concentrations required for maximum antioxidant activity of 1:1 mixture of α- and γ-tocopherol or natural soybean tocopherol mixtures (α:γ:β=13:64:21) were 250 and 500 ppm, respectively.

Hidiroglou *et al.* (1997b) compared the effects of feeding 1,000 IU of vitamin E activity from either dl- or d-α-tocopheryl acetate to dairy cows 8 weeks before calving through 8 weeks postpartum. Although plasma and red blood cell α-tocopherol concentrations of plasma and red blood cells were elevated by both sources, the dl-form resulted in higher values than the d-form. However, tocopherol concentrations of neutrophils and the production of both superoxide anion and hydrogen peroxide by blood neutrophils were not significantly different between the 2 sources, suggesting similar bioactivity of the 2 sources for neutrophil function.

Eicher *et al.* (1997) compared single oral doses of either d- or dl-α tocopherol in dairy calves and found higher vitamin E concentrations in plasma and the kidney with the d-isomer, while levels in red blood cells, spleen, liver, adipose tissue, muscle, gut, and heart were not significantly different between the 2 vitamin E sources.

The bioavailability of 3 physical forms of dl-(all-*rac*)-α-tocopheryl acetate was compared in dairy cows (Baldi *et al.*, 1997). The forms compared were adsorbate on silica, microencapsulated in stearic and palmitic acid, and vitamin E oil. Italian Friesian dairy cows were fitted with rumen cannulas. They fed a balanced lactation ration consisting of 62% forage (corn silage, alfalfa, and grass hays) and 38% grain (corn, barley, and soybean meal). Cows were administered 5,000 IU dl-α-tocopheryl acetate gelatin capsules in a 4×4 Latin Square experiment. An intraperitoneal injection of 5,000 IU vitamin E was used to compare to the intraruminal route. Overall, the kinetics of vitamin E absorption and decay were similar to published studies. Vitamin E adsorbate and microcapsules had a long half-life in plasma compared to vitamin E oil. Bioavailability tended to be higher for the adsorbate and microencapsulated forms of vitamin E.

Microencapsulation has emerged as an option to protect vitamin E. It allows its incorporation and controlled delivery into functional products for the food, feed, cosmetic, and pharmaceutical industries. This procedure can be performed using different techniques and materials, which should be selected according to the delivery system's final purpose (Ribeiro *et al.*, 2021).

Metabolism

In ruminants, there is little or no pre-intestinal absorption of dietary tocopherol. Rumen microbial destruction of tocopherol has been reported (McMurray and Rice, 1982; Weiss, 1998). An early report from Alderson *et al.* (1971) indicated ruminal degradation of a significant proportion of vitamin E, and degradability was greater the more concentrated the ration contained. However, the most recent studies using the stabilized form of vitamin E (dl-α-tocopheryl acetate) have reported little, if any, degradation of vitamin E in the rumen (Leedle *et al.*, 1993; Weiss *et al.*, 1995; Weiss, 1998). Hymøller and Jensen (2010b) showed no degradation of dl-α-tocopheryl acetate in the rumen using high-producing dairy cows. The vitamin E was added to the rumen contents through a rumen fistula and later was found at a constant level, indicating no degradation in the rumen. The discrepancy in results was attributed to the incomplete extraction of vitamin E from the digestive content in the methodology used by Alderson *et al.* (1971). Furthermore, as happens with vitamin A, the efficiency of α-tocopherol absorption depends on the diet's quantity and type of fat (Debier and Larondelle, 2005; Debier *et al.*, 2005).

In most species, including ruminants, vitamin E absorption is proportional to the animal's vitamin E status and requirement (Scherf *et al.*, 1996; Traber and Sies, 1996; Hidiroglou *et al.*, 1992). Vitamin E absorption ranges from 50 to 75% of intake in deficient animals, from 20 to 30% in animals with adequate vitamin E status, and from 1 to 5% in animals fed large excesses of vitamin E. However, this may not always be the case. Hidiroglou *et al.* (1988b) reported no correlation between vitamin E status and tocopherol absorption. Factors such as the dose, the form of presentation (physical and chemical), and the method of administration will affect its availability.

Absorption and transport

Early researchers investigated the effect of dietary fat on the intestinal absorption of tocopherol (Weiss *et al.*, 1994; Brigelius-Flohé, 2021). Various studies suggest that vitamin E is absorbed constantly when increasing doses are applied. Part of the vitamin E that is absorbed *de novo* can at least partially replace the vitamin E present in the circulating lipoproteins

(Baldi, 2005), which is an additional limiting factor if the plasma concentration of the vitamin is the parameter measured to evaluate the status of the animal (Bramley *et al.*, 2000; Ghaffari *et al.*, 2019). Furthermore, intestinal absorption is probably limited when the transporting capacity is reached (Weiss and Wyatt, 2003).

Vitamin E absorption is related to fat digestion and is facilitated by bile (liver function) and pancreatic lipase (Sitrin *et al.*, 1987). Jensen *et al.* (1997) found that the ileal digestibility of tocopherols varies based on the dietary fat source. The efficiency of digestion and absorption of vitamin E varies with dietary inclusion level. At 10 IU per kg, there is about 98% uptake of vitamin E, while at 100 and 1,000 IU per kg, efficiency declines to 80 and 70%, respectively. Vitamin E absorption can be impaired by various disorders associated with fat malabsorption (Han, 1998). A deficiency or an excess of dietary zinc may impair the absorption of vitamin E (Machlin, 1991; McDowell *et al.*, 1996; Campbell and Miller, 1998).

Tocopheryl acetate, the naturally occurring tocopherol form, is almost wholly hydrolyzed before absorption by duodenal pancreatic esterase, the enzyme that releases free fatty acids from dietary triacyl glycerides (Gallo-Torres, 1980a; Hidiroglou *et al.*, 1995). Tocopherol absorption occurs predominantly in the median portion of the small intestine through the portal vein to the liver. The ester bond, which increases stability, is hydrolyzed, and the resulting alcohol form is absorbed in the formation of bile salt micelles and lipids from the ration. Unlike vitamin A, tocopherol is not re-esterified during absorption.

Vitamin E is thus passively transferred into the micelle and absorbed through the brush border cells. The enterocytes of the upper and middle third of the small intestine absorb these micelles and transport them by the portomicrons and lipoproteins via lymph to the general circulation. Like all fat-soluble vitamins, carotenoids, and other fat-soluble dietary components, vitamin E is incorporated into chylomicrons. In healthy conditions, the efficiency of vitamin E absorption is variable from 35 to 50%, lower than that of vitamin A. In studies carried out with rats, Gallo-Torres (1980b) found that absorption of α-tocopherol and its esters, when ingested orally, was 20–40%.

As the dietary vitamin E level increases, the total amount of vitamin E absorbed will increase, but the relative amount absorbed will decline. Of the natural vitamin E compounds, approximately 32% of the α-, 18% of the β-, 30% of the γ-, and <2% of the δ-tocopherol forms are absorbed. Approximately 20 to 30% of orally ingested vitamin E is absorbed (Traber and Sies, 1996; Debier and Larondelle, 2005; Rigotti, 2007; Traber, 2013). Any ester form, *i.e.*, tocopheryl acetate, succinate, or propionate, to be absorbed into the body is converted to the alcohol form, and an α-tocopherol transfer protein has been identified (Traber, 2006, 2013).

The simultaneous digestion and absorption of dietary fats enhance the absorption of vitamin E. Most vitamin E is absorbed as alcohol, whether presented as free alcohol or as esters. Esters are hydrolyzed mainly in the intestinal wall, and the free alcohol enters the intestinal lacteals and is transported via the lymph to the general circulation. An α-tocopherol transfer protein has been identified (Traber, 2006, 2013).

Mammals and birds appear to prefer tocopherol versus other tocols. Rates and amounts of absorption of the various tocopherols and tocotrienols are in the same general order of magnitude as their biological potencies. α-tocopherol is absorbed best, with γ-tocopherol absorption slightly less than α-forms but with a more rapid excretion. Generally, the most vitamin E activity within plasma and other animal tissues is α-tocopherol (Jiang *et al.*, 2001; Hidiroglou *et al.*, 2003). The mechanisms for the uptake of vitamin E absorption into enterocytes are not well understood. Reboul and Borel (2011) believe that nonvitamin E-specific transporters like cholesterol and lipid transporters should be involved (Rigotti, 2007).

No plasma-specific vitamin E transport proteins have been described. Vitamin E in plasma is attached mainly to lipoproteins in the globulin fraction within cells and occurs mainly in mitochondria and microsomes. The liver takes the vitamin and releases LDL and VLDL (Rigotti, 2007; Traber, 2013).

Plasma vitamin E concentrations depend on α-tocopherol secretion from the liver (Kaempf-Rotzoli *et al.*, 2003). Additionally, rather than returning from the periphery, the newly absorbed vitamin E appears preferentially secreted into the plasma from the liver (Traber *et al.* 1998). Thus, the liver, not the intestine, discriminates between tocopherols (Traber, 2013). In contrast to α-tocopherol, the 7 other vitamers are not recognized by the α-tocopherol transfer protein (α-TTP) in the liver.

After hepatic uptake, the α-tocopherol form of vitamin E is preferentially resecreted into the circulation. The α-TTP is a critical regulator of vitamin E status that stimulates the movement of vitamin E between membrane vesicles *in vitro* and facilitates the secretion of tocopherol from hepatocytes. Recent studies have shown that the liver has a critical role in the bio discrimination of stereoisomers because of the presence of α-TTP, which preferentially transfers α-tocopherol, compared with other dietary vitamin E forms (Panagabko *et al.*, 2002). This protein preferentially selects RRR and 2R α-Toc for secretion into plasma (Leonard *et al.*, 2002). Some authors suggested that the metabolism of 2S stereoisomers in the liver may be faster than that of 2R stereoisomers; thereby, the reduced presence of 2S stereoisomers in the liver and other tissues could be caused by faster metabolism rather than the lower affinity of the α-TTC (Kiyose *et al.*, 1995; Kaneko *et al.*, 2000).

Specific receptors explain tissue distribution in tissues for lipoprotein carriers, passive diffusion from membrane lipoproteins to tissues, or lipoprotein lipase acting as a carrier protein (Parker, 1989; Rigotti, 2007). It has also been established that there is a negative interaction between vitamin E and vitamin A or β-carotene, as they interfere with each other in their absorption and deposition processes (Preś *et al.*, 1993 studied in sows; Schelling *et al.*, 1995; Goncalves *et al.*, 2015).

As the placental transfer of tocopherol from the dam to the fetus is minimal, milk's importance for enhancing the newborn's vitamin E status is greater (Debier and Larondelle, 2005). In ruminants, vitamin E does not cross the placenta in any appreciable amounts, with levels in the fetus generally lower than in the dam (Malone, 1975), making the neonate highly susceptible to vitamin E deficiency (Hidiroglou *et al.*, 1969; Van Saun *et al.*, 1989). Placental vitamin E transfer may decrease as gestation proceeds, possibly a dilution effect resulting from rapid fetal growth or a decrease in maternal vitamin E supply. Neonatal calves, lambs, and kids depend on colostrum as a source of vitamin E. Less than 1% of the dam's tocopherol intake is secreted in milk (Millar *et al.*, 1973). However, vitamin E concentration in colostrum is high (Table 4.1) and is directly affected by maternal vitamin E intake during gestation (Whitting and Loosli, 1948; Njeru *et al.*, 1994a,b; Quigley and Drewry, 1998).

Hidiroglou *et al.* (2003) reported a substantial transfer of 2H-labeled α-tocopherol across the placenta and through the MG in guinea pigs. The relative bioavailability (d3:d6) across fetal and neonatal tissues was, on average, 1.81:1.00, with a range from 1.62:1.00 to 2.01:1.00. Maternal tissues had a mean ratio of 1.77:1.00. A higher relative bioavailability ($P ≤ 0.05$) was observed with natural than synthetic α-tocopherol, as shown by a higher d3:d6 ratio in all tissues examined. Vitamin E was highest in colostrum on day 2 and then declined on the fifth day. Results from this experiment question the accepted biological potencies of natural:synthetic α-tocopheryl acetate of 1.36:1.00.

Storage and excretion

Vitamin E is stored throughout all body tissues, with the highest storage in the fat and liver (Traber and Head, 2021; Traber, 2013; Brigelius-Flohé, 2021). However, vitamin E is not indeed accumulated in the liver as it contains only a tiny fraction of total body stores, in contrast to vitamin A, for which about 95% of the body reserves are in the liver. Faustman *et al.* (1989) and Sales and Koukolová (2011) indicated that adipose tissue contained the highest concentrations of vitamin E, followed by liver, cardiac muscle, and *M. longissimus* in decreasing order. The liver preferentially secretes α-tocopherol into plasma under the control of haptic-α-transfer protein (Traber, 2006). Small amounts of vitamin E will persist tenaciously in the body during deficiency, particularly in neural tissues (Bjørneboe *et al.*, 1990).

Subcellular fractions (endoplasmic reticulum or the nuclear membrane) from differ-ent tissues vary considerably in their tocopherol content, with the highest levels found in membranous organelles, such as microsomes and mitochondria, which contain highly active oxidation-reduction systems (McCay *et al.*, 1981; Rigotti, 2007; Traber, 2013; Brigelius-Flohé, 2021). This indicates a specific cellular role of tocopherol, concentrated in sites of free-radical generation, the mitochondria, and microsomes of liver cells. Nevertheless, this distribution is not homogeneous in all animal cells.

Like erythrocytes, immune cells (neutrophils, macrophages, and lymphocytes) contain very high concentrations of vitamin E. Red blood cells contain significant amounts of vitamin E, which protects the erythrocytes from hemolysis. Marked differences have been observed in α-tocopherol deposition depending on the oxidative capacity of muscle fiber. Oxidative mus-cles present a greater concentration of vitamin E associated with a greater phospholipid con-tent, increased vascular development, and more significant activity of mitochondrial enzymes. Small amounts of vitamin E will persist tenaciously in the body for a long time. However, stores are exhausted rapidly by PUFA in the tissues. The rate of disappearance is proportional to the intake of PUFA. Other sources of oxidative stress, including disease and inflammation, deplete vitamin E (Celi, 2011).

The major excretion routes of absorbed vitamin E are feces and bile, in which tocopherol appears mainly in the free form (McDowell, 2000a). The tocopherols that pass through the intestinal tract occur from incomplete absorption, secretion from the mucosal cells into the lumen, desquamation of intestinal epithelial cells, and biliary excretion. Of the absorbed toco-pherols, some are converted to quinone and excreted. The biliary route can excrete tocopheryl acetates and tocopherol, but the amount is relatively small (~2.4%). Several oxidation products of vitamin E are also excreted in bile and urine, with tocopheryl quinone being the primary catabolite (Torquato *et al.*, 2019; Traber, 2013).

Biochemical functions

Vitamin E is essential for the integrity and optimum function of the reproductive, circulatory, nervous, immune, and muscular systems (Figure 4.23) (Hoekstra, 1975; Sheffy and Schultz, 1979; Bendich, 1987; Lehr *et al.*, 1998; McDowell, 2000a; Traber, 2013; Brigelius-Flohé, 2021). It is well established that some functions of vitamin E can be fulfilled in part or entirely by selenium or other antioxidants. The sulfur-bearing amino acids cystine and methionine affect the vitamin E requirement.

Vitamin C (ascorbic acid) has been shown to spare vitamin E in tissues by regenerating α-tocopherol from its oxidation products. It is one of the vitamins to which the greatest inves-tigative efforts have been dedicated to discovering its mechanism of action and requirements in all species, including ruminants (Traber, 2013; Hemingway, 2003; Kay *et al.*, 2005; Haga *et al.*, 2021).

Vitamin E:

- is the primary antioxidant in blood and, on a cellular level, it maintains the integrity of the cellular and vascular membranes
- it acts as a detoxifier and takes part in many other biochemical reactions
- is essential for the fertility
- it promotes the activity of immune system cells
- it can alleviate stress and increase immunocompetence (Jensen *et al.*, 1988 swine data; Baldi, 2005; Bouwstra *et al.*, 2010)
- is also involved in the prevention of cardiovascular and carcinogenic diseases.

Classical α-tocopherol functions of vitamin E
Antioxidant

Numerous studies have established the relationship between vitamin E consumed and the prevention of oxidation or oxidative distress in biological systems (Miller *et al.*, 1993; McDowell *et al.*, 1996; Azzi *et al.*, 2000; Singh *et al.*, 2005; Celi, 2011; Niki, 2016; Haga *et al.*, 2021; Brigelius-Flohé, 2021; Xiao *et al.*, 2021; Traber and Kamal-Eldin, 2022). Under physiological conditions, cells maintain redox homeostasis by producing oxidants, i.e., reactive oxygen species (ROS) and other free radicals, and their elimination by an antioxidant system. We have oxidative distress when the balance favors oxidants (Dunnett, 2003; Putman, 2023).

Free-radical reactions are ubiquitous in biological systems and are associated with energy metabolism, biosynthetic reactions, natural defense mechanisms, detoxification, and intra- and intercellular signaling pathways. Redox homeostasis is essential for aerobic organisms (bacteria, plants, animals, and humans). Highly reactive oxygen species such as the superoxide anion radical (O_2^-), hydroxyl radical (OH), hydrogen peroxide (H_2O_2), and singlet oxygen (O_2^-) are continuously produced in the course of normal aerobic cellular metabolism. Also, phagocytic granulocytes undergo respiratory bursts to produce oxygen radicals to destroy intracellular pathogens. However, these oxidative products can, in turn, damage healthy cells if they are

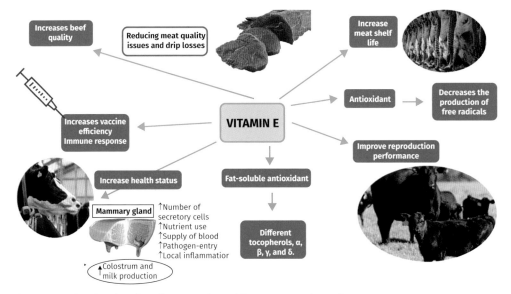

Figure 4.23 Vitamin E functions (Source: adapted from Haga *et al.*, 2021)

not eliminated (Celi, 2011) Antioxidants stabilize these highly reactive free radicals, thereby maintaining cells' structural and functional integrity (Chew, 1995; Singh *et al.*, 2005; Brigelius-Flohé, 2021). These processes are essential for resolution of all diseases (Bendich, 1993), development of immunity (Jin *et al.*, 2014; Doğan *et al.*, 2021), and mastitis in cows (Abd Ellah, 2013)

Vitamin E is a quenching agent for free-radical molecules with single, highly reactive electrons in their outer shells. Free radicals attract a hydrogen atom, along with its electron, away from the chain structure, satisfying the electron needs of the original free radical but leaving the PUFA short one electron. Thus, a fatty acid-free radical is formed that joins with molecular oxygen to form a peroxyl radical that steals a hydrogen-electron unit from yet another PUFA. This reaction can continue in a chain, destroying thousands of PUFA molecules (Gardner, 1989). Free radicals can highly damage biological systems (McCay, 1985).

Vitamin E has a crucial role within the cellular defense system in the face of oxidation at both intracellular and extracellular levels. α-tocopherol is integrated within the cellular membrane and protects lipids from oxidation, preventing them from being attacked by reactive oxygen and free radicals (Pascoe and Reed, 1989; Brigelius-Flohé, 2021). Tocopherols remove the peroxyl radical, donating a hydrogen atom and converting it to peroxide. Support for the antioxidant role of vitamin E *in vivo* also comes from observations that synthetic antioxidants can prevent or alleviate certain clinical signs of vitamin E deficiency diseases. Therefore, antioxidants are vital to humans' and animals' immune defense and health (Singh *et al.*, 2005).

Most vitamin E deficiency symptoms are related to disorders of the cellular membrane due to the oxidative degradation of PUFAs and phospholipids (Chow, 1979) and critical sulfhydryl groups (Schwarz, 1962; Brownlee *et al.*, 1977). The orientation of vitamin E within cell membranes appears to be essential to its functionality. Vitamin E interrupts free-radical damage at the initiation stage, thus preventing the chain reaction of cell damage. It has been demonstrated how the deposition of α-tocopherol in animal tissues increases in direct proportion to its supply in the diet and is accompanied by greater oxidative stability (Jensen *et al.*, 1997; Celi, 2011). On the other hand, it is known that susceptibility to oxidation increases as the number of double bonds of fatty acids increases (Gardner, 1989).

As the profile of fatty acids in the ration is reflected in the fatty acid composition of the different tissues of the animal, increasing the degree of unsaturation in the feed increases susceptibility to oxidation and reduces the quantity of α-tocopherol deposited in the tissues (Muggli, 1994). The type of fatty acid and tocopherol levels also vary between organs and can be modified by the diet. Hence, high levels of PUFA in the diet cause an increase in the susceptibility of tissues to lipid oxidation, increasing the requirements for vitamin E (Dutta-Roy *et al.*, 1994; Muggli, 1994). Vitamin E supplies become depleted when acting as an antioxidant, which explains the frequent observation that the presence of dietary unsaturated fats (susceptible to peroxidation) increases or precipitates a vitamin E deficiency. Consequently, vitamin E supplementation should increase parallel to the amount of unsaturated fatty acids and the degree of fat oxidation added to the feed (Luciano *et al.*, 2011; Traber, 2013).

Farm livestock requires 2.5–3.0 mg dl-α-tocopheryl acetate for each gram of PUFA in the diet. Using blended fats with an 18% PUFA, 5 mg of vitamin E should be added for every 1% blended fat. Requirements also depend on the presence or absence of other compounds intervening in the tissue oxidation defense system, such as Se. It should be borne in mind that depending on the feed ingredients and hence the content of tocopherols, carotenoids, and other antioxidants, there will be a variation in the oxidative state of the animal and, therefore, the requirements of antioxidants and specifically of vitamin E (Traber, 2013; Khan *et al.*, 2022). Interruption of fat peroxidation by tocopherol explains that dietary tocopherols protect or spare body supplies such oxidizable materials as vitamins A, C, and carotenes.

Relationship with selenium in tissue protection

Vitamin E and selenium (Se) share several molecular functions in regulating many genes encoding for proteins with potent antioxidant activity (Xiao *et al.*, 2021). Consequently, both have been included in the study of the selenogenome. Tissue breakdown occurs in most species receiving diets deficient in vitamin E and Se, mainly through peroxidation. Peroxides and hydroperoxides are highly destructive to tissue integrity and lead to disease development (Mohri *et al.*, 2005; Xiao *et al.*, 2021).

Se has been shown to act in aqueous cell media (cytosol and mitochondrial matrix) by destroying hydrogen peroxide and hydroperoxides via the enzyme glutathione peroxidase (GSH-Px), which is a cofactor (Miller *et al.*, 1995). This capacity prevents the oxidation of unsaturated lipid materials within cells, thus protecting fats within the cell membrane from breaking down. The various GSH-Px enzymes are characterized by different tissue specificities and are expressed from other genes. Different forms of GSH-Px perform their protective functions in concert, each providing antioxidant protection at various body sites.

Therefore, Se has a sparing effect on vitamin E and delays the onset of deficiency signs. Likewise, vitamin E and sulfur amino acids partially protect against or delay the onset of several forms of Se deficiency syndromes (Reffett *et al.*, 1988). Vitamin E in cellular and subcellular membranes appears to be the first line of defense against the peroxidation of vital phospholipids. Still, even with adequate vitamin E, some peroxides are formed. As part of the enzyme GSH-Px, Se is a second line of defense that destroys these peroxides before they can cause damage to membranes. Therefore, through different biochemical mechanisms, Se, vitamin E, and sulfur-containing amino acids can prevent some of the same nutritional diseases.

Membrane structure and prostaglandin synthesis

α-tocopherol may be involved in forming structural components of biological membranes, thus exerting a unique influence on the architecture of membrane phospholipids (Bourne *et al.*, 2007a; Xiao *et al.*, 2021). It is reported that α-tocopherol stimulated the incorporation of 14C from linoleic acid into arachidonic acid in fibroblast phospholipids. Also, it was found that α-tocopherol exerted a pronounced stimulatory influence on the formation of prostaglandins and thromboxanes from arachidonic acid, while a chemical antioxidant had no effect (Traber, 2013). Supplemental vitamin E has been reported to reverse the age-related decline in T-lymphocyte function by reducing prostaglandin production (Beharka *et al.*, 1997).

Meat quality

To improve oxidative stability and thus increase the shelf life of meat, antioxidants have been successfully added to animal feeds (Hidiroglou and Karpinski, 1987; Yang *et al.*, 2002a, b; Rather *et al.*, 2016). Different compounds such as carotenoids, vitamin E, vitamin C, and Se are known to have potent antioxidant effects on beef. Of them, α-tocopherol has demonstrated the highest biological efficiency in preventing lipid oxidation *in vivo* (Hill and Williams, 1995; Robbins *et al.*, 2003; Descalzo *et al.*, 2005; Descalzo and Sancho, 2008).

Myodystrophic tissue is common in cases of vitamin E-Se deficiency, with leakage of cellular compounds such as creatinine and various transaminase and dehydrogenase enzymes through affected membranes into plasma. The more active the cell (e.g., the cells of skeletal and involuntary smooth muscles), the greater the inflow of lipids for energy supply. The greater the risk of tissue damage if vitamin E is limited. Erythrocytes and capillary walls are also susceptible to damage in animals with marginal vitamin E status (Hidiroglou and Karpinski, 1987).

Certain deficiency signs of vitamin E (*i.e.*, muscular dystrophy) can be prevented by diet supplementation with other antioxidant nutrients, which helps validate the antioxidant role of tocopherols (Machlin, 1988; Traber, 2013). Chemical antioxidants are stored at shallow levels and thus are not as effective as tocopherol. To improve oxidative stability and thus increase the shelf life of meat, antioxidants have been successfully added to animal feeds. In the last few years, different compounds such as synthetic antioxidants such as ethoxyquin, carotenoids, vitamin C, Se, and plant extracts have been tested in various experiments to verify their potential antioxidant effect on beef quality (Kamal-Eldin and Appelqvist, 1996; Rather *et al.*, 2016; Salami *et al.*, 2016). Of them all, α-tocopherol demonstrated the highest biological efficiency in preventing lipid oxidation *in vivo* (Faustman and Cassens, 1989; Barouh *et. al.*, 2022). Ethoxyquin exhibits limited tissue storage and rapid clearance from the body and thus cannot replace tocopherol. Diets high in PUFA increase the vitamin E requirement.

Stress, immune response, and disease resistance

Vitamin E is perhaps the most studied nutrient related to the immune response (Meydani and Han, 2006). Evidence accumulated over the years and in many species indicates that vitamin E is an essential nutrient for the normal function of the immune system.

Considerable attention is being directed to vitamin E and Se's roles in protecting leukocytes and macrophages during phagocytosis, the mechanism whereby animals immunologically kill invading bacteria. Vitamin E and Se may help these cells survive the toxic products produced to kill ingested bacteria effectively (Badwey and Karnovsky, 1980). Macrophages and neutrophils from vitamin E-deficient animals have decreased phagocytic activity (Moriguchi and Kaneyasu, 2004).

Since vitamin E acts as a tissue antioxidant and aids in quenching free radicals produced in the body, any infection or other stress factor may exacerbate the depletion of the limited vitamin E stores in various tissues. The former 2 responses are generally used to determine a nutrient requirement.

During stress and disease, there is an increase in the production of glucocorticoids, epinephrine, eicosanoids, and phagocytic activity. Eicosanoid and corticoid synthesis and phagocytic respiratory bursts are prominent free-radical producers, challenging the animal's antioxidant systems. Duthie *et al.* (1987) proposed that stress-susceptibility syndrome may be associated with abnormal vitamin E metabolism.

Vitamin E also likely has an immunoenhancing effect by altering arachidonic acid metabolism and subsequent synthesis of prostaglandins, thromboxanes, and leukotrienes. Under increased stress conditions, levels of these compounds by endogenous synthesis or exogenous entry may adversely affect immune cell function (Hadden, 1987; Moriguchi and Kaneyasu, 2004). Thromboxane and interleukin II appear to exert a negative feedback effect on leukocyte function (Hadden, 1987). The protective effects of vitamin E on animal health may reduce glucocorticoids, which are known to be immunosuppressive (Golub and Gershwin, 1985).

Vitamin E and Se have stimulated humoral or cellular immune responses in ruminants. Vitamin E supplementation can enhance serum antibody synthesis, particularly IgG antibodies (Tengerdy, 1980). Increasing dietary vitamin E increases both antibody titers and phagocytosis of pathogens in calves (Cipriano *et al.*, 1982; Reddy *et al.*, 1985, 1987); lambs (Reffett *et al.*, 1988; Finch and Turner, 1989; Turner and Finch, 1990); and dairy cows (Politis *et al.*, 1995, 1996; Weiss *et al.*, 1997; Weiss, 1998). For example, the immune response was maximized in calves receiving 125 IU per day of vitamin E compared to calves receiving lower levels of dietary vitamin E (Reddy *et al.*, 1987). Stabel *et al.* (1992) reported that vitamin E increased immunoglobulin M (IgM) production by blood monocytes *in vitro* and increased interleukin-1 gene expression by monocytes isolated from vitamin E-supplemented steers. Vitamin E at high supplementation levels provides a robust immune response in livestock and enhances resistance to infectious diseases.

Garber *et al.* (1996) reported that mitogen-stimulated lymphocyte proliferation of dairy steers was maximized by feeding 1,000 IU of vitamin E daily compared to either lower or higher levels of supplementation. Vitamin E and selenium deficiency reduced *in vitro* lymphocyte proliferation in calves, while repletion restored the numbers and function of lymphocytes (Pollock *et al.*, 1994). Vitamin E and Se exerted specific and combined effects on immune cell function. Vitamin E affects cellular and humoral immune function; T-lymphocytes were increased (Ndiweni and Finch, 1995; Beharka *et al., 1997;* Meydani and Blumberg, 2020).

Vitamin E and Se supplementation in dairy cows reduced rates and duration of intramammary infections and incidence of clinical mastitis (Smith *et al.*, 1984, 1985, 1997; Batra *et al.*, 1992; Bouwstra *et al.*, 2010; Khan *et al.*, 2022).

Vitamin E and Se enhance host defenses against infections by improving phagocytic cell function. Both vitamin E and GSH-Px are antioxidants that protect phagocytic cells and surrounding tissues from oxidative attack by free radicals produced by the respiratory burst of neutrophils and macrophages during phagocytosis (Baboir, 1984; Baker and Cohen, 1983). Gyang *et al.* (1984) and Hogan *et al.* (1990, 1992) reported that dietary vitamin E supplementation increased the intracellular kill of *Staphylococcus aureus* and *Escherichia coli* by neutrophils.

Cows supplemented 4 weeks before calving through 8 weeks postpartum with 3,000 IU vitamin E per day, in the presence of adequate selenium (0.3 ppm), had increased neutrophil and macrophage function and reduced somatic cell count compared to controls (Politis *et al.*, 1995, 1996). Supplemental vitamin E was shown to specifically stimulate phagocytosis of *S. aureus* by bovine neutrophils (Ndiweni and Finch, 1995). Vitamin E and Se increased neutrophil chemotaxis and superoxide production in these studies.

High dietary vitamin E increased concentrations of α-tocopherol in blood neutrophils at parturition and cows with plasma concentrations of α-tocopherol <3.0 mg/ml at calving were 9.4 times more likely to have clinical mastitis during the first 7 days of lactation than were cows with plasma concentrations of α-tocopherol >3.0 mg/ml. Cows that received a dietary supplement with about 1,000 IU/day of vitamin E had 30% less clinical mastitis than did cows receiving a supplement of 100 IU/day of vitamin E. The reduction was 88% when cows were fed 4,000 IU/day of vitamin E during the last 14 days of the dry period (Weiss *et al.*, 1997).

Neutrophil function in dairy cattle is suppressed around the time of calving (Guidry *et al.*, 1976; Kehrli and Goff, 1989; Gilbert *et al.*, 1993a; Politis *et al.*, 2004), as are several other indices of immune function (Mallard *et al.*, 1998). High levels of vitamin E (3,000 IU per day) essentially prevented the suppression of blood neutrophil and macrophage function in dairy cows in the study by Politis *et al.* (1996). Gilbert *et al.* (1993b) found that impaired neutrophil function was associated with retained fetal membranes in dairy cows. This link is of interest in light of the studies showing that supplemental vitamin E during the dry period results in a decreased incidence of the retained placenta (Julien *et al.*, 1976a,b; Harrison *et al.*, 1984; Aréchiga *et al.*, 1994; Miller *et al.*, 1997; Erskine *et al.*, 1997; LeBlanc *et al.*, 2002).

The immune response in sheep has been improved with supplemental vitamin E. Vitamin E improved disease resistance in lambs challenged with *Chlamydia* (Stephens *et al.*, 1979). Reffett *et al.* (1988) reported that vitamin E and Se independently increased the immune response of lambs challenged with a viral pathogen. Myopathic lambs exhibit low lymphocyte responses when deficient in vitamin E and Se (Finch and Turner, 1989; Turner and Finch, 1990).

The poor lymphocyte responses of the lambs with nutritional myopathy were rapidly reversed by intramuscular administration of vitamin E–Se, with the prophylaxis most effective during the first 5 weeks of life (Finch and Turner, 1989). In a study of 1,300 lambings, supplementing 330 IU of vitamin E daily for 21 days before lambing significantly reduced lamb mortality for ewes lambing early in the season and increased the total weight of lambs weaned per ewe (Hatfield *et al.*, 2000). Late-lambing ewes did not show a significant response to vitamin E. Supplementing ewes for 28 days before and 28 days after lambing has been shown to significantly increase vitamin E concentration in colostrum in the serum of their nursing lambs (Njeru *et al.*, 1994a). Dairy ewes injected twice during the dry period with vitamin E and selenium (5 mg and 0.1 mg/kg BW) had significantly lower somatic cell counts, increased erythrocyte GSH-Px activity and enhanced neutrophil function compared to controls (Morgante *et al.*, 1999). Injection of 900 IU of vitamin E per week into ewes in late pregnancy increased lambs' survival and growth rate from birth through weaning (Ali *et al.*, 2004).

Vitamin E deficiency allows a usually benign virus to cause disease (Beck *et al.*, 1994). Antioxidants, including vitamin E, play a role in resistance to viral infection. In mice, enhanced virus virulence resulted in a myocardial injury that was prevented with adequate vitamin E. A selenium or vitamin E deficiency leads to a change in viral phenotype, such that a non-virulent strain of a virus becomes virulent, and a virulent strain becomes more virulent (Beck, 1997; 2007; Sheridan and Beck, 2008). Moriguchi and Muraga (2000) observed that vitamin E improved the immune system by enhancing host antiviral activity and the production of the antiviral cytokine interferon produced by activated T-cells.

Thus, host nutritional status should be considered a driving force for the emergence of new viral strains or newly pathogenic strains of known viruses.

The administration of LPS is a well-documented model for evaluating disease stress (Zebeli and Ametaj, 2009; Abaker *et al.*, 2017). The response to LPS can be attributed to events that include cytokine synthesis and release (Dinarello, 1996; Zebeli and Ametaj, 2009). Cytokines are released from activated macrophages in response to immunologic challenges and are primarily responsible for the subsequent metabolic effects (Gálvez *et al.*, 2022).

Reproduction

Early attempts to establish a beneficial role for vitamin E in ruminant reproduction were inconclusive (NRC, 2000) but currently, the effects of α-tocopherol in reproduction are well accepted (Brigelius-Flohé *et al.*, 2002; Brigelius-Flohé, 2021). In one experiment, 4 generations of male and female dairy cattle were fed low vitamin E diets (Gullickson, 1949). Although growth, reproduction, and milk production were average, several cattle died suddenly of apparent heart failure between 21 months and 5 years of age.

In the bull, supplemental vitamin E did not affect sperm or semen characteristics or fertility (Salisbury, 1944). However, large doses of vitamins A, D, E, and C have been reported to affect some characteristics of semen and sperm favorably (Kozicki *et al.*, 1981). Velásquez-Pereira *et al.* (1998) reported that feeding 4,000 IU per day of supplemental vitamin E to Holstein bulls reversed the adverse effects of feeding gossypol (14 mg free gossypol per day as cottonseed meal) on semen quality and reproductive performance. Supplemental vitamin E enhanced semen characteristics, plasma testosterone, and breeding performance of gossypol-fed bulls above that of the control group, which was not fed gossypol. This suggests a potential benefit of vitamin E for breeding bulls regardless of diet.

Laflamme and Hidiroglou (1991) reported that the pregnancy rate was improved (70 versus 33%) in beef heifers that had been fed supplemental vitamin E and Se starting from 8 months of age (weaning) and continuing for 6 months until breeding. In dairy cattle, supplementation with Se or both Se and vitamin E reduced the incidence of retained placenta in herds where the prevalence of retained placenta was high or when selenium or vitamin E were marginal in the diet (Hurley and Doane, 1989). Supplemental vitamin E–Se has also been reported to reduce metritis, cystic ovaries (Harrison *et al.*, 1984), and the time of uterine involution in cows with metritis (Harrison *et al.*, 1986).

Miller *et al.* (1997) summarized 7 years of experimental data (*n* = 602 cows) in which comparisons were made between cows fed either 200 or 1,000 IU of vitamin E per day for the last 42 days of the dry period. Statistical analysis revealed a highly significant effect of supplemental vitamin E in reducing the incidence of retained placenta (27.4% in controls versus 12.6% in vitamin E-supplemented; $P < 0.0001$). Cows fed 1,000 IU of supplemental vitamin E daily were 2.6 times less likely to develop retained placenta. In a trial with 126 cows fed 1,000 IU of supplemental vitamin E per day during the dry period, they significantly reduced the interval to first estrus (Miller *et al.*, 1997). Vitamin E increases plasma's fast-acting antioxidant capacity and may increase plasma estradiol by protecting the cytochrome P-450-dependent enzyme system required for estradiol synthesis (Miller *et al.*, 1993, 1997). These authors hypothesize that the ratio of corticosterone to estradiol in plasma indicates stress levels and predisposition toward reproductive disorders in dairy cattle.

Campbell and Miller (1998) fed 144 cows (64 primigravid heifers and 80 cows) either 0 or 1,000 IU of supplemental vitamin E per day in the presence or absence of excess iron and 800 mg added zinc for the last 42 days prepartum. Supplementation was discontinued after calving. Plasma vitamin E levels were low for all treatments (1.0–1.5 µg/ml), compared to levels considered minimal for periparturient cows (3.0–3.5 µg/ml), based on neutrophil function and udder health (Weiss, 1998). Despite the low levels of plasma vitamin E, cows supplemented with 1,000 IU vitamin E before calving significantly reduced days to first estrus, days to first breeding, and days open. Days open were reduced by 32% overall. The retained placenta was not affected by any treatment. Therefore, 1,000 IU of supplemental vitamin E fed for 42 days before calving had significant beneficial effects on reproduction after calving. In a research conducted in Ohio, the incidence of retained placenta was reduced from a mean of 51.2% in control cows to 8.8% in cows injected with a combination of selenium and vitamin E (Julien *et al.*, 1976b). Harrison *et al.* (1984) reported 17.5% retained placenta for control dairy cows, with no incidence for cows receiving both selenium and vitamin E.

Neither vitamin E nor selenium were as effective alone. From the same study, control versus Se administration reduced cystic ovaries (47 versus 19%) and incidence of metritis (84 versus 60%). Other research found no effect of a prepartum injection of selenium and vitamin E on the incidence of retained placenta (Gwazdauskas *et al.*, 1979; Schingoethe *et al.*, 1982; Kappel *et al.*, 1984; Hidiroglou *et al.*, 1988a). However, more recent studies have reported the positive effects of vitamin E or vitamin E + Se injection on dairy and beef cattle reproduction, especially under heat stress (LeBlanc *et al.*, 2002; Maldonado *et al.*, 2017).

Aréchiga *et al.* (1994), using 198 Holstein cows in Florida, found that a single injection of 50 mg selenium and 680 IU vitamin E at 21 days prepartum significantly reduced retained placenta (10.1 versus 3%) increased first service pregnancy rate (41 versus 25%), reduced services per conception and reduced days open (141 versus 121 days). Erskine *et al.* (1997) reported results of a trial with 420 Holstein cows, in which a single injection of approximately 4,000 IU vitamin E at 14 days prepartum significantly reduced retained placenta (6.4 versus 12.5%), metritis (3.9 versus 8.8%) and increased serum vitamin E up to 14 days after injection. Kim *et al.* (1997) compared cows injected 20 days before calving with a placebo, Se (40 mg), vitamin E (500 IU), or both Se and vitamin E. They reported significant reductions in retained placenta (13.3 versus 30%) and days to first service (59.5 versus 102.7) in cows injected with selenium and vitamin E.

Blood clotting
Vitamin E inhibits platelet aggregation (Steiner and Anastasi, 1976). It may play a role by inhibiting the peroxidation of arachidonic acid, which is required to form prostaglandins involved in platelet aggregation (Panganamala and Cornwell, 1982; Machlin, 1991; Traber, 2013). The antioxidant property of vitamin E also ensures erythrocyte stability and capillary blood vessel integrity maintenance.

Cellular respiration, electron transport, and deoxyribonucleic acid (DNA)
Vitamin E is involved in biological oxidation-reduction reactions (Traber, 2013). Vitamin E also appears to regulate the biosynthesis of DNA within cells. Vitamin E is essential in the cellular respiration of the heart and skeletal muscles (Olson, 1973). Vitamin E appears to enhance the activity of microsomal cytochrome P-450, which has multiple roles in detoxification and cell biosynthesis (Lehninger, 1982).

Relationship to toxic elements or substances
Both vitamin E and Se protect against the toxicity of various heavy metals (Whanger, 1981). Vitamin E is highly effective in reducing the toxicity of metals such as silver, arsenic, and lead and shows slight effects against cadmium and mercury toxicity. Vitamin E can be effective against other toxic substances (Al-Attar, 2011). This author reported that supplemental vitamin E partially prevented copper, lead, mercury, and cadmium toxicity. Based on the results of their study, Van Vleet and Ferrans (1992) suggested that increased amounts of Se and vitamin E might be needed to prevent the development of Se-vitamin E deficiency in animals fed rations containing large concentrations of several trace elements (silver, tellurium, cobalt, zinc, cadmium, or vanadium).

The cytochrome P450 system must detoxify mycotoxins, the activity of which appears related to vitamin E status. Adsorbents (bentonites, Ca aluminosilicates) used in research to alleviate symptoms of mycotoxicosis have been shown to reduce plasma vitamin E concentrations suggesting that vitamin E levels may need to be increased if these products are fed. Velásquez-Pereira et al. (1998) found that 4,000 IU of supplemental vitamin E per day significantly reduced bull sperm abnormalities caused by feeding 14 mg per day free gossypol occurring naturally in cottonseed meal. Likewise, Velásquez-Pereira et al. (1999) reported that feeding 4,000 IU vitamin E daily alleviated the harmful effects of gossypol on the growth and health of dairy calves and increased calf performance compared to the positive control ration.

Non-α-tocopherol functions of vitamin E
Although α-tocopherol has been the most widely studied form of vitamin E, other tocopherols and tocotrienols have been shown to have biological significance (Qureshi et al., 2001; Eder et al., 2002; McCormick and Parker, 2004; Schaffer et al., 2005; Nakagawa et al., 2007; Sun and Alkon, 2008; Freiser and Jiang, 2009; Traber, 2013; Comitato et al., 2017). The greater emphasis on α-tocopherol undoubtedly arises from observations that γ-tocopherol and δ-tocopherol are only 10 and 1% as effective as α-tocopherol in experimental animal models of vitamin E deficiency.

Research with tocotrienols and non-α tocopherols have been conducted with laboratory animals and in vitro studies. In humans, it has been well studied the use of supplemental vitamin E in chronic diseases such as ischemic heart disease, atherosclerosis, diabetes, cataracts, Parkinson's disease, and Alzheimer's disease (Traber and Sies, 1996). γ-tocopherol has beneficial properties as an anti-inflammatory and possibly antiatherogenic and anticancer agent (Brigelius-Flohé et al., 2002; Wolf, 2006). Tocotrienols have been shown to possess excellent antioxidant activity *in vitro* and have been suggested to suppress reactive oxygen substances more efficiently than tocopherols (Schaffer *et al.,* 2005; McDowell *et al.,* 2007). Studies have shown that tocotrienols exert more significant neuroprotective, anticancer, and cholesterol-lowering properties than tocopherols (Sun and Alkon, 2008).

Other functions
Additional functions of vitamin E that have been reported (Traber, 2013) include (1) normal phosphorylation reactions, especially of high-energy phosphate compounds, such as creatine phosphate and adenosine triphosphate (ATP); (2) a role in the synthesis of vitamin C (ascorbic acid); (3) a role in the synthesis of ubiquinone; and (4) a role in sulfur amino acid metabolism.

Pappu *et al.* (1978) have reported that vitamin E plays a role in vitamin B_{12} metabolism. A vitamin E deficiency interfered with converting vitamin B_{12} to its coenzyme 5' deoxy-adenosyl-cobalamin and, concomitantly, the metabolism of methylmalonyl-CoA to succinyl-CoA. For humans, Turley and Brewster (1993) suggested that cellular deficiency of adenosylcobalamin may be one mechanism by which vitamin E deficiency leads to neurologic injury. Recently, Chen C. *et al.* (2019) demonstrated in pigs the effect of vitamin E on small intestinal histomorphology, digestive enzyme activity, and the expression of nutrient transporters.

In rats, vitamin E deficiency has been reported to inhibit vitamin D metabolism in the liver and kidneys by interfering with the formation of active metabolites and decreasing the concentration of the hormone-receptor complexes in the target tissue. Liver vitamin D hydroxylase activity decreased by 39%, 1-α-hydroxylase activity in the kidneys decreased by 22%, and 24-hydroxylase activity by 52% (Sergeev *et al.,* 1990).

Nutritional assessment
Vitamin E has been assessed based on α-tocopherol concentrations in erythrocytes, lymphocytes, platelets, lipoproteins, adipose tissue, buccal mucosal cells, and LDL, and on α-tocopherol: γ-tocopherol in serum or plasma. Erythrocyte susceptibility to hemolysis or lipid oxidation, breath hydrocarbon exhalation, oxidative resistance of LDL, and α-tocopheryl quinone concentrations in cerebrospinal fluid have been used as functional markers of vitamin E status in humans. However, many of these tests tend to be nonspecific and poorly standardized.

The recognition that vitamin E has essential roles in platelet, vascular, and immune function and its antioxidant properties may lead to identifying more specific biomarkers of vitamin E status (Njeru *et al.,* 1994b, 1995; Morrissey and Sheehy, 1999). Vitamin E analyses encompass 8 naturally occurring vitamers, 4 tocopherols, and 4 tocotrienols. Still, only α-tocopherol is routinely measured and used for status determination since this form is preferably maintained in circulation.

α-tocopherol concentrations in plasma allow quantification by HPLC with fluorescence or UV detection. Using normal-phase HPLC, tocopherols and tocotrienols can also be separated. A recently introduced fast and sensitive reversed-phase HPLC method resolves the challenging separation of β- and γ-tocopherol. Separating and quantifying the 8 stereoisomers of α-tocopherol is much more challenging (Höller *et al.,* 2018).

Further research into functional markers of vitamin E status (e.g., products of lipid peroxidation) or assay systems would have more potential for point-of-care applications. Cell activity assays based on measuring hemolysis of erythrocytes under oxidative stress are another possible functional marker for α-tocopherol (Sauberlich, 1999).

There is a relatively high correlation between plasma and liver levels of α-tocopherol and the amount of dietary α-tocopherol administered and plasma levels. This has been observed in rats, chicks, pigs, lambs, and calves within relatively wide intake ranges. However, plasma tocopherol levels can be affected by blood lipid transport capacity. Plasma α-tocopherol concentration of 3.5 mg/l (8 µmol/l) is considered deficient in humans, with values of 9 mg/l (20 µmol/l) referred to as acceptable.

Deficiency signs
Specific vitamin E deficiency signs
Vitamin E displays a wide variety of deficiency signs, more than any other vitamin (Haga *et al.*, 2021). Deficiency signs differ among species and even within species. Blaxter (1962) reported that muscle degeneration and muscular dystrophy are the one vitamin E deficiency syndrome common to all species. White muscle disease (WMD), or nutritional muscular dystrophy or myodegeneration (NMD), is the primary clinical manifestation of a vitamin E or Se deficiency in newborn calves, lambs, and kids. Cardiac WMD, the equivalent of mulberry heart disease in pigs, is a common deficiency lesion in calves and lambs born to vitamin E-deficient dams. The young also tend to lack a normal suckling reflex and may be unable to stand or walk. White muscle disease occurs in all laboratory and farm animals, camels, buffalo, rhinos, and kangaroos. Muscular dystrophy is reported in several wild animals. For example, the condition in antelope is indistinguishable from WMD in cattle or sheep (NRC, 1983).

Fundamentally, WMD is a Zenker's degeneration of both skeletal and cardiac muscle fibers. Damaged muscle is replaced by connective tissue that is observable as gross white striations in the muscle fiber bundles. Lesions are usually symmetrical and bilateral (Blaxter, 1962), and affected muscles may tear easily and appear edematous. Necropsy may reveal generalized edema of the abdominal cavity and the lungs (Morrill and Reddy, 1987). Serum glutamic-oxalo-acetic transaminase (SGOT), lactic dehydrogenase (LDH), and creatinine phosphokinase (CPK) are elevated in vitamin E-deficient calves (Cipriano *et al.*, 1982; Reddy *et al.*, 1987) and yearling cattle (Allen *et al.*, 1975). The osmotic fragility of erythrocytes has been reported to increase in some instances of vitamin E deficiency (McDowell, 2000a).

NMD of ruminants occurs worldwide, but its incidence or at least diagnosis, particularly in a mild or subclinical form, varies widely between and even within countries (McDowell, 1985). The incidence of WMD in specific world regions is sporadic, with less than 1% of livestock herds affected. In other areas, such as Turkey and New Zealand, a 20–30% incidence of WMD may occur regularly. Considerable research has revealed an inverse relationship between the Se content of soil and the geographic occurrence of vitamin E–Se-responsive muscular dystrophy. Similarly, signs of vitamin E deficiency have been observed in zoo animals fed diets devoid of their natural forage or browse.

WMD occurs with 2 clinical patterns. The first is a congenital type of muscular dystrophy in which calves, lambs, or kids may be born dead or die within a few days of birth following sudden physical exertion, such as nursing or running. The second clinical pattern ("delayed white muscle disease") develops after birth; it is observed most frequently in lambs within 3 to 6 weeks of birth but may occur as late as 4 months after birth. The condition in calves generally manifests at 1 to 4 months of age. A vitamin E-responsive WMD has been observed in 4- to 6-month-old lambs kept on dry, poor-quality, late-season pasture. Godwin (1975) reported that the electrocardiogram of WMD-affected animals shows progressive development of a characteristic abnormality accompanied by a fall in blood pressure. Therefore, a fundamental change in vitamin E-Se deficiency is a circulatory failure linked to cardiac muscle degeneration and possibly to loss of blood vessel integrity. Muscle damage resulting from vitamin E and (or) Se deficiencies cause leakage of cell contents into the bloodstream. Thus, elevated levels of selected enzymes, above normal ranges, serve as diagnostic aids in detecting tissue degeneration. Serum enzyme concentrations used to monitor the incidence of nutritional muscular dystrophy include SGOT, LDH, CPK, aspartate aminotransferase (AST), and malic dehydrogenase (MDH). These enzymes may also be elevated by liver damage. Elevating serum enzyme activity usually precedes gross pathological changes or clinical signs (Sobel and Shell, 1972). In addition to the elevation of selected enzymes, serum and tissue concentrations of vitamin E and selenium decrease due to deficiencies and may be used to monitor the nutritional status of livestock at high risk of developing WMD (McDowell, 1992, 2000a).

Vitamin E deficiency in cattle

Typically, WMD in calves is characterized by generalized leg weakness, stiffness of gait, and myo-degeneration (Figure 4.24). Affected animals have difficulty standing, exhibit crossover walking, and have impaired suckling reflexes and ability. The tongue musculature may be affected in calves, explaining the poor suckling response (NRC, 2000). Calves may display a repeated extension and curling of the tongue (Morrill and Reddy, 1987). Death often occurs suddenly during exertion from heart failure due to severe damage to the heart muscle. Calves with WMD have chalky white striations, degeneration, and necrosis in the skeletal muscles and heart (Figure 4.25). In milder cases with calves, where the chief clinical signs are stiffness and difficulty standing, dramatic, rapid recovery can be achieved with vitamin E-Se injection followed by dietary fortification with vitamin E and Se.

The WMD in its acute, chronic, and peracute form can be distinguished in older calves, usually during the latter growth or early finishing period. Sudden stressors such as transport, regrouping, disease exposure, multiple vaccinations, severe weather, or abrupt changes

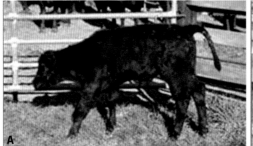
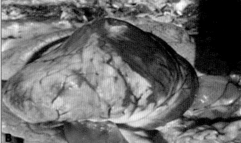
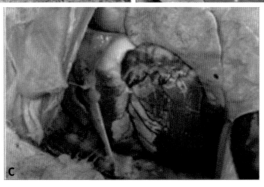

Figure 4.24 Vitamin E–selenium deficiency in cattle, white muscle disease. Top picture: calf of about 3 months old showing lameness and generalized muscle weakness can be seen. Bottom picture: fish flesh lesions in heart muscle which are abnormal white areas in heart muscles (source: http://www.flockandherd.net.au/sheep/reader/selenium-deficiency-monaro.html)

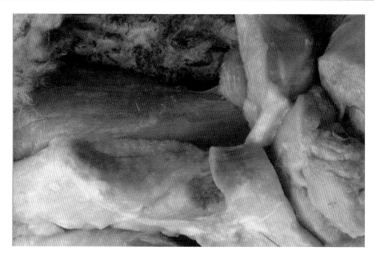

Figure 4.25 Vitamin E–selenium deficiency in cattle, white foci of fibrosis, and red inflammation grossly evident in hindlimb muscles (source: http://www.flockandherd.net.au/sheep/reader/selenium-deficiency-monaro.html)

in feed composition are generally considered precipitating factors. Sudden death without previous clinical signs of WMD is the main feature of the peracute condition. The cause is usually found by necropsy as advanced degeneration of the myocardium, with possible skeletal muscle lesions. In acute cases, motor disturbances, such as an unsteady gait or stiff-calf disease, stiffened muscles in the lumbar region, neck, and forelimb muscles, muscle tremors, perspiration, and sudden collapse, known as "buckling," are encountered.

Chronic marginal vitamin E deficiency is characterized by reduced disease resistance, reduced feed-to-gain ratio, and generally poor performance, especially under stress conditions. Feeder calves also display the vitamin E deficiency symptom known as buckling, in which stress, such as unloading at the feedlot or passage through the processing chute, triggers weakness of rear legs, buckling of fetlocks and, frequently, shaking or quivering of muscles (Figure 4.26). Calves often worsen until they cannot rise and may appear paralyzed. Frequently, affected calves will be down or continue to buckle for extended periods, and death loss is

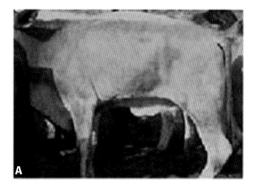
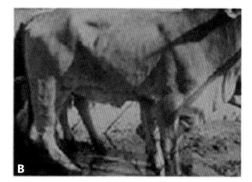

Figure 4.26 Vitamin E–selenium deficiency in cattle, white muscle disease. Flexion of hock and fetlock joints. Flexion is due to decreased support of the gastrocnemius muscle, which is severely affected by myodegeneration.

high in severe cases. Calvfe breeds with excitable temperaments appear to be most affected. Postmortem examination reveals pale, chalky streaks in the hamstring and back muscles, often damaging the heart, rib (intercostal) muscles, and diaphragm (McDowell, 1985).

Calves with experimentally induced vitamin E deficiencies have exhibited clinical signs of nutritional muscular dystrophy similar to those observed in calves under field conditions (Safford et al., 1954). The same symptoms also appeared in calves fed milk containing high levels of polyunsaturated oils but not in calves fed milk containing high levels of hydrogenated (saturated) oils (Adams et al., 1959). WMD can be easily induced in pre-ruminant calves by feeding polyunsaturated oils.

Initially, ruminating calves were thought to be protected from the vitamin E-depleting effect of PUFA because of the rumen microflora's apparent near 100% hydrogenation of all unsaturated fatty acids (Noble et al., 1974). However, research indicated that unsaturated fatty acids in grasses (e.g., linolenic acid) could produce oxidative damage and nutritional muscular dystrophy (NMD) in ruminating calves (McMurray and Rice, 1982; McMurray et al., 1983).

NMD in older calves occurs most frequently at the turnout to spring pasture (Anderson et al., 1976). McMurray et al. (1980) showed that PUFAs escape ruminal hydrogenation, resulting in a threefold increase of plasma linolenic acid within 3 days after turnout. Rice et al. (1981) showed that if protected from ruminal hydrogenation, linolenic acid rapidly reaches high levels in the blood and is associated with a rise in plasma creatine phosphokinase, indicating degenerative myopathy (muscle damage). Likewise, Walsh et al. (1993) reported that ruminating calves fed diets deficient in either vitamin E or both vitamin E and selenium had increased lipid peroxidation products in muscle tissue. Feeding rumen-protected (RP) linseed oil to vitamin E–selenium deficient calves further increased the level of lipid peroxidation in muscle.

Although most cases of WMD involve younger animals, degenerative myopathy has been reported in adult cattle (Tunca et al., 2009; Gitter et al., 1978; Hutchinson et al., 1982). Yearling Chianina heifers exhibited abortion, stillbirth, and periparturient recumbency (downer cow syndrome) (Hutchinson et al., 1982). Necropsy and tissue analysis revealed myodegeneration and a combined vitamin E and Se deficiency. Rapid growth in these heifers, coupled with the stresses of late pregnancy and parturition, may have contributed to this vitamin E deficiency. Marginal Se status would be a predisposing factor. Barton and Allen (1973) reported a myopathic condition affecting yearling cattle. It was associated with animals fed grains treated with propionic acid, which is known to destroy vitamin E. Depletion/repletion studies indicate that feedlot cattle require 50–100 IU per day of supplemental vitamin E (Hutcheson and Cole, 1985). The NRC (2000) states that receiving and starting feedlot cattle should be supplemented with 400 to 500 IU of vitamin E daily to optimize performance and health. The common factors in developing vitamin E-related WMD appear to be marginal vitamin E and selenium status, a sudden diet change to one high in PUFAs, and sudden animal stress. These factors, in combination, can precipitate vitamin E-responsive myopathy. Vitamin E should be supplemented at levels that ensure protection against marginal or outright deficiency.

In high-yield cows, most production diseases occur during transition periods. α-tocopherol declines in blood and reaches the lowest levels (hypovitaminosis E) around calving. Hypovitaminosis E is associated with the incidence of peripartum diseases (Haga et al., 2021). Therefore, many studies published over 30 years have investigated the effects of α-tocopherol supplementation. This α-tocopherol deficiency was thought to be caused by complex factors. However, until recently, the physiological factors or pathways underlying hypovitaminosis E in the transition period have been poorly understood. In the last 10 years, the α-tocopherol-related gene expression, which regulates the metabolism, transportation, and tissue distribution of α-tocopherol in humans and rodents, has been reported in ruminant tissues.

More recently, the incidence of reproductive disorders, predominantly retention of fetal membranes (RFM) and mastitis has been related to an insufficient vitamin E intake. The supplementation of approximately 1,000 IU/day of vitamin E (usually all-*rac*-α-tocopheryl acetate) to dry cows when adequate Se is supplemented reduces the incidence of RFM in some but not all studies. About one-half of the studies that examined the effect of injected vitamin E (usually in combination with Se) on RFM found no effect, and about one-half reported a positive response (Weiss, 1998).

Haga *et al.* (2021) summarized 6 physiological factors causing the hypovitaminosis E in high-yielding cows (Figure 4.27):

1. the decline in α-tocopherol intake from the close-up period
2. changes in the digestive and absorptive functions of α-tocopherol
3. the decline in plasma high-density lipoprotein as an α-tocopherol carrier
4. increasing oxidative stress and consumption of α-tocopherol
5. decreasing hepatic α-tocopherol transfer to circulation
6. increasing mammary α-tocopherol transfer from blood to colostrum, may be involved in α-tocopherol deficiency during the transition period.

However, the mechanisms and pathways are poorly understood, and further studies are needed to understand the physiological role of α-tocopherol-related molecules in cattle. Understanding the molecular mechanisms underlying hypovitaminosis E will contribute to preventing peripartum disease and high performance in dairy cows.

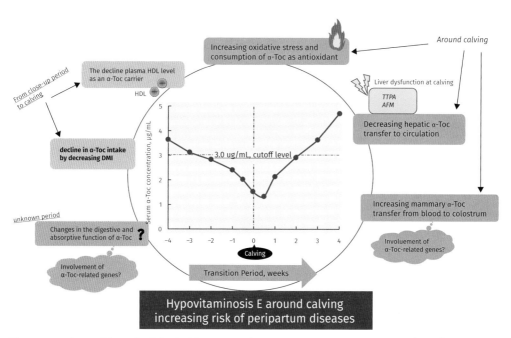

Figure 4.27 Six candidate physiological factors causing decreased blood α-tocopherol (α-Toc) level and hypovitaminosis E in transition high-yield dairy cows. Abbreviations: DMI, dry matter intake; TTPA, α-tocopherol transfer protein gene; AFM, afamin gene; HDL, high-density lipoprotein (source: Haga *et al.*, 2021).

Vitamin E deficiency in sheep and goats

In lambs, WMD, also known as stiff lamb disease, takes a course similar to that observed in calves. Motor disturbances such as unsteady gait (Figure 4.28), stiffness of the hindquarter muscles, neck, and forelimbs, arched back (Figure 4.29), muscle tremors, and perspiration are encountered in the acute form. On necropsy, white striations in cardiac muscle and bilateral lesions in skeletal muscles characterize the disease. A gradual but progressive swelling of the muscles, particularly in the lumbar region and rear legs, gives the erroneous impression of muscular development. Chronic cardiac muscle degeneration also occurs in the lamb, like the peracute deficiency encountered in calves (changes occur primarily in the myocardium). Affected lambs appear normal at birth but quickly lose weight after the third week of life. They also show an aversion to social stress and may stand apart from the flock. Cardiac arrhythmia and increased heart rate can result even after slight exercise. In the advanced stage, animals consume little, if any, feed, and rapid wasting occurs. Symptoms can be reversed by prompt administration of vitamin E and selenium (Hidiroglou and Karpinski, 1987).

For dystrophic lambs, an oral therapeutic dose of 500 IU dl-α-tocopheryl acetate is followed by 100 IU on alternate days until successful recovery (Rumsey, 1975). Vitamin E–selenium responsive conditions are not restricted to young animals and are manifested as a lack of thrift occurring in lambs at pasture (Underwood, 1981). Marginal vitamin E deficiency in yearling sheep can progress to WMD. In sheep of 9–12 months of age, the disease is frequently observed following the driving of the flock with the rapid onset of listlessness, muscle stiffness, inability to stand, prostration, and, in severe acute cases, death within 24 hours (Andrews *et al.*, 1968)

With selenium administration, Hartley and Grant (1961) reported that the incidence of WMD in barren ewes was reduced from over 30–5%. Farms in New Zealand have had lamb losses as high as 40–50%. The syndrome may respond to vitamin E, selenium, or both in these regions. Maas *et al.* (1984) described nutritional myodegeneration in lambs and yearling ewes with normal selenium status but deficiency of vitamin E. Deficiency of vitamin E and (or) selenium in the goat, as in other ruminants, results mainly in WMD. Goat kids are born with little or no reserves of the fat-soluble vitamins A, D, and E. Sudden death of young kids under 2 weeks of age may reveal postmortem evidence of muscle disease and degeneration in the heart muscle or the diaphragm. In older kids and mature animals, deficiency can occur after sudden exertion and stress. Affected animals exhibit bilateral stiffness, usually in the hind legs. In high-producing dairy goats, deficiency manifests itself in poor involution of the uterus, accompanied by retained placenta and metritis following kidding (Guss, 1977). Goat kids 4 to 5 weeks of age diagnosed with NMD had lower vitamin E and selenium concentrations in the liver,

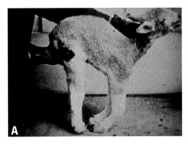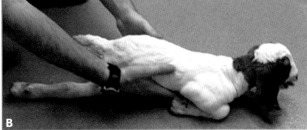

Figure 4.28 Vitamin E–selenium deficiency in sheep and goats due to white muscle or stiff lamb disease. Lambs and goats are unable to stand as a result of tissue degeneration (source: courtesy Muth, O.H., 1995 Oregon State University. https://www.msdvetmanual.com/musculoskeletal-system/myopathies-in-ruminants-and-pigs/nutritional-myopathies-in-ruminants-and-pigs)

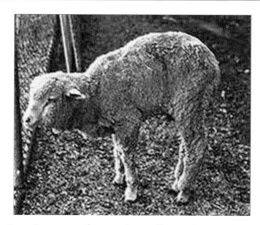

Figure 4.29 Maryland small ruminant page (source: https://www.sheepandgoat.com/wmd)

skeletal muscle, and myocardium (Rammell *et al.*, 1989). Vitamin E concentrations in the liver, skeletal muscle, and myocardium in NMD cases averaged 40, 43, and 30% of those in healthy goat kids, indicating vitamin E depletion.

Gut health issues related to vitamin E deficiency

Cows with left displaced abomasum (LDA), a costly disease occurring primarily in multiparous dairy cows during early lactation, have been reported to have 40% lower circulating concentrations of vitamin E. It is unknown, however, whether the lower circulating α-tocopherol concentrations precede LDA or remain after LDA. Qu *et al.* (2013) observed that until the last blood sampling before LDA diagnosis (49 days postpartum), cows had serum α-tocopherol concentrations 45% lower (5.0±0.9 vs. 9.1±0.9 µM) and α-tocopherol to cholesterol molar ratios 39% lower (1.90±0.19 vs. 3.09±0.26) than those of healthy cows. Serum α-tocopherol concentrations remained lower (<10 *vs.* ~15 µM) up to day 49 postpartum in cows with LDA. These findings indicated that lower serum α-tocopherol concentrations are a potential early indicator for developing LDA in multiparous cows.

Safety

Vitamin E has a wide margin of safety in animals, and toxicity of this vitamin has not been demonstrated in ruminants. Compared with vitamins A and D, acute and chronic studies in animals have shown that the toxicity risk is relatively lower with vitamin E. Still, excessively elevated levels can result in undesirable effects. Hypervitaminosis E studies in rats, chicks, and humans indicate maximum tolerable levels of 1,000–2,000 IU per kg of diet (NRC, 1987).

Excess dietary vitamin E was found to be too low in the activities of antioxidant enzymes in the red blood cells of rats fed salmon oil (Eder *et al.*, 2002). Although α-tocopherol has been the most widely studied, the other 3 tocopherols and 4 tocotrienols have recently been shown to have functions apart from α-tocopherol. Excess supplementation of α-tocopherol could be detrimental to the other vitamin E forms. In humans, excess supplementation of diets with α-tocopherol reduced serum concentrations of gamma and delta tocopherols (Haung and Appel, 2003; Wolf, 2006). The effects of high supplemental α-tocopherol levels on the other forms of vitamin E are unknown for livestock.

Vitamin K
Chemical structure and properties
The generic term vitamin K refers to different fat-soluble compounds of the quinone group that exhibits antihemorrhagic effect. The primary molecule is a naphthoquinone (2-methyl-1.4-naphthoquinone), and the various vitamers differ in the nature and length of the side chain (Figure 4.30):

- Vitamin K_1 or phylloquinone derived from plants.
- Vitamin K_2, or menaquinone, is the form of bacterial fermentation. Vitamin K_2 can be divided into subtypes indicated with MK-n, where n represents the number of isoprenoid residues in the aliphatic side chain: for example, short-chain for menaquinone-4 (MK-4) or long-chain for menaquinone-7 (MK-7). MK-4 is synthesized in the liver from ingested menadione or changed to a biologically active menaquinone by intestinal microorganisms (Suttie, 2013).
- Vitamin K_3, or menadione, is produced by chemical synthesis. This form, partially water-soluble and highly stable, is typically used in compound feeds for animal nutrition.

Natural sources
Naturally occurring sources of vitamin K are phylloquinone (vitamin K_1) from plants and menaquinones (vitamin K_2) produced by rumen and gut bacterial flora (Mladěnka et al., 2022). They are fat-soluble, stable to heat, and destabilized by oxidation, alkali conditions, strong acids, light, and irradiation. Vitamin K_1 is a golden yellow, viscous oil. It is slowly degraded by atmospheric oxygen but fairly rapidly destroyed by sunlight or ultraviolet light. Vitamin K_1 is present in fresh dark-green plants, e.g., dried alfalfa contains 10 mg/kg vitamin K_1, cereals around 0.2–0.3 mg/kg (NRC, 1998), and it is abundant in pasture and green roughages, thus providing high quantities of vitamin K to grazing livestock. Sunlight is essential for its formation, and parts of plants that do not usually form chlorophyll contain little vitamin K_1. However, the natural loss of chlorophyll as the yellowing of leaves does not bring about a corresponding change in vitamin K_1. Ruminant feedlot animals, swine, and poultry receive little vitamin K_1 from diets based on grains and oilseed meals.

Vitamin K_2 produced by bacterial flora would be considered the most crucial source for ruminants because massive quantities of vitamin K are commonly available from rumen synthesis. It can be found in all by-product feedstuffs of animal origin, including fish meal

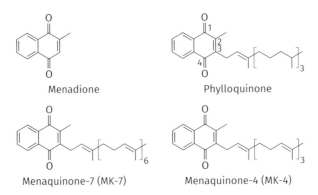

Menadione

Phylloquinone

Menaquinone-7 (MK-7)

Menaquinone-4 (MK-4)

Figure 4.30 Vitamin K structures

Table 4.4 Menadione salts used for diet supplementation

Vitamin K$_3$ salt	Menadione (K$_3$) concentration (%)	Amount of menadione salt to provide 1 g of menadione (K$_3$) (g)
Menadione sodium bisulfite (MSB)	50	2
Menadione dimethylpyrimidinol bisulfite (MPB)	45.4	2.2
Menadione nicotinamide bisulfite (MNB)	43	2.3
Menadione sodium bisulfite complex (MSBC)	33	3

(2 mg/kg) and fish liver oils, especially after they have undergone extensive bacterial putrefaction. The type of diet, independent of vitamin K concentration, will influence total K$_2$ synthesis.

Jiang et al. (2022) discovered that B and K$_2$ vitamin biosynthesis were mainly performed by microbes in the stomach and large intestine of ruminants that were predominantly distributed in the phyla of Bacteroidetes, Firmicutes, and Proteobacteria, suggesting that hindgut microbiota do contribute to the vitamin pool in the gastrointestinal tract (GIT) microbiome. Through this GIT vitamin-producing microbial gene catalog, 2,366 genomes assigned to multi-phyla predicted to *de novo* synthesize at least one B or K$_2$ vitamin were identified, wherein several imperative trophic metabolisms collaborated with vitamin biosynthesis. However, only 2.7% of the vitamin-producing genomes (VPGs) can synthesize 5 or more vitamins. Nearly half of the genomes can synthesize only one vitamin, indicating that most microbes in the GIT microbiome of ruminants are auxotrophs.

Commercial sources

Vitamin K supplementation in animal diets is provided by the synthetic product, namely menadione or vitamin K$_3$, in the form of various bisulfite complexes or water-soluble salts, which are more stable and potent (Huyghebaert, 1991; Hodges et al., 2017; Suttie, 2013). The feed industry does not utilize vitamin K$_1$ due to cost and lack of a stabilized form. Pure menadione is also not used because of poor stability and handling characteristics. Water-soluble derivatives of menadione, including menadione sodium bisulfite (MSB), menadione sodium bisulfite complex (MSBC), and menadione dimethylpyrimidinol bisulfite (MPB), are the principal forms of vitamin K, included in commercial diets. A more recently developed source of vitamin K is a complex of menadione and nicotinamide – menadione nicotinamide bisulfate (MNB) – that is 43.7% menadione and 31.2% nicotinamide. The various products used by the feed industry and their respective content in menadione are listed in Table 4.4.

Encapsulation techniques have been gradually applied to feed additives, which may improve the stability of vitamins. Mujica-Álvarez et al. (2020) reported that microencapsulation could enhance the stability of vitamins. The European Food Safety Authority (EFSA, 2014) reported that pelleting reduced crystal MSB to about 53% of the initial content (pelleting at 90°C, 6 mg MSB/kg feed) and reduced crystal MNB by about 52% of the initial content (pelleting at 70°C, 4.5 mg MNB/kg feed).

Moisture, choline chloride, trace elements, and alkaline conditions impair the stability of these K$_3$ supplements in premixes and diets. MSBC or MPB may lose almost 80% of bioactivity if stored in a vitamin-trace mineral premix containing choline for 3 months. Still, losses were considered far less if stored in a similar premix containing no choline. Coated K$_3$ supplements are generally more stable than uncoated supplements.

Metabolism
Absorption and transport
A recent review by Mladěnka *et al.* (2022) describes the metabolism of vitamin K in mammals. Like all fat-soluble vitamins, vitamin K is absorbed in association with dietary fats and requires the presence of bile salts and pancreatic juice for adequate uptake from the alimentary tract. The absorption of vitamin K depends on its incorporation into mixed micelles, and the optimal formation of these micellar structures requires the presence of both bile and pancreatic juice. Thus, any malfunction of the fat absorption mechanism (e.g., biliary obstruction, malabsorption syndrome) reduces the availability of vitamin K (Ferland, 2006). Menaquinone is absorbed by a passive process in the small intestine and colon. The digestibility of menaquinone is much greater than that of phylloquinone. Griminger and Donis (1960) observed in rats that around 60% of the phylloquinone had been eliminated in feces 24 hours after ingestion, while in the case of menaquinone, elimination was only 11%. Unlike phylloquinone and menaquinones, menadione salts, relatively water-soluble, are absorbed satisfactorily from low-fat diets. Male animals are more susceptible to dietary vitamin K deprivation than females due to a stimulation of phylloquinone absorption by estrogens. The administration of estrogens increases absorption in both male and female animals (Duello and Matschiner, 1971; Jolly *et al.*, 1977; Suttie, 2013).

The absorption of various forms differs significantly. In ruminants, the absorption occurs mainly in the small intestine, although it has been shown to also occur in the colon. The lymphatic system and portal circulation are the major transport routes of absorbed phylloquinone from the intestine. An energy-dependent process absorbs ingested phylloquinone from the proximal portion of the small intestine (Hollander, 1973). Shearer *et al.* (1970) demonstrated the association of phylloquinone with serum lipoproteins, but little is known about the existence of specific carrier proteins. In contrast to the active transport of phylloquinone, menaquinone is absorbed from the small intestine by a passive, noncarrier-mediated process. Menadione can be absorbed from both the small intestine and the colon by a passive approach and transformed into a biologically active form.

The measured efficiency of vitamin K absorption ranges from 10 to 70%, depending on the form of the vitamin administered. Some reports have indicated that menadione is wholly absorbed, whereas phylloquinone is absorbed only at a rate of 50%. The complete absorption of menadione may be due to the aqueous solubility of the menadione salts (Dubbs and Gupta, 1998).

Storage and excretion
The liver stores the vast majority of vitamin K. In other organs, menaquinones also exceed phylloquinone. As such, phylloquinone had biological activity upon prothrombin synthesis that was equal to that of menaquinone found in the chick's liver following the feeding of menadione. Therefore, MK-4 is most likely produced if menadione is fed or if the intestinal microorganisms degrade the dietary K_1 or K_2 to menadione. However, the formation of MK-4 is not required for the metabolic activity of vitamin K since phylloquinone is equally active in synthesizing the vitamin K-dependent, blood-clotting proteins (Bai *et al.*, 2021).

Menadione is widely distributed in all tissues and is very rapidly excreted. Although phylloquinone is quickly concentrated in the liver, it does not have a long retention time in this organ (Thierry *et al.*, 1970). The inability to rapidly develop a vitamin K deficiency in most species results from the difficulty in preventing the absorption of the vitamin from the diet or intestinal synthesis rather than from significant storage of the vitamin.

Rats were found to excrete about 60% of ingested phylloquinone in the feces within 24 hours of ingestion but only 11% of ingested menadione (Griminger, 1984). However, 38% of ingested menadione and only a tiny amount of phylloquinone were excreted via the kidneys during the same period. The conclusion was that although menadione is well absorbed, it is poorly retained in the liver, while the opposite is true for phylloquinone.

In humans, normal human subjects were found to excrete less than 20% of a large (1 mg) dose of phylloquinone in feces. Still, 70 to 80% of the ingested phylloquinone was excreted unaltered in the feces of patients with impaired fat absorption caused by pancreatic insufficiency or adult celiac disease. (Suttie, 2013). Some breakdown products of vitamin K are excreted in the urine. One of the main excretory products is a chain-shortened and oxidized derivative of vitamin K, which forms γ-lactone and is probably excreted as a glucuronide (Suttie, 2013).

Biochemical functions
Blood clotting
The principal function of vitamin K is to control the blood coagulation period since it activates plasmatic prothrombin (Tanaka *et al.*, 2008). A complex series of reactions convert circulating fibrinogen into a fibrin clot. Many proteins with different metabolic functions participating in the "cascade" of blood coagulation require vitamin K for their biosynthesis (Figure 4.31).

Vitamin K is required for the synthesis of the active form of prothrombin (factor II) and other plasma clotting factors, namely factor VII (proconvertin), factor IX (Christmas factor), and factor X (Stuart-Prower factor). These factors are synthesized as inactive precursors (zymogens) in the liver, and vitamin K is necessary for their conversion into biologically active proteins (Suttie and Jackson, 1977). Thus, in the case of vitamin K deficiency, blood coagulation time increases because of the lack of conversion of these factors. In deficiency, vitamin K administration produces a prompt response in 4 to 6 hours; without the liver, this response does not occur (Suttie, 2013).

Vitamin K-dependent proteins can be identified by γ-carboxyglutamic acid residues (Gla), an amino acid common to all vitamin K proteins. The discovery of this new amino acid clarified

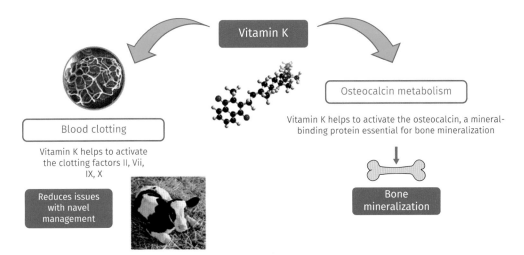

Figure 4.31 Vitamin K functions (source: adapted from Monegue, 2013)

the role of vitamin K in blood coagulation and led to the discovery of additional vitamin K-dependent proteins (e.g., bone proteins) (Ferland, 2006; Suttie, 2013).

Bleeding disorders result from an inability of a liver microsomal enzyme, currently called the vitamin K-dependent carboxylase (Esmon *et al.*, 1975), to conduct the average post-translational conversion of specific glutamyl residues in the vitamin K-dependent plasma proteins to γ-carboxy glutamyl residues (Nelsestuen *et al.*, 1974). Therefore, low vitamin K as a cofactor for this enzyme decreases thrombin generation.

Converting inactive precursor proteins to biologically active forms involve the carboxylation of glutamic acid residues in the inactive molecules. Carboxylation allows prothrombin and the other procoagulant proteins to participate in a specific protein-Ca phospholipid interaction necessary for their biological role (Suttie and Jackson, 1977; Suttie, 2013). Four other vitamin K-dependent proteins have also been identified in plasma: proteins C, S, Z, and M. Protein C and protein S play an anticoagulant rather than a procoagulant role in normal hemostasis (Suttie and Olson, 1990). Protein C inhibits coagulation and, stimulated by protein S, it promotes fibrinolysis. Also, a protein C–S complex can partially hydrolyze the activated factors V and VIII and thus inactivate them. Protein S can also regulate bone turnover (Binkley and Suttie, 1995). The function of proteins M and Z is unclear, and protein Z has been shown to have an anticoagulant role under some conditions (Suttie, 2013). When given to humans at pharmacological doses, menaquinone protects against fracture risk and bone loss in the spine (Shea and Booth, 2008).

The blood-clotting mechanism can be stimulated by either an intrinsic system, in which all the factors are in the plasma, or an extrinsic system. In the extrinsic coagulation system, tissue thromboplastin converts prothrombin in the blood to thrombin in the presence of various elements and Ca. The enzyme thrombin facilitates the conversion of the soluble fibrinogen into insoluble fibrin. Fibrin polymerizes into strands and enmeshes the blood-formed elements, especially the red blood cells, to create the blood clot (Griminger, 1984). The final active component in both the intrinsic and extrinsic systems activates the Stuart factor, which leads to prothrombin activation.

Continuing research has revealed that vitamin K-dependent reactions are present in most tissues, not just blood. A considerable number of proteins are subjected to this post-translational carboxylation of specific glutamate residues γ-carboxyglutamate residues (Vermeer, 1986). Atherocalcin is a vitamin K-dependent protein in atherosclerotic tissue. A vitamin K-dependent carboxylase system in the skin is related to Ca metabolism (de Boer-van den Berg *et al.*, 1986).

Bone mineralization and muscle metabolism

Two of the best-characterized vitamin K-dependent proteins not involved in hemostasis are osteocalcin or bone Gla protein (BGP), matrix Gla protein initially discovered in bone, and protein S. Vitamin K is a cofactor for the γ-glutamyl carboxylase enzyme needed to form γ-carboxyglutamate (Gla) residues in proteins such as osteocalcin and matrix Gla protein (Gallop *et al.*, 1980). Vitamin K is involved in bone and muscle homeostasis. In bone, it increases osteoblastogenesis while decreasing osteoclast formation and function. In muscle, it is associated with increased satellite cell proliferation and migration and might play a role in energy metabolism (Alonso *et al.*, 2023).

Proteins that undergo carboxylation reactions all participate in reactions that require Ca. Osteocalcin contains 3 Gla residues that give this protein its mineral-binding properties. Osteocalcin appears in bone matrix formation at the beginning of the mineralization of the bone and decreases osteoclast formation and function. It accounts for 15 to 20% of the non-collagen protein in the bone of most vertebrates and is one of the most abundant proteins in the body.

Osteocalcin is produced by osteoblasts, with synthesis controlled by $1,25(OH)_2D_3$-dihydroxy vitamin D. About 20% of the newly synthesized protein is released into circulation. It can be used to measure bone formation. As is true for other non-blood vitamin K-dependent proteins, the physiological role of osteocalcin remains largely unknown. However, reduced osteocalcin content of cortical bone (Vanderschueren *et al.*, 1990) and alteration of osteo-calcin distribution within osteons (Ingram *et al.*, 1994) are associated with aging. It remains unknown whether any of these findings are related to the age-related increased risk of frac-ture. Osteocalcin may play a role in the control of bone remodeling because it has been reported to be a chemoattractant for monocytes, the precursors of osteoclasts. Direct radi-oimmunoassay of adult bone powder extracts reveals that the content of intact osteocalcin ranges from 0.28 in humans to 2.0–2.5 mg/g dry bone in cows. The total concentration of circulating osteocalcin is elevated in cows and low in sheep (Hauschka *et al.*, 1989). Plasma osteocalcin is a good predictor of bone formation in cows (Liesegang *et al.*, 2000) and sheep (Farrugia *et al.*, 1989). This suggests a possible role for osteocalcin in bone resorption (Binkley and Suttie, 1995; Suttie, 2013).

Several cell types in the body secrete matrix Gla protein (matrix γ-carboxyglutamate-pro-tein) and protein S. However, matrix Gla protein is highly accumulated in bone and cartilage and is found in the calcification of blood vessels. It contains 5 vitamin-K-dependent γ-carboxyglu-tamic acid residues with high affinity to Ca and phosphate ions and can bind to hydroxyapatite crystals of mineralized tissue (Gallop *et al.*, 1980; Coen *et al.*, 2009). Matrix Gla protein-deficient mice have abnormal calcification, leading to osteopenia, fractures, and premature death owing to arterial calcification (Booth and Mayer, 1997). Potentially, vitamin K levels play a role in regulating the gene expression of these proteins essential for ossification. They could be asso-ciated with increased bone mineral density and reduced fracture risk (Alonso *et al.*, 2023). Clinical trials in sarcopenia also suggest that vitamin K supplementation could improve muscle mass and function (Alonso *et al.*, 2023).

Several observations in humans and animals have indicated that vitamin K could be involved in the pathogenesis of bone mineral loss (Binkley and Suttie, 1995; Cashman and O'Connor, 2008; Alonso *et al.*, 2023):

1. low blood vitamin K in patients with bone fractures
2. concentration of circulating under γ-carboxylated osteocalcin associated with age, low bone mineral density, and hip fracture risk
3. anticoagulant therapy is associated with decreased bone density; and
4. decreased bone loss and Ca excretion with vitamin K supplementation.

Nervous system

Another vitamin K-dependent protein is Gas 6 (growth arrest-specific gene 6). The function of this protein has a possible role in nervous system function, vascular cell function, and platelet activation (Suttie, 2007). To date, both *in vitro* and *in vivo* studies suggest a role of vitamin K in regulating multiple enzymes involved in sphingolipid metabolism within the myelin-rich regions in the brain (Denisova and Booth, 2005). The brain is enriched with sphingolipids, essential membrane constituents, and major lipid signaling molecules that have a role in motor and cognitive behavior.

Nutritional assessment

Traditional assessment of vitamin K status includes evaluation of blood-clotting time. As dis-cussed, the vitamin K family comprises K_1 (phylloquinone from plants) and K_2 (menaquinone from carnivorous and bacterial sources). Moreover, we must include the other vitamers indicated with MK-n, like MK-4 and MK-7. The various forms have quite different pharmacokinetics, with a half-life of 1–2 hours for MK-4 and K_1, 3 days or more for MK-7, and longer chain MKs (Schurgers and Vermeer, 2002).

Vitamin K status may be assessed by measuring the circulating concentration of each relevant vitamer or by measuring the circulating concentration of uncarboxylated Gla-proteins. Direct measurement of circulating K-vitamers is generally accomplished by reversed-phase HPLC or ultra-performance liquid chromatography (UPLC) with fluorescence or mass spectrometric detection. However, many menaquinones are not available as reference compounds. The concentration in circulation reflects recent dietary exposure rather than true status concentrations (Höller *et al.*, 2018). ELISA-based methods for measuring uncarboxylated Gla-proteins are currently the most reliable for assessing vitamin K status. These tests can determine tissue-specific proteins like uncarboxylated osteocalcin (ucOC) for bone.

Measurement of clotting time or prothrombin time has been used to evaluate vitamin K status and is considered a reasonably good measure of vitamin K deficiency. Prolonging the clotting time without liver disease indicates vitamin K deficiency. Further clarification of a deficiency can be provided by assays for specific vitamin K-dependent factors or by the rapid response to administration of vitamin K.

Currently, vitamin K status is assessed by measurement of the plasma concentration of one or more of the vitamin K-dependent clotting factors, prothrombin (factor II), factor VII, factor IX or factor X. More recently, plasma osteocalcin has been proposed as the most sensitive index of vitamin K status in animals and humans (Vermeer *et al.*, 1995).

Deficiency signs

Vitamin K deficiency is produced by ingesting the antagonist, dicumarol, or by feeding sulfonamides (in monogastric species) at levels sufficient to inhibit the intestinal synthesis of vitamin K. Supplementation of vitamin K will overcome the anticoagulation effect of dicumarol. Vitamin K antagonists increase the need for this vitamin. Mycotoxins are also antagonists that may cause vitamin K deficiency (Gentry and Cooper, 1981).

The primary clinical sign of vitamin K deficiency in all species is impairment of blood coagulation. Other clinical symptoms include low prothrombin levels, increased clotting time, and hemorrhaging. In its most severe form, a lack of vitamin K will cause subcutaneous and internal hemorrhages, which can be fatal or cause anemia, anorexia, and weakness.

Microorganisms in the rumen synthesize substantial amounts of vitamin K. A deficiency is seen only in the presence of a metabolic antagonist, such as dicumarol (Figure 4.32) from moldy sweet clover (*Melilotus officinalis, M. alba*). Dicumarol is a fungal (*Penicillium nigricans* and *Penicillium jensi*) metabolite produced from substrates in sweet clover hay, which is common in the Northern Plains of the USA and Canada. The coumarins in fresh sweet clover are inactive because they are bound to glycosides. They are activated when sweet clover is improperly cured (Vermeer, 1984). This condition, referred to as "sweet clover poisoning" or "hemorrhagic sweet clover disease," has been responsible for many animal deaths. Affected animals can die from bleeding following a minor injury or spontaneous bleeding.

Dicumarol passes through the placenta in pregnant animals, and newborn animals may become affected immediately after birth. All species of animals studied are susceptible, but cases of poisoning have involved mainly cattle and, to a minimal extent, sheep. Anti-vitamin K toxicity has been observed in sheep-fed *Ferula communis brevifolia* powder (Tligui and Ruth, 1994) and in cattle fed sweet vernal (*Anthoxanthum odoratum*) hay (Pritchard *et al.*, 1983). A low-coumarin variety of sweet clovers (*Melilotus dentata*) is available for use as forage.

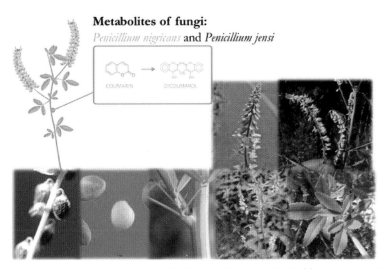

Metabolites of fungi:
Penicillium nigricans and *Penicillium jensi*

COUMARIN → DICOUMAROL

Figure 4.32 Dicumarol from moldy sweet clover (*Melilotus officinalis, M. alba*) (source: https://horsedvm.com/poisonous/sweetclover)

Clinical signs of dicumarol poisoning relate to the hemorrhages caused by blood coagulation failure. The first appearance of the clinical disease varies greatly and depends to a considerable extent on the dicumarol content of the particular sweet clover fed and animal age. If dietary dicumarol is low or variable, animals may consume the forage for months before signs of disease appear.

In an experiment with calves, dicumarol poisoning was produced by feeding naturally spoiled sweet clover hay that contained a minimum of 90 mg per kg dicumarol (Alstad *et al.*, 1985). The minimum time required to develop clinical signs of vitamin K deficiency in these calves was 3 weeks. A case of sweet clover poisoning in dairy cattle in California (Puschner *et al.*, 1998) was caused by feeding sweet clover silage that contained dicumarol produced by mold infestation. Symptoms included subcutaneous hemorrhage, bleeding from the reproductive tract, weakness, and death. Other reported symptoms are subcutaneous hemorrhage and clotting in the brisket, neck, and hips; stiffness and lameness; dull, listless behavior; and pale mucous membranes. Dicumarol has been reported to cause reproductive failure when fed at sub-clinically toxic levels.

Dicumarol poisoning can be reversed by administration of vitamin K. Parenteral vitamin K_1 was an effective treatment for calves at rates of 1.1, 2.2, and 3.3 mg per kg BW. Other researchers have reported that vitamin K_1 injections were effective in treating sweet clover poisoning in cattle but that vitamin K_3 (menadione) injections were not (Casper *et al.*, 1989). Pritchard *et al.* (1983) reported that large oral doses of vitamin K_1 were effective in treating sweet vernal poisoning of cattle but that vitamin K_3 gave less consistent results regarding prothrombin time. This may reflect a greater antagonism of dicumarol against menadione.

Another common cause of induced vitamin K deficiency in veterinary practice is accidentally poisoning animals with warfarin, a synthetic coumarin used as a rodent poison. Initial clinical signs may be stiffness and lameness caused by muscle and joint bleeding. Hematomas, epistaxis, or gastrointestinal bleeding may be observed. Death may occur suddenly with little preliminary evidence of disease and is caused by spontaneous massive hemorrhage or bleeding after injury, surgery, or parturition. DeHoogh (1989) reported 2 possible early embryonic deaths and 1 cow aborted from sweet clover poisoning.

In experimentally induced dicumarol poisoning, "hemorrhagic sweet clover disease," Alstad *et al.* (1985) reported that standard prothrombin time is equal to or less than 20 seconds. Vitamin K deficiency was characterized by prothrombin times more significant than 40–60 seconds, and with severe deficiency, prothrombin time can be as long as 5–6 minutes.

Even though inadequate dietary vitamin K alters bone osteocalcin, signs associated with the skeletal system are not as apparent as blood-clotting problems. Although blood clotting was impaired and there was a reduction in bone γ-carboxyglutamic acid concentrations, vitamin K deficiency did not functionally impair skeletal metabolism. Vitamin K-dependent γ-carboxylated proteins have been identified as ligands for a unique family of receptor tyrosine kinases with transforming ability. The involvement of vitamin K metabolism and function in 2 well-characterized birth defects, warfarin embryopathy, and vitamin K epoxide reductase deficiency, suggests that developmental signals from vitamin K-dependent pathways may be required for normal embryogenesis (Howe and Webster, 1994). Mycotoxins are also antagonists that may cause vitamin K deficiency; for example, their anticoagulant action is impaired by aflatoxins (Suttie, 2013).

Safety

Toxic effects of the vitamin K family are manifested mainly as hematologic and circulatory derangements. Not only is species variation encountered, but profound differences are observed in the ability of the various vitamin K compounds to evoke a toxic response (Barash, 1978).

Vitamin K_1 and Vitamin K_2 are nontoxic at very high dosage levels. Synthetic menadione compounds have shown toxic effects when fed to humans, rabbits, dogs, and mice in excessive amounts. However, the toxic dietary level of menadione is at least 1,000 times the dietary requirement (NRC, 2016; NASEM, 2021). Menadione compounds can safely be used at low levels to prevent the development of a deficiency but should not be used to treat a hemorrhagic condition. The parenteral LD50 of menadione or its derivatives is 200 to 500 mg per kg of BW in some species, and dosages of 2 to 8 mg per kg BW have been reported to be lethal in horses. Such data are not available for ruminants (NRC, 1989).

Finally, we must remember the vitamin K's interaction with other fat-soluble vitamins. Vitamin K activity is impaired by excessive levels of vitamins A (up to 100,000 IU/kg feed) and vitamin E (4,000 mg/kg feed), with repercussions on coagulation time (3 times longer). Some water-soluble menadiol sodium diphosphate and water-miscible formulations of phylloquinone may react with free tissue sulfhydryl groups when administered intramuscularly to neonates. Menadione compounds can safely be used at low levels to prevent the development of a deficiency but should not be used as a pharmacologic treatment for a hemorrhagic condition.

WATER-SOLUBLE VITAMINS

Water-soluble vitamins are made of the B complex vitamins plus choline and vitamin C. Most of them can be synthesized by the ruminal microflora in quantities that typically cover their requirements in different physiological situations. However, failures in ruminal physiology, high-grain diets, and stressful situations can reduce microbial production, and diet supplementation can have beneficial effects.

Vitamin B₁ (thiamine)
Chemical structure and properties

Thiamine consists of a pyrimidine molecule and a molecule of thiazole linked by a methylene bridge, and it contains both nitrogen and sulfur atoms (Figure 4.33). A hydroxyl (OH) group at one end allows it to form ester bonds with phosphoric acid, producing thiamine mono, di- or triphosphate. Thiamine is isolated in pure form as white, crystalline thiamine hydrochloride (89.2% thiamine) or thiamine mononitrate (91.9% thiamine). Most of the vitamin B₁ in animal tissues is thiamine diphosphate (TDP), also known as thiamine pyrophosphate (TPP) or cocarboxylase. Thiamine is isolated in pure form as white, crystalline thiamine hydrochloride. The vitamin has a characteristic sulfurous odor and a slightly bitter taste (Bettendorff, 2013).

Thiamine is predominately found in chloride hydrochloride ($C_{12}H_{17}N_4OSCl.HCl$, molecular mass 337.27 g/mol) that decomposes at 198°C (Bettendorff, 2013). Thiamine hydrochloride is a hydrophilic molecule: it can form a hydrate even under normal atmospheric conditions by absorbing nearly 1 mole of water and has a solubility of ~1 g/ml of water at 25°C. Under ordinary conditions, thiamine hydrochloride is more hygroscopic than mononitrate salt. However, both products should be kept in sealed containers to avoid deterioration.

Thiamine is highly soluble in water, sparingly soluble in alcohol, insoluble in fat solvents, and has a slightly bitter taste. It is susceptible to alkali, in which the thiazole ring opens at room temperature with a pH above 7. In a dry state, thiamine is stable at 100°C for several hours, but moisture accelerates destruction, and thus, it is much less stable to heat in fresh than in dry foods. It is destroyed by ultraviolet light.

Natural sources

Considerable amounts of thiamine are found in the primary raw materials of plant origin. Cereal grains and their by-products, soybean meal, cottonseed meal, and peanut meal, are relatively rich sources of thiamine. However, brewer's yeast is the richest known natural source of thiamine (usually between 3 and 6 mg/kg). Soy contains up to 7 mg/kg of whole soy, peas 2 mg/kg, and around 1.5 mg/kg of soy cake.

Since vitamin B₁ is present primarily in the germ and seed coats, by-products containing the latter are richer (7–20 mg/kg) than the whole kernel, while highly milled flour is deficient. In humans, beriberi was prevalent in Orient countries, where polished rice is the dietary staple.

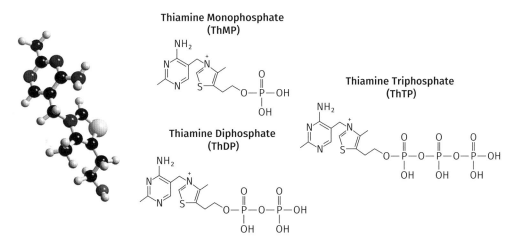

Figure 4.33 Vitamin B₁ chemical structures

Rice may have 5 mg per kg of thiamine, but the content is much lower for polished rice (0.3 mg per kg) and higher for rice bran (23 mg per kg) (Marks, 1975). Wheat germ ranks next to yeast in thiamine concentration. The level of thiamine in grain rises as the protein level rises it depends on species, strain, and use of nitrogenous fertilizers (Bettendorff, 2013).

Nevertheless, the frequent presence of mold or antagonists, such as mycotoxins, and high susceptibility to inactivation by heat must be considered. Analyses of moldy feed showed a thiamine content of less than 0.1 ppm, whereas the same feed that was not contaminated had a thiamine content of 5.33 ppm. Reddy and Pushpamma (1986) studied the effects of one year of storage and insect infestation on the thiamine content of feeds. Thiamine losses were high in several sorghums and pigeon peas (40% to 70%) and lower in rice and chickpeas (10% to 40%). Since thiamine is water-soluble and unstable to heat, significant losses may result during certain feed manufacturing processes (McDowell, 2000a; Bettendorff, 2013).

Commercial sources

Thiamine sources available for addition to feed are the thiamine chloride hydrochloride (337.28 g/mol; 98%) and thiamine mononitrate (327.36 g/mol; 98%) salts (Figure 4.34). Both are fine, granular, white to pale-yellow powders. Because of its lower solubility in water, the mononitrate salt has better stability characteristics in dry products than the hydrochloride, but both products should be kept in sealed containers (Bettendorff, 2013). Thiamine mononitrate is prepared from thiamine hydrochloride by dissolving the hydrochloride salt in a mildly alkaline solution. This process is followed by the precipitation of the nitrate half-salt with a stoichiometric amount of nitric acid. The concentration and requirements of vitamin B_1 are usually expressed in mg.

Metabolism
Absorption and transport
Thiamine is readily digested and released from naturally occurring sources. A precondition for normal thiamine absorption is sufficient stomach hydrochloric acid production. Phosphoric acid esters of thiamine are split in the intestine. The free thiamine formed is soluble in water and easily absorbed, especially in the jejunum.

The mechanism of thiamine absorption has yet to be fully understood, but active transport and simple passive diffusion are involved. There is active sodium-dependent transport of thiamine at low concentrations against the electrochemical potential, whereas, at high concentrations, it diffuses passively through the intestinal wall. Thiamine synthesized by the rumen and gut microflora in the cecum, or large intestine, is largely unavailable to animals except by coprophagy (Wang et al., 2014; Pan et al., 2018).

Specific proteins (transporters and carriers) in the cell membrane have binding sites for thiamine, allowing it to be solubilized within the cell membrane. This permits the vitamin to pass through the membrane and ultimately reach the aqueous environment on the other side

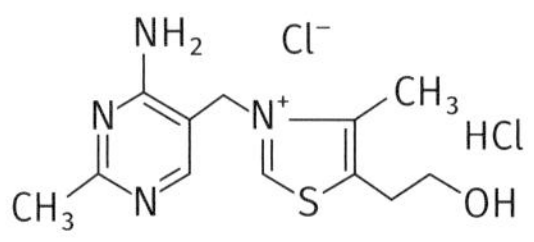

(a) Thiamine chloride hydrochloride 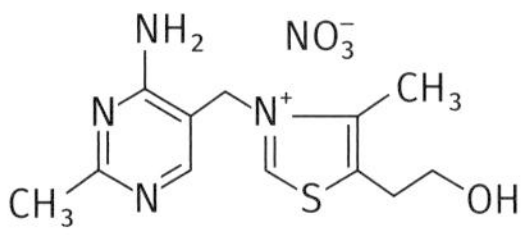 (b) Thiamine mononitrate

Figure 4.34 Vitamin B_1 forms used in animal nutrition

(Rose, 1990; Bates, 2006). Absorbed thiamine is transported via the portal vein to the liver with the carrier plasma protein. Thiamine is efficiently transferred to the embryo.

Thiamine phosphorylation can occur in most tissues, particularly in the liver. Almost 80% of thiamine in animals is phosphorylated in the liver under ATP to form the metabolically active enzyme form TPP (diphosphate or cocarboxylase). Of total body thiamine, about 80% is TPP, about 10% is TTP, and the remainder is thiamine monophosphate (TMP) and free thiamine. Up to 90% of whole-blood thiamine is concentrated in the erythrocytes and leukocytes (Mancinelli et al., 2003). Red blood cells and leukocytes accumulate thiamine partly due to their dependence on the pentose pathway and glycolysis.

Storage and excretion
Thiamine is one of the most poorly stored vitamins. However, thiamine is readily absorbed and transported to cells throughout the body. Most mammals on a thiamine-deficient diet will exhaust their body stores within 1–2 weeks, so a continuous thiamine supply is required (Ensminger et al., 1983). The thiamine content in individual organs varies considerably, and the vitamin is preferentially retained in organs with high metabolic activity. Thiamine is contained in the most significant quantities in major organs such as the liver, heart, brain, and kidneys during deficiencies. Although liver and kidney tissues have the highest thiamine concentrations, approximately 50% of the total thiamine body stores are in muscle tissue (Polegato et al., 2019).

Thiamine intakes above current needs are rapidly excreted. Absorbed thiamine is passed in urine and feces, with small quantities excreted in other secretions. Fecal thiamine may originate from feed, synthesis by microorganisms, or endogenous sources (i.e., via bile or excretion through the mucosa of the large intestine). When thiamine is administered in large doses, urinary excretion reaches saturation, and the fecal concentration increases considerably (Benevenga et al., 1966; Bräunlich and Zintzen, 1976). Most thiamine excess is excreted via feces (Amat et al., 2013).

Biochemical functions
Thiamine is one of the enzymes critical in the metabolism of lysine, branched-chain amino acids, carbohydrates, and lipogenesis (Bettendorff, 2013). The main functions of thiamine are illustrated in Figure 4.35 Primarily, thiamine is essential in carbohydrate and energy metabolism, especially in the heart and nervous system (Loew and Dunlop, 1972; Loew et al., 1975; Haven, 1982; Bâ, 2008; EFSA, 2010; Amat et al., 2013). For this reason, thiamine recommendations increase when the primary energy source supplied by the feed is carbohydrates.

The TPP or TDP is the coenzyme cocarboxylase, a thiamine derivative. TPP is the active thiamine derivative involved in the tricarboxylic acid cycle (TCA, citric acid, or Krebs cycle). Thiamine is the coenzyme for all enzymatic decarboxylations of α-keto acids. Thus, it functions in the oxidative decarboxylation of pyruvate to acetate, combined with coenzyme A (CoA) for entrance into the TCA cycle. Thiamine is essential in 2 oxidative decarboxylation reactions in the TCA cycle that take place in cell mitochondria and one reaction in the cytoplasm of the cells.

Decarboxylation in the TCA cycle removes carbon dioxide, and the substrate is converted into the compound having the next lower number of carbon atoms:

- pyruvate –> acetyl-CoA + CO_2
- α-ketoglutaric acid –> succinyl-CoA + CO_2.

These reactions are essential for the utilization of carbohydrates to provide energy. Vitamins B$_2$ (riboflavin), pantothenic acid, and niacin are also involved with thiamine in this biochemical process.

Thiamine plays a crucial role in glucose metabolism. TPP is a coenzyme in the transketolase reaction that is part of the direct oxidative pathway (pentose phosphate cycle) of glucose metabolism in the liver, brain, adrenal cortex, and kidney cell cytoplasm, but not skeletal muscle. The pentose phosphate cycle is the only mechanism known for ribose synthesis needed for nucleotide formation. This cycle also reduces nicotinamide adenine dinucleotide phosphate (NADPH), essential for lowering carbohydrate metabolism intermediates during fatty acid synthesis (Bettendorff, 2013).

Thiamine is, together with vitamin B$_6$ (pyridoxine) and vitamin B$_{12}$ (cobalamin), one of the commonly called "neurotropic" B vitamins, playing particular and essential roles both in the central nervous system (CNS) and the peripheral nervous system (PNS) (Muralt, 1962; Cooper *et al.*, 1963; Bâ, 2008; Calderón-Ospina and Nava-Mesa, 2020). The maintenance of nerve membrane function and the synthesis of myelin and several types of neurotransmitters (e.g., acetylcholine, serotonin, and amino acids) are essential in transmitting nervous impulses. Another thiamine function in the transmission of nervous impulses is due to its participation in the passive transport of sodium (Na$^+$) to excitable membranes, which is essential for the transmission of impulses at the membrane of ganglionic cells. However, thiamine's above-described role in energy metabolism explains a significant part of its activity in the nervous system by providing energy to nerve cells (Bâ, 2008).

Nutritional assessment

Thiamine nutritional status is typically determined by measuring the thiamine-dependent erythrocyte transketolase activity (ETKA) or thiamine (free or phosphorylated) concentrations.

The ETKA assay is the most acceptable for a functional assessment of thiamine deficiencies by measuring the relative increase of erythrocyte transketolase activity in response to *in vitro*

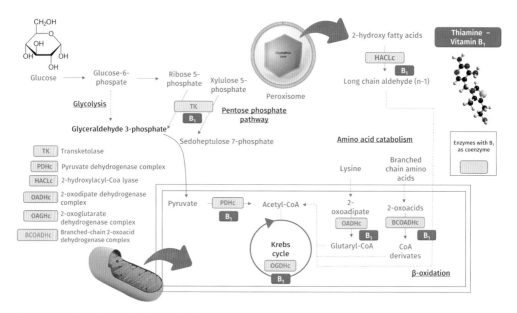

Figure 4.35 Vitamin B$_1$ roles in metabolism

addition of TDP. The best transketolase assay for assessing thiamine deficiency is based on the so-called TPP effect, which is the percentage increase in transketolase activity following the addition of excess TPP to the sample. However, analytical variability is reported due to standardization and sample stability issues (Sauberlich, 1999; Höller *et al.*, 2018). HPLC-based methods to quantify free thiamine and the phosphorylated form require further improvements.

Deficiency signs

Cereals and soy have a high thiamine content and are thus unlikely to lead to a deficiency; however, on occasion, deficiencies have been confirmed in the field, with symptoms such as anorexia, decreased body weight, vomiting, polyneuritis, and foot problems.

Clinical signs include an apparent weakness usually first characterized by poor leg coordination, especially of the forelimbs, and inability to rise and stand. The head is frequently retracted (*i.e.*, "stargazing") (Figure 4.36), and cardiac arrhythmia may occur. Affected animals may also display blindness and convulsions. Specific signs usually accompany growth depression, anorexia, severe diarrhea, dehydration, and death (McDowell, 2000a; NRC, 2000). Signs in calves can be either acute or chronic. Acutely affected calves displayed anorexia with severe diarrhea and died within 24 hours of onset. These signs appeared after 2–4 weeks on a low-thiamine diet (Johnson *et al.*, 1948).

Growing cattle display dullness and neural aberrations such as circling, head pressing, apparent blindness, excitability, and convulsions. These symptoms may be confused with those of certain bacterial or viral diseases (e.g., clostridial infections, listeriosis, encephalitis), heavy metal poisoning (e.g., lead), hypomagnesemia, or vitamin A deficiency. Mortality can be sudden and significant if animals are not treated. This condition, polioencephalomalacia (PEM) or cerebrocortical necrosis (CCN), cerebral necrosis, and forage poisoning, is also observed in sheep and goats (Amat *et al.*, 2013). The condition is often precipitated by feeding high-grain feedlot rations or the sudden introduction of livestock to lush pasture. Low copper status and high intakes of sulfur, especially sulfate, in feed or water are risk factors. In some instances, similar symptoms arise due to sulfur toxicity (Amat *et al.*, 2013) and the production and inhalation of hydrogen sulfide gas, a neurotoxin (Kandylis, 1984).

The extensive rumen synthesis of thiamine suggests that ruminants possessing a normally functioning rumen have no absolute dietary thiamine requirement. However, thiamine

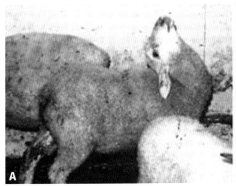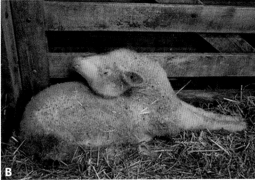

Figure 4.36 Thiamine deficiency in sheep: opisthotonos (head bent backward), cramp-like muscular contractions, balance disturbance, and aggressiveness (source: courtesy of Michel Hidiroglou, Animal Research Center, Ottawa, Canada. https://www.canr.msu.edu/sheep_goats/health/polioencephalomalacia)

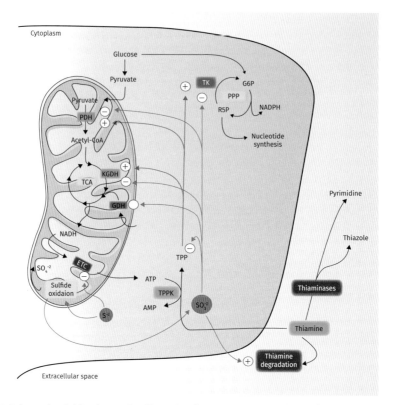

Figure 4.37 Schematic of thiamine and sulfite effect in some cellular activities (AMP, adenosine monophosphate; ATP, adenosine triphosphate; ETC, electron transport chain; GDH, glutamate dehydrogenase; G6P, glucose 6-phosphate; KGDH, α-ketoglutarate dehydrogenase; NADH, nicotinamide adenine dinucleotide; NADPH, nicotinamide adenine dinucleotide phosphate; PDH, pyruvate dehydrogenase; PPP, pentose phosphate pathway; R5P, ribose 5-phosphate; S^{2-}, sulfide; SO_3^{-2}, sulfite; SO_4^{-2}, sulfate; TCA, citric acid cycle; TK, transketolase; TPPK, thiamine pyrophosphokinase; TPP, thiamine pyrophosphate) (source: Amat *et al.*, 2013)

deficiencies do develop in ruminants under certain conditions. PEM is a disorder of the CNS and it refers to a laminar softening or degeneration of grain gray matter (Brent and Bartley, 1984; Amat *et al.*, 2013). The effects of sulfite on thiamine and some cellular activities are described in Figure 4.37. Thiamine deficiency blocks the glycolytic and pentose pathways in neural tissue, leading to inflammation and necrosis. PEM affects mainly calves and young cattle between 4 months and 2 years of age and lambs, young sheep, and goats between 2 and 7 months of age. The incidence of PEM is reported to be between 1% and 20%, and mortality may reach 100%. Clinical signs in mild cases include dullness, blindness, muscle tremors, especially of the neck, and opisthotonos ("stargazing").

Other progressive symptoms include circling, head pressing, and convulsions; in severe cases, collapse within 12–72 hours after the onset of the disease (Figure 4.38). In the final stages, the ears droop, and the limbs and head are extended, parallel to "stargazing" in thiamine-deficient chicks. Trembling and twitching of the musculature of the ears and eyelids, weaving of the head and neck, and grinding the teeth with groaning may be observed. Without treatment, death usually occurs within a few days. The primary lesions in these animals are necrotic areas in both cerebral hemispheres.

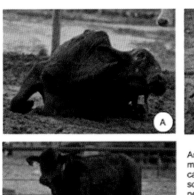
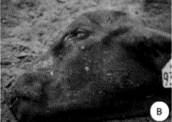
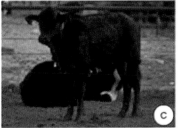

Animal (A and B) with polioencephalomalacia due to thiamin deficiency. Feedlot
cattle with this condition show dullness and
sometimes blindness, with a series of
nervous disorders such as circling, head
pressing and convulsions. After injections
of thiamin, this animal (C) returned to almost
normal with slight brain damage.

Figure 4.38 Polioencephalomalacia due to thiamine deficiency

PEM may appear as an acute disease with high mortality or in milder forms that run a more protracted course. Not all animals in a group will be affected. It is probable that, particularly in its mild form, the condition is often not diagnosed and may occur more frequently than is recognized. Clinical signs of CNS disorders associated with PEM are more readily recognized than nonspecific symptoms such as scouring, reduced growth, and anorexia. However, these signs are also exhibited at later stages of thiamine deficiency (Rammell and Hill, 1986). Thornber (1979) reported that lambs fed a thiamine-deficient diet may not show clinical signs of a CNS disorder for 3 to 5 weeks or longer. However, depressed blood thiamine levels and other clinical signs may be observed. Without treatment, mortality is about 50% in the mild form and may be up to 100% in the acute form of PEM. The incidence and death rates are highest in young animals from 2 to 5 months of age. Many experiments have shown that PEM can be caused by naturally occurring thiamine antagonists (thiaminase), reduced thiamine synthesis, or increased destruction of thiamine in the rumen. Several researchers report that most field cases of PEM result from a progressive thiamine deficiency, likely the result of bacterial thiaminases in the rumen or lower intestine (Loew *et al.*, 1975; Frye *et al.*, 1991). Clinical reports indicate that high-concentrate rations or sudden introduction of lush pasture produces rumen thiaminases and predisposes young cattle and sheep to PEM (Edwin and Lewis, 1971).

There is also evidence that disruptions of rumen function by sudden diet change can produce antithiamine analogs. Thiaminases can be produced by bacterial and fungal contamination of feeds (Davies *et al.*, 1968). *Clostridium sporogenes* and *Bacillus thiamineolyticus* have been isolated from the rumen of PEM-affected cattle and sheep (Loew *et al.*, 1975; Cushnie *et al.*, 1979; Haven *et al.*, 1983). Both organisms produce thiaminase type I. Thiaminases are found in certain plant species, such as the bracken fern. This is a particular problem in Australia where PEM occurs under pasture conditions, apparently due to grazing of certain fern species. Forage species suspected of causing PEM included *Sisymbrium irio* (London rocket), *Capsella bursa-pastoris* (shepherd's pulse), *Raphanus raphanistrum* (wild radish), and *Amaranthus blitoides* (Ramos *et al.*, 2005; McKenzie *et al.*, 2009).

In the study of McKenzie *et al.* (2009), the forages causing PEM were high in sulfur (0.62 and 10.1%), which is often associated with PEM. Furazolidone at high doses produces a thiamine-responsive neuropathology, including head tremors, ataxia, visual impairment, and convulsions (Adil *et al.*, 2024). The anticoccidial mode of action of amprolium is apparently through inhibition of thiamine phosphorylation. Loew and Dunlop (1972) found that elevated levels of amprolium (considerably above the levels needed to prevent coccidiosis) could produce the physical signs and the histological lesions of PEM. Amprolium-induced PEM produces abnormal changes in brain waves and is thiamine-responsive (Itabisashi *et al.*, 1990). Wernery *et al.* (1998) reported amprolium-induced PEM in dromedary camels when only a barley diet was fed and not when the camels were fed hay *ad libitum*. However, serum thiamine was depressed equally in both groups, indicating an interaction between amprolium and diet in producing PEM.

In Colombia, a wasting disease known as "secadera" or "drying up" (Figure 4.39) is alleviated by thiamine injections (Mullenax *et al.*, 1992). This author suggested that a fungus associated with native forage produces a thiaminase. On the contrary, Miles and McDowell (1983) report that the wasting disease secadera can be successfully controlled with a highly fortified complete mineral supplement. It is possible that supplementation of either thiamine or trace minerals can control this wasting disease through different mechanisms (McDowell, 1985). More recent data show an effect of copper on thiamine metabolism in cattle (Olkowski *et al.*, 1991), suggesting that marginal copper status is a factor in PEM and other related neural degenerative diseases (Frank *et al.*, 1992).

High-sulfur diets or water sources are associated with thiamine deficiency and PEM symptoms (Kandylis, 1984; Olkowski *et al.*, 1991; Gould, 1998; McKenzie *et al.*, 2009; Amat *et al.*, 2013). The toxicology of sulfur in ruminants has been reviewed in detail by Kandylis (1984) and Amat *et al.* (2013). Gould *et al.* (1991) reported that in steers, the highest rumen fluid sulfide concentrations coincided with the onset of clinical signs of PEM. McAllister *et al.* (1997) investigated a field case of PEM induced by high sulfate water and reported no reduction in blood thiamine in affected steers. Controlled studies have reported significant reductions (Goetsch and Owens, 1987) and small reductions (Alves de Oliveira *et al.*, 1997) in rumen thiamine production in response to high sulfate intakes. In a large field study, Olkowski *et al.* (1991) reported that beef cattle consuming high sulfate water sources had reduced blood thiamine status. Several cases

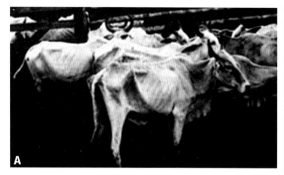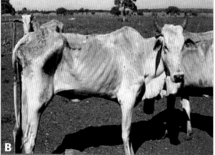

Figure 4.39 Thiamine deficiency in cattle. Wasting disease or "secadera" of cattle in the llanos of Colombia. Animals are characterized by an emaciated condition even with quality available forage. This condition has been reported as thiamine deficiency since it has been alleviated with thiamine injections. However, "secadera" has also been controlled with a highly fortified complete mineral supplement. (source: courtesy of L.R. McDowell, University of Florida)

of PEM have occurred when gypsum ($CaSO_4$) has been used as a feed intake-limiting factor. It would appear that the sulfate ion of gypsum, during its conversion to sulfide, must pass through sulfite, which may destroy thiamine or produce antithiamine analogs.

Feedlot cattle that received 0.72% sulfate had 50% less gain than controls, and some developed PEM (Sadler *et al.*, 1983). For sheep, high-sulfur intake was shown to have a detrimental effect on *in vitro* polymorphonuclear leukocyte function. Thus, ruminants consuming diets or water high in sulfur may have reduced immune function and increased disease risk (Olkowski *et al.*, 1990). Low copper status appears to play a role in sheep's PEM development (Olkowski *et al.*, 1991). High dietary sulfur and molybdenum can induce copper deficiency by forming thiomolybdates in the rumen (Maynard *et al.*, 1979). Thus, low dietary copper, high dietary or water sulfate, and molybdenum are predisposing factors for PEM. *Brassica* plant species contain high levels of sulfur and can produce low copper status in ruminants (Taljaard, 1993; Amat *et al.*, 2013).

The symptoms of PEM are not entirely specific to thiamine deficiency. However, thiamine deficiency is one of several causative factors, along with high-concentrate diets, excess sulfur intakes, and low copper status. Livestock grazing tall fescue infected by an endophyte (*Acremonium coenophiatum*) can suffer from tall fescue toxicosis. The symptoms resemble those caused by elevated rumen thiaminase activity, for example, PEM (Lauriault *et al.*, 1990), and are alleviated by thiamine supplementation (Dougherty *et al.*, 1991). Response to supplemental thiamine was more significant when cattle grazing endophyte-infected tall fescue were exposed to heat stress (Lauriault *et al.*, 1990). Results suggest that oral thiamine supplementation may alleviate tall fescue toxicosis of beef cattle during hot weather. An earlier study found that supplemental thiamine had no beneficial effect in cattle grazing fescue moderately infected by endophytes.

Diagnosis of thiamine deficiency initially depended upon recognition of the clinical signs in live animals, followed by confirmatory brain histopathology or clinical response to thiamine administration (Rammell and Hill, 1986). Moreover, affected animals react so promptly to treatment with thiamine (sometimes within hours) that prompt treatment with thiamine is used to confirm the diagnosis of PEM. Biochemical changes indicating that PEM is associated with thiamine deficiency include reduced blood, urine, and tissue thiamine concentrations, the dramatic elevation of blood pyruvate and lactate, and markedly reduced erythrocyte transketolase activity (Bräunlich and Zintzen, 1976; Karapinar *et al.*, 2010). Brin (1969) showed that blood transketolase activity (particularly in the red cells) is a reliable index of the availability of coenzyme TPP and thus is well correlated with the degree of deficiency in animals. ETKA indicates a marginal thiamine deficiency. Values of 120 to 250% have been reported for animals diagnosed with PEM (Edwin *et al.*, 1979).

Benevenga *et al.* (1966) performed a classical experiment on thiamine deficiency in Holstein calves fed a purified diet. Deficiency symptoms appeared 27 to 48 days after initiation of a thiamine-free diet. Anorexia, heart arrhythmia, respiratory distress, lacrimation, and teeth grinding were clinical symptoms. Blood pyruvate and lactate levels were elevated, hemoglobin and packed cell volume (PCV) depressed, and the activities of several liver enzymes were reduced by 30 to 50%. Re-feeding thiamine relieved all symptoms. Bräunlich and Zintzen (1976) concluded that PEM could be established if the following 4 situations exist.

1. *Case history*: animals on high-energy feeds rich in soluble carbohydrates died after showing central nervous system disorders.
2. *Biochemical evidence*: blood pyruvate has steeply increased, and erythrocyte transketolase activity has been reduced.

3. *Diagnostic therapy*: animals thought to have PEM will react promptly to initial treatment with thiamine.
4. *Pathological changes*: necropsy shows typical pathological anatomical changes, i.e., bilateral cortical necrosis in the brain.

Seasonal trends have been associated with PEM, possibly due to increased metabolic demands of gestation, lactation, and growth or changes in rumen microbial populations.

Additionally, feeding high-concentrate, low-fiber rations may induce PEM. It generally occurs in feedlot cattle about 3 weeks after a diet change. Thiamine deficiency in both chronic ruminal acidosis and acute ruminal lactic acidosis may occur because of inadequate synthesis of thiamine. Furthermore, a decrease in ruminal pH may result in the release of bacterial thiaminases. Research suggests that PEM is associated with lactic acid acidosis and adaptation to high-grain rations. Oltjen *et al.* (1962) reported that a reduction in rumen pH decreases thiamine in the rumen; a low ruminant pH is characteristic of cattle fed high-concentrate diets. However, this effect was not observed *in vitro* using rumen simulation techniques (Alves de Oliveira *et al.*, 1997).

PEM has caused significant economic losses in tropical countries, not only in feedlots where high-grain diets are fed but also where elevated levels of molasses are fed. When molasses is provided *ad libitum* together with diets containing little crude fiber, a disease referred to as "molasses toxicity" or "molasses drunkenness" appears (Losada *et al.*, 1971). Clinical signs of this condition closely resemble PEM, and some studies completed in Cuba have suggested that thiamine treatment and additional roughage may be an effective cure. Mella *et al.* (1976) induced PEM by feeding cattle a molasses-urea diet.

Substances with antithiamine activity, hence causing a deficiency, are common in nature and include structurally similar antagonists and structure-altering antagonists. For example, fish meal contains thiaminases. The synthetic compounds pyrithiamine, oxythiamine, and amprolium (an anticoccidial) are structurally similar antagonists. Their mode of action is competitive inhibition, interfering with thiamine at different points in metabolism.

Pyrithiamine blocks the esterification of thiamine with phosphoric acid, inhibiting the thiamine coenzyme cocarboxylase. Oxythiamine competitively inhibits thiamine's binding to the carboxylase complex, blocking critical metabolic reactions. The coccidiostat amprolium inhibits the intestinal absorption of thiamine and blocks the phosphorylation of the vitamin (McDowell, 2000a). Thiaminase activity destroys thiamine by altering the structure of the vitamin (Bettendorff, 2013). Two types of thiaminase enzymes, I and II, have been described. For thiaminase I, substitute a new base for the thiazole ring. This leads to less thiamine, but it also results in thiamine analogs consisting of the pyrimidine ring of the original thiamine and another ring from the "cosubstrate." This thiamine-analog may be absorbed, inhibiting thiamine-requiring reactions (McCandless, 2010). Thiaminase II cleaves the vitamin at the methylene bridge between the thiazole and the pyrimidine rings.

Sulfur has been shown to be antagonistic to thiamine enzymes. The sulfite ion has been shown to cleave thiamine from enzymes at the methylene bridge and, analytically, will imitate thiaminase. Tall fescue (*Festuca arundinacea Schreb.*) toxicosis resembles diseases caused by elevated rumen thiaminase activity (Lauriault *et al.*, 1990). Certain microorganisms (bacteria and molds) and plants (bracken fern) have produced thiaminases.

In premixes that include choline and trace minerals, thiamine stability is relatively low, and at ambient temperature, its content may be reduced by up to 50%. This occurs to a greater extent in feed contaminated by mycotoxin-producing fungi such as *Aspergillus* and *Fusarium*, where the B_1 concentration can drop by a factor of up to 10 (Nagaraj *et al.*, 1994). Thiamine content was reduced from 43 to 50% for 2 cultivars of wheat infested with *Aspergillus flavus* compared to the uncontaminated sound wheat (Kao and Robinson, 1973).

More detailed reviews of the role of thiaminases in induced thiamine deficiency in ruminants are available (Frye *et al.*, 1991; Harmeyer and Kollenkirchen, 1989). Thiamine-deficient animals have elevated plasma pyruvate concentrations (Molina *et al.*, 1994) since, with this vitamin deficiency, there is an accumulation of intermediates of carbohydrate metabolism.

Safety
Thiamine ingested in large amounts orally is not toxic; the same is true of parenteral doses. Dietary intake of thiamine up to 1,000 times the requirement is safe for most animal species (NRC, 1998). The effects of excessive intakes of thiamine have not been studied in ruminants (NRC, 1998).

Vitamin B$_2$ (Riboflavin)
Chemical structure and properties
Riboflavin exists in 3 forms in nature: free dinucleotide riboflavin and the 2 coenzyme derivatives, flavin mononucleotide (FMN) and flavin adenine dinucleotide (FAD) (Pinto and Rivlin, 2013; Merrill and McCormik, 2020). It is composed of a dimethylisoalloxazine nucleus combined with ribitol. Riboflavin is a water-soluble, odorless, bitter, orange-yellow compound that melts at about 280°C. The molecular structure of riboflavin is shown in Figure 4.40.

Riboflavin is only slightly soluble in water but readily soluble in dilute basic or strongly acidic solutions. It is pretty stable to heat in neutral and acid but not alkaline solutions, and a tiny amount (3–4%) is lost in feed processing (Pinto and Rivlin, 2013). Aqueous solutions are unstable to visible and ultraviolet light, and instability is increased by heat and alkalinity. Both light and oxygen have been found to induce riboflavin degradation (Miquel Becker *et al.*, 2003). When dry, riboflavin is appreciably less affected by light. Riboflavin plays a crucial role in problems related to light sensitivity and the photodegradation of milk and dairy products. Both light and oxygen have been found to induce riboflavin degradation (Miquel Becker *et al.*, 2003; Domingos *et al.*, 2011).

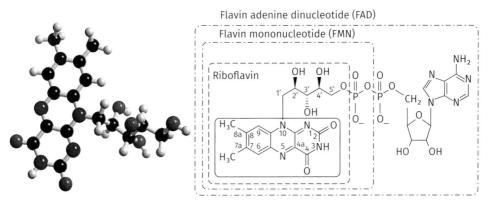

Figure 4.40 Vitamin B$_2$ chemical structure

Natural sources

Green plants, yeast, fungi, and some bacteria synthesize riboflavin. Rapidly growing, green leafy vegetables and forages, particularly alfalfa, are good sources, and the leaves have the highest riboflavin content. Cereals and their by-products have a relatively low riboflavin content, in contrast to their high thiamine content. Oilseed meals are fair sources, whereas grains and protein meals contain some riboflavin but should not be relied on as the sole sources of riboflavin.

Riboflavin is one of the more stable vitamins but can be rapidly destroyed by UV light or sunlight. Appreciable amounts may be lost upon exposure to light; up to one-half of the riboflavin content is lost in cooking, and most of the vitamin is lost in milk stored in transparent glass bottles (McDowell, 2000a). The riboflavin content of the milk of cows or goats is many times higher than in the diet due to rumen synthesis and probably also accumulation by the MG. Human milk contains about 0.5 mg of riboflavin per liter, while the riboflavin content of cow's milk is 3 times higher (i.e., 1.7 mg per liter).

Vitamin B$_2$ was first isolated from egg albumin in 1933 and subsequently detected in milk and liver. Riboflavin is found in appreciable quantities in green plants, by-products of animal origin (buttermilk 28 mg/kg, fishmeal between 5 and 10 mg/kg), and dehydrated alfalfa (alfalfa 15 mg/kg). Milling of rice and wheat results in considerable loss of riboflavin because most of the vitamin is in the germ and bran, which are removed during this process. About one-half of the riboflavin content is lost when rice is milled. Whole-wheat flour contains about two-thirds more riboflavin than white flour (McDowell, 2000a). Yeast, fungi, and some bacteria except *Lactobacilli*, including intestinal bacteria like *Faecalibacterium prausnitzii*, also synthesize riboflavin.

Commercial forms

Riboflavin is commercially available to the feed, food, and pharmaceutical industries as a feed-grade crystalline compound produced by chemical synthesis or fermentation, formulated in spray-dried powders containing 80% riboflavin. Riboflavin 5'-phosphate sodium salt (75–79% riboflavin) is available for applications requiring a water-dispersible source of riboflavin.

High-potency, USP, or feed-grade crystalline powders are electrostatic, hygroscopic, and dusty and, thus, do not flow freely and show poor distribution in feeds. In contrast, 80% of commercial spray-dried powders show reduced electrostaticity and hygroscopicity for better feed flowability and distribution (Adams, 1978).

Metabolism

Absorption and transport

Riboflavin covalently bound to protein is released by proteolytic digestion. Phosphatases hydrolyze phosphorylated forms (FAD, FMN) of riboflavin in the upper gastrointestinal tract to free the vitamin for absorption. Cells from deficient animals have a greater maximal absorption uptake of riboflavin (Rose *et al.*, 1986). At low concentrations, riboflavin absorption is an active carrier-mediated process. At high concentrations, however, riboflavin is absorbed by passive diffusion, proportional to concentration. Mucosal cells absorb free riboflavin via a dynamic, saturable transport system in all parts of the small intestine (Pinto and Rivlin, 2013). Free riboflavin is absorbed very efficiently throughout the small intestine. Riboflavin is phosphorylated to FMN in mucosal cells by the enzyme flavokinase (Rivlin, 2006). The FMN enters the portal system, is bound to plasma albumin, transported to the liver, and converted to FAD, the form most present in plasma and tissues.

Transport of flavin by blood plasma involves loose associations with albumin and tight associations with some globulins (McCormick, 1990). A genetically controlled riboflavin-binding protein is present in serum. Thyroid hormones, particularly triiodothyronine (T3), regulate the activities of the flavin biosynthetic enzymes, the synthesis of the apoflavoproteins, and the formation of covalently bound flavins (Pinto and Rivlin, 2013). Riboflavin-binding proteins have been reported to be present in the serum of pregnant cows (Merrill and McCormick, 2020).

Storage and excretion
Animals do not appear to be able to store appreciable amounts of riboflavin, with the liver, kidneys, and heart having the most significant concentrations. The liver, the primary storage site, contains about one-third of the total body riboflavin. Hepatic cells from deficient animals have a relatively greater maximal absorption uptake of riboflavin (Rose *et al.*, 1986). Hepatic cell riboflavin absorption occurs via facilitated diffusion.

Intakes of riboflavin above current needs are rapidly excreted in the urine, primarily as free riboflavin. Minor quantities of absorbed riboflavin are excreted in feces, bile, and sweat.

Biochemical functions
Riboflavin, in its phosphorylated form, FMN and FAD, or as a constituent of the flavoproteins, is a coenzyme and cofactor of more than 100 enzymes, namely flavoenzymes, involved in the transfer of electrons in redox reactions, in the metabolism of carbohydrates and amino acids and the synthesis and oxidation of fatty acids and transporting proteins (Pinto and Rivlin, 2013). Figure 4.41 shows the most critical functions of riboflavin.

The interaction of flavin coenzymes with their respective apoflavoproteins involves noncovalent and covalent associations, but only 25 have been identified as covalently linked. The conversion to FMN and FAD is regulated by nutritional status, particularly protein-calorie malnutrition, metabolic rate, hormones, and drugs. Flavoenzymes function within an eclectic array of cellular processes that involve (Pinto and Rivlin, 2013):

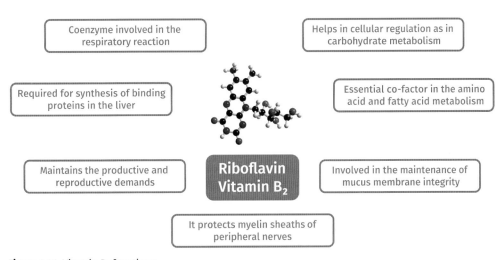

Coenzyme involved in the respiratory reaction

Helps in cellular regulation as in carbohydrate metabolism

Required for synthesis of binding proteins in the liver

Essential co-factor in the amino acid and fatty acid metabolism

Maintains the productive and reproductive demands

Riboflavin Vitamin B$_2$

Involved in the maintenance of mucus membrane integrity

It protects myelin sheaths of peripheral nerves

Figure 4.41 Vitamin B$_2$ functions

- electron transport, accepting and passing on hydrogen in the cytochrome system in the generations of ATP
- metabolism of lipids, drugs, and xenobiotic substances
- cell signaling
- protein folding.

If riboflavin levels are low, respiration becomes less efficient, and 10–15% more feed is required to meet energy needs (Christensen, 1983). The enzymes that function aerobically are called oxidases, and those that function anaerobically are called dehydrogenases. The general function is substrate oxidation and energy generation (*i.e.*, ATP). The flavoproteins show great versatility in accepting and transferring 1 or 2 electrons with various potentials in the mitochondria during the generation of ATP.

Many flavoproteins contain a metal (e.g., iron, molybdenum, copper, zinc). The combination of the flavin and metal ion is often involved in adjusting these enzymes in transfers between single- and double-electron donors. Xanthine oxidase contains the metals molybdenum and iron. It converts hypoxanthine to xanthine and the latter to uric acid. It also reacts with aldehydes to form acids, converting retinal (vitamin A aldehyde) to retinoic acid.

There is a close relationship between riboflavin and niacin because flavoproteins may accept a hydrogen ion (H^+) directly from the substrate, thus catalyzing the oxidation of the substrate, or it may catalyze the oxidation of some other enzyme by accepting a hydrogen ion from it. For example, from the niacin-containing coenzymes, nicotinamide adenine dinucleotide (NADH) and nicotinamide adenine dinucleotide phosphate (NADPH).

About 40 flavoprotein enzymes may be arbitrarily classified into 3 groups:

- NADH dehydrogenases: reduced pyridine nucleotide is a substrate, and the electron acceptor is either a member of the cytochrome system or some other acceptor besides oxygen
- dehydrogenases: accept electrons directly from the substrate and pass them to one of the cytochromes
- oxidases: accept electrons from the substrate and pass them directly to oxygen (O_2 is reduced to H_2O_2); they cannot reduce cytochromes.

Riboflavin functions in flavoprotein-enzyme systems to help regulate cellular metabolism, although they are also explicitly involved in the metabolism of carbohydrates. Riboflavin is also essential in amino acid metabolism as part of amino acid oxidases. These enzymes oxidize amino acids, which results in the decomposition of the amino acids, yielding ammonia and α-ketoacid. Distinct oxidized D-amino acids (prosthetic group FAD) and L-amino acids (prosthetic group FMN) are produced. In the methionine and homocysteine metabolism, riboflavin plays a coenzyme role in the same way as cobalamin, folate, and pyridoxine (Pinto and Rivlin, 2013).

Riboflavin not only is a critical link in the utilization of dietary folates and cobalamins but also controls homocysteine re-methylation and trans-sulphuration in association with methyl donor flavoenzymes within the one-carbon cycle as well as the FAD/FMN diflavin enzyme, MSR, the FAD-dependent N5, N10-methylenetetrahydrofolate reductase (MTHFR) necessary for methionine formation. This function affects cardiovascular disease and osteoporosis (Pinto and Rivlin, 2013).

In addition, riboflavin plays a role in fat metabolism (Rivlin, 2006), and a FAD flavoprotein is an essential link in fatty acid oxidation. This includes the acyl-coenzyme A dehydrogenases necessary for the stepwise degradation of fatty acids. An FMN flavoprotein is required for the synthesis of fatty acids from acetate. Thus, flavoproteins are needed to degrade and synthe-size fatty acids.

Riboflavin and other vitamins are essential in skin development, tensile strength, and heal-ing rates (Lakshmi *et al.*, 1989). A riboflavin deficiency can slow the epithelialization of wounds by 4–5 days (Lakshmi *et al.*, 1989), reduce collagen content by 25%, and decrease the tensile strength of injuries by 45%. Riboflavin deficiency can increase skin homocysteine by 2–4-fold, ultimately impairing collagen's crosslink formation (Lakshmi *et al.*, 1990). Marginal field defi-ciencies of riboflavin could increase skin tears, cause longer healing times, and ultimately increase costly downgrades.

Among the enzymes that require riboflavin is the FMN-dependent oxidase responsible for converting phosphorylated pyridoxine (vitamin B_6) to a functional coenzyme. Riboflavin defi-ciency also decreases the conversion of the vitamin B_6 coenzyme pyridoxal phosphate to the main vitamin B_6 urinary excretory product of 4-pyridoxic acid.

Riboflavin Coenzyme Q_{10} and niacin are associated with poly (ADP-ribose) polymer-ase (PARP), a family of proteins involved in several cellular processes, which function in post-translational modification of nuclear proteins. The poly ADP-ribosylated proteins func-tion in DNA repair, replication, and cell differentiation (Premkumar *et al.*, 2008; Pinto and Rivlin, 2013).

It plays a vital role in maintaining the integrity of mucous membranes and the nervous system (Pinto and Rivlin, 2013). It interacts with other vitamins: pyridoxine, niacin, and pan-tothenic acid. Riboflavin deficiency affects iron metabolism, with less iron absorbed and an increased rate of iron loss due to an accelerated rate of small intestinal epithelial turnover (Powers *et al.*, 1991; 1993).

Effects in ruminal fermentation

Dietary vitamins like riboflavin can stimulate ruminal cellulolytic microbial activity, improving growth performance and nutrient digestion. Wu *et al.* (2021) supplemented Holstein bulls with riboflavin at 0, 300, 600, and 900 mg/kg DM; Ren *et al.* (2022) supplemented lambs at 0, 15, 30, and 45 mg/kg DM; and Wang *et al.* (2022) supplemented Angus bulls with 0 or 60 mg riboflavin/kg DM and 0 or 35 mg pantothenate/kg DM in a factorial experiment. All research groups did not detect changes in voluntary feed intake. However, all of them observed improved BW daily gain and FCR. Total-tract DM, neutral-detergent fiber, acid detergent fiber, and crude protein digestibility increased linearly or quadratically. Rumen fermentation parameters were affected by dietary riboflavin in both experiments. Microbial enzymes and populations of fungi, proto-zoa, dominant cellulolytic bacteria, *Ruminobacter amylophilus*, and *Prevotella ruminicola* also increased linearly.

Nutritional assessment

The assessment of the riboflavin nutritional status is not simple, and it seems that the sensi-tivity to changes in riboflavin intake is relatively low. The typical functional test used the eryth-rocyte glutathione reductase activity coefficient (EGRac) assay, which allows for determining the degree of tissue saturation with riboflavin (Sauberlich, 1999).

The riboflavin vitamers – free riboflavin and the coenzymes FMN and FAD – can be analyzed directly in whole blood, serum (or homogenized erythrocytes), or urine (24 hour collection) using liquid chromatography coupled to tandem mass spectrometry (LC-MS/MS), and data can be compared with EGRac (Girard and Graulet, 2021). Correlations between plasma riboflavin and EGRac were good, and all vitamers but not FAD seem suitable to assess riboflavin status (Höller *et al.*, 2018).

Deficiency signs

Riboflavin is not required in the diet of adult ruminants *per se* because of rumen synthesis. Responses to supplemental riboflavin in animals with a functional rumen are smaller, but with present-day high-yield milk production and fast growth rates, the responses have been significant (Wu *et al.*, 2021; Ren *et al.*, 2022, 2023; Wang *et al.*, 2022; 2023). Miller *et al.* (1986) reported that cattle on a concentrate-silage diet would synthesize approximately 38 mg of riboflavin in the rumen. A dairy cow producing 42 kg of milk daily loses about 72 mg of riboflavin in milk alone, much more than consumed in the diet.

Riboflavin deficiencies have been demonstrated in young ruminants whose rumen flora is not yet established. Riboflavin deficiency results in redness of the mouth mucosa, lesions in the corner of the mouth and around the edges of the lips and navel, loss of hair, and excessive tear and saliva production (Radostits and Bell, 1970). Nonspecific signs are anorexia, chronic diarrhea, and reduced growth.

Riboflavin deficiency affects iron metabolism, with less iron absorbed and an increased rate of iron loss due to an accelerated rate of small intestinal epithelial turnover (Christensen, 1973; Powers *et al.*, 1991, 1993). A primary dietary riboflavin deficiency has broad implications for other vitamins, as flavin coenzymes participate in the metabolism of 5 vitamins: folic acid, vitamin B_6, vitamin K, niacin, and vitamin D (Pinto and Rivlin, 2013). Signs of lack of vitamin B_2 are pretty unspecific. Usually, they involve the tissues and functions most dependent on energy from carbohydrates: epithelial and nervous tissue and reproduction functions. Signs typically include loss of appetite, growth retardation, poorer feed conversion, vomiting, dermatitis, alopecia, inflammation of the anal mucosa, etc.

Safety

Much evidence has accumulated that supplementation with riboflavin over nutritional requirements has little toxicity for animals and humans (Pinto and Rivlin, 2013). Most data from rats suggest that dietary levels between 10 and 20 times the requirement (possibly 100 times) can be tolerated safely (NRC, 1998). When massive amounts of riboflavin are administered orally, only a tiny fraction of the dose is absorbed, the remainder excreted in the feces.

Lack of toxicity is probably because the transport system necessary for riboflavin absorption across the gastrointestinal mucosa becomes saturated, limiting riboflavin absorption (Christensen, 1973). Also, the capacity of tissues to store riboflavin and its coenzyme derivatives appears to be limited when excessive amounts are administered.

Vitamin B_6 (pyridoxine)
Chemical structure and properties

The term vitamin B_6 refers to a group of 3 pyridine derivatives named according to the functional group in the position 4 (Dakshinamurti and Dakshinamurti, 2013):

- pyridoxol or pyridoxine (PN), the alcohol form
- pyridoxal (PL), the aldehyde form
- pyridoxamine (PM), the amine form.

These 3 compounds have a similar vitamin activity and are interconvertible in the animal's body. Pyridoxine is the predominant plant form, whereas pyridoxal and pyridoxamine are vitamin forms generally found in animal products.

Three additional vitamin B_6 forms are the phosphorylated forms pyridoxine 5'-phosphate (PNP), pyridoxal-5'-phosphate, or codecarboxylase (PLP), and pyridoxamine 5'-phosphate

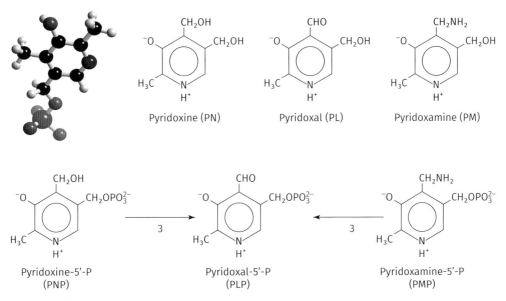

Figure 4.42 Vitamin B₆ chemical structure

(PMP). The natural, free forms of the vitamers could be converted to the critical coenzymatic form, PLP, by the action of 2 enzymes, a kinase, and an oxidase. Various forms of vitamin B₆ found in animal tissues are interconvertible, with vitamin B₆ metabolically active mainly as PLP and, to a lesser degree, as PMP (Figure 4.42).

Vitamin B₆ is stable to heat, acid, and alkali; however, exposure to light is highly destructive, especially in neutral or alkaline media. The free base and the commonly available hydrochloride salt are soluble in water and alcohol (Rosenberg, 2012).

Natural sources

Vitamin B₆ is widely distributed in feedstuffs. Most vitamin B₆ in animal products is in the form of pyridoxal and pyridoxamine phosphates, whereas in plants and seeds, the usual form is pyridoxine (McDowell, 2000a). The vitamin B₆ present in cereal grains (barley 3 mg/kg, corn 6 mg/kg, sorghum 3 mg/kg, oats 1 mg/kg) is concentrated mainly in bran, with the rest containing only tiny amounts. Most ingredients are reliable sources of this vitamin, but its bioavailability is relatively low (40–60%) in soybean meal is 65%, and in corn, it varies from 45 to 56% (Chen, Y.F. et al., 2019).

The principal source of vitamin B₆ for ruminants is microbial synthesis in the rumen. In an experiment in which sheep were fed a diet containing 1.5 mg of vitamin B₆ per kg McElroy and Goss (1939) measured 6–10 mg per kg of vitamin B₆ in dried rumen contents. Working on cattle, McElroy and Goss (1940) measured 8–10 mg of vitamin B₆ per kg of dried rumen contents in animals fed 1–1.5 mg per kg of vitamin B₆ in the diet. Ewes maintained on a diet containing little vitamin B₆ yielded milk that contained as much vitamin B₆ as the milk of ewes fed regular diets.

For young ruminants, milk is a useful source of vitamin B₆. Cow's milk contains approximately 0.30 mg of vitamin B₆ per liter (Gregory, 1975). Therefore, a 50-kg calf-fed milk at 10% of BW would receive approximately 1.75 mg of vitamin B₆. Both the NRC (2001) and NASEM (2021) recommend 6.5 mg of pyridoxine per kg of in calf milk replacer powder, providing the typical dairy calf with approximately 3 mg of vitamin B₆ daily.

Levels of vitamin B_6 contained in feedstuffs are also affected by processing and subsequent storage. Loss during processing, refining, and storage has been reported to be as high as 70% (Shideler, 1983) or in the range of 0 to 40% (Birdsall, 1975). Of the several forms, pyridoxine is far more stable than either pyridoxal or pyridoxamine. Therefore, the processing losses of vitamin B_6 tend to be highly variable (9 to 40%), with plant-derived foods (which mostly contain pyridoxine) losing little if any of the vitamin and animal products (mostly pyridoxal and pyridoxamine) losing large quantities (Ollilainen, 1999; Gregory and Ink, 1987). The bioavailability of feedstuffs can be as low as 40 to 50% after heating. There was slight difference in availability between corn samples not heated and those heated to 120°C. However, corn heated to 160°C contained significantly less available B_6. Losses may be caused, besides heat, also by light and various agents promoting oxidation. Blanching of rehydrated lima beans resulted in a loss of 20% of vitamin B_6, but, more significantly, the availability of the vitamin was reduced by almost 50% (Ekanayake and Nelson, 1990).

Pyridoxine-5'-β-D-glucoside (PNG), a conjugated form of vitamin B_6, is abundant in various plant-derived foods (McCormick, 2006). This form of B_6 may account for up to 50% of the total vitamin B_6 content of oilseeds such as soybeans and sunflower seeds. The utilization of dietary PNG relative to pyridoxine is 30% in rats and 50% in humans (Gregory et al., 1991a). The glycosylated PNG can quantitatively alter the metabolism of pyridoxine in vivo. Hence, it partially impairs the metabolic utilization of co-ingested non-glycosylated forms of vitamin B_6 (Nakano and Gregory, 1995; Nakano et al., 1997).

There are several vitamin B_6 antagonists, which either compete for reactive sites of apoenzymes or react with PLP to form inactive compounds. The presence of a vitamin B_6 antagonist in linseed meals is of particular interest to animal nutritionists. This substance was identified in 1967 as linatine, I-(N-γ-L-glutamyl) amino)-D-proline and was found to have antibiotic properties (Parsons and Klostermann, 1967). Pesticides (e.g., carbaryl, propoxur, or thiram) can be antagonistic to vitamin B_6. Feeding a diet enriched with vitamin B_6 prevented disturbances in the active transport of methionine in rats intoxicated with pesticides (Witkowska et al., 1992; Dakshinamurti and Dakshinamurti, 2013).

Commercial forms

Commercially, vitamin B_6 is available as a fine crystalline powder of pyridoxine hydrochloride 99% and in dilutions. Supplemental vitamin B_6 is reported to have higher bioavailability and stability than naturally occurring vitamins. Pyridoxine hydrochloride contains 82.3% vitamin B_6 activity. Dry premixes are used in feeds, and the crystalline product is used in parenteral and oral pharmaceuticals.

Metabolism
Absorption and transport

Little information is available on the digestion and absorption of vitamin B_6 in ruminants; however, significant quantities of the vitamin are synthesized in the rumen. Digestion of vitamin B_6 would first involve splitting the vitamin, as it is bound to the protein portion of the feed. The 3 vitamin B_6 compounds are absorbed from the diet in dephosphorylated forms, carried to the liver by enterohepatic circulation, where they convert mainly to pyridoxal phosphate. Both niacin and vitamin B_2 participate in this conversion. The small intestine is rich in alkaline phosphatases for the dephosphorylation reaction.

Sakurai et al. (1992) reported that a physiological dose of pyridoxamine was rapidly transformed into pyridoxal in the intestinal tissues and then released in the form of pyridoxal into the portal blood. Vitamin B_6 is absorbed mainly in the jejunum and the ileum by passive diffusion. Absorption from the colon is insignificant, even though colon microflora synthesizes the vitamin.

After absorption, B_6 compounds quickly appear in the liver, where they are mostly converted into PLP, considered the most active vitamin form in metabolism. Under normal conditions, most of the vitamin B_6 in the blood is present as PLP, which is linked to proteins, largely albumin in the plasma and hemoglobin in the red blood cells (McCormick, 2006). Both niacin, as MADPH-dependent enzyme, and riboflavin, as the flavoprotein pyridoxamine phosphate oxidase, are essential for the conversion of vitamin B_6 forms and phosphorylation reactions (Kodentsova et al., 1993).

Although other tissues also contribute to vitamin B_6 metabolism, the liver is responsible for forming PLP found in plasma. Pyridoxal and PLP found in circulation are associated primarily with plasma albumin and red blood cell hemoglobin (Mehansho and Henderson, 1980). Pyridoxal phosphate is the primary B_6 form in goat milk, accounting for 75% of the vitamin B_6 activity (Coburn et al., 1992). These authors disagree on whether pyridoxal or PLP is the transport form of B_6.

Storage and excretion
Vitamin B_6 is widely distributed in various tissues, mainly as PLP or pyridoxamine phosphate, with the majority stored principally in muscular tissue. Only small quantities of vitamin B_6 are stored in the body. Pyridoxal phosphate accounts for 60% of plasma vitamin B_6. Excess dietary vitamin B_6 increased whole-muscle total PLP. Pyridoxic acid is the major excretory metabolite of the vitamin, eliminated via the urine. Also, small quantities of pyridoxol, pyridoxal, pyridoxamine, and phosphorylated derivatives are excreted in urine (Henderson, 1984).

Vitamin B_6 metabolism is altered in renal failure, as observed in rats exhibiting plasma pyridoxal phosphate 43% lower than controls (Wei and Young, 1994). Bacterially fermentable substrates from wheat bran induced a higher bacterial vitamin B_6 synthesis than cellulose.

Biochemical functions
Vitamin B_6, primarily as PLP and, to a lesser extent, as PMP, plays an essential role in the amino acid, carbohydrate, and fatty acid metabolism and the energy-producing citric acid cycle, with over 60 enzymes known to depend on vitamin B_6 coenzymes. Pyridoxal phosphate functions in practically all reactions involved in amino acid metabolism, including transamination, decarboxylation, deamination, desulfhydration, and the cleavage or synthesis of amino acids. The largest group of vitamin B_6-dependent enzymes are transaminases. Aminotransferase participates in the interconversion of a pair of amino acids into their corresponding keto acids, e.g., amino groups transferred from aspartate to α-ketoglutarate forming oxaloacetate and glutamate (McCormick, 2006; Dakshinamurti and Dakshinamurti, 2013).

The minimum requirements of vitamin B_6 have been proposed for rations with moderate protein levels and a balanced amino acid relationship (Witkowska et al., 1992). The recommendations for vitamin B_6 supply increase with feeds with high protein levels or an amino acid profile distant from the ideal protein since more enzymes are needed to metabolize the excess amino acids, which depend on vitamin B_6.

Non-oxidative decarboxylations involve PLP as a coenzyme, e.g., converting amino acids into biogenic amines such as histamine, serotonin, γ-aminobutyric acid (GABA), and taurine.

Vitamin B_6 participates in functions that include (Marks, 1975; Driskell, 1984; McCormick, 2006; Dakshinamurti and Dakshinamurti, 2013):

- deaminases: for serine, threonine, and cystathionine
- desulfydrases and transulfurases: interconversion
- synthesis of niacin from tryptophan: hydroxykynurenine is not converted to hydroxyanthranilic acid but rather to xanthurenic acid due to a lack of the B_6-dependent enzyme, kynureninase (Miller *et al.*, 1957; Harmon *et al.*, 1969)
- formation of α-aminolevulinic acid from succinyl-CoA and glycine, the first step in porphyrin synthesis
- conversion of linoleic to arachidonic acid in the metabolism of essential fatty acids (this function is controversial)
- glycogen phosphorylase catalyzes glycogen breakdown to glucose-1-phosphate. Pyridoxal phosphate does not appear to be a coenzyme for the enzyme but rather affects the enzyme conformation
- synthesis of epinephrine and norepinephrine from either phenylalanine or tyrosine – both norepinephrine and epinephrine participate in carbohydrate metabolism and other body reactions
- racemases – PLP-dependent racemases enable certain microorganisms to utilize D-amino acids. Racemases have not yet been detected in mammalian tissues
- transmethylation involving methionine
- incorporation of iron in hemoglobin synthesis
- formation of antibodies – B_6 deficiency inhibits the synthesis of globulins that carry antibodies
- inflammation – higher vitamin B_6 levels were linked to protection against inflammation (Morris *et al.*, 2010)
- decarboxylation of tryptophan to serotonin (McDowell, 2000a).

Neurological functions

Pyridoxine is a coenzyme of several enzymes involved in the endogenous production of hydrogen sulfide, dopamine, norepinephrine, serotonin (5-hydroxytryptamine; 5-HT), and GABA, as well as taurine, sphingolipids, and polyamines, which are molecules involved in cell signaling in the central nervous system (Dakshinamurti and Dakshinamurti, 2013).

Neurological disorders, including states of agitation and convulsions, result from reduced B_6 enzymes in the brain, including glutamate decarboxylase and γ-aminobutyric acid transaminase. Dopamine release is delayed with a vitamin B_6 deficiency, contributing to motor abnormalities (Tang and Wei, 2004). Maternal restriction of B_6 in rats adversely affected synaptogenesis, neurogenesis, neuron longevity, and progeny differentiation (Groziak and Kirksey, 1987; 1990).

Effects on immunity and as an antioxidant

Animal and human studies suggest a vitamin B_6 deficiency affects both humoral and cell-mediated immune responses. In humans, vitamin B_6 depletion significantly decreased the percentage and the total number of lymphocytes mitogenic responses of peripheral blood lymphocytes to T- and B-cell mitogens and interleukin 2 production (Meydani *et al.*, 1991; Paul and Dey, 2015).

The role of PLP in affecting one-carbon metabolism is important in nucleic acid biosynthesis and immune system function. The PLP is also needed for gluconeogenesis by way of transaminases active on glucogenic amino acids and for lipid metabolism that involves several aspects of PLP function: for example, the production of carnitine needed to act as a vector for long-chain fatty acids for mitochondrial β-oxidation and of certain bases for phospholipid biosynthesis (McCormick, 2006).

Vitamin B$_6$ has antioxidant properties by inhibiting superoxide radicals, preventing lipid peroxidation, protein glycosylation, and Na$^+$, K$^+$-ATPase activity in high glucose–treated erythrocytes and hydrogen peroxide–treated monocytes and endothelial cells (Dakshinamurti and Dakshinamurti, 2013).

Metabolism of homocysteine and cardiovascular function

Vitamin B$_6$ has a significant role in the metabolism of amino acids, which includes essential interactions with endogenous redox reactions through its effects on the GPX system. In fact, B$_6$-dependent enzymes catalyze most reactions of the transsulfuration pathway, driving homocysteine (Hcy) to cysteine and further into GPX proteins. Hcy is a sulfur-containing amino acid formed during the metabolism of methionine. Pyridoxine is required as a coenzyme for the 2 key steps of the transsulfuration pathway catalyzed by cystathionine synthetase and cystathionine γ-lyase. In this metabolic pathway, several B vitamins are involved (Figure 4.43).

Since mammals metabolize sulfur- and seleno-amino acids similarly, this vitamin plays a vital role in the fate of sulfur-Hcy and its seleno counterpart between transsulfuration and one-carbon metabolism, especially under oxidative stress conditions. This is particularly important in reproduction because ovarian metabolism may produce excess ROS during the peri-estrus period, impairing ovulatory functions and early embryo development. Later in gestation, placentation raises embryo oxygen tension and may induce a higher expression of ROS markers and, eventually, embryo losses (Dalto and Matte, 2017).

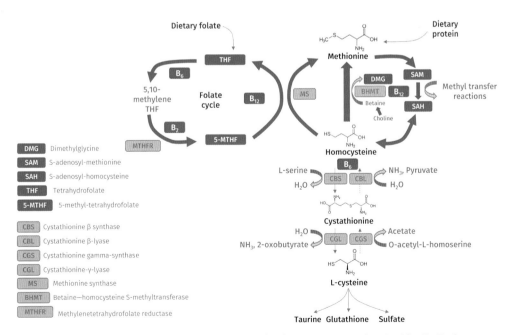

Figure 4.43 Folate, trans-sulphuration, and choline oxidation pathways are involved in riboflavin, pyridoxine, cobalamin, and choline

Pyridoxine deficiency may increase blood pressure by stimulating smooth muscle in the blood vessels, creating endothelial dysfunction, generating reactive oxygen species, and increasing susceptibility to oxidation. Hcy also enhances collagen synthesis, altering the elastin/collagen ratio, which contributes to the changes in the vessel wall that lead to systemic vascular resistance and hypertension (Dakshinamurti and Dakshinamurti, 2013).

As part of its role in amino acid metabolism, vitamin B_6 converts tryptophan to niacin, which again suggests the close relationship between different B complex vitamins and probably an association in the requirements of some of them. Vitamin B_6 is also involved in the formation of adrenaline and noradrenaline from phenylalanine and tyrosine, in the transmethylation sulphuration of methionine, and the incorporation of iron into the hemoglobin and myoglobin heme group. On the other hand, there is evidence to suggest the role of vitamin B_6 in the conversion of linoleic acid to arachidonic acid and forming antibodies.

Ruminal microbial metabolism
Numerous microorganisms require vitamin B_6 and appear to play a role in rumen metabolism. The saccharolytic rumen bacterium, *Butyrivibrio fibrisolvens*, requires vitamin B_6, biotin, and folic acid (Baldwin and Allison, 1983). Vitamin B_6 enhanced the *in vitro* production of phenylalanine from its precursors, phenyl pyruvic acid and phenylacetic acid, in mixed rumen bacteria and protozoa (Ruhul Amin and Onodera, 1998).

Nutritional assessment
The 6 interconvertible forms of vitamin B_6 can be measured in plasma to assess nutritional status. Still, PLP is the vitamer customarily used, and its measurement in erythrocytes seems to provide a more appropriate evaluation (Sauberlich, 1999).

However, considering the complex metabolic pathways in which vitamin B_6 is involved, ratios between metabolites, or the possibility of quantifying numerous amino acids and metabolites related to PLP-dependent pathways, may provide a better insight into nutritional status (Höller *et al.*, 2018). Parameters to evaluate vitamin B_6 metabolism include fecal and urinary vitamin B_6 concentration and excretion, vitamin B_6 concentration in blood, hematological criteria, the activity of aspartate aminotransferase in erythrocytes, and xanthurenic acid excretion in the tryptophan load test.

Deficiency signs
Vitamin B_6 deficiency gives rise to several unspecific signs, including appetite loss, growth retardation, dermatitis, hair loss, epileptic-like convulsions, and anemia (Rosenberg, 2012; Chawla and Kvarnberg, 2014). Given its leading role in amino acid metabolism, deficiency in this vitamin is associated with a decreased capacity to utilize protein and impairment of tryptophan and niacin metabolism, with a marked drop in the nitrogen balance.

Due to rumen microbial synthesis, vitamin B_6 deficiency in ruminants with a functioning rumen has not been reported in the literature. When selected experimental diets are used, vitamin B_6 is essential for the young calf. Calves reared on a milk replacer lost their appetite within 2 to 4 weeks, their growth was impaired, and they progressively showed apathy, diarrhea, anorexia, and incoordination. In the last stages, convulsions were soon followed by death (Johnson *et al.*, 1947). The convulsions included thrashing the legs and head and grinding the teeth (Johnson *et al.*, 1950).

Postmortem examination of vitamin B_6-deficient calves revealed hemorrhages in the epicardium and the kidneys, demyelination of the peripheral nerves, the proliferation of Schwann cells, desquamation of the intestinal mucosa, and pneumonia (Johnson *et al.*, 1950). Analyses of the urine from the vitamin B_6-deficient calves showed significantly reduced excretion of pyridoxine, pyridoxal, pyridoxamine, and pyridoxic acid (the major excretory metabolite).

In the preliminary stages of a vitamin B_6 deficiency in calves, animals fully recovered after an oral dose of 100 mg of vitamin B_6 (Johnson *et al.*, 1950). However, if this treatment was delayed until the occurrence of convulsive seizures, it was no longer possible to save the calf, even when the vitamin was administered by injection, indicating that irreparable damage had occurred.

An indication of a vitamin B_6 deficiency is elevated urinary levels of xanthurenic acid and kynurenic acid, indicating incomplete conversion of tryptophan. This evaluation is called the tryptophan-loading test. Vitamin B_6 participates in the incorporation of iron into hemoglobin and the synthesis of immunoglobulins, so its deficiency will cause blood alterations. For status evaluation, Driskell (1984) concluded that the best assessment parameter for vitamin B_6 status in clinical cases is the measurement of either the coenzyme stimulation or erythrocyte alanine aminotransferase activity or PLP level.

When vitamin B_6 deficiency reaches an advanced stage (probably due to degeneration of the peripheral nerves), disordered movement and ataxia appear. Finally, convulsions develop irregularly but are stimulated by excitement, as they are most often observed at feeding time. Between these convulsions, animals lie down and are apathetic and unresponsive (Bräunlich, 1974).

There are vitamin B_6 antagonists that either compete for reactive sites of apoenzymes or react with PLP to form inactive compounds. The presence of a vitamin B_6 antagonist in linseed is of particular interest to animal nutritionists. In 1967, this substance was identified as hydrazic acid and was found to have antibiotic properties (Parsons and Klostermann, 1967).

Safety

Insufficient data are available to support estimates of the maximum dietary tolerable levels of vitamin B_6 for ruminants. It is suggested, primarily from dog and rat data, that nutritional levels are at least 50 times the dietary requirements and are safe for most species (NRC, 1987).

Signs of toxicity, which occur most obviously in the peripheral nervous system, include changes in gait and peripheral sensation (Krinke and Fitzgerald, 1988; Xu *et al.*, 1989), ataxia, muscle weakness, and incoordination at levels approaching 1,000 times the requirement (Dakshinamurti and Dakshinamurti, 2013). Changes in central nervous system function were detected in rats fed excessive vitamin B_6, using measurement techniques of startle behavior (Schaeffer, 1993).

Vitamin B_{12} (cobalamin)
Chemical structure and properties

Nutritionists now consider vitamin B_{12} as the generic name for a group of compounds with vitamin B_{12} activity where the cobalt atom is in the center of the corrin nucleus (cobalt-containing corrinoids), containing 4 rings. When there is a cyanide group bound to cobalt, it is referred to as cobalamin. Cobalamin has a molecular weight of 1,355 and is the most complex structure and heaviest compound of all vitamins (Figure 4.44). The empirical formula of vitamin B_{12} is $C_{63}H_{88}O_{14}N_{14}PCo$, and its unusual feature is the content of 4.5% cobalt. The reference product is cobalamin, and requirements and concentrations are expressed in mass units (usually µg/kg).

Vitamin B_{12} is a dark-red crystalline hygroscopic substance, freely soluble in water and alcohol but insoluble in acetone, chloroform, and ether. Oxidizing and reducing agents and exposure to sunlight tend to destroy its activity. Losses of vitamin B_{12} during feed processing are

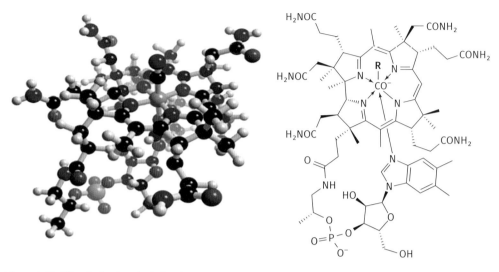

Figure 4.44 Vitamin B$_{12}$ chemical structure

usually not excessive because vitamin B$_{12}$ is stable at temperatures as high as 250°C, being the most stable vitamin during feed pelleting and storage processes (Lewis *et al.*, 2015).

Adenosylcobalamin and methylcobalamin are naturally occurring forms of vitamin B$_{12}$ in feedstuffs and animal tissues. Tissue metabolism converts cobalamin to the 2 primary coenzyme forms, adenosylcobalamin and methylcobalamin (Ellenbogen and Cooper, 1991). Cobalamin is not a naturally occurring form of the vitamin but is the most widely used form of cobalamin in clinical practice because of its relative availability and stability (Green and Miller, 2013). Structurally similar vitamin B$_{12}$ antagonists are produced by bacteria such as *Streptomyces griseus*, *E. coli*, and *Propionibacterium shermanii*. All these compounds contain a cobalt atom stabilized within a corrin ring structure similar to the porphyrin ring of hemoglobin and the cytochromes (Ellenbogen and Cooper, 1991).

Natural sources
Feedstuffs of animal origin, like meat, liver, kidney, milk, eggs, fish, or microorganisms, are reasonably good sources of vitamin B$_{12}$. The kidney and liver are excellent sources; these organs are richer in vitamin B$_{12}$ from ruminants than monogastrics. Vitamin B$_{12}$ presence in the tissues of animals is due to the ingestion of vitamin B$_{12}$ in animal feeds or from intestinal synthesis. The richest sources are fermentation residues, activated sewage sludge, and manure.

The concentration in fishmeal can reach more than 500 µg/kg, but in by-products of the dairy industry, it is much lower (for example, in whey, it barely reaches 10 µg/ kg). It is essential to point out the high variability in the concentration of this vitamin in the feedstuffs indicated. In a meat meal, the concentration is around 100 µg, while in bloodmeal, it exceeds 400 µg/kg.

The origin of vitamin B$_{12}$ in nature is bacterial synthesis. Yeast and fungi do not appear to synthesize vitamin B$_{12}$. Plant products are practically devoid of B$_{12}$. The vitamin B$_{12}$ reported in higher plants in tiny amounts may result from synthesis by soil microorganisms and excretion of the vitamin onto the soil, with subsequent absorption by the plant. The root nodules of certain legumes contain small quantities of vitamin B$_{12}$. Certain seaweed species (algae) have been reported to contain appreciable amounts of vitamin B$_{12}$ (up to 1 µg per gram of solids).

Seaweed does not synthesize vitamin B_{12}; it is synthesized by the bacteria associated with seaweed and then concentrated by the seaweed (Bito and Watanabe, 2022). Dagnelie *et al.* (1991) reported that vitamin B_{12} from algae is largely unavailable.

Unlike other B complex vitamins, cobalamin is synthesized almost exclusively by bacteria. It is, therefore, present only in foods that have been bacterially fermented or derived from animals that have obtained this vitamin from their gastrointestinal microflora or diet. There is no convincing evidence that the vitamin is produced in the tissues of animals. Microbial synthesis of vitamin B_{12} in the alimentary tract is of considerable importance to ruminants and species that practice coprophagy.

Evidence suggests that the amount and type of roughage in the diet affects the rumen synthesis of vitamin B_{12} even when cobalt is adequate. Restricted roughage rations have been reported to increase vitamin B_{12} levels in rumen fluid and serum, reduce milk and liver concentrations, and increase urinary excretion compared to cows fed roughage *ad libitum* (Walker and Elliot, 1972). Vitamin B_{12} levels in the rumen of dairy heifers fed corn silage are 1.4 to 2.7 times higher than when fed chopped or pelleted hay (Dryden and Hartman, 1970).

Jiang *et al.* (2022) identified 2,366 high-quality microbial genomes linked to vitamin B and K_2 synthesis. They found that only a few microbial genomes possessed complete *de novo* biosynthesis pathway of cobalamin. Yet, most genomes can utilize cobalamin via cobalamin transporters or cobalamin-dependent enzymes. Moreover, only cobalamin biosynthesis was reduced in the rumen microbiome of dairy cattle fed with the high-grain diet, suggesting that dietary fiber is vital for cobalamin biosynthesis. Therefore, these findings provided novel insights into regulating specific microflora, genes, and diet strategies for manipulation to improve the production of these essential vitamins in ruminants.

Cobalt is the primary dietary precursor of vitamin B_{12} in the ruminant. Although dietary cobalt of confined livestock is usually adequate, cobalt and secondary vitamin B_{12} deficiency are significant problems for grazing livestock worldwide (McDowell, 2000a; McDowell and Arthington, 2005). The concentration of cobalt in forages is affected by soil properties, plant species, stage of maturity, yield, pasture management, and climate. Soil levels of less than 2 ppm cobalt are considered deficient for ruminants (Correa, 1957). Liming soils increases the pH, reduces the uptake of cobalt by plants, and may increase the severity of a deficiency. Plants grown on soil containing 15 ppm cobalt with neutral or slightly acid pH can contain more cobalt than plants grown with 40 ppm cobalt and an alkaline pH (Latteur, 1962). Heavy rainfall tends to leach cobalt from the topsoil. This problem is often aggravated by the rapid growth of forage crops during the rainy season, further diluting the cobalt content of the diet. Plants have varying degrees of affinity for cobalt; some can concentrate the element much more than others. Legumes, for example, generally have an extraordinary ability to concentrate cobalt compared to grasses (Underwood, 1977). The nitrogen-fixing bacteria in the root nodules of legumes require cobalt. High dietary potassium levels induced a transient, 6-week reduction in plasma vitamin B_{12} concentrations (Smit *et al.*, 1999).

Commercial forms

Commercial sources of vitamin B_{12} are produced from fermentation products, available as cobalamin, the most stable form of this vitamin. Little is known about the bioavailability of orally ingested B_{12} in feeds. Vitamin B_{12} is produced by fermentation and is available commercially as cobalamin. Vitamin B_{12} is only slightly sensitive to heat, oxygen, moisture, and pH (Gadient, 1986). Vitamin B_{12} has good stability in premixes with or without minerals, regardless of the source of the minerals, and is little affected by pelleting (Scott, 1966; Verbeeck, 1975). However, Yamada *et al.* (2008) reported degradation of supplemental vitamin B_{12}; the vitamin was affected by storage time, light exposure, temperature, and vitamin C. It was determined that some vitamin B_{12} might have been converted into vitamin B_{12} analogs.

Metabolism
Ruminal metabolism
On average, 3% of dietary cobalt is converted to vitamin B_{12}, and only 1–3% of the vitamin B_{12} synthesized in the rumen is absorbed from the small intestine (Girard, 1998). Ruminal microflora also uses dietary cobalt to produce different molecules, called analogs, closely related to cobalamin but without biological activity for the host. Increasing dietary cobalt supply increases the production of these analogs in the rumen at the expense of the biologically active forms of the vitamin. Most analogs are inactive for the host, but a few studies indicate that some could have harmful effects. In addition to cobalamin, the only biologically active molecule for the cow, 7 analogs were identified in duodenal and ileal digesta (Girard et al., 2009). Although cobalamin was not the primary form synthesized by ruminal microflora, even if supplementary cobalamin was extensively destroyed by ruminal microflora, based on calculations of apparent intestinal disappearance, cobalamin seems to be the effective form absorbed in the small intestine.

Absorption and transport
The dietary vitamin B_{12} binds to salivary protein. As the salivary protein is digested, the B_{12} is freed and bound to an unknown intrinsic factor secreted by the gastric parietal cells. Digesting this vitamin first requires the release of the vitamin, frequently found in a protein matrix, by the action of digestive proteases, mainly trypsin.

The absorptive site for dietary or ruminal vitamin B_{12} is the ileum, the lower portion of the small intestine. Substantial amounts of B_{12} are secreted into the duodenum and then reabsorbed in the ileum. This is a process presumably needed for regulation based on the vitamin B_{12} status of the animal. Passing vitamin B_{12} through the intestinal wall is a complex procedure and requires the intervention of particular carrier compounds able to bind the vitamin molecule (McDowell, 2000a). In most species, for the absorption of vitamin B_{12}, the following is required (Green and Miller, 2013):

- adequate quantities of dietary cobalt, much of dietary vitamin B_{12} (e.g., cobalamin) is destroyed by ruminal microflora (Girard et al., 2009)
- a functional abomasum for digestion of food proteins, the release of vitamin B_{12}, and the production of the intrinsic factor for absorption of vitamin B_{12} through the ileum
- functional pancreas (trypsin secretion) is required for the release of bound vitamin B_{12} before combining the vitamin with the intrinsic factor
- functional ileum with receptor and absorption sites.

Gastric juice defects are responsible for most cases of food-vitamin B_{12} malabsorption in monogastrics (Carmel, 1994). Factors that diminish vitamin B_{12} absorption include protein, iron, vitamin B_6 deficiencies, thyroid removal, and dietary tannic acid (Hoffmann-La Roche, 1984).

There are structural differences in the vitamin B_{12} intrinsic factors among species. Intrinsic factor has been demonstrated in the cow but not the sheep. Factors that diminish vitamin B_{12} absorption include deficiencies of protein, iron, and vitamin B_6; thyroid removal/hypothyroidism; dietary tannic acid. Cobalamin analogs may compose up to 50% of the total plasma vitamin B_{12} in cattle but are undetectable in sheep (Halpin et al., 1984).

Therefore, intrinsic factor concentrates prepared from the stomach of one animal species do not always increase B_{12} absorption in other animal species or humans. Similarly, there are species differences in vitamin B_{12} transport proteins (Polak *et al.*, 1979; Green and Miller, 2013). Vitamin B_{12} is bound to transcobalamin (TC) and haptocorrin (HC) for transport in the blood, with about 20% being attached to TC and the rest to HC. The TC-bound cobalamin is the form most actively transported into tissues.

Storage and excretion

The storage of vitamin B_{12} is found principally in the liver, and other storage sites include the kidney, heart, spleen, and brain (Green and Miller, 2013). Even though vitamin B_{12} is water-soluble, Kominato (1971) reported a tissue half-life of 32 days, indicating considerable tissue storage. Cattle and sheep with regular liver stores can tolerate a cobalt-deficient diet for several months without showing vitamin B_{12} deficiency signs.

Andrews *et al.* (1960) reported that the proportion of liver cobalt that occurs as vitamin B_{12} varies with the cobalt status of the animal. In cattle or sheep grazing cobalt-adequate pastures, most of the cobalt in the liver is in the form of vitamin B_{12}. However, in cobalt deficiency, only about 33% of liver cobalt is vitamin B_{12}. This indicates that vitamin B_{12} is depleted during cobalt deficiency more rapidly than other forms of cobalt in the liver.

In ruminants, cobalt and vitamin B_{12} are excreted primarily in the feces, with smaller amounts excreted in urine (Smith and Marston, 1970). Urinary excretion of the intact vitamin B_{12} by kidney glomerular filtration is minimal. Biliary excretion via feces is the major excretory route. Lactating cows fed typical diets excrete 86–87.5% of all excreted cobalt in the feces (mainly associated with bile acids), 0.9–1.0% in the urine, and 11.5–12.5% in milk.

Biochemical functions

Vitamin B_{12} is essential to several enzyme systems that perform several basic metabolic functions. Although the essential tasks of vitamin B_{12} concern the metabolism of nucleic acids and proteins, it also functions in the metabolism of fats and carbohydrates. Overall, protein synthesis is impaired in vitamin B_{12}-deficient animals (Duncan and Webster, 1953; Friesecke, 1980). Moreover, the promotion of red blood cell synthesis and the maintenance of nervous system integrity are functions attributed to vitamin B_{12} (McDowell, 2000a; Green and Miller, 2013). Vitamin B_{12} is metabolically related to other essential nutrients, such as choline, methionine, and folic acid (Savage and Lindenbaum, 1995; Stabler, 2006).

A summary of vitamin B_{12} functions includes (Figure 4.45):

- purine and pyrimidine synthesis
- transfer of methyl groups
- formation of proteins from amino acids
- carbohydrate and fat metabolism.

Vitamin B_{12} is an essential cofactor in the following functions:

- the maintenance of normal DNA synthesis: failure of this metabolic pathway can lead to megaloblastic anemia
- the regeneration of methionine (methionine synthase and methylmalonyl-CoA mutase) for the dual purposes of maintaining protein synthesis and methylation capacity
- the avoidance of homocysteine accumulation, an amino acid metabolite implicated in vascular damage, thrombosis, and several associated degenerative diseases, including coronary artery disease, stroke, and osteoporosis (Green and Miller, 2013).

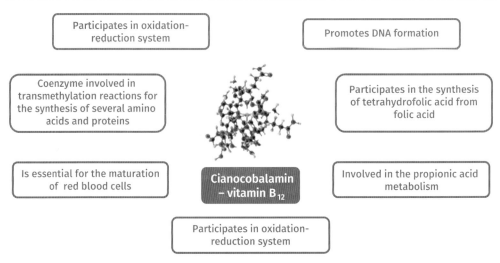

Figure 4.45 Vitamin B$_{12}$ functions

Gluconeogenesis and hemopoiesis are critically affected by cobalt deficiency, and carbohydrate, lipid, and nucleic acid metabolism depend on adequate B$_{12}$ and folic acid metabolism. Cobalamin participates in the metabolism of fatty acids, the synthesis of proteins, and reactions involving the transfer of methyl and hydrogenated/hydrogen groups (Green and Miller, 2013). Vitamin B$_{12}$ is a cofactor of 2 crucial metabolic reactions in the cells, one mitochondrial involving adenosylcobalamin and the other cytoplasmic, mostly related to methylcobalamin. Erythrocyte synthesis and maintenance of the integrity of the nervous system stand out among the many functions that are affected by and regulate this vitamin since it is in these functions that deficiency symptoms first present themselves.

In the mitochondrial reaction, B$_{12}$ in the form of 5'-deoxy-adenosylcobalamin is required for the enzyme methylmalonyl CoA mutase, a vitamin B$_{12}$-requiring enzyme (5´-deoxyadenosylcobalamin) that catalyzes the conversion of methylmalonyl-CoA to succinyl-CoA (Green and Miller, 2013). This is an intermediate step in transforming propionate to succinate during the oxidation of odd-chain fatty acids and the catabolism of ketogenic amino acids. In animal metabolism, propionate of dietary or metabolic origin is converted into succinate, entering the tricarboxylic acid (Krebs) cycle.

In the cytoplasmic reaction, B$_{12}$ in methylcobalamin is required in the folate-dependent methylation of the sulfur amino acid homocysteine to form methionine catalyzed by the enzyme methionine synthase. Apart from being necessary for adequate protein synthesis, methionine is also an essential precursor for maintaining methylation capacity through synthesizing the universal methyl donor S-adenosylmethionine. Additionally, the methionine synthase reaction is finally necessary for normal DNA synthesis. The methyl group transferred to homocysteine during methionine synthesis is donated by the folate derivative methyltetrahydrofolate (methyl-THF), forming THF. THF is later transformed to 5, 20-methylenetetrahydrofolate (methylene-THF) by a one-carbon transfer during serine conversion to glycine. Methylene-THF can be reduced again to form methyl-THF. Still, it also serves as the critical one-carbon source for the *de novo* synthesis of thymidylate from deoxyuridylate, which is required for DNA replication. Therefore, a vitamin B$_{12}$ deficiency reduces methionine supply and metabolic recycling of methyl groups. The latter effect interrupts the normal metabolism of folic acid and blocks its utilization. Thus, a vitamin B_{12} deficiency produces a secondary folic acid deficiency and a characteristic anemia (McDowell, 2000a).

Under intensive dairy systems, methionine may be limiting in specific diets. Under such circumstances, increasing methionine supply through feeding RP methionine can augment milk protein, fat concentrations, and yields in high-producing dairy cows, probably through increased protein synthesis (NRC, 2001). Methionine is not only an amino acid involved in the structure of proteins *per se*, but it also plays a unique role as the initiating amino acid for the synthesis of proteins (Brosnan *et al.*, 2007). Because of its role as a donor of preformed labile methyl groups, the supply of methionine affects the need for methyl neogenesis (Bailey and Gregory, 1999) and, consequently, for folic acid and vitamin B_{12}.

The nature of the ruminant digestive system imposes a significant dependence on gluconeogenesis because truly little glucose is being absorbed (Reynolds, 2006). In ruminants, the rate of gluconeogenesis increases with feed intake, and one of the major substrates for gluconeogenesis is propionate. Metabolic utilization of propionate after its absorption from the gastrointestinal tract depends on propionate's transformation into succinyl-co-enzyme A, requiring the subsequent actions of biotin- and vitamin B_{12}-dependent enzymes. Propionate is first transformed into propionyl-CoA, which is carboxylated to methylmal-onyl-CoA by a biotin-dependent enzyme, propionyl-CoA carboxylase. Methylmalonyl-CoA is then isomerized in succinyl-CoA under the action of the vitamin B_{12}-dependent enzyme methylmalonyl-CoA mutase. Succinyl-CoA finally enters the Krebs cycle, from which it can be directed toward gluconeogenesis (Le Grusse and Watier, 1993; McDowell, 2000b). Flavin and Ochoa (1957) established that for succinate production, the following steps are involved:

1. propionate + ATP + CoA → propionyl-CoA
2. propionyl-CoA + Coz + ATP → methylmalonyl-CoA (a)
3. methylmalonyl-CoA (a) → methylmalonyl-CoA (b)
4. methylmalonyl-CoA (b) → succinyl-CoA.

Methylmalonyl-CoA (a) is an inactive isomer. Its active form, (b), is converted into succinyl-CoA by a methylmalonyl-CoA isomerase (methylmalonyl-CoA mutase) (4th reaction above). Methylmalonyl-CoA also arises from metabolizing odd-chained fatty acids and certain amino acids (valine, isoleucine, methionine, and threonine) (Girard, 1998). The propionic acid pathway is essential in ruminants because they depend on propionic acid as the primary glucose precursor and propionic acid production in the rumen fermentation of dietary carbohydrates. Propionate production usually proceeds, but in cobalt or vitamin B_{12} deficiency, its clearance rate from blood is depressed, and methylmalonyl-CoA accumulates. This results in increased urinary excretion of methylmalonic acid and loss of appetite because impaired propionate metabolism leads to higher blood propionate levels, which are inversely correlated to voluntary feed intake (MacPherson, 1982; Kennedy *et al.*, 1995). Vitamin B_{12} is a metabolic essential for animal species studied, and vitamin B_{12} deficiency can be induced by adding high dietary levels of propionic acid.

The availability of vitamin B_{12} for methyl group transfer affects the supply and transfer rate of methyl groups in intermediary metabolism. Thus, vitamin B_{12} status affects the metabolism of choline and its derivatives and the synthesis of the purines and pyrimidines, components of DNA and RNA. As a result, rapidly dividing cells, particularly red blood cells, are sensitive to vitamin B_{12} status. The nervous system is also quite sensitive to the availability of vitamin B_{12}, possibly due to its high rate of metabolism. Reduction in the rate of protein synthesis is thought to be a principal cause of the growth depression frequently observed in vitamin B_{12}-deficient animals (Lassiter et al., 1953; Friesecke, 1980).

An additional function of vitamin B_{12} relates to immune function. In mice, vitamin B_{12} deficiency affected immunoglobulin production and cytokine levels (Mburu et al., 1993; Funada et al., 2001). Cobalt-deficient lambs had reduced concentrations of serum immunoglobulin G (IgG) and total protein (Fisher, 1991).

The deficiency of vitamin B_{12} induces a folic acid deficiency by blocking the utilization of folic acid derivatives. A vitamin B_{12}-containing enzyme removes the methyl group from methyl folate, thereby regenerating tetrahydrofolate (THF), made by the 5,20-methylene-THF required for thymidylate synthesis. It has been suggested that vitamin B_{12} status may affect the systemic metabolism of folic acid during early pregnancy (Girard and Matte, 2005a; Gagnon et al., 2015; Khan et al., 2020a). Numerous studies have also demonstrated the importance of vitamin B_{12} in reproduction (McDowell, 2000a).

Nutritional assessment
Historically, vitamin B_{12} was measured using microbiological assays such as the *Lactobacillus delbrueckii* method, which was later adapted for high-throughput use (Sauberlich, 1999). Measuring the total vitamin B_{12} concentration in serum is the first-line clinical test for determining vitamin B_{12} deficiency. The current assays are primarily based on the competitive binding of the serum vitamin to intrinsic factor, followed by radiometric or fluorescence-based detection (Höller et al., 2018).

TC-bound cobalamin, the form most actively transported into tissues, can be measured and considered a relevant marker of vitamin B_{12} status. A newer method estimates holotranscobalamin (holoTC) as a fraction of vitamin B_{12} carried by TC in serum and, therefore, available for tissue uptake (Höller et al., 2018).

Deficiency signs
Lassiter et al. (1953) demonstrated vitamin B_{12} deficiency in calves under 6 weeks old that received no dietary animal protein. Clinical signs characterizing the deficiency included poor appetite and growth, lacrimation, muscular weakness, demyelination of peripheral nerves, and emaciation.

Lambs
Young lambs (up to 2 months of age) require vitamin B_{12} supplementation, especially with early weaning programs (NRC, 1985). In vitamin B_{12}-deficient lambs, there is a sharp decrease of vitamin B_{12} concentrations in blood and liver before gross deficiency signs such as anorexia, weight loss, and a decrease in blood hemoglobin concentration. At necropsy, the body of a severely deficient animal is highly emaciated, often with a total absence of body fat. Fatty liver, hemosiderized spleen, and hypoplasia of the erythrogenic tissue of bone marrow are also characteristic (Filmer, 1933). The anemia in lambs is normocytic and normochromic, but the anemia is mild and is not responsible for the primary deficiency signs of cobalt deficiency. Anorexia and marasmus invariably precede any considerable degree of anemia.

The first discernible response to feeding cobalt or parenteral vitamin B_{12} is a rapid appetite and body weight improvement. Metabolically, vitamin B_{12} deficiency is characterized by decreases in the activity of methylmalonyl-CoA mutase, with a resultant increase in plasma and urinary methylmalonic acid (MMA), and by decreased activity of methionine synthase with a concomitant rise in plasma homocysteine (Kennedy et al., 1992, 1995). The reduction in methionine synthase activity, in turn, reduces the availability of methylated compounds, including methylated phospholipids (Kennedy *et al.*, 1992). The latter effect may be a cause of nerve demyelination. A recent study has associated high blood concentrations of methyl-malonic acid and Hcy with symptoms of acute and chronic hepatitis in vitamin B_{12}-deficient twin lambs (Vellema *et al.*, 1999). That study also observed brain lesions in vitamin B_{12}-deficient lambs (Vellema *et al.*, 1999).

White liver disease

Vitamin B_{12} deficiency is often caused by a cobalt deficiency in ruminating cattle and sheep. The syndrome is also known as "white liver disease." The signs mimic pre-ruminant vitamin B_{12} deficiency and are reversible by either cobalt or vitamin B_{12} supplementation (Ulvund and Pestalozzi, 1990; Kennedy *et al.*, 1997).

Vitamin B_{12}-deficient lambs exhibit a reduced lymphocyte response to *Mycobacterium para-tuberculosis* vaccination and higher fecal egg counts from nematode infection than lambs supplemented with adequate cobalt (Vellema *et al.*, 1996). Likewise, Paterson and MacPherson (1990) reported that cattle fed a cobalt-deficient diet for 10 weeks or longer significantly reduced the neutrophil killing of *Candida albicans* yeast and more significant weight loss when infected experimentally with brown stomach worm (*Ostertagia ostertagi*).

Cobalt deficiency in beef cattle resulted in reduced appetite and weight gain, reduced vitamin B_{12} status, decreased triiodothyronine in serum, reduced folate levels in the liver, and a significant increase in liver accumulation of iron and nickel (Stangl *et al.*, 1999). Liver vitamin B_{12} concentrations of 0.10 µg or less per gram wet weight are "clearly diagnostic of cobalt deficiency disease" (Underwood, 1979). Liver cobalt concentrations in the range of 0.05–0.07 mg per kg DM or below are critical levels indicating deficiency (McDowell, 1985).

Average concentrations of serum methylmalonic acid (MMA) are tentatively suggested as being less than 2 µmol per liter. In comparison, subclinical cobalt deficiency is indicated by serum MMA concentrations of 2 to 4 µmol per liter and outright cobalt deficiency by more than 4 µmol per liter of serum (Paterson and MacPherson, 1990). Marca *et al.* (1996) reported blood vitamin B_{12} concentrations greater than 0.2 µg/ml in sheep, in agreement with previous deficiency studies. Plasma MMA concentrations remained below 2 µmol/liter, considered average for sheep. Milk vitamin B_{12} concentrations were 10 µg/ml in colostrum and early milk and declined after that to 50% or less than the original value by 21 days of lactation (Marca *et al.*, 1996). However, some more recent reports (Playford and Weiser, 2021) have indicated lower concentrations (Table 4.1).

Other histological and biochemical signs of cobalt/vitamin B_{12} deficiency in ruminants include cardiovascular lesions resembling arteriosclerosis in sheep (Mohammed and Lamand, 1986); accumulation of odd-number, branched-chain fatty acids in tissues (Kennedy *et al.*, 1994); and accumulation of succinate in rumen fluid due to the blockage in propionic acid synthesis (Kennedy *et al.*, 1996).

Vitamin B_{12} deficiency induced by exposure to nitrous oxide resulted in almost complete inhibition of methionine synthase activity in sheep's liver, heart, and brain tissue (Xue *et al.*, 1986). The results led the authors to conclude that methyl group transfer via methionine synthase is required for the adequate supply of methionine and methylated compounds. Amino acid concentrations are altered by cobalt deficiency in cattle, as described by Stangl *et al.* (1998). In that study, feeding a cobalt-deficient diet reduced appetite, growth, and vitamin B_{12} status and significantly reduced plasma methionine (by 53%) as well as the concentrations of valine, leucine, isoleucine, threonine, arginine, tyrosine, and taurine. Conversely, plasma serine and Hcy were significantly increased by 2.7 and 4.8 times, respectively. Liver amino acid content was not affected.

Cobalt deficiency

Cobalt deficiency has been reported to reduce lamb survival and increase susceptibility to parasitic infection in cattle and sheep (Ferguson *et al.*, 1988; Suttle and Jones, 1989). Cobalt deficiency has been associated with the photosensitization of lambs characterized by a swollen head (Hesselink and Vellema, 1990). The condition responded to 2 injections of vitamin B_{12} 3 weeks apart. Cobalt deficiency in pregnant ewes reduced lamb numbers and increased stillbirths and neonatal mortality (Fisher, 1991). Lambs born from cobalt-deficient ewes were slower to nurse. They had reduced serum immunoglobulin G (IgG) and total protein concentrations, lower serum vitamin B_{12}, and elevated serum MMA concentrations compared to normal lambs (Fisher, 1991).

In African goats, cobalt deficiency reduced serum vitamin B_{12} and erythrocyte counts. However, the growth rate was not significantly affected, suggesting that goats, like cattle, are more resistant to cobalt/vitamin B_{12} deficiency than sheep (Mburu *et al.*, 1993). Goats depleted of cobalt and thus vitamin B_{12} exhibited irregular estrus cycles, macrocytic anemia, decreased plasma progesterone and luteinizing hormone, and high plasma corticosteroids compared to normal animals (Mgongo *et al.*, 1984).

Except for P and copper, cobalt is the most common mineral deficiency for grazing livestock in tropical countries (McDowell *et al.*, 1984; McDowell, 1992). Cobalt deficiency signs are nonspecific, and distinguishing between a cobalt deficiency and primary malnutrition or parasitization is often tricky. Acute clinical signs of cobalt deficiency mimic those of vitamin B_{12} deficiency (Figure 4.46) and other vitamin B deficiencies (Figure 4.47).

The incidence of cobalt deficiency can vary significantly from year to year, from an undetectable mild deficiency to an acute stage. Lee (1963) illustrated this variation in a 14-year experiment with sheep in southern Australia. Half the ewes, replacements, and progeny received supplemental cobalt and remained healthy (in no particular order by years). The undosed half had the following performance for the 14 years: in 2 years, lambs were unhealthy, but there were no deaths; in 3 years, the growth rate of the lambs was slightly retarded; in 4 years, 30 to 100% of the lamb crop was lost; in 5 years, the performance of the remaining stock was as good as that of dosed animals. The conclusion would be that if there was no benefit from cobalt supplementation in a particular year, there was no guarantee that a moderate to severe cobalt deficiency would not occur (McDowell, 2000b). McDowell and Arthington (2005) have extensively reviewed cobalt nutrition.

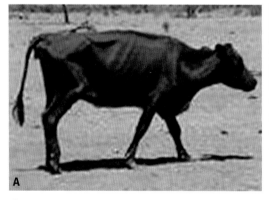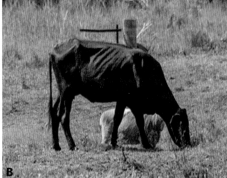

Figure 4.46 Cobalt deficiency in cattle, wasting disease

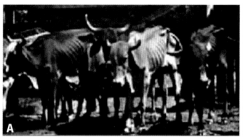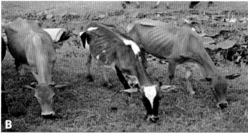

Figure 4.47 Cobalt deficiency in cattle, wasting disease (source: courtesy of L.R. McDowell, University of Florida)

Safety
A dietary level of at least several hundred times the requirement is considered safe for most species (NRC, 1987): vitamin B_{12} is reported to be toxic with around 5 mg per kg diets. Adding vitamin B_{12} to feeds in amounts far above requirement or absorbability appears to be without hazard. Signs of toxicity are unclear, especially with many older reports, since results are likely confounded with toxic effects of fermentation residues inadvertently included with vitamin B_{12} during manufacture. Cobalt also has low toxicity, with 10 mg per kg, the maximum dietary tolerable level for the common livestock species (NRC, 1980). Becker and Smith (1951) concluded that 150 mg per kg DM, or 1,000 times normal levels, can be tolerated by sheep for many weeks without visible toxic effects. Characteristic signs of chronic cobalt toxicity in most species are reduced feed intake and BW, emaciation, anemia, hyperchromenia, and increased liver cobalt (NRC, 1980). Cobalt toxicity in cattle is characterized by mild polycythemia, excessive urination, defecation, salivation, shortness of breath, and increased hemoglobin, red cell count, and packed cell volume (NRC, 2000).

Niacin (vitamin B_3)
Chemical structure and properties
The 2 forms of niacin or vitamin B_3, nicotinic acid (pyridine-3-carboxylic acid) and nicotinamide (or niacinamide; pyridine-3-carboxylic acid amide), are functional parts of the coenzymes nicotinamide adenine dinucleotide (NAD and NADH in the reduced form) and nicotinamide adenine dinucleotide phosphate (NADP and NADPH in the reduced form), involved in the cellular respiration processes (Kirkland, 2013). As conversion takes place quickly and very efficiently, it is considered that both forms possess the same vitamin activity. The term niacin is frequently used for both the free acid form and the amide form.

The empirical formula is $C_6H_3O_2N$ (Figure 4.48). Nicotinic acid and nicotinamide correspond to 3-pyridine carboxylic acid and its amide. Both are white, odorless, crystalline solids soluble in water and alcohol. They are resistant to heat, air, light, alkali, and oxidation and thus are stable in feeds. Niacin is also stable in the presence of the usual oxidizing agents; however, it will undergo decarboxylation at a high temperature in an alkaline medium. There are antivitamins or antagonists for niacin. These compounds have the basic pyridine structure; 2 important antagonists of nicotinic acid are 3-acetyl pyridine and pyridine sulfonic acid.

Nicotinic acid and nicotinamide generally possess the same activity, although one report with lactating cows suggested that the nicotinamide form has slightly higher activity (Jaster and Ward, 1990). An additional source of supplemental niacin would be the vitamin K supplement

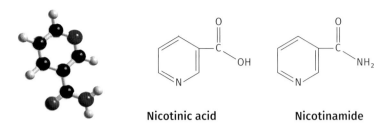

Nicotinic acid   Nicotinamide

Figure 4.48 Niacin chemical structure

Menadione Nicotinamide Bisulfite (MNB), with a content ≥31% nicotinamide. Results with chicks suggest MNB is fully effective as a source of vitamin K and niacin activity.

Natural sources

The supply of niacin to the ruminant comes from 3 primary sources: (1) dietary niacin, (2) conversion of tryptophan to niacin, and (3) ruminal synthesis of niacin. Niacin is widely distributed in feedstuffs of both plant and animal origin. Good sources are animal and fish by-products (50–150 mg/kg), distiller grains, yeast, peanut meal (150–200 mg/kg), various distillation and fermentation solubles, cereals, and certain oilseed meals.

Niacin is reasonably stable under normal conditions, but its bioavailability is low, at least in monogastric animals, especially in wheat and sorghum (10–15%) and in corn (0% to 30%), as it is found in combination with a peptide or a carbohydrate (Luce *et al.*, 1966; 1967). In oilseeds, bioavailability is 40%. Oilseeds contain about 40% of their total niacin in bound form, while only a tiny proportion of the niacin in pulses, yeast, crustacean, fish, animal tissue, or milk is bound.

Two types of bound niacin were initially described: (1) a peptide with a molecular weight of 12,000–13,000, the so-called niacinogens, and (2) a carbohydrate complex with a molecular weight of approximately 2,370 (Darby *et al.*, 1975). The name niacytin has been used to designate this latter material from wheat bran. Using a microbiological assay, Ghosh *et al.* (1963) reported that 85 to 90% of the total nicotinic acid in cereals is in a bound form. Using a rat assay procedure, for 8 samples of mature cooked cereals (corn, wheat, rice, and milo), only about 35% of the total niacin was available (Carter and Carpenter, 1982).

Therefore, in calculating the niacin content of formulated diets, all the niacin from cereal grain sources should probably be ignored or given a value no greater than one-third of the total. In immature seeds, niacin is part of biologically available coenzymes necessary for seed metabolism. Niacin binding to carbohydrates by ester linkages may cause it to be retained in the mature seed until utilized. Hence, the availability of vitamins for man and animals is impaired. In rats, growth assays for available niacin, corn harvested immaturely ("milk stage") gave values from 74 to 88 µg per gm. In contrast, corn harvested at maturity gave assay values of 16–18 µg per gm (Carpenter *et al.*, 1988).

Most species can use the essential amino acid tryptophan, from which niacin can be synthesized. However, tryptophan is preferably used for protein synthesis (Kodicek *et al.*, 1974), and ruminant feedstuffs tend to be low in tryptophan.

There is little doubt that niacin synthesis can occur in the rumen (Panda *et al.*, 2017). Still, the extent to which it occurs, particularly with commercial feedstuffs, and its contribution to the niacin supply are controversial. Niacin is often present in higher concentrations in rumen DM than in the diet, and this has been interpreted as evidence of net synthesis in the rumen

(Hollis *et al.*, 1954). Nevertheless, the positive response of ruminants to supplemental niacin in some studies indicated that the niacin supply is sometimes suboptimal.

Commercial forms

Crystalline products are used in feeds and pharmaceuticals, and dry dilutions in feeds. Nicotinic acid and niacinamide are commercially available as granular powder formulations containing 99% activity. Positive response to supplementation has been noted with either source. Campbell *et al.* (1994) noted only minor differences in dairy cows' nicotinic acid and niacin metabolism.

Metabolism

Ruminal production

Synthesis of niacin in the rumen has been demonstrated in sheep (Rérat *et al.*, 1959), cattle (Hungate, 1966), and goats (Porter, 1961). This synthesis has also been suggested to be under metabolic control, e.g., more is synthesized when small amounts are provided in the ration and vice versa (Porter, 1961; Abdouli and Schaefer, 1986). Niacin stimulates microbial protein synthesis (Arambell *et al.*, 1982), the production of propionic acid (Ridell *et al.*, 1981, 1989; Arambell *et al.*, 1982; Hannah and Stern, 1985), and digestion of cellulose (Hannah and Stern, 1985).

Absorption and transport

Niacin in foods and feed occurs mainly in its coenzyme forms. Nicotinic acid is converted to the amide form in the tissues, and Erickson *et al.* (1991) suggested this occurs in the rumen. Pyrophosphatase activity in the upper small intestine metabolizes NAD and NADP to yield nicotinamide, which is then hydrolyzed to form nicotinamide riboside and eventually free nicotinamide, which is hydrolyzed during digestion, yielding nicotinamide, which seems to be absorbed as such without further hydrolysis in the gastrointestinal tract (Kirkland, 2013).

In the gut mucosa, nicotinic acid is converted to nicotinamide (Stein *et al.*, 1994). Nicotinic acid and nicotinamide are rapidly absorbed from the stomach and the intestine by diffusion at either physiological or pharmacologic doses (Nabokina *et al.*, 2005; Jacob, 2006). At low concentrations, absorption appears to be via sodium-dependent high-affinity transporters. In animals, absorption from the small intestine seems to be the primary route by which niacin is made available to the host. Although direct absorption from the rumen is possible, it is usually limited because only a tiny portion (3–7%) of the vitamin is in the supernatant fraction of rumen fluid; most is bound within the microbes themselves (Rérat *et al.*, 1959).

Once absorbed from the lumen into the enterocyte, nicotinamide may be converted via the Preiss–Handler pathway to NAD or released into the portal circulation. Although some nicotinic acid moves into the blood in its native form, the enterocyte's bulk of nicotinic acid is converted to NAD. The intestinal mucosa contains niacin conversion enzymes such as NAD glycohydrolase (Henderson and Gross, 1979). As required, NAD glycohydrolases in the enterocytes release nicotinamide from NAD into the plasma, as the principal circulating form of niacin, for transport to tissues that synthesize NAD as needed.

Blood transport of niacin is associated mainly with red blood cells. Erythrocytes effectively absorb nicotinic acid and nicotinamide by facilitated diffusion, converting them to nucleotides to maintain a concentration gradient. However, niacin rapidly leaves the bloodstream and enters the kidney, liver, and adipose tissues.

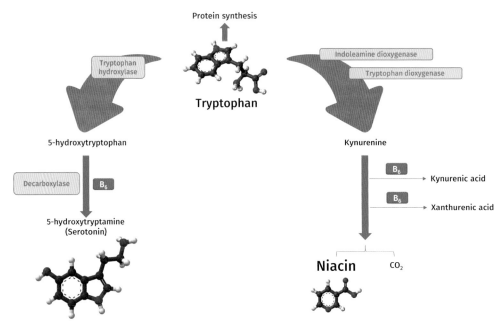

Figure 4.49 Overview of tryptophan metabolism to produce niacin

Niacin from tryptophan

The amino acid tryptophan is a precursor for niacin synthesis in the body. There is considerable evidence that synthesis can occur in the intestine, and there is also evidence that synthesis can take place elsewhere within the body. The extent to which the metabolic requirement for niacin can be met from tryptophan will depend first on the amount of tryptophan in the diet and second on the efficiency of conversion of tryptophan to niacin (Panda *et al.*, 2017; Petrović *et al.*, 2020). The kynurenine pathway of tryptophan conversion to nicotinic acid and, finally, NAD in the body is shown in Figure 4.49.

This reaction is irreversible (Kirkland, 2013). Protein, energy, vitamin B_6, and vitamin B_2 nutritional status and hormones affect one or more steps in the conversion sequence and hence can influence the yield of niacin from tryptophan. Two enzymes require iron to convert tryptophan to niacin, with a deficiency reducing tryptophan utilization. At low levels of tryptophan intake, the conversion efficiency is high, and it decreases when niacin and tryptophan levels in the diet are increased.

Animal species differ widely in their ability to synthesize niacin from tryptophan, but all are relatively inefficient. From various experiments, approximately 60 mg of tryptophan is estimated to be equivalent to 1 mg of niacin in humans. In comparison, the rat is more efficient at a conversion rate of 35 to 50 mg of tryptophan required. The conversion efficiency of tryptophan to niacin in the chick is estimated to be 45:1 (Baker *et al.*, 1973) and relatively efficient. Ruminants would be less efficient in this conversion than most species.

The variability in the conversion efficiency of tryptophan to niacin among species is probably due to inherent differences in liver levels of picolinic acid carboxylase. This enzyme diverts one of the intermediates (2-amino, 3-acroleylfumaric acid) to the picolinic acid pathway instead of allowing this compound to condense to quinolinic acid, the immediate precursor of nicotinic acid (Kirkland, 2013).

Picolinic acid carboxylase activity in livers of various species has a positive correlation to experimentally determined niacin requirements. The rat diverts truly little of its dietary tryptophan to carbon dioxide and water and, thus, is relatively efficient in converting tryptophan to niacin. In practice, the production of niacin from tryptophan is minimal since this amino acid is not typically found in excess in diets. Moreover, high levels of fat in feed, especially saturated fat, will inhibit this reaction (Kirkland, 2013). Finally, tryptophan is preferably used for protein synthesis (Panda *et al.*, 2017; Kodicek *et al.*, 1974; Kirkland, 2013).

Storage and excretion
Although niacin coenzymes are widely distributed in the body, no proper storage occurs. The liver is the site of the greatest niacin concentration in the body, but the amount stored is minimal. The tissue content of niacin and its analogs, NAD and NADP, is a variable factor, dependent on the diet and several other factors, such as strain, sex, age, and treatment of animals (Hankes, 1984).

The liver is a central processing organ for niacin. Aside from its role in converting tryptophan to NAD, it receives nicotinamide and some nicotinic acid via the portal circulation, and nicotinamide is released from other extrahepatic tissues. In the liver, nicotinic acid and nicotinamide are metabolized to NAD or to yield compounds for urinary excretion, depending on the niacin status of the organism.

Urine is the primary pathway of excretion of absorbed niacin and its metabolites, methylated or oxidized derivatives. The excretion of these metabolites is measured in studies of niacin requirements and niacin metabolism. The main excretory products in humans, dogs, rats, and pigs are the methylated metabolite N1-methyl nicotinamide or 2 oxidation products of this compound, 4-pyridone or 6-pyridone of N1-methylnicotinamide. On the other hand, in herbivores, niacin does not seem to be metabolized by methylation, but substantial amounts are excreted unchanged. In the chicken, however, nicotinic acid is conjugated with ornithine as either α- or δ-nicotinyl ornithine or dinicotinyl ornithine. The excretion of these metabolites is measured in studies of niacin requirements and niacin metabolism.

Biochemical functions
Several metabolic reactions in which niacin participates, forming part of the NAD and NADP coenzymes. Therefore, it is essential to metabolize carbohydrates, amino acids, and fatty acids and obtain energy through the Krebs cycle. NAD and NADP coenzymes are essential in the metabolic reactions that furnish energy to the animal. Like the riboflavin coenzymes, the NAD and NADP-containing enzyme systems play a key role in biological oxidation-reduction, including more than 200 reactions in the metabolism of carbohydrates, fatty acids, and amino acids due to their capacity to serve as hydrogen-transfer agents. Hydrogen is effectively transferred from the oxidizable substrate to oxygen through a series of graded enzymatic hydrogen transfers. Nicotinamide-containing enzyme systems constitute one such group of hydrogen-transfer agents.

Important metabolic reactions catalyzed by NAD and NADP are summarized as follows (McDowell, 2000a; Kirkland, 2013):

1   carbohydrate metabolism:
    ○   glycolysis: anaerobic and aerobic oxidation of glucose
    ○   TCA or Krebs cycle

2 lipid metabolism:
   ○ glycerol synthesis and breakdown
   ○ fatty acid oxidation and synthesis
   ○ steroid synthesis
3 protein metabolism:
   ○ degradation and synthesis of amino acids
   ○ oxidation of carbon chains via the TCA cycle
4 photosynthesis
5 rhodopsin synthesis.

Niacin, riboflavin, and coenzyme Q_{10} are associated with PARP synthesized in response to DNA strand breaks and are involved in the post-translational modification of nuclear proteins (Kirkland, 2013). The PARP proteins function in DNA repair, replication, and cell differentiation (Carson *et al.*, 1987; Premkumar *et al.*, 2008). These functions may be necessary for tissues with high turnover rates, like the skin, intestines, central nervous system (Kirkland, 2013; Gasperi *et al.*, 2019), and the immunological system. Rat data have shown that even a mild niacin deficiency decreases liver PARP concentrations, which are also altered by feed restriction (Rawling *et al.*, 1994). Zhang *et al.* (1993) suggested that a severe niacin deficiency may increase the susceptibility of DNA to oxidative damage, likely due to the lower availability of NAD.

Niacin-dependent PARP participates in the post-translational modification of nuclear proteins. For ruminants, niacin is mainly required for unique protein and energy metabolism features, including liver detoxification of portal blood NH_3 to urea and liver metabolism of ketones in ketosis. Niacin can increase microbial protein synthesis (Girard, 1998). This may result in an increased molar proportion of propionate in rumen volatile fatty acids and may cause an increased rate of flow of material through the rumen. The function of primary interest for lactating dairy cows deals with the role of niacin in fatty acid oxidation and glucose synthesis, particularly as a preventive and possible treatment for clinical and subclinical ketosis.

Nutritional assessment
Niacin and its metabolites can be measured in plasma via gas chromatography (GC), HPLC, or simultaneously via LC-MS/MS. However, the central gap is the lack of reliable ranges, even in humans, making the assessment extremely complicated. Determination of the activity of erythrocyte nicotinic acid mononucleotide pyrophosribosyl transferase has been used as a possible method to assess the nutritional status of niacin (Höller *et al.*, 2018).

Deficiency signs
In the pre-ruminant calf, a diet free of niacin and low in tryptophan produced deficiency signs of sudden anorexia, severe diarrhea, ataxia, and dehydration, followed by sudden death. Supplementation with 2.5 mg of nicotinic acid per liter of milk, offered *ad libitum* twice daily, prevented the deficiency (Hopper and Johnson, 1955). On this basis, the daily niacin requirement for calves from all sources would be 10–15 mg daily. Niacin may increase microbial protein synthesis; however, several studies indicate no effects. Differences between these studies, all utilized *in vitro* systems, may reflect the amount and availability of niacin in the unsupplemented diet, the niacin status of the microbes, or both (NRC, 2001).

Niacin could be higher in feedlot cattle, during heat stress, in dairy cows during early lactation, or in ketotic cows. Endogenous niacin synthesis is decreased by ketones and increased by corticosteroids, leading to the hypothesis that the beneficial effect of adrenal corticoids on ketosis is derived from increased niacin synthesis. This suggests that niacin may be a helpful adjunct to glucocorticoid therapy for ketosis. Supplemental niacin has been reported to increase plasma insulin and glucose response to β-agonists (Chilliard and Ottou, 1995). Insulin resistance in periparturient ruminants prioritizes glucogenic nutrients for vital functions, fetal growth, and lactose production and enhances the mobilization of fatty acids and glycerol from adipose tissue (Bell and Bauman, 1997). However, exaggerated insulin resistance in adipose tissue can potentially lead to further increases in plasma non-esterified fatty acid (NEFA) concentrations and the onset of metabolic disorders. Increased plasma NEFA concentration has been associated with insulin resistance in Holstein cows. Reduction of plasma NEFA concentration by nicotinic acid enhanced the response to insulin in feed-restricted Holstein cows (Pires and Grummer, 2007). Impaired insulin signaling due to elevated NEFA may affect various cell functions in different tissues, with important repercussions on the physiology and productivity of the periparturient dairy cow. Erickson *et al.* (1990) reported a trend for reduced lipolysis (area under the curve for NEFA) in response to epinephrine challenge in cows fed 12 g per day of either nicotinic acid or nicotinamide. Skaar *et al.* (1989) found no effect of niacin on hepatic lipidosis during the periparturient period in dairy cows.

Supplementation of encapsulated niacin to Holstein cows (Zimbelman *et al.*, 2010) during heat stress increased DM intake, sweating rates, and lower body core temperatures. Supplemental niacin (500 ppm) to lambs (Mizwicki *et al.*, 1975) fed a high concentrate diet containing urea: (1) increased nitrogen utilization; (2) improved the percentage of absorbed nitrogen retained; (3) reduced urinary nitrogen excretion; and (4) reduced the percentage of nitrogen found as urea nitrogen. All of these positive responses indicated improved protein metabolism with high-concentrate diets. Comparable results were observed when supplementing 100 ppm niacin to growing and finishing lambs (Shields *et al.*, 1982).

Safety
Niacin has a wide margin of safety. The toxic effects of nicotinic acid occur only at levels far above requirements. Limited research indicates that nicotinic acid and nicotinamide are toxic at dietary intakes greater than 350 mg per kg BW per day (NRC, 1987). The intravenous LD_{50} of niacin in mice is 2.5 g per kg BW. The oral LD_{50} and subcutaneous LD_{50} in mice are 4.5 and 2.8 g per kg, respectively. Nicotinamide is 2 to 3 times more toxic than free acid (Waterman, 1978). The nicotinic acid and niacinamide tolerance for ruminants has not been determined.

Pantothenic acid (vitamin B$_5$)
Chemical structure and properties
Pantothenic acid is also referred to as vitamin B$_5$, though the origin of this designation is obscure (Rucker and Bauerly, 2013). Pantothenic acid is an amide consisting of pantoic acid joined to β-alanine (3-[(2,4-dihydroxy-3, 3-dimethyl-1-oxobutyl) amino]propanoic acid) found forming part of the coenzymes, especially CoA, containing the vitamin as an essential component, and the acyl groups carrier protein (ACP). The structural formula and crystalline structure are shown in Figure 4.50.

The free acid of the vitamin is a viscous, pale-yellow oil readily soluble in water and ethyl acetate. It crystallizes as white needles from ethanol and is reasonably stable to light and air. The oil is highly hygroscopic and easily destroyed by acids, bases, and heat. Maximum heat stability occurs at pH 5.5–7.0 (Rucker and Bauerly, 2013).

Pantothenic acid is optically active (characteristic of rotating a polarized light). It may be prepared as the pure dextrorotatory (d) or racemic mixture (dl) form. The racemic form has approximately one-half the biological activity of d-Ca pantothenate, the commercial form used in animal nutrition. Only the dextrorotatory form, d-pantothenic acid, is effective as a vitamin.

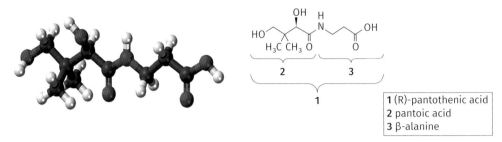

Figure 4.50 Structure of pantothenic acid

The most common pantothenic acid antagonist is omega-methyl-pantothenic acid, which has been used to produce a vitamin deficiency in humans (Hodges *et al.*, 1958). Other antivitamins include pantoyltaurine; phenylpantothenate hydroxocobalamin (c-lactam), an analog of vitamin B_{12}; and antimetabolites of the vitamin containing alkyl- or aryl-ureido and carbamate components in the amide part of the molecule (Fox, 1991; Brass, 1993).

Natural sources

Pantothenic acid is widely distributed in feedstuffs of animal and plant origin. Alfalfa hay, peanut meal, cane molasses, yeast, rice bran, green leafy plants, wheat bran, brewer's yeast, fish solubles, and rice polishings are good sources of vitamins for animals. Millin Corn and soybean meal diets are low in pantothenic acid. g by-products, such as rice bran and wheat bran, are useful sources, 2 to 3 times higher than the respective grains.

The concentration in cereals is around 10 mg/kg, ranging 5–6 mg in corn to 15 mg in oats. According to Southern and Baker (1981), the availability of pantothenic acid in barley, wheat, and soy is high but much lower in sorghum. By-products of cereals generally have a much higher concentration (rice bran 22 mg/kg, wheat bran 18–30 mg/ kg, etc.). However, it has not been possible to find information on its availability. Amounts in vegetable protein concentrate vary. While peanut meal contains 47 mg/kg, soy and linseed contain around 15 mg, and sunflower only 10 mg/kg. Legumes have a lower concentration (peas, 5 mg/kg). The concentration of milk by-products is between 20 and 45 mg/kg, and fish-meal between 10 and 20 mg/kg. Finally, fibrous foods such as alfalfa concentration are around 30 mg/kg.

The biological availability of pantothenic acid is high in corn and soybean meal but low in barley, wheat, and sorghum, approximately 60%. (Bowland and Owen, 1952; Southern and Baker, 1981). Changing processing methods can significantly alter vitamin feed levels. For example, with changes in sugar technology, literature values for the pantothenic acid content of beet molasses have decreased from 50 to 100 mg per kg in the 1950s to about 1–4 mg per kg (Palagina *et al.*, 1990).

Pantothenic acid is relatively stable in feedstuffs during long storage periods (Chen *et al.*, 2019). Heating during processing may cause considerable losses, especially if temperatures attain 100 to 150°C for prolonged periods and pH values above 7 or below 5. Gadient (1986) considers pantothenic acid to be slightly sensitive to heat, oxygen, or light but overly sensitive to moisture. As a general guideline, pantothenic acid activity in regular pelleted feed over 3 months at room temperature should be 80 to 100%. Although this vitamin is found in practically all ruminant feedstuffs, complementary supplementation is advisable in rations for high-yielding dairy cows and fast-growing cattle fed concentrated rations to ensure a high production level.

Higher concentrations of pantothenic acid are found in the rumen than in the dietary components, indicating microbial synthesis of the vitamin. For young ruminants, milk from the dam is a reliable source of this vitamin, with colostrum and whole milk from cows containing about 1.73 and 3.82 µg of pantothenic acid per ml, respectively (Foley and Otterby, 1978).

Commercial forms

Pantothenic acid is available as a commercially synthesized product for feed, known as D- or DL-Ca pantothenate. Because livestock and poultry can biologically utilize only the d-isomer of pantothenic acid, nutrient requirements for the vitamin are routinely expressed in the d-form.

One gram of d-Ca pantothenate equals 0.92 g of d-pantothenic acid activity. Therefore, 1.087 g of d-Ca pantothenate is required to achieve the activity of 1 g of d-pantothenic acid. Sometimes, a racemic mixture – i.e., equal parts d- and dl-Ca pantothenate – is offered to the feed industry. The racemic mixture of 1 g of the dl-form has 0.46 g of d-pantothenic acid activity. Hence, with this product, 2.174 g is needed to get the activity of 1 g of d-pantothenic acid. Products sold based on racemic mixture content can be misleading and confusing to a buyer not fully aware of the biological activity supplied by d-Ca pantothenate. To avoid confusion, the label should clearly state the grams of d-Ca pantothenate or its equivalent per unit weight and the grams of d-pantothenic acid. Moreover, the racemic mixture can create handling problems because of its hygroscopic and electrostatic properties.

Losses of Ca pantothenate may occur in premixes that are highly acidic. Verbeeck (1975) reported Ca pantothenate to be stable in premixes with or without trace minerals, regardless of the mineral form.

Metabolism
Absorption and transport
Pantothenic acid is found in feeds inbound (primarily as CoA) and free forms. It is necessary to liberate the pantothenic acid from the bound forms in the digestive process before absorption. Work with chicks and rats indicated that pantothenic acid, its salt, and the alcohol are absorbed primarily in the jejunum by a specific transport system that is saturable and sodium ion dependent (Fenstermacher and Rose, 1986; Miller *et al.*, 2006). The alcohol form, panthenol, oxidized to pantothenic acid *in vivo*, appears to be absorbed somewhat faster than the acid form.

After absorption, pantothenic acid is transported to various tissues in the plasma. Most cells take it up via another active-transport process involving the cotransport of pantothenate and sodium in a 1:1 ratio (Olson, 1990). Pantothenic acid is converted to CoA and other compounds within tissues, where a vitamin is a functional group (Sauberlich, 1985). Coenzyme A is synthesized by cells from pantothenic acid, ATP, and cysteine. Pantothenic acid kinase, a cytosolic enzyme, is rate-limiting for the overall pathway of coenzyme A biosynthesis (Brass, 1993).

Storage and excretion
Livestock does not appear to be able to store appreciable amounts of pantothenic acid; organs such as the liver and kidneys have the highest concentrations. Most pantothenic acid in blood exists in red blood cells as CoA, but free pantothenic acid is also present. The serum does not contain CoA but does contain free pantothenic acid.

Urinary excretion is the primary route of body loss of absorbed pantothenic acid, and excretion is prompt when the vitamin is consumed in excess. Most pantothenic acid is excreted as a free vitamin, but some species (e.g., dogs) pass it as β-glucuronide (Taylor *et al.*, 1972). Pearson *et al.* (1953) and Smith and Song (1996) described that pantothenic acid's urinary and fecal excretion was 4 to 6 times the intake when semi-synthetic diets were fed. Pantothenic acid excretion increased with increased crude protein intakes. An appreciable quantity of pantothenic acid (~15% of daily intake) is wholly oxidized and excreted across the lungs as CO_2.

Biochemical functions

Pantothenic acid participates in several metabolic pathways critical in endogenous metabolism energy exchange in all tissues. The coenzymes are involved in more than 100 metabolic pathways involving the metabolism of carbohydrates, proteins, and lipids and the synthesis of lipids, neurotransmitters, steroid hormones, porphyrins, hemoglobin, heme, cholesterol, and acetylcholine. Its main functions include (Rucker and Bauerly, 2013):

- utilization of nutrients
- synthesis of fatty acids, cholesterol, and steroid hormones
- synthesis of neurotransmitters, steroid hormones, porphyrins, and hemoglobin
- participation in the citric acid cycle or Krebs cycle as a constituent of acetyl-coenzyme A (3-phospho-adenosine-5-diphospho-pantothene) and other enzymes and coenzymes
- energy-yielding oxidation of fats, carbohydrates, and amino acids
- involved in the production of antibodies, the adrenal glands' activity, and the acetylation of choline for nervous impulse transmission
- relationship with vitamin B_{12}; if the latter is deficient, it accentuates the lack of pantothenic acid
- interactions with folic acid, biotin, and copper.

CoA's most critical function is acting as a carrier mechanism for carboxylic acids (Lehninger, 1982; Miller *et al.*, 2006; Rucker and Bauerly, 2013). When bound to CoA, such acids have a high potential for transfer to other groups, and such carboxylic acids are typically referred to as "active." The most important of these reactions is the combination of CoA with acetate to form "active acetate" with a high-energy bond that renders acetate capable of further chemical interactions. Combining CoA with two-carbon fragments from fats, carbohydrates, and certain amino acids to form acetyl-CoA is essential in their complete metabolism because the coenzyme enables these fragments to enter the TCA cycle.

For example, acetyl-CoA is utilized directly by combining with oxaloacetic acid to form citric acid, entering the TCA cycle. Coenzyme A and ACP are a carrier of acyl groups in enzymatic reactions involved in synthesizing fatty acids, cholesterol, sphingosine, porphyrins, and other sterols; oxidation of fatty acids, pyruvate, and a-ketoglutarate; and biological acetylations. Decarboxylation of a-ketoglutaric acid in the TCA cycle yields succinic acid, which is then converted to the "active" form by linkage with CoA. Active succinate and glycine participate in the first step of heme biosynthesis.

In acetyl-CoA, acetic acid can also combine with choline to form acetylcholine, a chemical transmitter at the nerve synapse. It can be used to detoxify various drugs, such as sulfonamides. Pantothenic acid also stimulates the synthesis of antibodies, increasing animal resistance to pathogens. It appears that when pantothenic acid is deficient, the incorporation of amino acids into the blood albumin fraction is inhibited, which would explain why there is a reduction in the titer of antibodies (Axelrod, 1971).

Nutritional assessment

Early assays use pantothenic acid-dependent microorganisms such as *Lactobacillus plantarum* for quantification (Sauberlich, 1999). This assay is prone to various interferences, and therefore, more specific RIA or ELISA tests have been developed (Sauberlich, 1999) and used to measure it in blood plasma to determine body status (Höller *et al.*, 2018).

Deficiency signs

Pantothenic acid is not typically required in the diet of adult ruminants because ruminal microorganisms synthesize this vitamin in adequate amounts. Pantothenic acid deficiency has been produced experimentally in calves (Johnson *et al.*, 1947; Sheppard and Johnson, 1957; Roy, 1980). Significant clinical signs include anorexia, reduced growth, weakness of legs, rough hair coat, dermatitis, diarrhea, and eventual death. The most characteristic pantothenic acid deficiency sign in the calf is scaly dermatitis around the eyes (spectacle eye) and muzzle. Anorexia and diarrhea follow after 11–20 weeks on a deficient diet. Calves become weak and unable to stand and may develop convulsions. They are susceptible to mucosal infection, especially in the respiratory tract. Postmortem studies have shown moderate sciatic and peripheral nerve demyelination. There is some edema in the muscular tissue. When deficient calves received Ca pantothenate, they responded with increased appetite, weight gains, and subsequent reversal of dermatitis and other symptoms.

Safety

No data have been reported for pantothenic acid toxicity studies with ruminants: however, it is regarded as nontoxic. Dietary levels of at least 20 g of pantothenic acid per kg diet can be tolerated by most species (NRC, 1987). These levels are around 100 times the recommended supplementation for all species. Ca pantothenate, sodium pantothenate, and panthenol are not mutagenic in bacterial tests.

Biotin (vitamin B$_7$)
Chemical structure and properties

The chemical structure of biotin includes a sulfur atom in its ring (like thiamine) and a transverse bond across the ring (Figure 4.51). Biotin is a bicyclic compound, a monocarboxylic acid with sulfur as a thioether linkage or described in another way as a monocarboxylic acid with a carboxybutyl side chain that forms an amide linkage with lysine (called biocytin) in the biotin-requiring enzymes.

One of the rings contains a ureido group (-N-CO-N-), and the other is a tetrahydrothiophene ring. The tetrahydrothiophene ring has a valeric acid side chain. With its rather unique structure, biotin contains 3 asymmetric carbon atoms; therefore, 8 different isomers are possible (5-[(3aS,4S,6aR)-2-oxohexahydro-1H-thienol[3,4-d]imidazol-4-yl] pentanoic acid). Of these isomers, only d-biotin has vitamin activity (Mock, 2013).

The nitrogen atom opposite the side chain acts as a transfer point for carboxyl groups in enzymatic carboxylation reactions, the primary function of biotin enzymes (Bonjour, 1991).

Previously, biotin has been known as vitamin H or coenzyme R. Biotin crystallizes from water as long, white needles. Its melting point is 232–233°C. Free biotin is soluble in dilute alkaline solutions and hot water and practically insoluble in fats and organic solvents. Biotin is relatively stable under ordinary conditions. It is destroyed by nitric acid, other strong acids, strong bases, and formaldehyde and is inactivated by oxidative rancidity reactions. It is gradually destroyed by ultraviolet (UV) radiation (Camporeale and Zempleni, 2006; Said, 2012).

Structurally related biotin analogs can vary from no activity to partial replacement of biotin activity to antibiotin action. Mild oxidation converts biotin to sulfoxide, and strong oxidation converts it to sulfone, which is metabolically inactive. Potent agents result in sulfur replacement by oxygen, resulting in oxybiotin and desthiobiotin. Oxybiotin has partial biotin activity

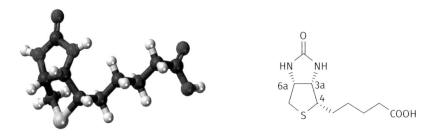

Figure 4.51 D-biotin chemical structure

in chicks (one-third) and rats (one-tenth). Besides these biotin analogs, other compounds can bind biotin to form a stable complex, thus preventing the utilization of the vitamin by animals and microorganisms. The microorganism *Saccharomyces avidinii* produces a biotin-binding protein, streptavidin, and other compounds that can inactivate free biotin and inhibit biotin synthesis in susceptible microorganisms. A prominent nutrient-drug interaction is that biotin-dependent enzymes are reduced with the epilepsy drug carbamazepine (Rathman *et al.*, 2002). Requirements and concentrations are usually expressed in mass units (mg or µg/kg) (Camporeale and Zempleni, 2006; Said, 2012).

Natural sources
Biotin is present in feedstuffs in both bound and free forms, and much of the bound biotin is unavailable to animal species. For poultry, swine, and presumably for ruminants, often less than half of the microbiologically determined biotin in a feedstuff is biologically available (Table 4.5). Of all the vitamins present in feed ingredients of plant origin, biotin is the one that presents the most variable content and bioavailability, being affected by numerous environmental factors (Frigg, 1976, 1984; Misir and Blair, 1984; Mock, 2013; Chen Y.F. *et al.*, 2019). Soybean meal, for instance, contains a mean biotin content of 270 µg per kg with a range of 200 to 387 µg per kg (Frigg and Volker, 1994). Milling wheat or corn reduced biotin concentrations (Bonjour, 1991).

Biotin is present in feedstuffs and yeast in both bound and free forms; therefore, it is crucial to know the form of biotin, i.e., bound or unbound, and its overall content in the feed. Much of the bound biotin to protein or lysine (biocytin) is unavailable to animal species as covalent bonds hinder its digestion and availability for the animal. Less than one-half of the microbiologically determined biotin in a feedstuff is biologically available (Frigg, 1984).

The bioavailability of biotin is estimated at 100% for alfalfa, corn, cottonseed, and soybean meal. However, biotin availability is variable for other feedstuffs, for example, 11–50% in barley, 62% in corn gluten meal, 30% in fish meal, 10–60% in sorghum, 32% in oats, and 0–62% in wheat (Kopinski *et al.*, 1989; McDowell, 2004; Chen Y.F. *et al.*, 2019). Diets based on these cereals without biotin supplementation led to higher mortality and slower growth rates.

Other factors influencing biotin availability (and requirement) are some nutrients, such as fiber, which interfere with its intestinal absorption (Misir and Blair, 1984), protein level – with higher requirements at 18% than at 22% of crude protein in the diet – the level of choline and the other water-soluble vitamins – which at high levels reduce the bioavailability of biotin – and the proportion and the composition in fatty acids of added fats.

Biotin is unstable to oxidizing conditions and, therefore, is destroyed by heat, especially under conditions that support simultaneous lipid peroxidation by solvent extraction and

Table 4.5 Biotin content in the Feedstuffs (source: adapted from Frigg, 1984)

Feedstuffs	Mean bioavailable biotin content (ug/kg)	Feedstuffs	Mean bioavailable biotin content (ug/kg)
Barley	14	Safflower seed meal	305
Corn	79	Sunflower seed meal	346
Corn gluten meal	189	Fish meal	135
Oats	86	Meat meal > 50% CP	88
Rye	0	Meat and bone meal < 50% CP	76
Rice polishings	74	Skim milk powder	165
Sorghum	58	Whey powder	316
Wheat	0	Cassava meal	3
Wheat bran	72	Grass meal	238
Wheat middlings	17	Alfalfa	407
Wheat germ	150	Molasses, beet	331
Rapeseed meal	68	Molasses, cane	1080
Soybean meal	270	Brewer's yeast	634

improper storage conditions. At the same time, steam pelleting does not affect the stability of biotin (McGinnis, 1986b), and there has even been an increase of 10% measured in its bioavailability (McGinnis, 1986a,b).

Information is lacking on the biotin availability of feedstuffs in ruminants. Experiments with the rumen simulation technique (RUSITEC) indicated that rumen availability of biotin from barley/hay rations of varying forage to grain ratio ranged from 65 to 77% with a mean of 70% (Da Costa Gomez et al., 1998). The primary source of biotin for ruminants is that synthesized by microorganisms in the rumen. Although biotin synthesis occurs across a wide range of diets (Hayes et al., 1966), increasing the proportion of grain in the ration reduces net synthesis by over 50% (Da Costa Gomez et al., 1998). Miller et al. (1986) found that rumen biotin synthesis varied with the cereal grain source fed. Frigg and Volker, (1994) estimated from bio-kinetic data that net ruminal biotin synthesis of mature Holstein cattle was negligible. Available data suggest that 1–5 mg of biotin are synthesized per day in the rumen of cattle, and 1–3 mg per day are absorbed.

Milk from ruminants is an excellent source of biotin. Cow colostrum contained 1.0–2.7 µg biotin per 100 ml (Foley and Otterby, 1978). Milk biotin levels can go from 8 to 9 µg per 100 ml (Midla et al., 1998; Fitzgerald et al., 2000). In these same studies, feeding 20 mg per day of supplemental biotin increased milk biotin levels to 16.2–22.6 µg per 100 ml. A ewe's milk is reported to contain over twice as much biotin as a cow's (NRC, 1985).

Commercial forms

Biotin is commercially available as a 100% crystalline product or as various dilutions, premixed, and low-potency spray-dried preparations. The d-form of biotin is the biologically active form. It is the form that occurs in nature and is also the commercially available form. A 2% spray-dried biotin product with a carrier (triturate) is commercially available for feed or drinking water use. Spray-dried biotin has more uniform biotin activity and higher numbers of particles per gram than the triturates. These properties enhance the mixing and distribution of biotin in feeds and supplements.

Supplemental d-biotin was reported to have a net bioavailability in mature Holstein cattle of 50–60% with a half-life in the body of 6–18 hours (Frigg *et al.*, 1993; Frigg and Volker, 1994). Steinberg *et al.* (1994) reported an apparent bioavailability of 40% in lactating dairy cows. Kluenter and Steinberg (1993) and Steinberg *et al.* (1996) fed graded oral doses of d-biotin in a stabilized, spray-dried form and studied the effects on plasma and milk biotin levels in lactating dairy cows. Biotin was supplemented between 0 and 80 mg per day. Plasma biotin was significantly higher in dry cows than in lactating cows. Significant diurnal variation occurred in plasma biotin, which increased within 1 hour of feeding supplemental biotin and continued to increase until 4 hours after the second daily feeding (Kluenter and Steinberg, 1993). In both studies, a highly significant linear regression was found between oral biotin intake and both plasma output in milk (r^2 = 0.96). Therefore, it is clear that orally supplemented biotin is absorbed proportionately to doses up to 80 mg daily. The short systemic half-life of biotin concentrations and biotin output in milk (r^2 = 0.96). Therefore, like most water-soluble vitamins, it is clear that orally supplemented biotin requires daily supplementation if plasma and tissue levels are to be consistently increased in ruminants.

Metabolism
Absorption and transport
After feed ingestion, biotinidase, present in pancreatic juice and intestinal mucosa, catalyzes the hydrolysis of biocytin, the biotin-bound form, to biotin and free lysine during the luminal phase of proteolysis. In most species that have been investigated, physiological concentrations of biotin are absorbed from the intestinal tract by a sodium-dependent active-transport process, which is inhibited by dethiobiotin and biocytin (Said and Derweesh, 1991).

Absorption of biotin by a Na^+-dependent process was noted to be higher in the duodenum than in the jejunum, which was, in turn, more elevated than that in the ileum. It was concluded that the proximal part of the human small intestine was the site of maximum biotin transport (Said *et al.*, 1988; Said, 2011). Biotin is absorbed intact in the first third to half of the small intestine (Bonjour, 1991).

Biotin exits the enterocyte across the basolateral membrane. This transport is also carrier mediated. However, this carrier is Na+ independent, is electrogenic, and cannot accumulate biotin against a concentration gradient (Said, 2011). Biotin transport is regulated by multiple factors, including biotin nutritional status, enterocyte maturity, anatomic location, and ontogeny (Said, 2011). Biotin transport is more active in the villus than in the crypt cells. Transport is most active in the upper small intestine and progressively less active aborally into the colon.

Biotin appears to circulate in the bloodstream free and bound to a serum glycoprotein, which also has biotinidase activity and catalyzes biocytin's hydrolysis. In humans, 81% of biotin in plasma was free, and the remainder was bound (Mock and Malik, 1992; Mock, 2013). In chicken plasma, 2 biotin-binding proteins have been detected, which appear to be functionally different. Information on biotin transport, tissue deposition, and storage in animals and humans is minimal. Mock (1990) reported that biotin is transported as a free water-soluble component of plasma, is taken up by cells via active transport, and is attached to its apoenzymes (Lane *et al.*, 1964). Said *et al.* (1992) reported that biotin is transported via a specialized, carrier-mediated transport system into the human liver. This system is Na^+ gradient-dependent and transports biotin via an electroneutral process (Mock, 2013). The placenta has a Na^+-dependent transporter that transports biotin, pantothenic acid, and lipoic acid (Prasad *et al.*, 1997).

Storage and excretion

All cells contain some biotin, with larger quantities in the liver, brain, placenta, white blood cells, and kidney. The intracellular distribution of biotin corresponds to known locations of biotin-dependent carboxylase enzymes, especially the mitochondria (Mock, 2013). Investigations of biotin metabolism in animals are difficult to interpret, as biotin-producing microorganisms are present in the intestinal tract distal to the cecum.

The amount of biotin excreted in urine and feces often exceeds the total dietary intake, whereas urinary biotin excretion is usually less than the intake (Pour *et al.*, 2017). The efficient conservation of biotin and the recycling of biocytin released from the catabolism of biotin-containing enzymes may be as crucial as the intestinal bacterial synthesis of the vitamin in meeting biotin requirements (Bender, 1992). ^{14}C-labeled biotin showed the major portion of intraperitoneally injected radioactivity to be excreted in the urine and none in the feces or as expired CO_2 (Lee *et al.*, 1973).

Biochemical functions

Biotin is a coenzyme essential for gluconeogenesis, lipogenesis, and the elongation of essential fatty acids. It converts carbohydrates to protein and vice versa, transforming protein and carbohydrates into fat. Biotin is a cofactor of various enzymes that allow CO_2 to be fixed or eliminated in organic molecules (pyruvate carboxylase, propionyl coenzyme A carboxylase, acetyl coenzyme A carboxylase, among others). All the enzymes involved in biotin require ATP and magnesium for activation. Biotin is vital for the normal functioning of the reproductive and nervous systems and the thyroid and adrenal glands.

Biotin also plays a vital role in maintaining normal blood glucose levels from the metabolism of protein and fat when the dietary intake of carbohydrates is low. As a component of 5 carboxylating enzymes, it can transport carboxyl units and fix carbon dioxide (bicarbonate) in tissue (Camporeale and Zempleni, 2006; Mock, 2013).

The 5 biotin-dependent carboxylases are:

- propionyl-CoA carboxylase (PCC)
- methylcrotonyl-CoA carboxylase (MCC)
- pyruvate carboxylase (PC)
- acetyl-CoA carboxylase 1 (ACC1)
- acetyl-CoA carboxylase 2 (ACC2).

All except ACC2 are mitochondrial enzymes. In carbohydrate metabolism, biotin functions in both carbon dioxide fixation and decarboxylation, with the energy-producing citric acid cycle dependent upon the presence of this vitamin. The hydrolysis of ATP drives the reaction to ADP and inorganic phosphate. Specific biotin-dependent reactions in carbohydrate metabolism are:

- carboxylation of pyruvic acid to oxaloacetic acid
- conversion of malic acid to pyruvic acid
- interconversion of succinic acid and propionic acid
- conversion of oxalosuccinic acid to α-ketoglutaric acid. Biotin enzymes are essential in protein synthesis, amino acid deamination, purine synthesis, and nucleic acid metabolism.

Biotin is required for transcarboxylation in the degradation of various amino acids. Vitamin deficiency in mammals hinders the standard conversion of the deaminated chain of leucine to acetyl-CoA. Depleting hepatic biotin reduces the hepatic activity of methylcrotonyl-CoA carboxylase, which is needed for leucine degradation (Mock and Mock, 1992; Mock, 2013). Likewise, the ability to synthesize citrulline from ornithine is reduced in liver homogenates from biotin-deficient rats. The urea cycle enzyme ornithine transcarbamylase was significantly lower in the livers of biotin-deficient rats (Maeda *et al.*, 1996).

Fatty acid metabolism
Acetyl-CoA-carboxylase catalyzes the addition of CO_2 to acetyl-CoA to form malonyl CoA, the first reaction in synthesizing fatty acids. Biotin is required for normal long-chain unsaturated fatty acid synthesis and is vital for essential fatty acid metabolism. Deficiency in rats and chicks inhibited arachidonic acid (20:4) synthesis from linoleic acid (18:2) while increasing linolenic acid (18:3) and its metabolite (22:6). The reduced synthesis of arachidonic acid (20:4) in chicks reduces plasma prostaglandin E_2 (PGE_2) since arachidonic acid is a precursor of prostaglandin (20:4) (Watkins and Kratzer, 1987). The characteristic dermatitis of biotin deficiency may be partly due to aberrations of essential fatty acid metabolism (Zempleni and Mock, 1999).

Immunity and cell signaling
Biotin is also required for the normal function of immune cells that actively accumulate biotin (Bonjour, 1991; Zempleni and Mock, 1999). Populations of T- and B-lymphocytes depend on biotin supply, and marginal biotin status reduces antibody production (Zempleni and Mock, 1999). Evidence has emerged that biotin plays unique roles in cell signaling, epigenetic control of gene expression, and chromatin structure (Rodríguez-Meléndez and Zempleni, 2003; Riveron-Negrete and Fernandez-Mejia, 2017). In rats, biotin regulates the genetic expression of holocarboxylase synthetase and mitochondrial carboxylases (Rodríguez-Meléndez *et al.*, 2001). Manthey *et al.* (2002) report that biotin affects the expression of biotin transporters, biotinylation of carboxylases, and the metabolism of interleukin-2 in Jurat cells. These cells are an immortalized line of human T-lymphocyte cells used to study acute T cell-related diseases like leukemia, T cell signaling, and the expression of various chemokine receptors susceptible to viral entry, particularly HIV.

The 3 primary species of rumen cellulolytic bacteria are required for biotin (Baldwin and Allison, 1983). Biotin is a cofactor in the microbial enzyme methylmalonyl-CoA-carboxyl transferase, which catalyzes a step in propionic acid synthesis. The omission of biotin from *in vitro* rumen fermentations reduces propionic acid production (Milligan *et al.*, 1967). Biotin is involved with gluconeogenesis, propionate metabolism, fatty acid synthesis, and amino acid degradation. The nature of the ruminant digestive system imposes a significant dependence on gluconeogenesis because truly little glucose is being absorbed (Reynolds *et al.*, 2007). In ruminants, the rate of gluconeogenesis increases with feed intake, and one of the major substrates for gluconeogenesis is propionate. Metabolic utilization of propionate after its absorption from the gastrointestinal tract depends on propionate's transformation into succinyl-coenzyme A, requiring the subsequent actions of biotin- and vitamin B_{12}-dependent enzymes. Propionate is first transformed into propionyl-CoA, which is carboxylated to methylmalonyl-CoA carboxylase. Biotin supplementation increased the activity of liver pyruvate carboxylase (Ferreira *et al.*, 2007). Sone *et al.* (1999) reported that biotin enhances glucose-stimulated insulin release from the rat pancreas.

Hoof formation
The biomechanical properties of a hoof horn are determined by its structural characteristics. These characteristics, which include intra- and extracellular biochemical composition and

arrangement of horn cells, are determined during keratinization and cornification. Any disturbance of this process, such as interrupting nutrient supply because of circulatory abnormalities or essential nutrient deficiency, may adversely affect horn structure and quality (Mülling
et al., 1999). The claw horn is a modified skin derivative and contains significant quantities of
the structural protein keratin. Biotin is an essential nutrient in keratin synthesis and lipogenesis, the 2 major metabolic pathways in keratinization (Lischer et al., 2002). It participates in
the differentiation of epidermal cells and the production of keratin and intracellular cementing substances (Mülling et al., 1999). The intracellular cementing substance binds together
the keratin leaflets of the hoof horn. However, the main action of biotin supplementation is
on the reduction of wear of the horny tissue more than the growth of the hoof (Vermunt and
Greenough, 1995).

Vermunt and Greenough (1994) compiled data that are associated with the etiology of
hoof issues. Among them, individual cow factors stand out, such as: lactation stage, age and
number of births, occurrence of systemic infection, limb conformation and genetic inher-
itance. In relation to herd factors, nutrition, management, level of physical activity, comfort
and environment.

Hoof problems constitute a group of conditions that have a major impact on the dairy
cow productivity. It represents a serious animal welfare issue and causes significant economic
losses (Collick et al., 1989; Esslemont, 1990; Potter and Broom, 1990; Bargai and Levin 1993;
Shearer and Van Amstel, 1997) and it is a limiting factor for the animals health that inappro-
priate use of the locomotor system (Roest, 1993) changing animals behavior and productivity.

Nutritional assessment

Biotin status analysis can be measured in plasma using different methods, including microbiological, GC, avidin binding, colorimetric, polarographic, and isotope dilution assays (Sauberlich,
1999). Research on several markers of biotin status is ongoing in humans, but more clinical
validation is needed (Höller et al., 2018).

Deficiency signs

Because it is a required cofactor in 4 critical metabolic enzymes, biotin deficiency adversely
affects many tissues, especially those with high metabolic activity or cell division rates. Biotin
is required for the thyroid and adrenal glands' normal function and reproductive and nervous
systems. Its effect on the cutaneous system is most dramatic. The classic sign of biotin deficiency in animals and humans is a characteristic red, scaly dermatitis, especially around the
eyes, nose, and mouth. Metabolic changes include lactic acidosis, aciduria, and increased urinary excretion of 3-hydroxy isovaleric acid, a metabolite of leucine (Zempleni and Mock, 1999).

The blockage in propionic acid metabolism results in the accumulation of 3-hydroxy propionic acid in the urine (Zempleni and Mock, 1999). Production of essential fatty acids is abnormal in biotin deficiency (Watkins, 1989), which may be the mechanism by which skin lesions are
produced (Mock, 1991). Immune function is compromised by biotin deficiency, with reductions
in plasma immunoglobulins and both T- and B-lymphocytes (Zempleni and Mock, 1999).

Biotin deficiency in calves is characterized by paralysis of the hind legs, generalized weakness, and reduced urinary excretion of biotin (Wiese et al., 1946). The parenteral administration
of biotin corrected the condition. Flipse et al. (1948) reported a potassium-biotin interrelationship in calves. Calves fed purified diets low in potassium and biotin developed progressive
paralysis of the hind legs that spread to the forelegs, neck, and respiratory system. Death
resulted within 12–24 hours of the first symptoms. The parenteral administration could cure
the condition of either potassium salts or biotin. A more recent study (Mülling et al., 1999)

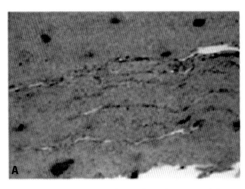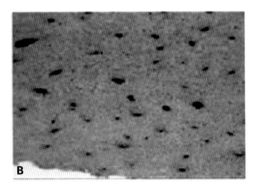

Figure 4.52 Biotin deficiency in dairy cows: (a) before and (b) 12 months after biotin supplementation (source: Distl and Schmid, 1994)

produced biotin deficiency in a calf to study its effects on hoof growth and keratinization. The calf displayed the classic biotin deficiency dermatitis symptoms around the muzzle and eyes. The hoof epidermis displayed several specific abnormalities, including a marked decrease in keratin production, a reduced intracellular cementing substance, a very thin germinative cell layer, and a thin hoof sole with a brittle and crumbly consistency. The typical border of cornification between live and dead horn layers had disappeared entirely in the biotin-deficient calf. Based on their observations, the authors concluded that biotin is essential for normal keratinization and hoof horn quality (Figure 4.52).

A study of biotin deficiency in Angora and Cashmere goats (Mengal *et al.*, 1998) reported that biotin deficiency significantly reduced hoof growth and concentration of cysteine and lysine in hoof horn, which participate in the cross-linking of protein. No significant breed-by-treatment interactions were reported. The consistent reduction in hoof disorders observed experimentally in response to supplemental biotin in dairy and beef cattle and improvement in milk production suggest that marginal biotin deficiency occurs for these animals under intensive management with high production levels. Lischer *et al.* (2002) concluded that 40 mg of biotin per day positively influenced the healing of hoof sole ulcers during 50 days of supplementation. Bergsten *et al.* (2003) evaluated supplementation of 20 mg/day of biotin in dairy cows during 2 lactations and observed diverse claw lesions (Figure 4.53). These authors observed that biotin-supplemented cows had a 24% incidence of sole hemorrhages in the final hoof trimming. In comparison, control cows without supplementation had a 50% incidence of this claw lesion. Similar responses or lesions in poultry, horses, and swine have been interpreted as marginal biotin deficiency (McDowell, 2000a).

Biotin deficiency adversely affects cellular and humoral immune function (Camporeale and Zempleni, 2006). The synthesis of antibodies is reduced in biotin-deficient rats. Biotin deficiency in mice decreases the number of spleen cells and the percentage of B-lymphocytes in the spleen.

Safety
Given the rapid metabolic turnover of biotin, toxicity is unlikely to occur in livestock. Studies in humans and laboratory animals have shown a high tolerance level for oral biotin and few, if any, toxicity symptoms (Bonjour, 1991). Relatively elevated levels of supplementation have been used in humans to combat weak fingernails, dermatitis, and hair loss and as a therapy for diabetes without noticeable adverse reactions (Bonjour, 1991).

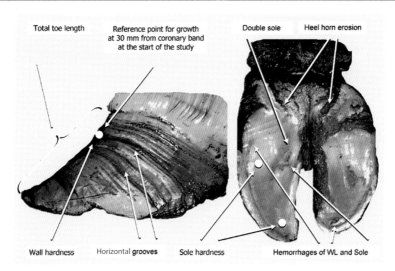

| Total toe length | Reference point for growth at 30 mm from coronary band at the start of the study | Double sole | Heel horn erosion |

| Wall hardness | Horizontal **grooves** | Sole hardness | Hemorrhages of WL and Sole |

Figure 4.53 Claw lesions observed in dairy cows: biotin supplementation (20 mg/day) reduced in half the sole hemorrhages (source: Bergsten *et al.*, 2003)

Folic acid (vitamin B$_9$)
Chemical structure and properties
Folacin is the generic descriptor for the original vitamin folic acid and related compounds that qualitatively show folic acid activity. The terms folacin, folate, and folic acid can be used interchangeably and refer to many compounds that possess folic acid's biological activity. Folic acid is structurally one of the most complex vitamins. Folic acid has the most significant number of biologically active forms of any vitamin.

The pure substance is designated pterylomonoglutamic acid. It consists of one pteridine nucleus, one molecule of para-aminobenzoic acid, and one glutamic acid moiety. The basic folate molecule is 5,6,7,8-tetrahydropteroylglutamate, also referred to as tetrahydrofolate (THF) monoglutamate, which consists of a 2-amino-4-hydroxy-pteridine (pterin) moiety linked via a covalent bond, methylene group at the C-6 position to a p-aminobenzoyl-glutamic acid. Its chemical structure contains 3 distinct parts: glutamic acid, a para-aminobenzoic acid (PABA) residue, and a pteridine nucleus (Figure 4.54). Over 100 active forms have been identified, varying according to the reduction state of the pteridine nucleus (di- or tetrahydrofolate), the presence or absence of methyl or other single-carbon groups on the N5 and N10 atoms, and the number of glutamic acid residues present (Girard, 1998).

In most naturally occurring folates, the number of glutamate units in the side chain of peptides varies from 5 to 8. The PABA portion of the vitamin structure was once considered a vitamin. Research has shown that if the folic acid requirement of the organism is met, there is no need to add PABA to the diet. Folic acid is a synthetic, fully oxidized monoglutamate form of the vitamin used commercially in supplements, fortified/enriched foods, and feeds (Bailey *et al.*, 2013).

Folic acid is a yellowish-orange crystalline powder that is tasteless, odorless, and insoluble in alcohol, ether, and other organic solvents. It is slightly soluble in hot water in the acid form but quite soluble in the salt form. It is relatively stable to air, oxygen, and heat in neutral and alkaline solutions but unstable in acid solutions. From 70 to 100% of the folic acid activity is destroyed on autoclaving at pH 1 (Frieden *et. al.*, 1944). It is readily degraded by light and

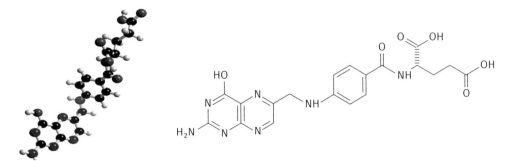

Figure 4.54 Folic acid chemical structure

ultraviolet radiation, and heating can considerably reduce folic acid activity, particularly under oxidative conditions (Gregory, 1989).

However, feed additives can reduce this source. Sulfonamides are the folic acid biosynthetic intermediate PABA analogs widely used as antibacterial agents (Brown, 1962). By competing with PABA, sulfonamides prevent folic acid synthesis so that microorganisms cannot multiply, reducing or eliminating an important source of folic acid to the animal.

Natural sources

Much of the naturally occurring folic acid in feedstuffs is conjugated with varying numbers of different glutamic acid molecules, reducing its absorption efficiency. Folic acid is present in most of the ingredients, almost exclusively THF acid derivatives, especially in those of animal origin, but in insufficient quantity (Lindemann, 1988; Chen *et al.*, 2019).

Good sources are soybeans, other beans, nuts, and cereal grains (1.8 mg/kg). It is also found in oilseeds (2.5 mg/kg), especially in whole seeds (soybean 3.5 mg/kg compared with 0.5 mg/kg in soy meal). Products of animal origin also have moderate concentrations (blood meal 0.8 mg/kg, fishmeal between 0.2 and 1.0 mg/kg, whey 0.9 mg/kg, etc.). The stable THF acid derivatives have a methyl or formyl group in the 5-position and generally possess 3 or more glutamic acid residues in glutamyl linkages. Only limited amounts of free folic acid occur in natural products, and most feed sources contain predominantly polyglutamyl folic acid. The abundance of folic acid in green forages is confirmed by greater folic acid concentrations in milk from grazing herds than in herds fed dry hay (Dong and Oace, 1975).

The mean availability of folic acid in 7 separate food items was close to 50%, ranging from 37 to 72% in the monoglutamate form (Babu and Srikantia, 1976). The bioavailability of orally administered 5-methyl folic and 5-formyl folic acid was equal to folic acid for rats (Bhandari and Gregory, 1992). Folic acid bioavailability in various foods generally exceeded 70% (Clifford *et al.*, 1990). The bioavailability of monoglutamate folic acid is substantially greater than polyglutamyl forms (Gregory *et al.*, 1991b; Clifford *et al.*, 1990). Polyglutamyl folates must be hydrolyzed to monoglutamates before absorption (Seyoum and Selhub, 1998). Additionally, the amount available for each animal varies depending on differences in intestinal pH or general living conditions.

Most naturally occurring folates are relatively unstable. Thus, folates exhibit a significant loss of activity during harvesting, storage, and processing, but measured folate concentrations are also highly influenced by the method used for sample preparation. The synthetic form, folic acid, is more resistant to chemical oxidation (Scott, 1999). A considerable loss of folic acid (50–90%) occurs during feed manufacturing. Folic acid is sensitive to light and heating, particularly in acid solutions. Under aerobic conditions, the destruction of most folic acid forms is significant with heating.

Concentrations of folic acid in ruminal DM range from 0.3 to 0.6 mg/kg (Lardinois *et al.*, 1944). Corresponding values for strained rumen fluid ranged from 0.08 to 0.19 mg/kg (Hayes *et al.*, 1966). Rumen microbial synthesis of folic acid begins with the onset of a functional rumen. Some bacterial species can synthesize folates, and others need them. Different amounts of folates can be synthesized and used in the rumen depending on the feed composition. For steers, Girard *et al.* (1994) and Hayes *et al.* (1966) described a relationship between the proportion of concentrates in the diet and the quantity of folates in the rumen. High-concentrate diets increased folates. The authors hypothesized that this increase is due to enhanced microbial activity in the rumen caused by rapidly degradable carbohydrates.

Commercial forms
Spray-dried folic acid and dilutions of crystalline folic acid are the most widely used product forms in animal feeds. Several lines of evidence indicate higher bioavailability of added folic acid than naturally occurring folates in many foods, with approximately 50% lower availability (Gregory, 2001). Synthesized folic acid is the monoglutamate form.

Supplementation with synthetic pteroylmonoglutamate form (MG), N5-formyl-5,6,7,8,-tetrahydrofolic acid (THFA), or commercial bacterial cell powder sources rich in reduced folates had similar biopotency (Harper *et al.*, 2003). Although folacin is only sparingly soluble in water, sodium salt is quite soluble and is used in injections and feed supplements (McGinnis, 1986a, b).

Metabolism
Absorption and transport
Polyglutamate forms of folic acid are digested via hydrolysis to pteroylmonoglutamate before transport across the intestinal mucosa. The enzyme responsible for the hydrolysis of pteroyl-polyglutamate is a carboxy peptidase known as folate conjugase (Baugh and Krumdieck, 1971). Most likely, several conjugase enzymes are responsible for the hydrolysis of the long-chain folate polyglutamate to the mono glutamates, which then enter the mucosal cell.

Pteroylmonoglutamate is absorbed predominantly in the duodenum and jejunum, apparently by an active process involving sodium. Folates are also absorbed by a simple diffusion mechanism when concentrations are at pharmacological levels or when the intestinal pH is above 6.0. The uptake of folic acid in the cecum raises the likelihood of absorption of bacterial-derived folic acid.

Most folacin is reduced to THFA and can be methylated. Kesavan and Noronha (1983) suggested using rat results. That luminal conjugase is a secretion of pancreatic origin. The hydrolysis of folic acid polyglutamate forms occurs in the lumen rather than at the mucosal surface or within the mucosal cell. Studies showed that about 79–88% of labeled folic acid is absorbed, and absorption is rapid since serum concentrations usually peak about 2 hours after ingestion.

After hydrolysis and absorption from the intestine, dietary folates are transported in plasma as monoglutamate derivatives, predominantly as 5-methyltetrahydrofolate. The monoglutamate derivatives then enter cells by specific transport systems. The pteroylpolyglutamates, the primary folic acid form in cells, are built up stepwise by an enzyme, folate polyglutamate synthetase. Polyglutamates keep folic acid within the cells since only the monoglutamate forms are transported across membranes, and only monoglutamates are found in plasma and urine (Wagner, 1995).

Storage and excretion

Folic acid is widely distributed in tissues, mainly in the conjugated polyglutamate forms of folic acid, usually containing 3 to 7 glutamyl residues linked by peptide bonds. The natural coenzymes are abundant in every tissue examined (Wagner *et al.*, 1984). Specific folate-binding proteins (FBPs) that bind folic acid mono- and polyglutamate are known to exist in many tissues and body fluids, including the liver, kidney, small intestinal brush border membranes, leukemic granulocytes, blood serum, and milk (Tani and Iwai, 1984). Giguère *et al.* (1998) reported a high-affinity FBP in cow, pig, and sheep serum. The physiological roles of these FBPs are unknown. However, it has been suggested that they play a role in folic acid transport analogous to the intrinsic factor in the absorption of vitamin B_{12}.

Folate is actively and passively transported across the placenta during late gestation, and the vitamin is stored primarily in the liver of the developing fetus (Narkewicz *et al.*, 2002). The folate status of the newborn kid is relatively low. Folic acid content is the greatest in the colostrum and declines precipitously with the onset of copious milk production (Girard *et al.*, 1996). Starting at parturition, folate concentrations in milk decrease until 4 weeks after parturition, when folate concentrations reach a stable plateau until lactation's end (Girard *et al.*, 1995). The folate balance of the kid may be more precarious than that of lambs because the concentration of folic acid in goat's milk is at least 5 times less than that of ewe's milk.

Studies have shown that 79–88% of labeled folic acid is absorbed and absorption rapidly, with serum concentrations usually peaking about 2 hours after ingestion. The mean availability of folic acid in 7 different foods was close to 50%, varying from 37 to 72% (Babu and Srikantia, 1976). Folic acid is widely distributed in tissues, mainly in the conjugated polyglutamate forms.

Urinary excretion of folic acid represents a small fraction of total excretion. However, fecal folic acid concentrations are pretty high, often higher than intake, representing undigested folic acid and, more importantly, many bacterial syntheses in the large intestine. Bile contains elevated levels of folic acid due to enterohepatic circulation, with most biliary folic acid reabsorbed from the small intestine. This suggests a physiologic mechanism exists to regulate folate re-uptake based on tissue requirements (Bailey *et al.*, 2013).

Biochemical functions

The principal functions of folic acid are related to:

- the synthesis of protein and purines, and pyrimidines, which make up the nucleic acids needed for cell division (Bailey *et al.*, 2013)
- the interconversions of various amino acids
- the maturation process of red corpuscles and the functioning of the immune system.

This means multiple coenzyme forms transfer one-carbon activity (Bailey *et al.*, 2013). In form of THFA, folic acid is indispensable in transferring single-carbon units in various reactions, a role analogous to that of pantothenic acid in the transfer of 2-carbon units (Bailey and Gregory, 2006; Bailey *et al.*, 2013). The 1-carbon unit can be formyl, methylene, or methyl groups. Some biosynthetic relationships of one-carbon units are shown in Figure 4.55.

The major *in vivo* pathway providing methyl groups involves the transfer of a one-carbon unit from serine to THF to form 5,10-methylenetetrahydrofolate, which is subsequently reduced to 5-methyltetrahydrofolate. Methyl tetrahydrofolate then supplies methyl groups to remethylate homocysteine in the activated methyl cycle, providing methionine for synthesizing the critical methyl donor agent S-adenosylmethionine (Krumdieck, 1990; Jacob *et al.*, 1994; Bailey *et al.*, 2013).

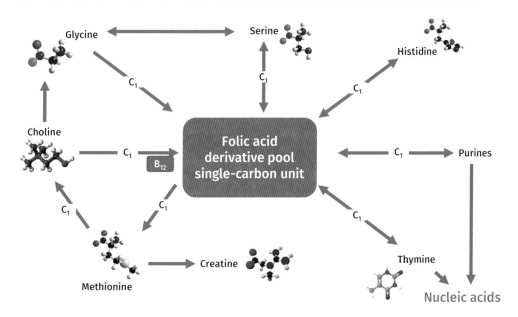

Figure 4.55 Folic acid metabolism requires single-carbon units

The critical physiological function of THF consists of binding the single-carbon (C_1) units to the vitamin molecule, thus transforming them to "active formic acid" or "active formaldehyde." These are interconvertible by reduction or oxidation and transferable to appropriate acceptors. Folic acid polyglutamates work at least as well as or better than the corresponding monoglutamate forms in every enzyme system examined (Wagner, 1995). It is now accepted that the pteroylpolyglutamates are the acceptors and donors of one-carbon units in amino acid and nucleotide metabolism, while the monoglutamate is merely a transport form.

Specific reactions involving single-carbon transfer by folic acid compounds are:

- purine and pyrimidine synthesis for nuclei acids
- interconversion of serine and glycine
- glycine–carbon as a source of C_1 units for many synthetic pathways (glycine cleavage system)
- histidine degradation
- synthesis of methyl groups for such compounds as methionine, choline, and thymine (a pyrimidine base)
- methionyl-tRNA transformylase is a required step in initiating all protein synthesis.

As folacin is involved in the interconversion of serine and glycine, in the degradation of histidine, and in the addition of methyl groups to compounds such as methionine from homocysteine, choline from ethanolamine, and thiamine, inadequate levels of other methyl group donors – such as vitamin B_{12}, serine, methionine, betaine, and choline – increase folic acid requirements (Bailey *et al.*, 2013). Logically, high protein levels in the diet raise the dietary recommendations for folate.

Purine bases (adenine and guanine), as well as thymine, are constituents of nucleic acids. With a folic acid deficiency, there is a reduction in the biosynthesis of nucleic acids essential for cell formation and function. Hence, deficiency of the vitamin leads to impaired cell division and alterations of protein synthesis; these effects are most noticeable in rapidly growing tissues such as red blood cells, leukocytes, intestinal mucosa, and embryonic and fetal tissues. In rats, an adequate supply of folic acid and related methyl donors can benefit fetal development directly by improving lipid metabolism in fetal and maternal tissues (McNeil *et al.*, 2009). Without adequate folate, the normal maturation of primordial red blood cells in bone marrow is arrested at the megaloblast stage. As a result, characteristic macrocytic anemia develops. White blood cell formation is also affected, resulting in abnormalities such as thrombopenia, leukopenia, and multilobed neutrophils.

Folic acid is needed to maintain the immune system. The blastogenic response of T-lymphocytes to certain mitogens is decreased in folic acid-deficient humans and animals, and the thymus is preferentially altered (Dhur *et al.*, 1991). Its function in metabolism is closely linked to that of vitamin B_{12}, choline, and vitamin C, but also to vitamin B_6 because of its role in reassembling the profile of amino acids circulating in plasma on explicit demand by ribosomes, which regulate the process of protein synthesis.

Nutritional assessment

Serum/plasma folate is a good indicator of current folate status and is used as a first-line clinical indicator of folate deficiency (Sauberlich, 1999). Folates can be measured using HPLC-MS/MS, electrochemical or fluorescence-based techniques, radio- and immuno-based assays, and the traditional *Lactobacillus casei* growth assay. This microbiological approach measures all biologically active folate species, including di- and triglutamates of the species, but cannot differentiate between the species (Höller *et al.*, 2018).

As folate and cobalamin jointly participate in one-carbon metabolism and thus have close biological links, both are usually measured concurrently since the deficiency will interact with the blood status markers of the other (Höller *et al.*, 2018).

Deficiency signs

Folacin deficiency produces unspecific symptoms, such as megaloblastic anemia, leucopenia, and growth retardation. Deficiency symptoms are uncommon as microorganisms can synthesize this vitamin in the rumen. However, special attention must be paid to young animals, where intestinal flora is still insignificant, and when substances with antimicrobial action are administered in the feed. Vitamin degradation during storage can also reduce its bioavailability (Yang *et al.*, 2021b) and consequently cause a reduction in plasma levels.

Tissues that have a rapid rate of cell growth or tissue regeneration, such as the epithelial lining of the gastrointestinal tract, epidermis, and bone marrow, are most affected (Hoffbrand, 1978). Li *et al.* (2020) demonstrated the effect of folic acid supplementation in developing the intestinal mucosa in newborn lambs (Figure 4.56). The intestinal muscle layer in the lamb offspring was enhanced significantly with increasing maternal folic acid supplementation.

A folic acid deficiency has not been demonstrated in the calf, but Draper and Johnson (1952) reported a deficiency in lambs fed synthetic diets. The disease was characterized by leukopenia, followed by diarrhea, pneumonia, and death. Folic acid therapy promoted the regeneration of white cells, and 0.39 mg per liter of diet prevented the deficiency. Folic acid deficiency has been reported in sheep experiencing a vitamin B_{12} deficiency. The vitamin B_{12} deficiency was severe enough to decrease voluntary feed intake to less than 200 g per day (NRC, 2007).

The efficiency of folic acid synthesis by rumen microflora and whether this is adequate at weaning and later have not yet been established. For example, in an experiment in which

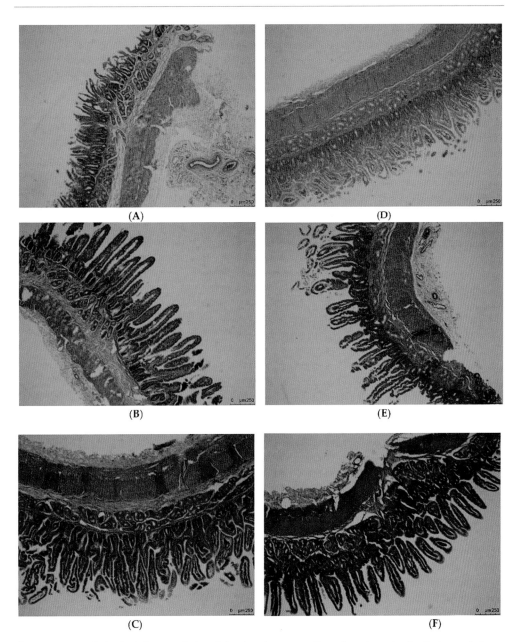

Figure 4.56 Morphological characteristics of duodenal cross-section of newborn lambs that were fed folic acid by the mother during pregnancy. (A–C) are cross-sections from twin-born lambs from ewes fed 0, 16 or 32 mg·(kg DM)–1 folic acid in the basal diet, respectively; (D–F) are cross-sections from triplet-born lambs from ewes fed 0, 16 or 32 mg·(kg DM)–1 folic acid in the basal diet, respectively (source: Li et al., 2020)

supplemental folic acid was administered to dairy heifers intramuscularly weekly during the first 4 months of life, the average daily gain increased by 8% during the 5 weeks following weaning (Dumoulin *et al.*, 1991). This supplementation also increased serum and hepatic folates, blood hemoglobin, and packed cell volume. These results suggest that marginal folic acid deficiency may develop in calves or lambs post-weaning until full rumen function is achieved. The effects of folic acid supplementation on milk production have been variable.

For gestating primiparous and multiparous cows, Girard *et al.* (2005) found a non-significant increase in milk production of 14% in the last part of lactation due to an intramuscular injection of 160 mg folic acid once per week. However, they could not find an effect on milk production immediately after calving. In contrast, Girard and Matte (1998) found a 6% increase in milk production during the first 100 days of lactation for multiparous cows receiving 4 mg folic acid per kg BW and a 10% increase from day 100 to day 200. Supplementary folic acid and vitamin B_{12} increased milk production from 34.7 to 38.9 kg per day and increased milk lactose, protein, and total solids yields (Preynat *et al.*, 2009).

Safety
Folic acid is generally considered a nontoxic vitamin (NRC, 1998). Excess folates are rapidly excreted in the urine. No adverse responses to ingestion of folic acid have been documented in any species.

Vitamin C
Chemical structure and properties
Vitamin C is named ascorbic acid (2-oxo-L-threo-hexono-1,4-lactone-2,3-enediol), and there are 4 stereoisomers: D- and L-ascorbic acid and D- and L-isoascorbic acid (with the D-form also named erythorbic acid). Vitamin C is structurally similar to glucose. However, the term vitamin C refers only to the compounds with L-ascorbic acid activity, which are biologically active, and it includes 2 forms (Figure 4.57):

- L-ascorbic acid: reduced form
- dehydro-L-ascorbic acid: oxidized form.

Although in nature, the vitamin is primarily present as ascorbic acid, and both forms are biologically active, but not the D-isomers. In nature, the reduced form of ascorbic acid may reversibly oxidize to the dehydroxidized form, i.e., dehydroascorbic acid (Johnston *et al.*, 2013), and dehydroascorbic acid is irreversibly oxidized to the inactive diketogulonic acid. The latter can be further oxidized to oxalic acid and L-threonic acid. Since this change occurs readily, vitamin C is susceptible to destruction through oxidation, accelerated by heat and light. Reversible oxidation-reduction of ascorbic acid with dehydroascorbic acid is vitamin C's most important chemical property and the basis for its known physiological activities and stabilities (Moser and Bendich, 1991).

Vitamin C is a white to yellow-tinged crystalline powder. It crystallizes out of the water, like square or oblong crystals. It is slightly soluble in acetone and has lower alcohol. A 0.5% solution of ascorbic acid in water is strongly acid with a pH of 3. The vitamin is more stable in acid than in an alkaline medium. Crystalline ascorbic acid is relatively stable in the air without moisture. However, vitamin C is the least stable and, therefore, most easily destroyed of all the vitamins. Several chemical substances, such as air pollutants, industrial toxins, heavy metals, and some pharmacologically active compounds, are antagonistic to vitamin C and can increase vitamin requirements (Johnston *et al.*, 2013).

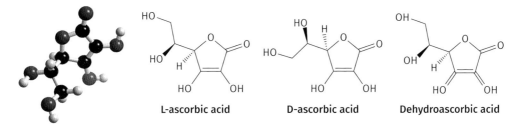

Figure 4.57 Vitamin C chemical structure

Natural sources

The primary sources of vitamin C are fruits and green plants, but some foods of animal origin contain more than traces of the vitamin. Vitamin C occurs in significant quantities in animal organs, such as the liver and kidney, but in only tiny amounts in meat. Post-harvest storage values vary with time, temperature, damage, and enzyme content (Zee *et al.*, 1991; Johnston *et al.*, 2013).

Commercial forms

Ascorbic acid is commercially available as:

- 100% crystalline L-ascorbic acid
- sodium ascorbate
- 97.5% L-ascorbic acid – ethyl cellulose-coated (EC)
- 35% phosphorylated Na/Ca salt of L-ascorbic acid (Ca or Na ascorbyl-2-phosphate; $C_6H_9O_9P$ molecular mass 256.11 g/mol)
- 50% phosphorylated Na salt of L-ascorbic acid (Ca or Na ascorbyl-2-phosphate; $C_6H_6O_9Na_3P\cdot H_2O$ molecular mass 358.08 g/mol).

When providing supplemental ascorbic acid in heat-treated feeds, using a stabilized form like EC-coated or phosphorylated forms is strongly advisable. In storage experiments, ascorbic acid protected in this manner was 4 times more stable than untreated ascorbic acid crystals (Kolb, 1984). Adams (1978) reported that EC ascorbic acid retained more after processing than the crystalline form, 84 versus 48%. Retention of ascorbic acid in mash feed was reasonably good, but stability was poor in crumbled meals with elevated storage time and temperature.

The ascorbyl-2 polyphosphate is more rumen-stable than crystalline vitamin C and is effective in elevating plasma ascorbic acid concentrations in ruminating dairy cattle. The average plasma ascorbic acid concentration was approximately 4.0 µg/ml and was increased by 22% in cattle supplemented with 20 g/day stabilized in vitamin C (MacLeod *et al.*, 1996). The effect persisted over a 31 day experimental period, indicating that vitamin C supplementation did not reduce endogenous synthesis. However, a wide variation has been observed in the level of these responses and, therefore, in the zootechnical results obtained, which may be due to diverse factors:

- low stability of vitamin C in feed, which improves significantly in phosphorylated forms and also in drinking water, especially if alkaline and unchlorinated
- dietary energy level
- level and duration of dosage

- the age of the animals
- the intensity and combination of stress factors, disease, immunological challenge, or injury.

Hidiroglou (1999) reported that cows dosed orally with 40 g/day ethylcellulose-coated vitamin C had higher plasma vitamin C levels than when dosed with crystalline vitamin C. Interestingly, cows dosed with vitamin C via the abomasum had only slightly higher plasma vitamin C levels than cows dosed orally. In sheep, Hidiroglou et al. (1997a) found that duodenal administration of vitamin C did result in higher plasma levels than oral dosing. However, they found slight difference among crystalline vitamin C, ethylcellulose-coated vitamin C, ascorbyl-2-polyphosphate, and sodium ascorbate in effect on plasma vitamin C and the level above basal plasma levels. These studies conflict with early experiments showing rapid and extensive ruminal destruction of crystalline vitamin C (Cappa, 1958; Itze, 1984). Garrett et al. (2007) evaluated rumen-protected encapsulation of vitamin C as it related to fermentation by rumen bacteria. Rumen bacteria extensively degraded raw ascorbic acid (unencapsulated) in less than 6 hours. Two different encapsulation methods proved effective in protecting 50% or more of the ascorbic acid exposed to rumen bacterial fermentation through 24 hours. Padilla et al. (2007) supplemented cows with a vitamin C preparation coated with hydrogenated soybean oil. Cattle likely absorbed more than half of this protected product. Further studies are needed in this area. Black and Hidiroglou (1996) reported that intramuscular injection produced a greater level above basal plasma vitamin C than intravenous administration of vitamin C.

Through modern technological advances, a form of ascorbic acid is currently being marketed as a phosphate ester, which is stable in heat processing and storage conditions. The product L-ascorbyl-2-monophosphate (Rovimix Stay-C 35®) contains 35% ascorbic acid (Schultze and Willy, 1997). The phosphate ester allows the ascorbic acid to withstand heat processing. When entering the digestive tract, the phosphate ester is cleaved off, and the ascorbic acid is available for adsorption.

Metabolism
Synthesis
Ruminants synthesize ascorbic acid. Humans, other primates, guinea pigs, invertebrates, some insects, fish, bats, and birds lack this enzyme and cannot synthesize vitamin C (Sauberlich, 1990). Endogenous production of vitamin C depends on the presence or absence of the liver microsomal enzyme L-gulono-γ-lactone oxidase (GLO, which imparts the ability to synthesize ascorbic acid from monosaccharides) (Lehninger, 1982). In ruminants, this enzyme is present in the microsomes of liver cells and is responsible for ascorbic acid biosynthesis. The enzyme converts L-gulono-γ-lactone to L-keto-gulono-γ-lactone, which produces L-ascorbic acid through isomerization.

Absorption and transport
Vitamin C is absorbed like carbohydrates (monosaccharides) in the small intestine. The bioavailability of vitamin C in feeds is limited, but 80 to 90% appears to be absorbed (Kallner et al., 1977). Intestinal absorption in vitamin C-dependent animals requires sodium-dependent vitamin C transporters (SVCT1 and SVCT2) at low digesta concentrations (Johnston, 2006; Johnston et al., 2013). It is assumed that those not scurvy-prone species like ruminants have an absorption mechanism by diffusion at higher concentrations, mainly in the duodenum and jejunum (Spencer et al., 1963; Tsukaguchi et al., 1999; Johnston, 2006). Slight variations on the leading site of absorption have been observed. The absorption site in the guinea pig is in

the duodenal and proximal small intestine, whereas the rat showed the highest absorption in the ileum (Hornig *et al.*, 1984). However, the presence of SCTV1 in the chick renal proximal tubule has been identified. Ascorbic acid is readily absorbed when quantities are small, but limited intestinal absorption occurs when excess ascorbic acid is ingested. Considerable quantities of ascorbic acid are secreted into the gastrointestinal tract and then reabsorbed as dehydroascorbate (Dabrowski, 1990).

Absorbed vitamin C readily equilibrates with the body pool of the vitamin. Several enzymes or non-enzymatic processes first convert ascorbic acid to dehydroascorbate in its metabolism. In a glutathione-dependent reaction, it can then be reduced back to ascorbic acid in cells (Johnston *et al.*, 2013). Elevated levels of dietary iron, zinc, copper, and pectin reduce the utilization of ascorbic acid, either by direct oxidation of vitamin C or by reducing its absorption (Sauberlich, 1990).

Dehydroascorbic acid is the preferred vitamin C for uptake by erythrocytes, lymphocytes, and neutrophils (Sauberlich, 1990). Recycling between dehydroascorbate and ascorbate is a prominent feature of vitamin C metabolism in erythrocytes and white blood cells and appears to aid in maintaining antioxidant reserves (Mendiratta *et al.*, 1998). The Se enzyme glutathione peroxidase participates in the regeneration of ascorbic acid from dehydroascorbic acid in bovine erythrocytes (Washburn and Wells, 1999). Ascorbic acid is also stabilized by the antioxidant enzymes superoxide dismutase and catalase (Miyake *et al.*, 1999), which require copper, zinc, manganese, and iron. No specific binding proteins for ascorbic acid have been reported, and it is suggested that the vitamin is retained by binding to subcellular structures.

Storage and excretion

Ascorbic acid is widely distributed throughout the tissues in animals capable of synthesizing vitamin C and in those dependent on an adequate dietary amount of the vitamin. In experimental animals, the highest concentrations of vitamin C are found in the pituitary and adrenal glands, and high levels are also found in the liver, spleen, brain, and pancreas (Sauberlich, 1990). Tissue levels are decreased by virtually all forms of stress, which also stimulates the biosynthesis of the vitamin in those animals capable of synthesis.

Vitamin C tends to be concentrated in tissues during wound healing. In calves, the major reservoirs of ascorbic acid are in the lungs, liver, and muscle tissue (Toutain *et al.*, 1997). Based on radioisotope measurements of ascorbic acid kinetics, the lungs appear to be a smaller but rapidly mobilized vitamin C pool. At the same time, the liver and muscle are more significant, more slowly mobilized reserves (Toutain *et al.*, 1997).

Ascorbic acid is metabolized to 2,3-diketogulonic acid and oxalate and excreted in the urine, with small amounts in sweat and feces (Sauberlich, 1990). In guinea pigs, rats, and rabbits, oxidation to CO_2 is the primary excretory mechanism for vitamin C. Primates do generally not utilize the CO_2 catabolic pathway, with significant loss occurring in the urine. Urinary excretion of vitamin C depends on body stores, intake, and renal function.

Biochemical functions

Unlike other species, ruminants, as previously discussed, can synthesize ascorbic acid from glucose in the liver (Matsui, 2012), depending on the animal's weight (Johnston, 2006). Evidence suggests that in some circumstances, this endogenous synthesis may be insufficient (Ranjan *et al.*, 2012). The capacity for vitamin C synthesis varies with age and hereditary predisposition.

Ascorbic acid participates in fundamental biological and metabolic processes, and its function is related to its reversible oxidation and reduction characteristics (Table 4.6). Thus, its action is essential in the following:

- calcification processes
- immune response
- adaptation to stress
- maintenance of electrolytic balance.

Biochemical and physiological functions of vitamin C have been reviewed by several authors (Moser and Bendich, 1991; Padh, 1991; Gershoff, 1993; Johnston, 2006; Johnston *et al.*, 2013). However, the exact role of this vitamin in the living system is not entirely understood since a coenzyme form has not yet been reported.

In more detail, the main biochemical functions of vitamin C are (Figure 4.58):

- antioxidant and immune role (stimulation of phagocytic activity)
- biosynthesis of collagen
- control of glucocorticoid synthesis
- conversion of vitamin D_3 to its active form
- absorption of minerals
- metabolism, detoxification, wound healing, and reproduction.

Antioxidant and immune role (stimulation of phagocytic activity)

One of the most interesting properties of vitamin C is its ability to function as a reducing agent or electron donor. Ascorbic acid converts to dehydroascorbic acid and is subsequently reduced in the cell cytoplasm, essential to electron transfer (oxidation-reduction). It reacts rapidly with free radicals and acts synergistically with vitamin E, facilitating the regeneration of the reduced form of α-tocopherol in biological systems (Kornegay, 1986), hence accounting for the observed sparing effect on this vitamin (Jacob, 1995). In the process of sparing fatty acid oxidation, tocopherol is oxidized to the tocopheryl free radical. Ascorbic acid can donate an electron to the tocopheryl free radical, regenerating the reduced antioxidant form of tocopherol.

Table 4.6 Enzymes depending on ascorbic acid for maximum activity

Enzymes	Function
Proline hydroxylase (EC 1.14.11.2)	Trans-4-hydroxylation of proline in procollagen biosynthesis
Procollagen-proline 2-oxoglutarate 3-dioxygenase (EC 1.114.11.7	Trans-4-hydroxylation of proline in procollagen biosynthesis
Lysine hydroxylase (EC1.14.11.4)	5-hydroxylation of lysine in procollagen biosynthesis
Gamma-butyrobetaine, 2-oxyglutarate 4-dioxygenase (EC 1.14.11.1)	Hydroxylation of a carnitine precursor
Trimethyllysine-2 oxoglutarate dioxygenase (EC 1.14.11.8)	Hydroxylation of a carnitine precursor
Dopamine β-monooxygenase (EC 1.14.27.1)	Dopamine β-hydroxylation in norepinephrine biosynthesis
Peptidyl glycine alpha-amidating monooxygenase activity	Carboxyterminal alpha-amidation of glycine-extended peptides in peptide hormone processing
4-hydroxypenylpyruvate dioxygenase (EC 1.13.11.27)	Hydroxylation and decarboxylation of a tyrosine metabolite

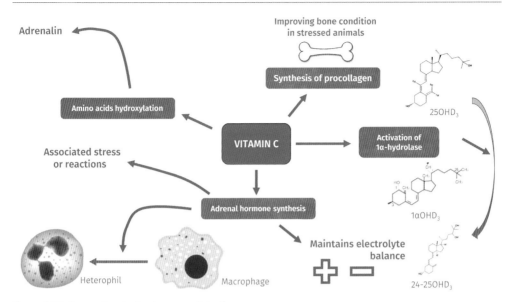

Figure 4.58 Some vitamin C roles on metabolism

Tissue defense mechanisms against free-radical damage generally include vitamin C, E, and β-carotene as the primary vitamin antioxidant sources. In addition, several metalloenzymes that include glutathione peroxidase (Se), catalase (iron), and superoxide dismutase (copper, zinc, and manganese) are also critical in protecting the internal cellular constituents from oxidative damage.

The dietary and tissue balance of all these nutrients is vital in protecting tissue against free-radical damage (Benito and Bosch, 1997; Cadenas *et al.*, 1998). Both *in vitro* and *in vivo* studies showed that antioxidant vitamins enhance cellular and noncellular immunity. The antioxidant function of these vitamins could, at least in part, enhance immunity by maintaining the functional and structural integrity of critical immune cells and erythrocytes. Extensive recycling of vitamin C occurs in neutrophils, monocytes, and macrophages (Washko *et al.*, 1993), and the presence of bacteria stimulates this process (Wang *et al.*, 1997). Ascorbic acid enhances macrophage production of nitric oxide, which is involved in bactericidal reactions (Mizutani *et al.*, 1998). Vitamin C and E supplementation potentiates white blood cell function in healthy adults (Jeng *et al.*, 1996). Camarena and Wang (2016) discussed the epigenetic role of vitamin C in health and disease. A compromised immune system will reduce animal production efficiency through increased disease susceptibility, increasing animal morbidity and mortality (Bronzo *et al.*, 2020).

Ascorbic acid is reported to have a stimulating effect on the phagocytic activity of leukocytes, the function of the reticuloendothelial system, and the formation of antibodies. Ascorbic acid levels are very high in phagocytic cells, with these cells using free radicals and other highly reactive oxygen-containing molecules to help kill pathogens that invade the body. Ascorbic acid, as an effective scavenger of reactive oxygen species, minimizes the oxidative stress associated with the respiratory burst of activated phagocytic leukocytes, thereby functioning to control the inflammation and tissue damage associated with immune responses with antihistamine, anti-endotoxin, and anti-inflammatory properties (Rojas *et al.*, 1996; Chien *et al.*, 2004).

Vitamin C has an antihistamine effect (Johnston and Huang, 1991; Johnston *et al.*, 1992), reducing plasma histamine levels, possibly enhancing neutrophil chemotaxis, and improving bronchial dilation during infection (Gershoff, 1993). In related findings, vitamin C has been shown to attenuate the damaging effects of bacterial *Escherichia coli* endotoxin on the lungs of sheep (Dwenger *et al.*, 1994) and guinea pigs (Benito and Bosch, 1997). Vitamin C has also been shown to impart protection against *E. coli* LPS endotoxin damage to the liver (Cadenas *et al.*, 1998) and heart (Rojas *et al.*, 1996), possibly by induction of the mixed-function oxi-dase system. High concentrations of endotoxin inhibit the uptake of vitamin C by the adrenal cortical cells (Garcia and Municio, 1990).

In ruminants there is evidence of the effect of vitamin C on immune function. Researchers at Auburn University reported both positive effects (Blair and Cummins, 1984) and no effect (Cummins and Brunner, 1989) on plasma immunoglobulin concentration of colostrum-de-prived dairy calves. Hidiroglou *et al.* (1995) reported no effect of vitamin C alone (0–2 g per day) on immunoglobulin concentrations or lymphocyte response to mitogen in dairy calves. However, the same authors reported a trend for increased immunoglobulin M (IgM) in plasma when calves received both vitamin C and vitamin E. Roth and Kaeberle (1985) reported that parenteral administration of 20 mg per kg ascorbic acid reversed the suppressive effects of dexamethasone on neutrophil function and tended to enhance neutrophil phagocytosis of *S. aureus* bacteria. Ascorbic acid supplementation reduced respiratory rate, rectal temperature, and serum cortisol level and increased serum thyroid hormone (T_4) in heat-stressed lambs (Kobeisy *et al.*, 1997). High environmental temperature has been reported to reduce plasma vitamin C concentrations in Holstein cattle, especially above 26.6°C (Singh, 1957).

Biosynthesis of collagen

The beneficial effects of ascorbic acid in collagen biosynthesis are extensively documented and represent the most clearly established role for vitamin C. Collagens are the tough, fibrous, intercellular materials (proteins) that are the principal components of skin and connective tissue, the organic matrix of bones and teeth and the ground substance between cells (Moser and Bendich, 1991; Padh, 1991; Gershoff, 1993; Tsuchiya and Bates, 1997; Johnston, 2006; Johnston *et al.*, 2013).

In the case of vitamin C deficiency, the impairment of collagen synthesis appears to be due to a lowered ability to hydroxylate lysine and proline, which constitutes the basis for the cross-over of tropocollagen molecules, giving rise to structures of great size and consistency. Also, its hydroxylation capacity is essential in carnitine synthesis and may be indirectly involved in fatty acid and cholesterol metabolism. In addition to the relationship of ascorbic acid to hydroxylase enzymes, Franceschi (1992) suggests that vitamin C is required for the differen-tiation of connective tissue such as muscle, cartilage, and bone derived from mesenchyme (embryonic cells capable of developing into connective tissue). Ascorbic acid was proposed to contribute to the prevention of muscle degeneration affecting meat color and other qual-ity parameters (Oohashi *et al.*, 2000; Nam and Ahn, 2003). The collagen matrix produced by ascorbic acid-treated cells is proposed to provide a permissive environment for tissue-specific gene expression. A common finding in all studies is that vitamin C can alter the expression of multiple genes as cells progress through specific differentiation programs (Ikeda *et al.*, 1997).

Beneficial effects result from ascorbic acid synthesizing "repair" collagen. Alteration of base-ment membrane collagen synthesis and its integrity in the mucosal epithelium during vitamin C restriction might explain how the capillary fragility is induced in scurvy and the increased incidences of periodontal disease under vitamin C deprivation. Failure of wounds to heal and gum and bone changes resulting from vitamin C undernutrition are direct consequences of reducing insoluble collagen fibers. Ascorbic acid is a cofactor in extracellular matrix metabolism because it affects collagen, laminin, various cell-surface integrins, and elastin. Vitamin C is a cofactor for enzymes key to the post-translational modification of matrix proteins (Johnston *et al.*, 2013).

Control of glucocorticoid synthesis

Vitamin C controls the synthesis of glucocorticoid norepinephrine in the adrenal gland. The protective effects of vitamin C (also vitamin E) on health may partially result from reducing glucocorticoid circulating levels (Nockels, 1990). During stress conditions (e.g., heat stress, weaning), glucocorticoids, which suppress the immune response, are elevated (Farooq *et al.*, 2010). Vitamin C reduces adrenal glucocorticoid synthesis, helping to maintain immunocompetence.

In addition, ascorbate can regenerate the reduced form of α-tocopherol, perhaps accounting for the observed sparing effects of these vitamins (Jacob, 1995). In the process of sparing fatty acid oxidation, tocopherol is oxidized to the tocopheryl free radical. Ascorbic acid can donate an electron to the tocopheryl free radical, regenerating the reduced antioxidant form of tocopherol.

Conversion of vitamin D_3 to its active form

Because of its relationship to hydroxylation enzymes, vitamin C directly affects the C-1 hydroxylation of $25OHD_3$ to the active form $1,25(OH)_2D_3$ (Suter, 1990; Cantatore *et al.*, 1991).

Absorption of minerals (iron)

Ascorbic acid has a role in metal ion metabolism due to its reducing and chelating properties. This results in enhanced absorption of minerals from the diet and their mobilization and distribution throughout the body. Ascorbic acid promotes non-heme iron absorption from food (Olivares *et al.*, 1997; Kontoghiorghes *et al.*, 2020). It reduces the ferric iron at the acid pH in the stomach and forms complexes with iron ions that stay in solution at alkaline conditions in the duodenum (Kontoghiorghes *et al.*, 2020). In hematopoiesis, ascorbic acid facilitates the transfer of iron from transferrin (a plasma protein) to ferritin (an organ protein), which stores iron in the bone marrow, spleen, and liver. Ascorbic acid can also be involved in the metabolism of zinc, copper, and manganese in the reduced state.

Some other functions of ascorbic acid are the following.

- **Effect on oxidative enzymes.** Due to the ease with which ascorbic acid can be oxidized and reversibly reduced, it probably plays an essential role in reactions involving electron transfer in the cell. Almost all terminal oxidases in plant and animal tissues can directly or indirectly catalyze the oxidation of L-ascorbic acid. Such enzymes include ascorbic acid oxidase, cytochrome oxidase, phenolase, and peroxidase. In addition, its oxidation is readily induced under aerobic conditions by many metal ions and quinones.
- **Metabolism of amino acids.** Ascorbic acid has a role in the metabolic oxidation of specific amino acids, including tyrosine, histidine, and tryptophan.
- **Synthesis of carnitine.** Carnitine is synthesized from lysine and methionine and depends on 2 hydroxylases containing ferrous iron and L-ascorbic acid. Vitamin C participates in the hydroxylation of trimethyl lysine. Vitamin C deficiency can reduce the formation of carnitine, resulting in the accumulation of triglycerides in the blood and the physical fatigue and lassitude associated with scurvy (Ha *et al.*, 1994). About 98% of total body carnitine is in muscle; skeletal and heart muscle carnitine concentrations are reduced by 50% in vitamin C-deficient guinea pigs compared with controls (Johnston *et al.*, 2013).

- **Induction of the gluconeogenic** through liver enzyme phosphoenolpyruvate carboxykinase (Maggini and Walter, 1997).
- **Interrelationships of vitamin C to B vitamins:** tissue levels and urinary excretion of vitamin C are affected in animals in case of deficiencies of thiamine, riboflavin, pantothenic acid, folic acid, and biotin.
- **Detoxification of toxins:** natural compounds, and other xenobiotics by live microsomes. Vitamin C has been demonstrated to inhibit nitrosamines, which are potent carcinogens (Mirvish, 1986).
- **Drug metabolism.**
- **Biological role in keratinocytes.** Because the skin must provide the first line of defense against environmental free-radical attack (e.g., sunburn, skin aging, and skin cancer), it has developed a complex antioxidant network that includes enzymatic and non-enzymatic components (Duarte and Almeida, 2012). The epidermis is composed of several layers of keratinocytes supplied with enzymes (superoxide dismutase, catalase, thioredoxin reductase, and glutathione reductase) and low-molecular-weight antioxidant molecules (tocopherol, glutathione, and ascorbic acid) (Podda and Grundmann-Kollmann, 2001). Since ascorbic acid is essential in collagen formation, its presence increases the capacity to heal skin wounds (Pullar *et al.*, 2017; Vaxman *et al.*, 1995; Duarte and Almeida, 2012). In keratinocytes, vitamin C counteracts oxidative stress via transcriptional and post-translational mechanisms. Vitamin C can: 1) act directly by scavenging reactive oxygen species (ROS) generated by stressors; 2) prevent ROS-mediated cell damage by modulating gene expression; 3) regulate keratinocyte differentiation by maintaining a balanced redox state; and 4) promote cell cycle arrest and apoptosis in response to DNA damage (Catani *et al.*, 2005). Pullar *et al.* (2017) reviewed the roles of vitamin C in skin health.
- **Hormone activation.** Vitamin C is also involved in many hormone activation processes. Hormones like melanotropins, calcitonin, growth hormone-releasing factors, corticotrophin and thyrotropin, vasopressin, oxytocin, cholecystokinin, and gastrin undergo amidations where ascorbic acid serves as a reductant to maintain copper in a reduced state at the active site of the enzyme (Johnston *et al.*, 2013).
- **Reproduction.** Ascorbic acid is found in up to a ten-fold concentration in seminal fluid compared to serum levels and decreasing levels have caused nonspecific sperm agglutination (Mittal *et al.*, 2014). In a review of ascorbic acid and fertility, Luck *et al.* (1995) suggested 3 of ascorbic acid's principal functions: its promotion of collagen synthesis, its role in hormone production, and its ability to protect cells from free radicals, which may explain its reproductive actions. The high concentration of vitamin C in the testicle and ovarian *corpus luteum* (Petroff *et al.*, 1996) suggests a physiological role linked to reproduction.

Nutritional assessment

Several biological compartments, such as whole blood, erythrocytes, leucocytes, and plasma or serum, can be used to assess vitamin C status. However, serum or plasma ascorbate concentration is the most reliable marker (Rojas *et al.*, 1996). Analysis of ascorbic acid in biological samples is complicated by the high susceptibility of this compound to oxidation, which requires the use, for example, of EDTA (Höller *et al.*, 2018).

Several approaches have been developed to measure vitamin C in biological materials: HPLC provides an efficient means to quantify vitamin C with good selectivity and sensitivity (Höller *et al.*, 2018).

Deficiency signs

Classic symptoms of scurvy, the vitamin C deficiency, are marked deterioration of mucosal integrity and health and subsequent loss of disease resistance. Because ruminants possess the metabolic pathway to synthesize ascorbic acid, they are only likely to experience outright deficiency symptoms in the neonatal period before synthesis reaches total capacity.

Cummins (1992) cites several published reports of vitamin C deficiency signs in young calves. The signs included oral cavity and skin lesions, low plasma ascorbate levels, increased susceptibility to disease, and evidence of muscle pain and subcutaneous hemorrhage. Ascorbic acid appears to play a prominent role in collagen synthesis related to the intracellular hydroxylation of proline and lysine during the formation of tropocollagen. Therefore, some of the effects of vitamin C deficiency in mucosa lesions and capillary fragility are due to collagen failing to crosslink correctly and the lack of hydroxyproline and hydroxylysine. Ascorbic acid deficiency disrupts iron transport between blood plasma and storage organs.

The death of cows and calves due to scurvy was characterized by changes in the oral cavity mucosa, muzzle, skin, weight loss, and general unhealthiness (Cole *et al.*, 1944; Duncan, 1944). In calves, extensive dermatosis was observed in animals receiving insufficient milk, accompanied by hair loss and skin thickening. Blood ascorbic acid was low, and the condition was successfully treated with parenteral vitamin C administration. Studies of blood vitamin C concentrations in calves fed a typical diet revealed significant individual differences, with variations related to the genetic background.

Immunity, stress, and disease

In other species, vitamin C deficiency results in impaired neutrophil and macrophage chemotaxis and depressed T-lymphocyte response to respiratory disease (Beisel, 1982; Sauberlich, 1994; Hemila and Douglas, 1999). Disease conditions have been found to affect vitamin C metabolism. Vitamin C can protect tissues by enhancing humoral and cellular immune responses to disease (Nockels, 1988). With a vitamin C deficiency, impaired chemotaxis in macrophages and depressed T-lymphocyte response have been reported (Beisel, 1982). Vitamin C deficiency impairs the bactericidal activity of neutrophils (Goldschmidt, 1991).

Stress caused by housing, disease, weather changes, transport, or other factors is the most probable cause of marginal vitamin C deficiency in ruminants (Cummins and Brunner, 1991; Mackenzie *et al.*, 1997). However, studies have not established a clear basis for the level of vitamin C required for optimal health and performance of calves, lambs, or goat kids. Supplementation of milk replacer with vitamin C at levels similar to whole milk would appear advisable.

Studies with bulls indicated reduced vitamin C status during cold stress (Hidiroglou *et al.*, 1977). Hypovitaminosis C has been observed primarily in winter and early spring and, most commonly, in calves (Soldatenkov and Suganova, 1966). Jagos *et al.* (1977) found considerably lower plasma vitamin C content in calves with bronchopneumonia than in healthy animals. A relationship has been reported between hypovitaminosis C, skeletal muscle pain, and subcutaneous hemorrhages in calves (Pribyl, 1963). Dobsinska *et al.* (1981) studied the relationship between ascorbic acid status and body weight gain of calves in a large commercial facility. They found a negative correlation between the 2 parameters in 2–22-week-old bull calves. Calves from herds characterized by poor health status generally had reduced ascorbic acid status during the critical period from birth to 2 weeks of age. Supplementation with 1.25–2.5 g of vitamin C per day reportedly reduced the incidence of respiratory disease (Itze, 1984; Palludan and Wegger, 1984; Hemingway, 1991).

Reproduction

According to Chatterjee (1967), degeneration of the ovaries and testes occurs in guinea pigs on an ascorbic acid-free diet, but the effects are associated with general inanition. There is evidence for reduced testosterone synthesis by Leydig cells of the testes of vitamin C-deficient male guinea pigs. The precise role of ascorbic acid in sex steroid biosynthesis has not been established. In females, there are considerable demands for collagen synthesis and degradation during pregnancy as uterine growth, placental development, and fetal development depend on rapid increases in connective tissue components, of which ascorbic acid plays a critical role.

The establishment and maintenance of pregnancy in all farm animals depend upon maintaining a corpus luteum that produces progesterone and, in some species, estrogen production by the placenta. Since adequate ascorbic acid concentrations in tissue may be essential for normal sex steroid metabolism by ovarian and fetal-placental tissue, vitamin C would appear crucial to the reproductive process. Petroff *et al.* (1996) measured total ascorbate and oxidized ascorbate levels in the ovarian stroma, follicles, and *corpora lutea* throughout the estrus cycle and during pregnancy. They reported that maximal luteal and follicular function periods are associated with elevated concentrations of total ascorbate within these tissues. In addition, aging of the corpora lutea was associated with a high partitioning of reduced ascorbate. Petroff *et al.* (1996) demonstrated that prostaglandin (PGF2) depletes the porcine corpus luteum of vitamin C by inducing the secretion of the vitamin into the bloodstream. Thus, these findings support the hypothesis that vitamin C depletion contributes to the demise of the porcine corpus luteum.

Mastitis

Positive effects of ascorbic acid supplementation on milk yield and quality have been reported (Kucmyj, 1955). Even though cows can synthesize vitamin C and vitamin C is not a required nutrient for dairy cows, data are accumulating that show a considerable reduction in plasma vitamin C for lactating cows with mastitis (Naresh *et al.*, 2002; Weiss *et al.*, 2004; Kleczkowski *et al.*, 2005; Ranjan *et al.*, 2005) and in heat-stressed cows (Padilla *et al.*, 2006). The severity of clinical signs of mastitis is correlated with the magnitude of the decrease in plasma vitamin C concentration (Weiss *et al.*, 2004). Vitamin C supplementation stimulated recovery from acute mammary inflammation with reduced somatic cell counts (Weiss and Hogan, 2007).

Neutrophils are a primary host defense mechanism against mastitis, and the responsiveness of neutrophils is related to the incidence and severity of mastitis in dairy cows. Vitamin C concentrations in neutrophils isolated from milk were about 3 times greater than in blood neutrophils (Weiss and Hogan, 2007). The duration of clinical mastitis, peak body temperature, number of colony-forming units of *E. coli* isolated from the infected gland, and loss in milk yield were associated with a change in concentration of vitamin C in milk from the challenged quarter (Weiss *et al.*, 2004).

In conclusion, young ruminants appear susceptible to vitamin C deficiency during the first few weeks of life, particularly when subjected to stress, disease exposure, or limited colostrum intake. Vitamin C is not an essential dietary nutrient for adult ruminants. However, supplemental vitamin C benefits for animals under stress or disease conditions, such as mastitis, have been shown.

Safety

Several studies with poultry, swine, and laboratory animals have shown no deleterious effect when the animals are fed elevated levels of vitamin C (NRC, 1998). Data on the tolerance and toxicity of ascorbic acid for ruminants are unavailable. In guinea pigs, extremely high levels (8.7%) fed for 6 weeks caused decreased bone density and decreased urinary hydroxyproline compared to control animals fed 0.2% of ascorbic acid (Bray and Briggs, 1984). However, no significant bone changes were observed. One sign is an excess accumulation of iron in the liver. It would appear extremely difficult to produce vitamin C toxicity from dietary sources in ruminants due to the apparent rumen destruction of the vitamin.

Choline
Chemical structure and properties
Choline is considered a vitamin, although it does not fulfill some of the prerequisites of this definition. It can be synthesized in the liver of ruminants from serine and methyl groups, requiring 3 moles of methionine for each mole of choline synthesized. However, for most metabolic processes, the quantity and rate of synthesis are insufficient to cover requirements, especially when the supply of precursors such as methionine, vitamin B_{12}, or folacin is limited.

Choline is a β-hydroxyethyl-trimethyl-ammonium hydroxide (Figure 4.59). Pure choline is a colorless, viscous, strongly alkaline liquid that is notably hygroscopic. Choline is soluble in water, formaldehyde, and alcohol and has no definite melting or boiling point. The chloride salt of this compound, choline chloride, is produced by chemical synthesis for use in the feed industry, although there are other forms. Choline chloride consists of deliquescent white crystals, which are very soluble in water and alcohol. Aqueous solutions are almost pH neutral (Jiang X. *et al.*, 2013).

Natural sources
All naturally occurring fats contain some choline, and thus, it is supplied by all feeds that contain fat. Egg yolk, glandular meats, and the brain are the richest animal sources, whereas the germ of cereals, legumes, and oilseed meals are the best plant sources (DuCoa, 1994). Corn is low in choline, with wheat, barley, and oats containing approximately twice as much choline as corn.

Since betaine can spare the choline requirements, knowing betaine concentrations in feeds would be helpful. Unfortunately, most feedstuffs contain only small amounts of betaine. However, wheat and wheat by-products contain over twice as much betaine as choline. Sugar beets are also high in betaine.

Little is known about the biological availability of choline in natural feedstuffs. Using a chick assay method, soybean, canola, and peanut meals obtained a substantial proportion of unavailable choline (Emmert and Baker, 1997). In bioavailability, soybean lecithin products are equivalent to choline chloride (Emmert *et al.*, 1997). Although 3 times as rich in total choline as soybean meal, canola meal has less bioavailable choline (Emmert and Baker, 1997).

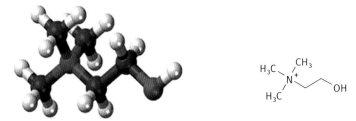

Figure 4.59 Choline structure

Endogenous choline synthesis makes bioavailability challenging to quantify. The bioavailability of choline for ruminants is of minor importance because both naturally occurring choline in feeds, predominantly found in phospholipids (lecithin), and dietary choline from supplements, such as choline chloride, is extensively degraded in the rumen (Sharma and Erdman, 1988, 1989a). Choline supplements are only of value if they are resistant to rumen degradation. The RP choline products have been available since the 1990s (Erdman and Sharma, 1991).

Commercial forms

Commercially, choline is produced by chemical synthesis, and choline salts are used in dietary supplementation. The available forms are:

- choline chloride 75% solution in water
- choline chloride on a carrier (50–70 wt. %)
- choline chloride crystals (>95%)
- rumen-protected choline chloride (RPC).

The 75% liquid is very corrosive and requires special storage and handling equipment. It is unsuitable for inclusion in concentrated vitamin premixes but is most economical to add directly to concentrate feed mixtures. The physical properties of choline chloride should be considered for mixing and storing vitamins and vitamin-trace mineral premixes, especially if they will be stored for several months. Choline chloride is highly hygroscopic and can attract moisture to vitamin and vitamin-trace mineral premixes.

Yang *et al.* (2021c) reported that after 6 months of storage, the loss of vitamin in a vitamin premix without choline chloride was 1–5%. But, with choline chloride in the premix, the vitamin loses up to 32% of its activity. In a vitamin-trace mineral premix, the impacts were even more harmful. Without the choline in the vitamin-trace mineral premix, after 6 months of storage, the loss of vitamins was 12–30%, but with the choline chloride, the number of vitamins lost was 23–52%. These values are lower than previously reported in the literature about vitamin stability in the presence of chloride, Cu, and Zn. The reason is that most vitamin products have improved in stability in the past few years (Yang *et al.*, 2021c).

Metabolism
Synthesis

Most animals can significantly synthesize choline (Chan, 1991; Garrow, 2007). Therefore, absorption from the intestine may not be critical to the animal under normal conditions. The biosynthesis of choline results from the decarboxylation of the amino acid serine to ethanolamine in a pyridoxal-dependent reaction. Ethanolamine is then progressively methylated to form choline. Excess dietary methionine is one of the primary sources of the methyl groups used in the biosynthesis of choline (Ardalan *et al.*, 2010; Jiang *et al.*, 2013; Potts *et al.*, 2020).

Absorption and transport

Choline is present in the unsupplemented diet, mainly in phosphatidylcholine or lecithin, with less than 10% as the free base or sphingomyelin. In ruminants, dietary choline is rapidly and extensively degraded in the rumen from studies with both sheep (Neill *et al.*, 1979) and cattle (Atkins *et al.*, 1988; Sharma and Erdman, 1988). Estimates of rumen degradation have ranged from 85 to 99% (Sharma and Erdman, 1989a). In *in vivo* studies with dairy cows, in which choline intake was increased up to 303 g per day over controls, there was only a 1.3 g per day increase in choline flow to the duodenum (Sharma and Erdman, 1988).

Trials with sheep (Neill *et al.*, 1979) and goats (Emmanuel and Kennelly, 1984) suggested that ruminants metabolize and utilize choline differently than monogastric animals. Choline absorption must be very limited in all ruminants because of (1) the almost complete degradation of dietary choline in the rumen, (2) only limited supplies from any rumen protozoa that might escape rumen degradation, and (3) the complete absence of choline in rumen bacteria. However, RPC containing choline chloride covered by a protective layer of fatty acids can be used as a feed additive to enhance its absorption with positive effects on DM intake and milk yield (Humer *et al.*, 2019).

Choline is released from lecithin and sphingomyelin by hydrolysis by digestive enzymes of the gastrointestinal tract, although 50% of ingested lecithin enters the thoracic duct intact (Chan, 1991). Choline is released from lecithin by hydrolysis in the intestinal lumen. Pancreatic secretions and intestinal mucosal cells contain enzymes capable of hydrolyzing lecithin in the diet. Phospholipase A$_2$ cleaves the α-fatty acid within the gut mucosal cell, and phospholipase B cleaves both fatty acids. Quantitatively, digestion by pancreatic lipase is the most crucial process (Zeisel, 1990). The net result is that most ingested lecithin is absorbed as lysophosphatidyl-choline.

These lipid components are incorporated into mixed micelles and enter the enterocytes, mainly within the duodenum and jejunum, by passive diffusion. Choline is also absorbed primarily in the jejunum and ileum by the energy and sodium-dependent carrier mechanism. Only one-third of ingested choline in monogastric diets appears to be absorbed intact (Hegazy and Schwenk, 1984). Choline seems to be absorbed through a transport system in the small intestine that is not dependent on cellular energy (Jiang *et al.*, 2013). Intestinal microorganisms metabolize the remaining two-thirds of choline to trimethylamine, which is excreted in the urine between 6 and 12 hours after consumption (De La Huerga and Popper, 1952).

The extent to which choline is absorbed from raw materials is doubtful. Absorbed choline is transported into the lymphatic circulation primarily in lecithin bound to chylomicron and is transported to the tissues predominantly as phospholipids associated with the plasma lipoproteins (De La Huerga and Popper, 1952).

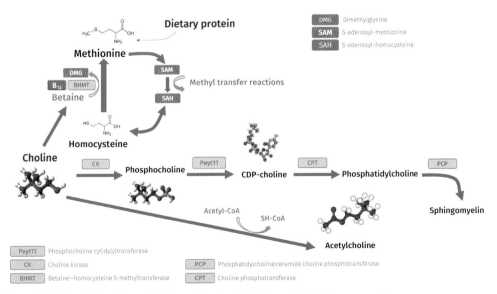

Figure 4.60 Metabolic pathway for the synthesis of choline and related compounds

Phospholipase C cleaves lecithin, yielding a diglyceride and phosphorylcholine. Free choline can be oxidized in the mitochondria to yield betaine aldehyde, which is further converted into betaine, the methyl group source. The small fraction of choline acetylated provides the vital neurotransmitter acetylcholine. Various metabolic functions and synthesis of choline are depicted in Figure 4.60.

Storage and excretion
Most choline deposited in tissues exists in esterified forms, particularly phosphatidylcholine and phospholipids, accounting for 90% of all choline in the liver. Free choline accounts for only 0.5–1% of the total choline deposited. Glycerophosphocholine and betaine are overrepresented in the kidney, whereas acetylcholine is found in relatively high amounts in the brain (Jiang *et al.*, 2013).

Dietary choline is the main factor governing excretion. Two-thirds of ingested choline is metabolized by microbiota to trimethylamine and excreted in the urine within 6–12 hours after ingestion (De La Huerga and Popper, 1952). When an equivalent amount of choline is ingested as lecithin, trimethylamine excretion is lesser and appears within 12–24 hours after intake.

Biochemical functions
Choline is ubiquitously distributed in all plant and animal cells, mainly in the form of the phospholipids phosphatidylcholine (lecithin), also-phosphatidylcholine, choline plasmalogens, and, to a lesser extent, in free form or as sphingomyelin–essential components of all membranes (Zeisel, 1990).

Lecithin contains the predominant phospholipid (>50%), phosphatidylcholine, in most mammalian membranes. In the lung, desaturated lecithin is the primary active component of surfactant (Brown, 1964), a lack of which results in respiratory distress syndrome in premature infants. Endotoxic shock with *Escherichia coli* LPS, simulating an infection, induces impaired pulmonary phosphatidylcholine biosynthesis and associated respiratory illness (Benito and Bosch, 1997). Choline is a precursor for the biosynthesis of the neurotransmitter acetylcholine. Glycerophosphocholine and phosphocholine are storage forms for choline within the cytosol and principal forms found in milk (Rohlfs *et al.*, 1993). The antioxidant protective effects of ascorbic acid reduce these effects. The main functions of choline can be grouped into 8 categories (Zeisel, 2006; Garrow, 2007; Jiang *et al.*, 2013):

- **It is a metabolic essential for building and maintaining cell structure.** As a phospholipid component, choline is a structural part of lecithin, certain plasmalogens, and sphingomyelins. Lecithin is a part of animal cell membranes and lipid transport moieties in cell plasma membranes. Both phosphatidylcholine and sphingomyelin are preferentially localized to the outer leaflet of the lipid bilayer, thereby contributing to the lipid asymmetry of cellular membranes. These choline-containing phospholipids undergo dynamic *trans-* and intermembrane movements, facilitating membrane trafficking (Jiang *et al.*, 2013). Choline is required as a constituent of the phospholipids needed for the normal maturation of the cartilage matrix of the bone, which facilitates its growth.
- **Choline plays an essential role in fat metabolism in the liver.** It prevents abnormal accumulation of fat (fatty livers) by promoting its transport as lecithin or increasing the utilization of fatty acids in the liver (Weiss and Fereira, 2006a; Zempleni *et al.*, 2007; Xu *et al.*, 2010). Phosphatidylcholine is the major phospholipid on the surface of VLDLs: it is packaged with triglyceride droplets in the Golgi cisternae, producing VLDLs that are exported out of the liver. Choline is thus referred to as a "lipotropic" factor because it acts on fat metabolism by

hastening removal or decreasing fat deposition in the liver. Phosphatidylcholine is also the major phospholipid (>95%) in bile and is derived primarily from HDL-phosphatidylcholine (Jiang *et al.*, 2013).

- **Choline is essential for forming acetylcholine.** Acetylcholine is a substance that allows the transmission of nerve impulses. It is the agent released at the termination of the parasympathetic nerves. With acetylcholine, nerve impulses are transmitted from presynaptic to postsynaptic fibers of the sympathetic and parasympathetic nervous systems.
- **Choline metabolites as second messengers.** Phosphatidylcholine and sphingomyelin contained in cellular membranes are sources of choline-derived second messengers, including lysophosphatidylcholine, lysosphingomyelin, arachidonic acid, DAG, phosphatidic acid, ceramide, and sphingosine. These second messengers influence signaling pathways involved in inflammation, growth, differentiation, eicosanoid generation, cell cycle arrest, and apoptosis.
- **Choline to form platelet-activating factor.** The platelet-activating factor (PAF) is produced from phosphatidylcholine. PAF participates in processes like platelet activation, blood pressure regulation, and inflammation. PAF releases arachidonic acid to form eicosanoids (Jiang *et al.*, 2013).
- **Choline is a source of labile methyl groups or methyl group donors** for transmethylation reactions important in forming many substances. Choline furnishes labile methyl groups to form methionine from homocysteine and creatine from guanidino acetic acid (Nesheim and Johnson, 1950). It shares this role with methionine and betaine, which means that all these substances can partially substitute for each other. However, their interrelations, reviewed by Simon (1999), are complex.

Folic acid and Vitamin B_{12} also play a part in these reactions. Thus, their requirements increase with an insufficient supply of choline (demonstrated in poultry by Ryu *et al.*, 1995). Methyl groups function in synthesizing purine and pyrimidine, which are used to produce DNA. Methionine is converted to S-adenosylmethionine in a reaction catalyzed by methionine adenosyl transferase. S-adenosylmethionine is the active methylating agent for many enzymatic methylations. A disturbance in folic acid or methionine metabolism changes choline metabolism and vice versa (Zeisel, 1990). The involvement of folic acid, vitamin $B_{12,}$ and methionine in methyl group metabolism and *de novo* choline synthesis may allow these substances to substitute partly for choline. A severe folic acid deficiency has been shown to cause secondary liver choline deficiency in rats (Kim *et al.*, 1994).

The demand for choline as a methyl donor is probably the primary factor determining how rapidly a diet deficient in choline will induce pathology. The pathways of choline and 1-carbon metabolism intersect at the formation of methionine from homocysteine. Methionine is regenerated from homocysteine in a reaction catalyzed by betaine: homocysteine methyltransferase (BHMT), in which betaine, a metabolite of choline, serves as the methyl donor (Finkelstein *et al.*, 1982). To be a source of methyl groups, choline must be converted to betaine, which has been shown to perform methylation functions and choline in some cases. However, betaine fails to prevent fatty livers and hemorrhagic kidneys. Emmert *et al.* (1997) detected elevations in liver activity by adding choline and betaine, whereas choline does not affect the renal enzyme. Although statistically significant changes in hepatic and renal BHMT activity occurred in both experiments conducted by Emmert *et al.* (1997), the magnitude of the responses was probably not physiologically significant.

Since choline contains biologically active methyl groups, methionine can partly be spared by choline and homocysteine (Zeisel and Caudill, 2018; Jiang *et al.*, 2013; Potts *et al.*, 2020).

Research with lactating dairy cattle suggests that a high proportion of dietary methionine is used for choline synthesis (Erdman and Sharma, 1991; Benoit *et al.*, 2010). The amino acid methionine is the source of the methyl donor S-adenosyl methionine. This metabolite provides methyl groups in various reactions, including the *de novo* synthesis of choline from phosphatidylethanolamine. When choline is oxidized irreversibly to betaine, betaine can provide methyl groups that recycle homocysteine to methionine. Because of these metabolic relationships, the dietary supply of either choline or betaine affects requirements, and methionine supply can affect betaine and choline metabolism.

- **Choline has been shown to influence brain structure and function.** For rodents, choline was critical during fetal development, affecting stem cell proliferation and apoptosis, thereby altering brain structure and function. Memory is permanently enhanced in rodents exposed to choline during the latter part of gestation (Zeisel and Niculescu, 2006).
- **Choline supplementation alters carnitine homeostasis** (Daily and Sachan, 1995). Lower urinary excretion of carnitine has been observed in humans and guinea pigs supplemented with choline.

Nutritional assessment

Plasma choline (and betaine) concentrations are strongly correlated with choline intake amounts, but in severe deficiency, choline concentrations do not fall according to the low nutritional intake (Hongtrakul *et al.*, 1997).

Deficiency signs

Although animals can synthesize choline internally, the young ruminant may require supplementation, at least in milk replacers. An apparent choline deficiency syndrome was produced in calves with a synthetic milk diet containing 15% casein (Johnson *et al.*, 1951). Within 6–8 days, calves developed extreme weakness, labored breathing, and could not stand. Supplementation with 260 mg of choline per liter of milk replacer prevented these deficiency signs.

Some studies have reported improved performance of feedlot cattle in response to supplemental choline. Several reports from Washington (Swingle and Dyer, 1970) and Maryland (Rumsey, 1975) have shown increased gains by 6–7% and improved feed efficiency by 2.5–8% in finishing cattle when supplemented with 500–700 ppm dietary choline. In other experiments with growing cattle, no response to choline occurred (Wise *et al.*, 1964; Harris *et al.*, 1966).

Research has indicated a positive influence of RPC on blood metabolites in beef finishing heifers (Bindel *et al.*, 1998) and dairy cattle (Humer *et al.*, 2019). Several RPC choline products vary in their rumen stability and intestinal release of choline (Figure 4.61). The RPC has improved the growth performance of finishing cattle without negatively affecting carcass characteristics (Drouillard *et al.*, 1998; Bryant *et al.*, 1999; Bindel *et al.*, 2000). Drouillard *et al.* (1998) observed an interaction between dietary fat and supplemental choline, but the results of Bindel *et al.* (2000) contradicted this finding. Feeding RPC to lambs has increased live weight gain by 10% (Bryant *et al.*, 1999). Nunnery *et al.* (1999) compared 2 levels of 2 sources of RPC in finishing beef steers and found no effect of either source or level of RPC on feedlot performance. However, choline reduced carcass fatness and yield grade.

Two studies with Angora goats found no effect on the performance of doelings but an increase in growth rate in weathers in response to feeding 3 g per day of RPC (Puchala *et al.*, 1999; Shenkoru *et al.*, 1999). A study of the effects of choline on rumen function in sheep found that 0.5–2 g per day of choline reduced rumen volatile-fatty-acid concentrations with either a roughage or high-concentrate diet (Flachowsky *et al.*, 1988).

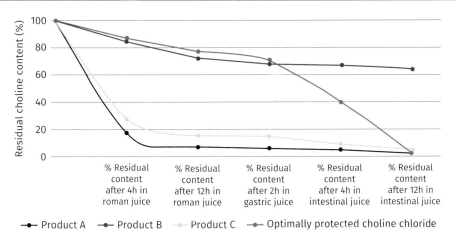

Figure 4.61 *In vitro* rumen stability and intestinal release of protected choline chloride products (source: https://www.srpublication.com/understanding-the-role-of-protected-choline-to-reduce-ketosis-and-support-transition-cows/)

Choline may be a limiting nutrient for fat milk synthesis. Lactating cows fed supplemental choline showed an increase in fat milk percentage and fat-corrected milk (Erdman *et al.*, 1984). However, a subsequent experiment found no effect of supplemental choline (Atkins *et al.*, 1988). In another experiment, Erdman and Sharma (1991) could not show a positive effect on fat milk percentage from choline by post-ruminal infusion. Grummer *et al.* (1987) reported no effect of abomasal infusion of choline on fat milk synthesis in lactating cows. Still, they found that fat milk yield was increased significantly by infusion of soy lecithin compared to soy oil.

In dairy cattle, choline supplementation has improved lactational performance (Sharma and Erdman, 1989b; Erdman and Sharma, 1991; Pinotti *et al.*, 2003; Emanuele *et al.*, 2007; de Ondarza *et al.*, 2007; Toghdory *et al.*, 2007). Supplementing betaine in goats' diet has increased milk yield by 12–36%. However, production responses to supplemental choline or betaine have been inconsistent. Feeding RPC at 0.078, 0.156, or 0.234% of ration DM increased milk yield from 1–2.6 kg per day in dairy cows with no consistent effect on milk fat yield (Erdman and Sharma, 1991).

Feeding RPC for 28 days before calving had variable effects on DM intake and milk production (Hartwell *et al.*, 1999). Cows were fed 0, 6, or 12 g of RPC daily with either a 12 or 14% crude protein diet. In cows fed the 12% protein diet prepartum, feeding 6 g per day of RPC decreased milk yield over 120 days postpartum, while feeding 12 g per day with the same prepartum diet increased milk yield. Conversely, when fed the 14% crude protein diet prepartum, cows fed 6 g per day of RPC had increased 120-day milk yield, while cows fed 12 g per day of RPC had significantly lower milk production (Hartwell *et al.*, 1999). In a study with the same RPC product in primiparous dairy heifers, feeding 15 g of RPC per day during lactation did not affect dry matter intake or milk yield. However, there was a tendency for an increase in milk fat yield (Vasquez *et al.*, 1999). Deuchler *et al.* (1998) reported that RPC used in several other cited studies was effective in elevating milk choline secretion when fed to lactating dairy cows.

Limited research indicates that supplemental choline may reduce fatty liver in transitional dairy cows (Jurlin, 1965; Hartwell *et al.*, 2001; Cooke *et al.*, 2007; Zom *et al.*, 2010). Feeding RPC was very effective in increasing milk production in fat cows (Zahra *et al.*, 2006) and for those receiving a methionine-limited diet (Davidson *et al.*, 2008). Overall, cows that received RPC produced 1.2 kg per day more milk in the first 60 days of lactation. Still, this effect was attributable to an increase in milk production of 4.4 kg per gram among cows with a body condition score ≥4 at 3 weeks before calving; fat cows that received RPC ate 1.1 kg DM per day more from week 3 before calving through week 4 after calving (Zahra *et al.*, 2006). Multiparous cows fed RPC on a diet low in methionine had higher milk yields and increased milk protein yield than controls, but not cows that also received additional methionine (Davidson *et al.*, 2008).

Feeding dairy cows RPC and methionine indicated an improved reproductive performance (Ardalan *et al.*, 2010). The RPC and methionine-fed cows had the lowest open days, days to first estrus, and services per conception compared with other groups.

Carnitine is partially synthesized from methyl groups derived from choline and other donors via S-adenosylmethionine (Lehninger, 1982). Carnitine is a component of carnitine-acyltransferases I and II, 2 molecules required to transport long-chain fatty acids into the mitochondria for oxidation. Choline may affect lipid metabolism indirectly by influencing the synthesis of carnitine. A series of studies with lactating dairy cows found that plasma and liver carnitine could be increased by feeding or abomasal infusion of carnitine. Still, carnitine supplementation did not affect milk yield and dry matter intake (LaCount *et al.*, 1995, 1996a,b). However, total-tract digestibility of lipids and energy increased in response to carnitine supplementation by either route (LaCount *et al.*, 1995).

Safety
Limited data with poultry and pigs indicated a high tolerance for choline (NRC, 1998). The tolerance of ruminants to native choline would be expected to be high due to extensive rumen degradation.

Chapter 5

Optimum vitamin nutrition in beef cattle

INTRODUCTION

The determination of vitamin recommendations for beef production is highly complex due to the diversity of production systems (extensive, semi-intensive, intensive), the different categories of animals (beef cows, weaner calves, feedlot calves, etc.), the weather influencing on animal behavior and welfare (summer, winter, tropical and temperate zones), feed ingredients and forage available, the variety of breeds (native, imported, *Bos taurus* and *B. indicus*) and animal and feeding management. This diversity hinders the standardization of nutritional requirements in general and of vitamins in particular. Additionally, the scientific literature is more limited for vitamins than for other nutrients (NRC, 2016; NASEM, 2021).

The concept of vitamin supplementation has undergone an essential change in the last few years and has moved from minimum supplementation, which guarantees the metabolic and physiological functions, to necessary supplementation, which also reduces the incidence of pathological problems, enhances ruminal and metabolic efficiency for better growth, maintains optimum reproduction, and improves the quality of the final product. Under the conditions of stress frequently associated with intensive production systems (weaning, poor adaptation to the feeder, confinement, restricted voluntary intake, the presence of pathogenic agents in the environment, transport, etc.), it may be advisable to increase vitamin supply to above the established requirements to improve the immune status of the animals.

Vitamins are either fat-soluble or water-soluble. Fat-soluble vitamins (A, D, E, and K) are essential and should be supplied in the ration. Water-soluble vitamins (B group vitamins, vitamin C, and choline) have traditionally been considered non-essential for bovine livestock due to their vital provision through synthesis by rumen microorganisms. Nevertheless, the availability of specific water-soluble vitamins may be limited in some situations, and their supplementation can improve the state of health or production of the herd. In the past decades, B vitamin supplementation has received more attention to improving ruminal metabolism efficiency.

In this chapter, we will review and update the vitamin recommendations for beef herds to supply appropriate vitamin levels according to specific conditions. When making recommendations on the necessary vitamin supply in the diet of finishing calves, we will also be considering the presence of these vitamins in the final product for human consumption, the meat.

The recommended vitamin supplementation for calves during suckling and starter/grower phases are provided in Table 5.1a and 5.1b. In Table 5.2 we have calculated, based on NRC (2016), the recommended vitamin supplementation levels for beef cattle and beef cows at different body weights and feed intake based on the NRC recommended vitamin level per kg/feed. Finally, in Table 5.3 we have summarized the levels recommended by NRC (2016) and those proposed by OVN™ dsm-firmenich (2022b) for similar weight ranges.

Whereas NRC (2016) recommended supplementing diets with fat-soluble vitamins A, D, and E, dsm-firmenich (2022b) suggested the supplementation with vitamin B_1 and biotin for all beef categories, β-carotene for beef cows and the first metabolite of vitamin D_3 – $25OHD_3$ (commercial name HyD®) – for beef cattle during fattening and finishing phase. dsm-firmenich (2022b), in elaborating its recommendations, is also considering industry practice in different geographies and the benefits provided by vitamins on parameters other than performance like animal health (e.g., immune modulation), and meat quality.

FAT-SOLUBLE VITAMINS

As mentioned above, the different production systems make it quite complicated to establish a consensus among investigators over the minimum and maximum levels recommended for beef cattle. Consequently, there are still extensive margins of use between the recommendations and customary practice. It must be noted that there are also differences among sources of information on the vitamin content of meat, according to origin or cut (Table 5.4).

Table 5.1a Vitamin level in natural milk and vitamin inclusion level in milk replacers for calves according to research committees and feed industry organizations (units/kg DM)

Vitamin	Units	NRC (2001)[1]	NASEM (2021)[2]	OVN™ 2022 (dsm-firmenich, 2022b)[3]
Vitamin A	IU	9,000	11,000	20,000–32,000
Vitamin D_3	IU	600	3,200	2,000–4,000
Vitamin E	mg	50	200	150–200
Vitamin K	mg	–[4]	–[4]	1–1.5
Vitamin B_1	mg	6.5	6.5	2.5–5
Vitamin B_2	mg	6.5	6.5	2.5–4.5
Vitamin B_6	mg	6.5	6.5	2.5–4.5
Vitamin B_{12}	mg	0.07	0.07	0.04–0.08
Niacin	mg	10	10	9–18
d-pantothenic acid	mg	13	13	7–9
Folic acid	mg	0.5	0.5	0.2–0.3
Biotin	mg	0.1	0.1	0.05–0.1
Vitamin C	mg	–	–	250–500
Choline	mg	1,000	1,000	500–750
β-carotene	mg	–	–	100

Note: [1] These values assume a 45 kg calf consuming 0.53 kg of milk replacer solids (DM)/day. Concentrations should be reduced if calves are fed substantially more significant amounts of milk replacer (e.g., ≥1 kg/day of solids).
[2] These values assume a 60 kg calf consuming 0.6 kg of milk replacer solids. Concentrations should be reduced if calves are fed substantially more significant amounts of milk replacer (e.g., ≥1 kg/day of solids).
[3] OVN™ 2022 is based on current industry practices.
[4] Microbial synthesis of vitamin K within the intestines appears adequate, and supplemental vitamin K is usually unnecessary (Nestor and Conrad, 1990).

Table 5.1b Vitamin inclusion level for calves during starter and grower phases[1] according to research committees and feed industry organizations (units/kg DM)

Vitamin	Units	NRC (2001)	NASEM (2021)	OVN™ 2022 (dsm-firmenich, 2022b)
Vitamin A	IU	4,000	3,700	7,500–10,000
Vitamin D₃	IU	600	1,100	2,200–3,000
Vitamin E	mg	25	67	135–200

Note: [1] These values assume during starter phase an 80 kg calf consuming 2.4 kg of starter DM and during grower phase a 110 kg calf consuming 3.3 kg of grower DM.

Vitamin A

Vitamin A is a family of molecules grouped under the name retinol. Vitamin A is measured in international units (IU) or retinol equivalents (RE). One IU is equivalent to 0.3 µg of all-*trans*-retinol, its more active isomer of the same name. In Chapter 4, we described the relationships of IU with other sources of vitamin A. Retinol is obtained from the β-carotene (or provitamin A) in forage, which is converted to vitamin A in intestinal mucosa. Bovine livestock can store some β-carotene in fat reserves. One milligram of β-carotene has an activity equivalent to 400 IU of vitamin A.

Feedstuffs for beef cattle vary in vitamin A composition (Pickworth *et al.*, 2012b). The concentration of β-carotenes in plants diminishes as they mature and also due to the oxidation processes that take place during storage once plants have been cut, so the concentration in hay and silage is much lower than that in a pasture with fresh plants (Table 5.5). However, industrial dehydration conserves β-carotenes better than drying on the ground. Similarly, increased storage time reduces β-carotene concentration (Bruhn and Oliver, 1978). Retinol is sensitive to oxidation, light, acids, humidity, and microminerals (NRC, 2000, 2016). Prolonged storage of the vitamin in premixes containing minerals, raised temperature and humidity, pelleting, processing in blocks or by extrusion, or rancid fats in the ration all reduce the stability of vitamin A.

Of all the vitamins required in beef cattle feed, vitamin A is of the most practical importance for production since it is essential for average growth and development, tissue maintenance, and bone development (NRC, 1996, 2000, 2016; CSIRO, 2007; INRA, 2018). Vitamin A fulfills many functions in the body. The most important being involvement in vision, embryo development, reproduction, immunity, maintenance of homeostasis, and differentiation of a wide range of MG cells (Goodman, 1980, 1984). In productive herds, symptoms of deficiencies are infrequent. However, there are periods when the availability of vitamins is less than optimum, which may affect reproductive performance and immune competence. A vitamin A deficiency is most likely to occur during the winter, in rations with a high proportion of concentrates, and when the feed provided has been exposed to sunlight and high temperatures or stored for long periods. On the other hand, toxicity due to an excess of vitamin A is not very likely in ruminants since its high degree of microbial degradability in the rumen limits the quantity available to the animal (NRC, 2000, 2016).

Recommendations

Beef cows (gestation/lactation) and breeding bulls

According to the latest NRC (2016) report on beef cattle, the vitamin A requirement for gestating beef heifers and cows is 2,800 IU/kg DM feed or 28,000–33,600 IU/head day (Table 5.2). This value did not change compared to previous reports (NRC, 1996, 2000). The NRC Committee (NRC, 2016) opted to express requirements in both IU/kg BW and IU/kg DM to provide more flexibility in feed formulation. Compared to other sources given in IU/kg BW (Table 5.6), these levels are

Table 5.2 Estimated vitamin supplementation level for beef cattle, beef cows, and breeding bulls

	Weaned calves	Yearling steers/heifers	Slaughter weight	Gestating beef cows	Lactating beef cows	Breeding bulls
Body weight, kg	200–270	320–400	590–680	550–650	550–650	800–900
Feed intake, kg/head/day	6.0–8.0	9.0–11.0	14.0–16.0	10–12	14–16	17–18
Vitamin A, IU/kg feed[1]	2,200	2,200	2,200	2,800	3,900	3,900
Vitamin D, IU/kg feed[1]	275	275	275	275	275	275
Vitamin E, mg/kg feed[1]	35	35	35	35	35	35
Vitamin A, IU/head/day	13,200–17,600	19,800–24,200	30,800–35,200	28,000–33,600	54,600–62,400	66,300–70,200
Vitamin D, IU/head/day	1,650–2,200	2,475–3,025	3,850–4,400	2,750–3,300	3,850–4,400	4,675–4,950
Vitamin E, mg/head/day	210–280	315–385	490–560	350–420	490–560	595–630

Note: [1] Vitamin recommended level according to NRC (2016).

Table 5.3 Vitamin inclusion level (units per head per day) for beef cattle and beef cows according to research committees or feed industry organizations

Vitamin	Units	NRC (2016)	OVN™ (dsm-firmenich, 2022b)
BEEF CATTLE			
Growing			
Vitamin A	IU	19,800–24,200	25,000–50,000
Vitamin D$_3$	IU	2,475–3,025	6,000–9,000
Vitamin E	mg	315–385	200–300
Vitamin B$_1$	mg	–	60–250[1]
Biotin	mg	–	10–20[2]
Fattening and finishing			
Vitamin A	IU	30,800–35,200	40,000–80,000
Vitamin D$_3$	IU	3,850–4,400	5,000–7,000
25OHD$_3$ (HyD®)	mg	–	1
Vitamin E	mg	490–560	500–2,000[3]
Vitamin B$_1$	mg	–	60–250[1]
Biotin	mg	–	10–20[2]
BEEF COWS			
Gestation			
Vitamin A	IU	28,000–33,600	40,000–70,000
Vitamin D$_3$	IU	2,750–3,300	5,000–10,000
Vitamin E	mg	350–420	350–500
Biotin	mg	–	20[2]
β-carotene	mg	–	300–500[4]
Lactation			
Vitamin A	IU	54,600–62,400	40,000–70,000
Vitamin D$_3$	IU	3,850–4,400	5,000–10,000
Vitamin E	mg	490–560	350–500
Biotin	mg	–	20[2]
β-carotene	mg	–	300–500[4]
BREEDING BULLS			
Vitamin A	IU	66,300–70,200	50,000–80,000
Vitamin D$_3$	IU	4,675–4,950	5,000–10,000
Vitamin E	mg	595–630	300–500
Biotin	mg	–	20[2]

Note: [1] Upper level for cattle on high concentrate rations.
[2] For optimum hoof health and meat marbling.
[3] Upper level for improved color case-life, 100 to 120 days pre-slaughter.
[4] 6-8 weeks before 1st insemination/mating when intake of green forages is low.

Table 5.4 Nutritional values of beef meat by country and cuts

	Unit	South Africa (2010)[1] Cooked				USA (2011)[2] Raw			South America (2014)[3] Raw	UK (2018)[4] Raw	
		Rump	Silverside	Brisket	Hind shin	Western griller	Fillet mignon	Tender medallions	Beef meat	Calf loin	Beef loin
Moisture	g	48.9	57.4	45.2	58.1	73	61	73	–	–	–
Protein	g	24.5	28.5	20.79	29.6	22	19	21	–	20	20.9
Lipids	g	25.28	12.85	32.6	11.99	4	18	6	–	7.3	3.2
Energy	KJ	–	–	–	–	539.73	1041.81	594.12	–	610.86	481.16
Cholesterol	mg	90.8	87.66	87.54	85.84	61	68	58	–	–	62
Vitamin A	mg	–	–	–	–	0	0	0	–	–	Trace
β-carotene	mg	–	–	–	–	–	–	–	0.045–0.078	–	–
Vitamin D	µg	–	–	–	–	–	–	–	–	–	Trace
Vitamin E	mg	–	–	–	–	–	–	–	0.210–0.46	–	–
Vitamin K	mg	–	–	–	–	–	–	–	–	–	–
Vitamin B$_1$	µg	112	197	94	102	90	70	90	–	–	60
Vitamin B$_2$	µg	108	110	101	103	240	110	270	–	–	210
Vitamin B$_3$	mg	42.7	52.5	36.7	3.83	6.4	5.2	5.6	–	–	5.1
Vitamin B$_6$	mg	0.369	0.351	0.383	0.375	0.72	0.54	0.52	–	–	0.2
Vitamin B$_{12}$	mg	2.16	2.04	1.95	2.11	0.0036	0.0009	0.0051	–	0.0011	0.002
d-pantothenic acid	mg	–	–	–	–	0.77	0.55	0.92	–	–	0.5
Folic acid	µg	–	–	–	–	–	–	–	–	–	–
Vitamin C	mg	–	–	–	–	0	0	0	2.5	–	–

Note: [1]Schonfeldt *et al.* (2010); [2]Patterson *et al.* (2011); [3]Cabrera and Saadoun (2014); [4]Rabia *et al.* (2018).

Table 5.5 Provitamin A carotenoid composition in common beef cattle feedstuffs (source: Pickworth et al., 2012a)

	β-carotene[1,2]		Vitamin A equivalents[3,4]		DM, %		OM, %		NDF, %		ADF, %		CP, %		Ether extract, %	
	Mean	SEM	Mean	SEM	Mean	SEM	Mean	SEM	Mean	SEM	Mean	SEM	Mean	SEM	Mean	SEM
Alfalfa hay	728.3	336.3	2,913	1345.3	84	0.19	91	0.44	42	2.59	37.8	1.66	17.2	0.31	1.74	0.36
Fescue hay	730.7	132.9	2,923	531.7	85.2	0.51	93.4	1.15	65.6	4.24	40.2	3.26	8.3	1.05	2.05	0.38
Orchard grass hay	777.2	137.8	3,109	550.8	85.2	0.51	93	0.21	65.1	2.1	40.9	4.16	8.84	0.18	1.79	0.14
Wheat x ryegrass hay	496.3	–	1,985	–	85	–	94.4	–	70.6	–	44.4	–	10.6	–	1.01	–
Wheat straw	15.1	–	60.4	–	84.3	–	96.2	–	90.3	–	66.1	–	1.2	–	1.02	–
Fescue pasture	9,966	661.6	39,865	2,646	32.5	1.41	95.7	1.5	66.1	1.94	40	2.62	10.8	1.05	2.72	0.23
Corn silage	1,722	257.9	6,900	1,032	39.4	2.48	95.8	0.32	43.6	1.79	28.8	1.55	7	0.4	2.68	0.12
Corn products																
Whole shelled corn	29.5	2.5	170	17.3	87.8	0.94	98.7	0.04	–	–	–	–	8.1	0.18	1.29	0.03
Steam–flaked corn	30.8	1.9	137.4	9.3	78.9	0.13	99.1	0.04	–	–	–	–	8.1	0.29	2.51	0.13
Cracked–corn	36.1	1.2	149.8	21.3	86	0.85	98.8	0.09	–	–	–	–	8.8	0.28	2.55	0.34
High–moisture corn	72.9	7.6	359.1	38.1	71.5	0.62	98.7	0.05	–	–	–	–	8.3	0.2	3.26	0.24

Notes: [1]Expressed as micrograms per 100 g of DM.
[2]Includes cis–9 and all–trans β–carotene.
[3]Expressed as international units per kilogram of DM.
[4]Calculated as follows: 1 mg of β–carotene = 400 IU of vitamin A.

lower than NASEM (2021) for dairy cattle, NRC (2007) for small ruminants, and CSIRO (2007) and INRA (2018) for beef cattle. It is essential to understand that the NRC (2016) requirements did not consider the contributions of vitamin A precursors. These needs must be adjusted depending on changes in feed intake or feed sources. The CVB (2022) recommended between 2,000 and 3,500 IU/kg DM for adult dairy cattle, with the highest value fed at a high daily milk yield.

The NRC (2016) has considered it is advisable to increase vitamin A levels in dry cows to boost immune competence and reduce mammary health and postpartum reproduction problems. However, it must be remembered that the vitamin A concentration in colostrum depends on the vitamin A received by cows during the dry period. This affects the quantity of vitamin A weaner calves consume during the first days of life. If the cow calves after a long winter-feeding period during which they have ingested low-quality hay, colostrum will have a low vitamin A content. It may prove helpful to supplement calves with this vitamin.

A particular case where the same recommendation would apply is that of primiparous cows. These are prone to producing colostrum with lower levels of vitamin A (INRA, 2018), which may not be sufficient to meet the requirements of the calves, sometimes before being put out to pasture, as it occurs in the middle of winter in many European and North American countries. Under these circumstances, the β-carotene reserves accumulated by the animal may be helpful. Still, if the feed has been composed of low-quality hay or corn silage for a prolonged period, there is a risk that these reserves may become practically exhausted, leading to a shortfall, especially if the feed has been stored for an extended period. For this reason, INRA (1988, 2018) recommends a regular supply of at least 30,000–40,000 IU of vitamin A/day for lactating cows and those in late gestation.

Both the NRC (1996, 2000, 2016) and INRA (1988, 2018) recommended a vitamin A supply of 3,900 IU/kg DM feed or 84 IU/kg BW for beef cows in lactation and bulls. These levels equal approximately 54,600–62,400 IU/head per day for lactating beef cows and 66,300–70,200 IU/head per day for breeding bulls (Table 5.2). However, to maximize productivity, promote calf growth and take possible stressful situations into account CSIRO (2007) and INRA (1988, 2018) suggested that an optimum vitamin A intake should be around 223 and 200 IU/kg BW (Table 5.6). These requirements are not always met in the case of lactating cows, which calve indoors and are fed hay, silage, or straw.

In its recent OVN™ dsm-firmenich (2022b) recommended a supplementation of 40,000–70,000 IU/head per day across gestation and lactation and 50,000–80,000 IU/head per day for breeding bulls (Table 5.3). For all these categories there's quite a good alignment between these 2 sources of recommendation. dsm-firmenich (2022b) recommended the supplementation with ß-carotene at 300–500 mg/head per day (Table 5.3) for its benefits on reproduction performance, which are discussed in detail in Chapter 6.

Table 5.6 Vitamin A requirements for beef cattle in IU/kg BW according to different sources

	Units	Gestating heifers and cows	Lactating cows and bulls	Beef feedlot cattle
Beef cattle (NRC, 2016)	IU/kg BW	60	84	47
Dairy cattle (NASEM, 2021)	IU/kg BW	110	110	–
Small ruminants (NRC, 2007)	IU/kg BW	151	178	–
CSIRO (2007)	IU/kg BW	150	223	100
INRA (2018)	IU/kg BW	130	200	50

According to the BR Corte (2023), addressing the nutritional requirements of purebred zebu and crossbred animals, the supplementation of non-castrated Nelore males with fat-soluble vitamin blends (ADE) in high-concentrate diets under brazilian conditions increased the total apparent digestibility of starch. The committee of the current edition of BR Corte (2023) is suggesting using the vitamin supplementation levels for beef cattle recommended by NRC (2016) and OVN® (DSM, 2016).

Calves: suckling, starter, and grower

The most recent recommendation on vitamin A supplies for suckling calves or those on artificial feed is 110 IU/kg BW (NRC, 2016). This is equivalent to incorporating around 9,000 IU/kg DM milk replacer. A higher supplementation level of 20,000–32,000 IU/kg is indicated in the OVN™ guidelines (dsm-firmenich, 2022b) (Table 5.1a). However, feeding weaner calves milk replacers containing vitamin A levels of 20,000–40,000 IU/kg DM is a standard practice, hence significantly above the NASEM (2021) recommendation (Erdman, 1992).

In starter and grower feed, NASEM (2021) recommends providing 3,700 IU/kg DM starter feed, whereas a level of 7,500–10,000 IU/kg DM is recommended by dsm-firmenich (2022b) (Table 5.1b).

It must be remembered that adverse effects have been observed when giving an overdosage of vitamin A to young calves supplemented with 30,000 IU/day during the first weeks of life (Franklin et al., 1998). These effects were attributed to interference by vitamin A with the vitamin E status of the animals, so in this case, the vitamin E level should be raised as well. McGill et al. (2019) showed that vitamin A deficient calves are unable to respond to the mucosal bovine respiratory syncytial virus BRSV-polyanhydride nanoparticle (NP)-based vaccine, are afforded no protection from BRSV challenge and have significant abnormalities in the inflammatory response in the infected lung.

Beef cattle

Recommended levels for beef cattle from the post-weaning phase to slaughter weight are given in Tables 5.2 and 5.3. The NRC (2016), confirming the recommendations previously given (NRC 1996, 2000), indicated vitamin A levels per animal per day are calculated based on the suggested level of 2,200 IU/kg feed and an average feed intake. The resulting ranges are 13,200–17,600, 19,800–24,200, and 30,800–35,200 IU/head day, respectively, for weaned calves, yearling steers/heifers, and up to slaughter weight. In its recent OVN™ guidelines, dsm-firmenich (2022b) suggested 25,000–50,000 IU/head per day during the growing phase and 40,000–80,000 IU/head per day during fattening and finishing periods.

Dosages higher than those given would be justifiable for animals under stress, for example, after weaning or on arrival at the feedlot after a long journey, when one of the more common symptoms is reduced appetite. In these conditions, the vitamin A supply may increase from 4,000 to 6,000 IU/kg DM (NRC, 1996, 2016).

The results of a descriptive analysis based on surveys carried out among US nutritionists (Vasconcelos and Galyean, 2007) indicated that the average recommended for diets in the final stage of fattening is 5,215 IU/ kg DM (range 2,205–11,023). This was far above the values recommended by the NRC for fattening beef cattle (NRC, 2000, 2016). However, they were similar to the FEDNA (2018) recommendation for vitamin premix in concentrate diets for growing calves in all phases (5,000–10,000 UI/kg).

The specific feeding conditions in each feedlot must be considered. Rations containing around 90% concentrate, mainly hay or silage, and no fresh forage should consider supplementation. More recently, Samuelson et al. (2016) reported that the average concentration of vitamin A recommended by nutritionists was approximately 4,796 and 4,715 IU/kg for receiving and finishing diets, respectively.

The ruminal degradability of vitamin A can be 67% (Rode *et al.*, 1990; McDowell, 2000a,b). This degradation is higher when feeding higher-concentrate rations than rations rich in forage, so it seems reasonable to suggest a need to increase vitamin A supply for feedlot steers. Gorocica-Buenfil *et al.* (2007a,b,c, 2008) conducted 4 experiments, 3 with beef cattle, demonstrating that 2,200 or 2,700 IU supplemental vitamin A/kg improved gains in one experiment (Gorocica-Buenfil *et al.*, 2007b) and improved feed efficiency in 2 of the experiments (Gorocica-Buenfil *et al.*, 2007c, 2008) compared to non-supplemented cattle.

However, this increase in supplementation should never exceed 100% of standard recommendations, considering the total intake of vitamin A or carotenes. Considering the possibility of adverse effects, the recommendation should be cautiously applied and requires a review of the total intake. For example, Bryant *et al.* (2010) fed 360 black yearling steers with a 91% concentrate diet, based on steam-flaked corn, to evaluate the effects of supplemental vitamin A (0, 1,103, 2,205, 4,410, or 8,820 IU/kg dietary DM) on performance and carcass quality. However, performance did not improve after 2,205 IU/kg dietary DM.

It should be noted that using excessive dosages of vitamin A, for example, 3 times higher than levels recommended by the NRC, has resulted in a drop in the daily live weight gain and a poorer conversion index for feedlot calves (Hill *et al.*, 1995; Zinn *et al.*, 1996; Pyatt *et al.*, 2005), which could be linked to an interaction with the availability of vitamin E, restricting its oxidative capacity. Park *et al.* (2018) in a review of factors affecting intramuscular fat deposition in beef cattle, defined the appropriate age and duration of Vitamin A depletion or supplementation appearing as important factors affecting marbling score. Restricting Vitamin A in 15-month-old cattle until the final finishing phase (29 month of age) increased marbling score, but not in 23 months old cattle prior to finishing. Continuous dietary Vitamin A restriction during the late fattening phase is not recommended because prolonged Vitamin A restriction may lead to health problems and retard growth rate.

High levels of vitamin A in finishing feed cattle and meat quality

Excessive supplementation with vitamin A to feedlot steers, especially in the finishing phase, can reduce beef cattle's meat quality and may affect the location of fat deposition (Pyatt and Berger, 2005; Arihara, 2006). The molecular mechanisms causing this effect are described in Figure 5.1. Increased vitamin A concentrations have been shown to limit adipocyte differentiation *in vitro* (Pickworth *et al.*, 2012b). In fact, it is recommended that the supply of vitamin A in the diet be reduced during this period as a mechanism to favor the intramuscular fat (IMF) deposition (Priolo *et al.*, 2002; Siebert *et al.*, 2006; Gorocica-Buenfil *et al.*, 2007a, b, c; 2008), which in addition favors the preservation of the meat color and reduces the oxidative capacity of lipids in the meat (Daniel *et al.*, 2008). Kruk *et al.* (2008) evaluated vitamin A supplementation to a low β-carotene and vitamin A cereal-based ration on a feedlot for 308 days. Ten of the 20 steers were supplemented with vitamin A (retinyl palmitate, 60 IU of vitamin A/100 kg body weight/day), and the other 10 received no supplement. The results demonstrated that restriction of vitamin A intake changed IMF deposition without changing subcutaneous fat depots. Angus steers that had been depleted of vitamin A showed IMF in the longissimus thoracis (LT) et lumborum by 35% ($P < 0.026$) and seam fat area at the quartering site by 33% ($P < 0.027$) when compared with cattle supplemented with vitamin A. There were no changes in IMF in the semitendinosus. Visually assessed marbling scores were also higher (19%; $P < 0.094$) in the non-supplemented, depleted group. There was no effect of vitamin A depletion on cattle growth and other meat traits (eye muscle area, meat color, pH, meat cut weight), meat-eating attributes (tenderness, cooking loss),

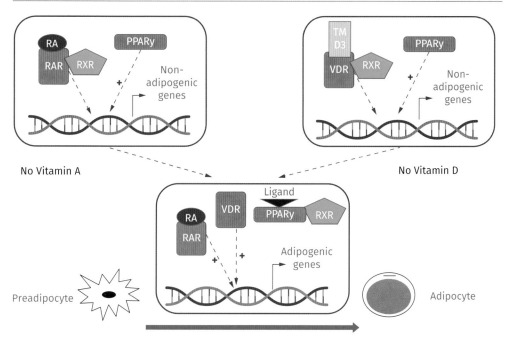

Figure 5.1 Transcriptional regulation of adipogenesis gene expression by retinoic acid (RA) and vitamin D. RA (an active form of vitamin A) binds to the retinoic acid receptor (RAR), and vitamin D₃ (Vit D₃) binds to the vitamin D receptor (VDR) (source: adapted from Pyatt and Berger, 2005)

or muscle fiber diameter. Fat color was the only difference ($P < 0.01$) among the meat traits. Vitamin A-depleted animals had whiter fat than the controls. Moreover, the fat from the vitamin A-depleted group was softer with a lower melting point. It was concluded that the reduced vitamin A consumption, leading to vitamin A depletion, increased IMF. On the other hand, vitamin A depletion did not increase subcutaneous fat depth or change other meat quality traits, suggesting that marbling and these other traits are not invariably related.

Pickworth *et al.* (2012b) conducted a feedlot trial at the Ohio State University feedlot in Wooster, OH. One hundred sixty-eight Angus crossbred steers with initial BW 284±0.4 kg were blocked by initial BW into 3 BW block groups. They were allotted to 24 pens, resulting in calves in each block with similar initial BW (238±0.5, 284±0.7, and 330±0.9 kg for light, moderate, and heavy BW blocks, respectively). Pens within each BW block were randomly assigned to 1 of 4 treatments. A 2 × 2 factorial arrangement of treatments was utilized. The main effects were dietary supplementation of vitamins A and D: the vitamin A treatments were no supplemental vitamin A (NA) or 3,750 IU/kg of dietary DM supplemental vitamin A (SA), and the vitamin D treatments were no supplemental vitamin D (ND) or 1,860 IU/kg of dietary DM supplemental vitamin D (SD). Therefore, the 4 dietary treatments were NAND (neither supplemental vitamin A nor D), NASD (no supplemental vitamin A with vitamin D supplementation), SAND (supplemental vitamin A without vitamin D supplementation), and SASD (supplemental vitamin A and vitamin D). This study showed increased backfat thickness and performance grades associated with diets without vitamin A supplementation, resulting in better marbling scores. It is important to note that in in this study the vitamin A and D supplementation were much above the recommended levels.

Strategic vitamin A restriction but not decreasing plasma concentration below 30 IU/dl (or 90 μg/l) during weeks 15–23 can be an essential factor in improving metabolizable energy (ME), reducing health-related problems, and improving marbling or IMF deposition in steers

(Park *et al.*, 2018). Excessive retinol can inhibit adipocyte differentiation and has a negative relationship with adipogenesis. Therefore, controlled restriction of vitamin A intake increases IMF (Park *et al.*, 2018). This study evaluated this effect in 450 black Angus crossbred steers. After 24 hours of arrival, a blood sample was collected from each bovine for its genotypic classification. Then, 130 steers were selected and randomly distributed among 4 pens. Steers were equally divided between 2 vitamin A treatments: supplemented (750,000 IU/month) and unsupplemented (0 IU/month). Vitamin A was in the form of 1,000,000 IU/g microencapsulated retinyl palmitate. The supplemented treatment was designed to approximate the NRC (2016) recommendation of 2,200 IU/kg DM for vitamin A supplementation. Results indicated restricting vitamin A supplementation in finishing diets can significantly increase marbling and IMF scores. In addition, the ADH1C c.-64T>C TT genotype was associated with higher IMF than the CC genotype when vitamin A was limited (Ward *et al.*, 2012).

Salinas-Chavira *et al.*, (2014) found higher feed intake and average daily gain when Holstein steers in feedlot were fed 30,000 IU of vitamin A as retinyl propionate and retinyl palmitate versus animals not fed vitamin A. Jin *et al.* (2015) observed that supplementary β-carotene (0, 600, 1200, or 1800 mg/day) for 90 days to steers increased blood and tissue β-carotene and vitamin A (retinol) levels after withdrawing the supplementation for 60 days. The IMF content, meat color, and retinol in blood, muscle, or adipose tissues were unaffected. Backfat thickness decreased slightly with increasing β-carotene supplementation and significantly differed between groups during depletion.

Using a proteomic approach, Campos *et al.* (2020) conducted a study to assess the molecular mechanisms involved in the IMF deposition in beef cattle supplemented with vitamin A during the finishing phase. Vitamin A supplementation during the finishing phase decreased IMF deposition in beef cattle. Proteome and phospho-proteome analysis, together with biological and networking analysis of the protein differentially abundant between treatments, indicated that vitamin A supplementation affects the overall energy metabolism of skeletal muscle, impairing lipid biosynthesis in skeletal muscle.

Wagyu animals have a high marbling characteristic due to their genetic deposition for fat accumulation. Oka *et al.* (1997) working with castrated wagyu steers with or without vitamin A found high vitamin A supplementation delivered higher average daily gain and carcass weight and good marbling score compared to low vitamin A supplementation. In this case, lower vitamin A levels the marbling score was also rated as good, 5.3 for high vitamin A versus 7.8 for low vitamin A. However, the same authors (Oka *et al.*, 2018) found no differences in marbling scores in a sequence of 3 experiments with Japanese black animals finished at 15 months of age, when animals got high or low vitamin A intramuscular injection.

Peng *et al.* (2019) did not observe differences on marbling scores when Korean Hanwoo animals fed for 240 days with (8,000 IU/kg DM) or without vitamin A supplementation. Both treatments reached good marbling scores (5.2 for animals supplemented with 8,000 IU of vitamin A versus 5.4 non-supplemented).

Similar results were reported by Bryant *et al.* (2010) working with 360 Angus steers fed high concentrate diet for 147 days with 3 levels of vitamin A supplementation (1,103, 2,205 and 4,410 IU/kg of DM) versus non-supplemented animals: no differences were observed on marbling scores, corroborated by Pyatt *et al.* (2005) who also did not find differences in marbling scores when crossbreed Simmental/Angus animals were fed low vitamin A (2,350 IU/kg DM) or high vitamin A (7,250 IU/kg DM).

The scientific evidence indicates that dietary vitamin A restriction increases marbling in feedlot cattle; however, this practice negatively affects antibody responses to vaccines. These effects were observed in an experiment conducted by Jee *et al.* (2013) with 40 feedlot Angus calves receiving either a high (HVA; 3,300 U of vitamin A/kg of dietary DM) or a low (LVA; 1,100 U of vitamin A/kg of dietary DM). Calves receiving the LVA diet between days 112 and 140 compromised the serum Immunoglobulin G1 (IgG1) titer responses against inactivated bovine coronavirus vaccine (BCoV), which suggested suppressed T-helper 2-associated antibody (IgG1) responses (Figure 5.2). Thus, low vitamin A diets may compromise the effectiveness of viral vaccines and make calves more susceptible to infectious diseases. The significant reduction

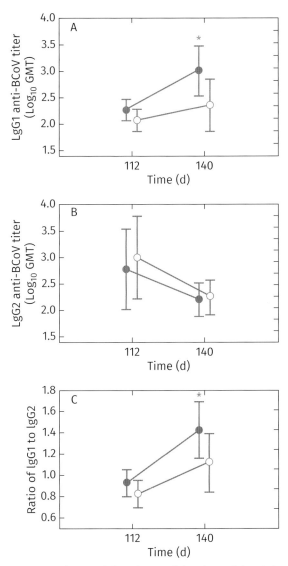

Figure 5.2 Serum retinol concentrations and titers for IgG1 (A) and IgG2 (B) and the ratio of IgG1 to IgG2 (C) before (day 112) and after (day 140) intramuscular (IM) administration of 2 doses of an inactivated BCoV vaccine (administered on days 112 and 126) to calves in the HVA (filled circles; n = 18) and LVA (open circles; 17) groups. Values reported are the geometric mean titer (panels A and B) and mean (panel C) ± 95% confidence interval (panels A-C). *Within a day for each variable, the value differs significantly (*P* < 0.05; repeated-measures ANOVA followed by the Duncan multiple range test) between the HVA and LVA groups. (Source: Jee *et al.*, 2013).

in serum retinol concentrations was observed only at 140 days, after 4 weeks of feeding the low vitamin A diet. Wellmann *et al.* (2020) working with finishing steers and systematic depletion and repletion of Vitamin A and its effect on animal performance and carcass characteristics concluded, throughout the duration of the study, that dry matter intake of the steers not receiving vitamin A supplementation was depressed ($P = 0.01$). Differences were not observed across treatments for hot carcass weight, rib eye area, back fat thickness, kidney–pelvic–heart fat percentage, marbling score, or dressing percent ($P \geq 0.10$). The current NASEM (2021) indicates that the vitamin A requirement of 2,200 IU/kg is adequate for repletion of vitamin A status of feedlot steers.

Vitamin A parenteral administration at birth
In contrast to the effects of vitamin A in the finishing phase, parenteral administration of vitamin A at birth in steer calves destined to feedlots has shown positive effects on IMF at slaughter age. Harris *et al.* (2018) administered vitamin A (0, 150,000, or 300,000 IU) at birth in Angus steer calves ($n = 30$). Results (Table 5.7) indicated that weaning weight and weight during the following weighing times increased linearly according to vitamin A level, but no BW difference was observed at harvest. However, the IMF and ribeye marbling score quadratically increased with vitamin A at 308 days before switching to a finishing diet. The effects were explained by increased zinc finger protein (ZNFP423) gene expression stimulating adipogenic processes.

Vitamin A administration to neonatal calves can also promote muscle growth by promoting myogenesis, increasing satellite cell density, and causing a shift to oxidative muscle fibers. Wang *et al.* (2018) injected 150,000 IU of vitamin A (retinyl palmitate in glycerol) per calf at birth and 1 month of age. Vitamin A increased cattle growth at 2 months. Vitamin A also increased myogenesis measured as increased PAX7 positive cells and higher gene expression of myogenic markers PAX7, MYF5, MYOD, and MYOG in a biopsy of the biceps femoralis muscle. PAX7 plays an essential role in regulating muscle satellite cells' myogenic potential and function. Muscles of injected calves had more myotubes and a higher degree of myogenesis. Consistently, vitamin A increased latissimus dorsi (LATD) muscle fiber size at harvest. In addition, vitamin A increased the ratio of oxidative type I and type IIA fibers and reduced the glycolic type IIX fibers. Furthermore, we found that RA, a critical bioactive metabolite of vitamin A, activated the PPARGC1A promoter, which explains the upregulated expression of PPARGC1A in skeletal muscle. PPARGC1A promotes intramuscular fatty acid oxidation, transforms fast-twitch to slow-twitch myofibers, and increases skeletal muscle mass.

Maciel *et al.* (2022) observed similar vitamin A stimulation of this key adipogenic marker (ZNF423) and angiogenic genes in bovine LT muscle. They injected intramuscularly male ($n = 10$)

Table 5.7 Effect of vitamin A intramuscular injection at birth on Angus steers growth performance (source: Harris *et al.*, 2018)

Vitamin A (IU)	Age (days)			
	Birth	210	308	438
	Body weight (kg)			
0	35.1	219.2[b]	312.1[b]	581.8
1,50,000	35.6	248.7[ab]	333.0[ab]	610.4
3,00,000	35.6	246.0[a]	339.7[a]	588.3

Note: Figures on the column with different letters are statistically different $P < 0.05$.

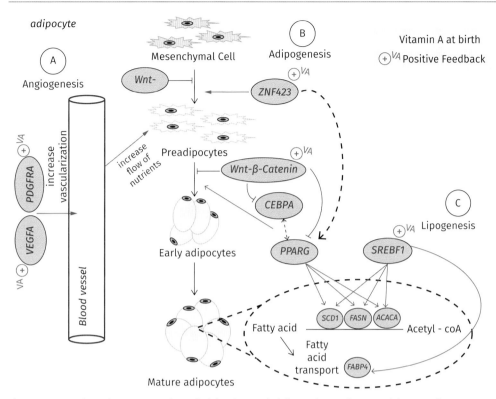

Figure 5.3 Relationship among angiogenic (A) adipogenic (B) and lipogenic genes (C) on ruminant adipose tissue. The transcription factors/regulated are in red font, and their target gene is in blue font. In addition, the blue arrow shows positive feedback, and the red arrow shows negative feedback. Vitamin A at birth can increase the deposition of marbling since it performs positive feedback on genes related to angiogenic (VEGFA and PDGFRA), adipogenic (ZNF423), and lipogenic (SREBF1, ACACA, SCD1, and FABP4). ACACA = acetyl-CoA carboxylase; CEBPA = CCAAT enhancer-binding protein α; FASN = fatty acid synthase; FABP4 = fatty acid-binding protein 4; PDGFRA = platelet-derived growth factor receptor A; PPARG = peroxisome proliferator-activated receptor γ; SCD1 = stearoyl-CoA desaturase-1; VEGFA = vascular-endothelial growth factor A; WNT = wingless-type MMTV integration site family member 10B; ZNF423 = protein zinc fingers 423. (Source: Maciel *et al.*, 2022).

and female (n = 7) Montana × Nellore calves at birth with 300,000 IU of vitamin A. This experiment observed no significant effects of vitamin A on BW gain. However, vitamin A increased the IMF content more in males than females. The authors explained the mechanisms of these vitamin A effects, as depicted in Figure 5.3. In conclusion, the neonatal parenteral administration of vitamin A in beef calves can improve cattle's meat quality, as expressed by IMF at harvesting.

Vitamin D

Vitamin D, also known as an antirachitic vitamin, regulates Ca (and P) metabolism and maintains correct Ca levels in the blood. This vitamin can be obtained from sterols converted by ultraviolet irradiation from the sun. A good amount of vitamin D is produced in the skin of animals through the photoconversion of 7-dehydrocholesterol to vitamin D_3 (cholecalciferol). Similarly, vitamin D_2 (ergocalciferol) is obtained from sun-dried forage.

The 2 forms (D_2 and D_3) have the same theoretical potency in ruminants with 1 IU corresponding to 0.025 μg. However, from a metabolic point of view, D_2 is cleared from circulation faster than D_3 (Hymøller and Jensen, 2010b), probably due to a lower affinity of the plasma based VBP (Horst *et al.*, 1982). To become completely functional, these vitamins must be activated, first in the liver, where they are hydroxylated to 25 hydroxycholecalciferol (25OHD$_2$ and 25OHD$_3$), and then in the kidneys, where they are converted to 1,25-dihydroxycholecalciferol [1,25(OH)$_2$D$_2$ and 1,25(OH)$_2$D$_3$]. The plasmatic concentration of 25OHD is generally recommended to evaluate the status of vitamin D in the animal (Horst *et al.*, 1994). Nevertheless, there is seasonal sunlight-associated variation in vitamin D status in beef cattle. Serum 25OHD$_3$ concentrations above 20 ng/ml have traditionally been considered adequate for the growth and development of cattle. Still, recent evidence has indicated that concentrations below 30 ng/ml are largely insufficient for immunity. Cattle monocytes produce the active form of the vitamin 1,25(OH)$_2$D$_3$ in response to bacterial challenge through toll-like receptor signaling, and this locally produced 1,25OH$_2$D$_3$ upregulated genes are involved in the innate immune system (Rhodes *et al.*, 2003; Nelson *et al.*, 2010; Merriman *et al.*, 2015). However, circulating precursors are necessary. Rhodes *et al.* (2003) reported that 1,25(OH)$_2$D$_3$ plays a role at the onset of infection and in developing the granuloma of *Mycobacterium bovis*-infected cattle. Corripio-Miyar *et al.* (2017) evaluated the effects of 1,25OH$_2$D$_3$ on cattle monocyte-derived dendritic cells (MoDCs) phenotype. These authors reported that vitamin D-conditioned MoDCs showed a reduced expression of co-stimulatory – lower interleukin 12 (IL-12) and higher interleukin 10 (IL-10) – and antigen-presenting molecules, as well as a reduced capability of endocytose ovalbumin. These results indicated a significant positive impact of vitamin D on immune responses against diseases such as tuberculosis or paratuberculosis. Recently, Wherry *et al.* (2022) demonstrated that vitamin D$_3$ compounds, but mainly 1,25(OH)$_2$D$_3$, modulate both pro- and anti-inflammatory immune responses in dairy cattle infected with *M. avium* subspecies *paratuberculosis*, impacting the bacterial viability within the macrophage.

Casas *et al.* (2015) measured the blood concentration of 25OHD in crossbred animals born from March to May in 2011 and 2012 in Nebraska. In period 1 animals had serum 25OHD concentrations of 26.3±1.5 ng/ml. The 25OHD concentrations for late summer (period 2) were 46.6±1.4 and 51.0±1.5 ng/ml for 2011 and 2012, respectively. Serum concentrations of 25OHD in early fall (period 3) were 63.8±1.4 ng/ml and 55.2±1.5 ng/ml for calves in 2011 and 2012, respectively. Values observed for late summer and early fall indicated vitamin D sufficiency ($P < 0.001$) compared with period 1. With diminishing exposure to ultraviolet B rays and consuming ~800 IU or 1,800 IU (2011 and 2012, respectively) of supplemental vitamin D, the calves' midwinter (period 4) 25OHD concentrations fell to 15.2±1.6 ng/ml and 16.7±1.5 ng/ml for 2011 and 2012, respectively, after 4 to 5 month on a finishing diet ($P < 0.0001$). This is considered vitamin D insufficiency in most species. Without sufficient UVB exposure, the dietary vitamin D requirements for rapidly growing beef cattle may need to be increased.

Nelson *et al.* (2016a) observed similar results in 43 cow–calf pairs plus an additional 54 calves in herds located in Florida, Idaho, and Minnesota in the spring calving season and summer months. This group concluded that the lower serum 25OHD of cows in spring compared with summer and the prevalence of vitamin D deficiency of calves (10–15 ng/ml) observed here indicate that increased vitamin D supplementation of cows over the winter months or vitamin D supplementation of newborn calves would be beneficial. These authors verified that subcutaneous injection at birth of vitamins A, D (40,000 IU vitamin D$_3$), and E improved the vitamin status of calves. Still, it was also reported that very few herds receive supplementation.

Flores-Villalva *et al.* (2021) determined that the mean circulating concentration of 25OHD at calf birth was 7.64±3.21 ng/ml, indicating vitamin D deficiency. Neither the injection of vitamin D$_3$ at birth nor the elevated levels in milk replacer (6,000 or 10,000 IU/kg) yielded discernible changes to the pre-weaning circulating concentration of 25OHD. The milk replacers had 6,000 IU/kg for the control calves and 10,000 IU/kg in the vitamin D calves. The controls received a ration with 2,000 IU/kg of vitamin D_3, and the vitamin D calves had 4,000 IU/kg of vitamin D_3 in the ration. In a factorial experiment, half of the calves in each dietary treatment were indoors, and the other half outdoors. In this experiment, no calf reached the recommended vitamin D immune sufficiency level of 30 ng/ml of 25OHD until at least 3 months of age. Increasing dietary vitamin D_3 via ration in the post-weaning period significantly elevated 25OHD concentrations in serum in calves maintained indoors. Maximal levels of circulating 25OHD were achieved in calves maintained outdoors, reaching 60.86±7.32 ng/ml at 5 months of age. The most significant divergence in hematology profile was observed between control indoors and vitamin D groups indoors with control indoor calves showing an elevated count of neutrophils, eosinophils, and basophils associated with reduced 25OHD concentrations. Neither interleukin 18 (IL-8) expression nor reactive oxygen production (free radicals) in serum significantly differed between calves with high and low 25OHD, indicating that other vitamin D-dependent mechanisms may contribute to the observed divergent circulating cellular profiles. This novel data on the vitamin D status of neonatal calves identifies a significant window of vitamin D insufficiency, which is associated with significant differences in circulating immune cell profiles. Vitamin D insufficiency may, therefore, exacerbate pre-weaning disease susceptibility.

Recommendations
Estimating optimum vitamin D requirements is challenging due to the difficulties of measuring body stores and determining the amount of *in vivo* synthesis, the limited information on Ca and P total intake, and the potential interactions with many other nutrients. The BR Corte (2023) recommends the OVN® (DSM, 2016) and NRC (2016) vitamin D levels for calves, growing, finishing and cows, for both Zebu cattle and for *Bos taurus* crossbred animals.

The NRC (1996, 2000, 2016) recommended to supply 275 IU of vitamin D/kg DM feed for beef cattle in general for all phases of gestating or lactating cows and grower or finisher calves. This equals approximately 5.7 IU/kg BW.

This value is similar to the NRC (2007) recommendation of 5.6 IU/k BW for ewes in late pregnancy and lactating ewes. The CSIRO (2007) recommended 10 IU/kg for this class of ewes. The NASEM (2021) set a 30 IU/kg BW requirement for dairy cattle. The INRA (2018) gives a similar recommendation (300 IU/ kg of DM) that would be valid for most growing and fattening cattle. The CVB (2022) recommended between 300 and 500 IU/kg DM for dairy cows. The highest value should be fed during the dry-off period.

In the case of suckling calves (Table 5.1a), a supply of 600 IU/kg DM milk replacer was recommended by NRC (2001) and this level has been increased to 3,200 IU/kg of milk replacer by NASEM (2021). Finally, dsm-firmenich (2022b) suggests a range 2,000–4,000 IU/kg milk replacer, which is quite consistent with NASEM (2021). In starter and grower feed NRC (2001) 600 IU/kg DM, a level which has been increased by NASEM (2021) to 1,100 IU/kg DM. Also, for this phase dsm-firmenich (2022b) recommends a higher level 2,200–3,000 IU/kg DM (Table 5.1b).

In Table 5.2, we calculated the NRC (2016) suggested levels for weaned calves, beef cattle, beef cows and breeding bulls based on the recommended level of 275 IU/kg feed. Finally, in Table 5.3 we have summarized the NRC (2016) and the dsm-firmenich (2022b) recommendations for the different cattle categories. Overall, the range of recommendation of the latter source is higher compared to NRC (2016), reflecting the higher level of feed in practice and the opportunity offered by vitamin D_3 to modulate immune response. dsm-firmenich (2022b) also suggested feeding the first metabolite $25OHD_3$ (commercial name HyD®) to beef cattle at 1 mg/head day in the fattening and finishing phases for enhancing growth performance.

Data obtained from a descriptive study (Vasconcelos and Galyean, 2007) indicated that in the US, supplies of vitamin D in finishing cattle diets are higher than the NRC (2016) recommendations (averaging 329.9 IU/kg of DM), but with a wide range of variation (0.0 to 1.102 IU/kg of DM).

In a more recent survey, Samuelson et al. (2016) stated that vitamin D recommendations by nutritionists in the USA ranged between 271 and 142 IU/kg for receiving and finishing diets, respectively. No vitamin D was added for receiving and finishing diets, indicating that most nutritionists did not provide supplemental sources of vitamin D. However, it is also possible that vitamin D was included as a component of another supplement, such as vitamin A, and therefore was not considered in the respondents' answers.

Because vitamin D is synthesized easily in animals exposed to sunlight or eating sun-dried feed (e.g., alfalfa hay), much bovine livestock (e.g., cows and calves in the field or open sheds with sunny yards) may not require additional supplementation of this vitamin under tropical conditions or constant sunlight exposure (NRC 1996, 2000, 2016). Differences have been observed in storage capacity, tissue concentration, and supplementation requirements of vitamin D between *B. indicus* and *B. taurus* cattle, which may be associated with a greater capacity for adaptation in the former (Montgomery et al., 2004). However, systematic addition is needed for animals permanently housed indoors. According to INRA (1988, 2018), increasing vitamin D levels in animals receiving significant amounts of β-carotene or suffering from metabolic acidosis would also be appropriate. Still, these must always be within tolerance limits to avoid toxicity caused by excess.

Acedo et al. (2018) and Carvalho et al. (2019) working with finishing beef cattle fed 1 mg 25OHD$_3$/head/day, found higher carcass dressing by 0.55% and 4.2 kg higher hot carcass weight confirming that 25OHD$_3$ is a better source of vitamin D$_3$ that can support beef cattle performance.

In beef cattle finishing feedlot diet, Niehues et al. (2020) supplemented 25OHD$_3$ at a dose of 1 mg/animal/day in crossbred Angus-Nellore steers for 105 days. The carcass average daily gain and hot carcass weight were higher than control animals fed monensin at 25 mg/kg/DM. This data corroborates the gene expression activation for muscle development as observed by Martins et al. (2020).

Supplementation and meat quality

Studies conducted worldwide demonstrated no impact of vitamin D$_3$ administered for a short period before slaughter (10 days) on the production rates, such as feed intake, daily weight gain, and FCR (Półtorak et al., 2017). However, higher vitamin D supplementation (between 0.5 and 7.5 × 10⁶ IU) during the week before slaughter improves the meat's tenderness (Swanek et al., 1999; Montgomery et al., 2000, 2002; Foote et al., 2004; Carnagey et al., 2008a,b). This improvement in the meat quality may be associated with increased Ca concentration, which would cause more significant proteolysis in the days following slaughter (Montgomery et al., 2000, 2002; Półtorak et al., 2017). This tenderness leads to a shorter aging process, from 21 to 14 days, depending on the type of muscle, and prolonged shelf life (Półtorak et al., 2017). The effects of vitamin D on tenderness seem to be less pronounced in mature beef cows (Carnagey et al., 2008a,b).

Foote et al. (2004) conducted 3 experiments to determine whether feeding 25OHD$_3$ or 1,25(OH)$_2$D$_3$ improves the tenderness of longissimus dorsi (LD), semimembranosus (SM), and infraspinatus (IF) muscles without leaving residual vitamin D$_3$ and its metabolites in the muscle. In the first 2 experiments, 24 crossbred steers were used to determine the effects of different oral amounts of 1,25(OH)$_2$D$_3$ (Exp. 1; $n = 12$) and 25OHD$_3$ (Exp. 2; n = 12) on plasma Ca²⁺ concentrations. In the third experiment, crossbred steers were allotted randomly to 1 of 4 treatments: (1) control placebo ($n = 7$); (2) 5 × 10⁶ IU of vitamin D$_3$/day ($n = 9$) for 9 days and harvested 2 days after last treatment; (3) single, 125-mg dose of 25OHD$_3$ ($n = 8$) 4 days before harvest; or (4) single, 500-μg dose of 1,25(OH)$_2$D$_3$ ($n = 9$) 3 days before harvest. In summary, feeding supplemental 25OHD$_3$ to beef cattle before harvest may result in more tender LD and semimembranosus steaks without generating a large vitamin D$_3$ residue, as observed in muscle from vitamin D$_3$-treated cattle.

Increased vitamin D concentrations have been shown to limit adipocyte differentiation *in vitro* (Pickworth *et al.*, 2012b) and *in vivo* (Roudbari *et al.*, 2020), affecting marbling in the skeletal muscle of beef cattle. Vitamin D also inhibits adipogenesis *in vitro*. 1,25(OH)$_2$D$_3$, the active vitamin D metabolite, inhibits preadipocyte differentiation and suppresses adipogenic PPARG gene expression in 3T3 L1 cells. Park *et al.* (2018) conducted a feedlot trial at the Ohio State University feedlot in Wooster, OH. The 168 Angus crossbred steers were blocked by initial BW (284±0.4 kg) into 3 groups. They were allotted 24 pens, resulting in calves in each block with similar initial BW (238±0.5, 284±0.7, and 330±0.9 kg for light, moderate, and heavy BW blocks, respectively). Pens within each BW block were randomly assigned to 1 of 4 treatments. A 2 × 2 factorial arrangement of treatments was utilized. The main effects were dietary supplementation of vitamins A and D: the vitamin A treatments were no supplemental vitamin A (NA) or 3,750 IU/kg of dietary DM supplemental vitamin A (SA), and the vitamin D treatments were no supplemental vitamin D (ND) or 1,860 IU/kg of dietary DM supplemental vitamin D (SD). Therefore, the 4 dietary treatments were NAND (neither supplemental vitamin A nor D), NASD (no supplemental vitamin A with vitamin D supplementation), SAND (supplemental vitamin A without vitamin D supplementation), and SASD (supplemental vitamin A and vitamin D). Dietary restriction of vitamin D alone had little impact on adipose accretion.

Duffy *et al.* (2017) evaluated vitamin D supplementation in 30 continental (Charolais × Limousine) heifers blocked based on BW and age and randomly allocated to 1 of 3 dietary treatments: T1: basal + 0 IU of vitamin D$_3$/kg diet; T2: basal + 2,000 IU of vitamin D$_3$/kg diet; T3: basal + 4,000 IU of vitamin D$_3$/kg diet. Additionally, dietary treatments were offered for the final 30-day period pre-slaughter. The basal diet consisted of a standard *ad libitum* finishing regime of concentrates and forage (straw) offered at a ratio of 90:10. The vitamin D$_3$ levels in the experimental diets were chosen to comply with EU regulations. Moreover, diets were formulated to meet the nutrient requirements of finishing beef heifers, and the primary diet contained 110 g/kg crude protein and 11.4 MJ/kg metabolizable energy. In conclusion, this study has shown that short-term dietary supplementation of heifer diets, and within allowable EU inclusion levels (4,000 IU of vitamin D$_3$ kg/feed), can successfully enhance beef vitamin D content and improve beef tenderness of muscles.

In a second experiment, Duffy *et al.* (2018a) evaluated supplementing vitamin D with 3 different sources. (1) basal diet + 4,000 IU of vitamin D$_3$ (Vit D$_3$); (2) basal diet + 4,000 IU of vitamin D$_2$ (Vit D$_2$); and (3) basal diet + 4,000 IU of vitamin D$_2$-enriched mushrooms (Mushroom D$_2$) for a 30-day pre-slaughter period for 30 heifers. The supplementation of heifer diets with Vit D$_3$ yielded higher ($P < 0.001$) LT total vitamin D activity (by 38–56%; $P < 0.05$) and serum 25OHD concentration (by 20–36%; $P < 0.05$), compared to that from vitamin D$_2$ and mushroom D$_2$ supplemented animals. Irrespective of vitamin D source, carcass characteristics, sensory, and meat quality parameters were unaffected ($P > 0.05$) by the dietary treatments. However, it was confirmed that vitamin D$_3$ supplementation in cattle diets is the most productive way to enhance total beef vitamin D activity. The benefits of enriching meat with vitamin D were reviewed by Duffy *et al.* (2018b).

Vitamin D$_3$ may exert 2 contrasting functions on adipogenesis: inhibiting adipocyte differentiation and promoting fat accumulation in adipocytes. Depending on the animals' growth phase, low dietary intake of Ca leads to increased plasma 1α,25-dihydroxy vitamin D$_3$ that suppresses adipocyte differentiation and reduces marbling (Pyatt and Berger, 2005; Nguyen *et al.*, 2021).

Vitamin D supplementation and mineral metabolism

Vitamin D is an essential modulator of Ca homeostasis and has several effects on the immune system. However, there is considerable genetic variability in the vitamin D metabolism. Casas *et al.* (2013) conducted a study to estimate the heritability of vitamin D status and identify genomic regions associated with the concentration of circulating 25OHD in beef cattle. Vitamin D status was measured in crossbred animals from Cycle VII of the United States Meat Animal Research Center (USMARC) Germplasm Evaluation Project. Progeny was born from March through May 2008 and 2010. Heritability was estimated, and a genome-wide association study was conducted on the 25OHD concentration measured in 1,432 animals at preconditioning and 1,333 animals at weaning. Genotyping of the population was done by attributing from the parental generation genotyped with a high-density array (777,000 single nucleotide polymorphism, SNP) to a target population genotyped with a medium-density SNP array (50,000 SNP). After imputation, 675,018 SNP were used in the genome-wide association study. Results from this study suggested that CYP2J2 is a gene controlling cattle serum 25OHD concentrations. CYP2J2 should be considered a prime candidate for understanding genetic and physiological factors affecting serum $25OHD_3$ concentrations and, therefore, vitamin D status in cattle.

Improving the absorption of P for the animal by influencing metabolic pathways controlled by vitamin D can potentially improve the productivity and profitability of extensive livestock enterprises. McGrath *et al.* (2012; 2013) indicated that supplementation of $25OHD_3$ in sufficient doses (3.25 mg/head day) has been shown to increase active absorption of both Ca (3 g/day) and P (4 g/day). Tomkins *et al.* (2020) evaluated the efficacy of rumen bolus containing $25OHD_3$, commercially available as Hy-D®, and monensin on blood P and Ca concentrations in young cattle. A total of 84 heifers, initial live weight 184±2.0 kg (mean ± SEM), were allocated to 4 groups, dosed with 1 of 4 slow-release boluses: (1) placebo (control), (2) monensin (120 mg/day), (3) Hy-D® (6 mg/day), or (4) monensin (120 mg/day) and Hy-D® (6 mg/day), and managed on a common unimproved native pasture from August 2012 to February 2013. Postdosing, liveweight, hip height, and body condition scores were recorded 4 times, and individual fecal and jugular blood samples were collected. The study demonstrated that sustained and elevated plasma concentrations of $25OHD_3$ and P can be achieved compared with control animals. The slow-release rumen bolus maintained an elevated $25OHD_3$ plasma concentration. It indicated a target plasma concentration of $25OHD_3$ for increasing P absorption in beef cattle is between 200 and 300 ng/ml.

Vitamin E

Vitamin E is a group of molecules with α-tocopherol as vegetables' most biologically active form and form used to supplement animals' diet. One IU vitamin E equals 1 mg of all-racemic-α-tocopherol acetate. In the text, we use IU (e.g., IU/kg DM) with the meaning of its equivalence to mass units (mg/kg DM). The vitamin E content of the feed is very variable. Depending on its maturity state, forage contains between 80 and 200 IU of vitamin E per kg DM (Tramontano *et al.*, 1993; Jukola *et al.*, 1996). The α-tocopherol concentration reduces rapidly once the plant is cut. Prolonged exposure to oxygen or sunlight increases the speed of degradation (Thafvelin and Oksanen, 1966). Silage and hay, frequently used in winter feed for beef cattle, have between 20 and 80% less tocopherol than fresh forage. Cereals and oilseeds are low in vitamin E, except for whole soybean and cotton seeds.

Vitamin E is an important antioxidant agent in rations rich in unsaturated fatty acids. It stimulates the production of antibodies and enhances immune response (Craven and Williams, 1985; Hogan *et al.*, 1993; Rivera *et al.*, 2002). An optimum intake of vitamin E brings about a lower incidence of retained placentas and metritis, improvements in MG health, the health of the reproductive system (Smith *et al.*, 1985; Hogan *et al.*, 1993; Harrison *et al.*, 1984; Lacetera *et al.*, 1996), and improvements in immune competence and meat quality (McDowell *et al.*, 1996, McDowell, 2000a; Rivera *et al.*, 2002). However, it is challenging to discuss vitamin E without considering the role of selenium since the effects of both micronutrients are closely related to animal productivity (Hoekstra, 1975; Droke and Loerch, 1989; Hemingway, 2003; Khan *et al.*, 2022; Jung *et al.*, 2023).

The animals require both elements and fulfill a metabolic role in the animal in addition to their antioxidant effect. In some cases, although not always, vitamin E can be substituted by selenium to a certain extent or vice versa. Although selenium cannot wholly replace vitamin E as a nutrient, it does reduce its requirements and delays the appearance of symptoms of vitamin E deficiency in the animal (Spears, 2000; Hemingway, 2003).

Recommendations
Beef cows (gestation/lactation) and breeding bulls

INRA (1988, 2018) indicated that generally, in ruminants, the vitamin E requirement would be around 5–10 IU (or mg)/kg DM feed, recommending in the case of dairy cows (gestating and lactating) a supply of 15 IU/kg DM feed, a value that could probably be extrapolated and used directly for beef cows. The NRC report on beef cattle (1996, 2016) provided a wide range of 15 to 60 IU/kg DM feed for beef cattle, including beef cows during both gestation and lactation cows. The NASEM, in its report on dairy cows (2021), increased vitamin E recommendations for lactating cows considerably, by 30%, to 20 IU/kg DM, and increased its recommendation for dry cows even more markedly (1.6 IU/kg BW), equivalent to 80 IU/ kg DM.

In Table 5.2, we calculated, using a dose of 35 IU/kg DM, a daily vitamin E dietary supplementation of 350–420 and 490–560 IU/head per day for beef cows in gestation and lactation, respectively. Both levels are very close to 350–500 IU/kg DM indicated by dsm-firmenich (2022b) (Table 5.3).

The usefulness of applying the recommendations given by NASEM (2021) for dairy cows to beef cattle is debatable since the increment recommended is based on improving immune competence in animals subjected to very demanding production conditions. However, the evidence of its effect on the health of the MG and the reproductive function should be considered, given that the vitamin E reserves in a suckling calf are low. Some investigators recommend supplementing prepartum gestating cows with vitamin E to increase the concentration of vitamin E in the colostrum (Weiss *et al.*, 1994; Quigley and Bernard, 1995; Weiss, 1998). The dose recommended for the supplementation of cows is 1,000 IU/d of vitamin E (Zobell *et al.*, 1995; Quigley and Bernard, 1995), and it has been proposed as an alternative for increasing blood levels of vitamin E in the cow and the colostrum and minimizing the incidence of postpartum metabolic disorders. Adopting this practice is also recommended to maximize resistance to diseases in calves during the first weeks of life (Quigley and Drewry, 1998; Debier *et al.*, 2005).

In breeding bulls, the calculated recommendation using the same level of 35 IU/kg DM gives a supplementation of 595–630 IU/head day (Table 5.2) which is similar to 300–500 IU/head day given by dsm-firmenich (2022b) (Table 5.3).

Calves: suckling, starter, and grower

According to the NRC (1996, 2000, 2016), vitamin E requirements have not been well established, although young calves are considered to be between 15 and 60 IU/kg DM. In milk replacers, NASEM (2021) recommended 200 IU/kg DM, indicating a significant increase compared to

50 IU/kg DM recommended in its previous report (NRC, 2001). dsm-firmenich (2022b) is close to NASEM (2021), recommending a range of 150–200 IU/kg DM (Table 5.1a). During the starter and grower phase NRC (2001) suggested 25 IU/kg DM, whereas NASEM (2021) increased to 67 IU and dsm-firmenich (2022b) proposed 135–200 IU/kg DM. This higher level considers the benefits of this vitamin in counteracting stress and modulating the immune system (Table 5.1b).

The tendency to provide higher levels of vitamin E than those recommended is based on increased requirements of animals in the stress situations typical of current production systems, especially in feedlots, which are becoming more and more intensive. In such a case, a higher vitamin E supplementation can better modulate the immune system and decrease medical costs (Hidiroglou *et al.*, 1995; Reddy *et al.*, 1986, 1987; Carter *et al.*, 2005). However, the presence of unsaturated fatty acids in milk replacers can increase the risk of oxidation of the ration, increasing the need for antioxidants. Stobo (1983) suggested that vitamin E concentration in milk replacers should be formulated according to the unsaturated fatty acid content of the ration and suggested a ratio of 1.5–2.5 IU of vitamin E per gram of linoleic acid. In regular milk replacers, this ratio is achieved with a daily intake of between 25 and 63 IU/kg DM.

Although there is no solid evidence to justify the need to use levels above those recommended for vitamin E, 2 situations merit special consideration. First, frequent digestive disorders in young calves reduce vitamin E absorption. Second, as previously indicated, supplementation with high quantities of vitamin A interferes with vitamin E absorption. For these reasons, and because of the comprehensive safety margin of vitamin E, it seems reasonable to consider a possible increase in the supply of this vitamin above recommended levels in certain situations.

Beef cattle
The NRC (1996, 2000, 2016) recommended a vitamin E supply within a range of 15 and 60 IU/kg DM in concentrate for feedlot calves. Calves in stressful conditions should be provided with 400 to 500 IU/calf daily during the receiving period for a 250 kg calf, which is equal to 1.6 to 2.0 IU/kg BW. However, vitamin E dietary concentrations of regular healthy finishing cattle should fall between 25 and 35 IU/kg DM or 0.52 to 0.74 IU/kg BW. The INRA (1988, 2018) recommended 25 IU of vitamin E/kg of DM. Using a dose of 35 IU/kg DM, we have calculated the recommended vitamin E level per animal per day during the grow-out phases from post-weaning to slaughter weight (Table 5.2). In Table 5.3, comparing the recommendations of NRC (2016) – 315–385 IU/head day – and dsm-firmenich (2022b) – 200–300 IU/head day – we can observe a substantial agreement. During the fattening and finishing phases, NRC (2016) recommended 490–560 IU/head per day, whereas dsm-firmenich (2022b) suggested a higher level of 500–2,000 IU/head per day, but the latter includes the effect of the higher levels on immunity, stress, and meat quality traits.

As said above, these levels should be increased during stressful situations since vitamin E participates actively in the immune system. It is known that stress caused by weaning, transport, mixing with animals from other farms, and adapting to the feedlot leads to the rapid depletion of reserves of this vitamin (Hill and Williams, 1995). Vitamin E supplementation (400 IU/head per day) during the feedlot's first 3–4 weeks can positively affect growth, conversion index, and disease incidence (Lee *et al.*, 1985; Droke and Loerch, 1989; Galyean *et al.*, 1999). For this reason, the NRC (1996, 2016) recommended a supplemental supply of 400–500 IU/day of vitamin E in these critical periods. Some reports demonstrated the favorable effect of supplementation with vitamin E in stress situations associated with the transfer of animals to feedlots. Elam (2006) analyzed bibliographical data to evaluate the effect of the quantity of ingested vitamin E (range 0 to 2,000 IU/head/day) on the effective response and health of calves that had just arrived at the feedlots. The results indicated that, although no positive effects were observed in daily weight gain or the ingestion of food, the provision of vitamin E did reduce the incidence of respiratory diseases. The average reduction was 0.35% for each 100 UI of vitamin E ingested daily.

Vasconcelos and Galyean (2007) reported in their feedlot survey that the mean vitamin E concentrations in feedlot diets were 25.7 IU/kg DM. In a more recent survey, this group (Samuelson *et al.*, 2016) reported that receiving diets contain 29.8 IU/kg, and finishing diets contain 25.1 IU/kg. The vitamin E supplementation was 20 and 0 IU/kg for receiving and finishing diets, respectively. This indicates that although nutritionists often add vitamin E to receiving diets, most choose not to provide additional vitamin E to finishing cattle.

Supplementing with vitamin E during finishing to improve product yield has had varied responses. In general, positive responses have been observed in animals that had previously suffered from vitamin E deficiency (Hutcheson and Cole, 1985) but were not observed in those that had always been well-fed (Carrica *et al.*, 1986; Schaefer *et al.*, 1989; Arnold *et al.*, 1992). Growth rate and conversion index improvements are generally found in young animals with good growth potential who have undergone stress conditions (Hill and Williams, 1995).

Rivera *et al.* (2002) conducted 3 experiments to evaluate the effect of dietary vitamin E on the reception performance and health and the finishing performance of beef cattle. 120 beef steers (Experiment 1; baseline BW = 173 kg) and 200 beef heifers (Experiment 2; baseline BW = 204 kg) were randomly assigned to 1 of 3 treatment diets formulated to supply 285, 570 or 1,140 IU/animal daily of supplemental vitamin E during the reception period. Furthermore, in Experiment 3, 17 steers were used to study the effects of the same 3 levels of vitamin E on the humoral immune response to an ovalbumin vaccine administered on days 0 and 14. During this experiment 3, jugular blood samples were collected on days 0, 7, 14, and 21. Supplemental vitamin E had limited effects on performance. However, statistically significant effects were found on the humoral immune response and possible recovery from respiratory diseases (Rivera *et al.*, 2002). Rivera *et al.* (2003) reported that receiving calves fed supplemental vitamin E (570 IU/d for 5 days) were treated more often for respiratory disease than calves drenched or injected with vitamin E (2,850 IU) on feedlot arrival.

Supplementation of vitamin E to reduce lipid meat oxidation

Another possible reason for supplementing higher vitamin E levels in rations for beef calves in the finishing phase is to reduce the oxidation of lipids, improve the color of the meat, and, as a consequence, obtain a product with a longer shelf life (Descalzo and Sancho, 2008). The supply of high quantities of vitamin E in the final fattening period (500–2,000 mg/head day) improves the color stability of refrigerated or frozen meat (McDowell *et al.*, 1996). This allows the display period of the fresh meat to be lengthened from 1 to 3 days without loss of color and is essential in meat destined for export. The loss of color in meat, which in the case of red meat production changes from bright to dark red, is due to the high potential for myoglobin oxidation (Faustman and Cassens, 1990). Oxidation of muscle pigments is one of the leading causes of deterioration in meat quality (Faustman *et al.*, 1989). Supplementation with a high dosage of vitamin E improves color and also inhibits fat oxidation, reducing the risk of rancidity (Schaefer *et al.*, 1991; Arnold *et al.*, 1992; Hill and Williams, 1993 and 1995) and lengthening the shelf life of salable meat (McDowell *et al.*, 1996).

According to these latter authors, the α-tocopherol concentration in muscular tissue should reach 0.30–0.35 mg/100 g of meat to obtain this kind of result. This is possible by employing supplementation with 500 IU/day of vitamin E during about 100–125 days before calves slaughter (Schaefer *et al.*, 1991; Stubbs *et al.*, 2002; Rowe *et al.*, 2004). In some countries, a quick and cheap spectrophotometric method in slaughterhouses has been proposed, which allows the identification of meat from animals supplemented with vitamin E (Smith, 1994), intending to pay a better price to the farmer according to the quality of meat produced. However, Luciano et al. (2011) concluded that vitamin E in muscle alone does not explain the resistance of meat to oxidative deterioration because there is an interaction with highly peroxidizable polyunsaturated fatty acids (PUFA).

Supplementation and meat tenderness and quality

Supplementation with vitamin E in a dose of 1,000 IU/day 125 days before slaughter improves the meat's tenderness. It protects the calpain, the enzyme responsible for softening the meat, from oxidation (Rowe et al., 2004). It has also been suggested that supplementation with vitamin E during the finishing phase in feedlots constitutes an effective method to increase the stability of lipids during cooking (Lanari et al., 1994). However, this effect is not always evident (Robbins et al., 2003). Descalzo and Sancho (2008) reviewed the effect of including antioxidants in the diet on the characteristics and quality of the meat. They concluded that the magnitude of the beneficial effect of supplementing the finishing diet with vitamin E is very variable and dependent on the basal diet offered, i.e., forage vs. concentrate, silage, nature of the supplement, etc.

In conclusion, the available data suggest current recommendations for feedlot animals of 15–60 IU/kg DM may be increased during the receiving period and adaptation to the feedlot to 400–500 IU/day to improve their immune competence and at the finishing period to 500–1,000 IU/day, for about 3 months, if an economic profit may be obtained from an improvement in the quality of the meat produced.

Grass-fed beef may have a higher demand for endogenous antioxidants due to its high content of PUFA. However, many pasture-fed cattle receive synthetic vitamin E (Röhrle et al., 2011). Yang et al. (2002b) evaluated the effect of vitamin E in pasture-fed cattle. Thirty-two Hereford cross steers (mean BW 294 + 9.5 kg) were divided into 4 equally sized groups and assigned to 1 of 4 treatments for 132 days before slaughter. Treatments were grass-fed supplemented with 0 or 2,500 IU dl-α-tocopherol acetate/head/day (vitamin E) or grain-fed in a sorghum-based grow-out ration supplemented with 0 or 2,500 IU/head/day of vitamin E. α-tocopherol acetate intakes were estimated to be 2,200, 4,700, 300, and 2,800 IU/head/day for the grass-fed control and supplemented cattle and the grain-fed control and supplemented cattle, respectively. Pasture feeding with and without supplementation increased lipid oxidation of aged beef. Vitamin E supplementation did not improve pasture-fed beef's color and lipid stability.

Juárez et al. (2011) evaluated the effects of dietary vitamin E with or without flaxseed on beef fatty acid composition. Eighty feedlot steers were blocked by initial weight and housed in 8 feedlot pens balancing by weight within treatment (2 pens per dietary treatment, 10 animals per pen, and 20 animals per dietary treatment) and fed ad libitum. Steers (381±7.10 kg) were blocked by weight and assigned to 1 of the 4 diets in a 2 × 2 factorial experiment, with 2 levels of dietary vitamin E, with and without flaxseed: control-E (451 IU dl-α-tocopherol acetate/head/day), control + E (1,051 IU dl-α-tocopherol acetate/head/day), flaxseed-E (10% ground) and flaxseed + E. Feeding both flaxseed and vitamin E showed positive effects on total omega–3 fatty acid levels. However, accumulating atypical hydrogenation products and their potential bioactivity requires further study.

Camagey et al. (2008b) conducted a trial on 48 Angus crossbred heifers to determine whether a single bolus of 25OHD$_3$ (500 mg administered as a one-time oral bolus 7 days before slaughter), vitamin E (1,000 IU/kg DM administered daily as a top-dress for 104 days before slaughter), or a combination of the 2 would improve the tenderness of steaks from the LM of beef heifers. Results indicate that the use of 500 mg of 25OHD$_3$ or 1,000 IU of vitamin E alone but not in combination, effectively improved tenderness of steaks from the LM of beef heifers. Additionally, results from the current study indicate that vitamin E also enhances the effect of aging on tenderness of beef.

It has been observed that beef cattle fed wet distillers grains plus solubles (WDGS) are tenderer than beef from steers fed corn. Meat from WDGS-fed steers contains more PUFA in the sarcoplasmic reticulum membrane. As a result, the membrane integrity is altered post-mortem, resulting in more rapid Ca leakage and improved tenderness through early activation of Ca-dependent proteases. Chao *et al.* (2017) reported that 450 mg (1,000 IU) of vitamin E per head daily could mitigate these effects.

The effects of vitamin E on lipid metabolism were evaluated by Ladeira *et al.* (2020). The study aimed to analyze the expression of the PPARA, SREBF1 genes, and other genes involved in lipid metabolism in the LT muscle of cattle fed diets containing soybean or cottonseed with or without vitamin E. Twenty-eight Red Norte (¼ Angus, ¼ Nellore, ¼ Senepol, ¼ Caracu) young bulls with an average of 20 months of age and 343 ± 10.1 (SEM) kg of initial liveweight (LW) were used in a completely randomized design using a 2 × 2 factorial arrangement, with 4 treatments and 7 replicates (animals) per treatment. The animals were housed in pens with 30 m² per animal with permanent access to fresh water. The inclusion of soybean in the diets provided 64.8 g/kg of ether extract, while cottonseed provided 65.6 g/kg of ether extract on a DM basis. Half of the animals that received each type of concentrate (cottonseed or soybean) were supplemented with 2,500 IU of vitamin E per head per day (all-*rac*-α-tocopherol acetate) during the experimental period. In conclusion, supplementation with vitamin E altered the expression of genes involved in lipid metabolism in LT muscle, indicating that α-tocopherol is probably a cell-signaling molecule.

Vitamin K

Vitamin K has antihemorrhagic effects, as it is necessary to synthesize a series of blood coagulation factors (Combs and McClung, 2022). Vegetables (K$_1$) and ruminal bacteria (K$_2$) are essential sources of this vitamin. K$_2$ is the principal source of vitamin K in ruminants, and deficiencies in ruminants are seldom detected. They are only reported when anticoagulant substances have been consumed, such as when forage contaminated with fungal dicumarol is consumed. Vitamin K recommendations is only given for veal calves 1–1.5 mg/kg DM by dsm-firmenich (2022b). No recommendation was given by NRC (2016) and NASEM (2021), considering that microbial synthesis in the intestine of young animals sufficiently covers their requirement (Table 5.1a).

WATER-SOLUBLE VITAMINS

Newborn calves have limited stores of water-soluble vitamins and depend on milk until the rumen microflora synthesize these vitamins. Milk contains abundant amounts of B vitamins. Recommendations are focused on milk replacers. Requirements for beef cattle have not been set because ruminal bacteria provide adequate amounts under most common situations. However, there is already interest in estimating B vitamin status in dairy cows (Girard and Graulet, 2021), and some of that information will help improve beef cattle feeding (Ashwin *et al.*, 2018).

Diet and feed additives can modify B vitamin microbial synthesis. In feedlots, when concentrate in the diet increases, thiamine declines, whereas niacin increases substantially in the rumen, and the duodenal concentration of thiamine, niacin, riboflavin, and biotin does not change (NRC, 2016). Monensin (22 mg/kg diet) can indirectly decrease niacin in the duodenum and ileum, but other B vitamins remain unaffected. Out of the different sources of information, only dsm-firmenich (2022b) recommended the supplementations of a few B group vitamins.

Thiamine (vitamin B₁)

Thiamine is a coenzyme in many metabolic reactions (EFSA, 2010). The quantity of thiamine synthesized in the rumen (between 28 and 72 mg/day) is the same as or higher than that ingested in the ration (Breves et al., 1981). No requirements have been laid down for ruminants in good health and with a functional rumen. Supplies from microbial synthesis and the diet are sufficient to meet the requirements of cows and calves, even considering the ruminal degradation of dietary thiamine of 48% (Zinn et al., 1987). For ruminants, thiamine is not toxic, and the safety margins in monogastric are 1,000 times the recommended dose (NRC, 1987), although no safety limits have been established for ruminants.

The requirements of thiamine for feedlot ruminants have not been determined, and it is assumed that ruminal microorganisms provide a sufficient quantity (INRA, 1988, 2018; NRC, 1996, 2016).

In the case of veal calves, both NRC (2001) and NASEM (2021) recommended the incorporation of 6.5 mg/kg DM thiamine in milk replacer, and dsm-firmenich (2022b) suggested a supplementation of 2.5–4.5 mg/kg DM (Table 5.1a). By extrapolating the requirements for pigs (NRC, 1979), Zinn (1992) estimated the requirements for feedlot calves to be 0.14 mg/kg $BW^{0.75}$.

dsm-firmenich (2022b) proposed thiamine supplementation of 60–250 mg/head day in beef cattle (Table 5.3). This recommendation is mainly driven by industry practice but supported by some papers showing the impact of thiamine in alleviating oxidative stress and protecting ruminal epithelial barrier function. Ma et al. (2021) reported that supplementing 200 mg thiamine/kg DM to goats fed a high-concentrate diet (concentrate: forage, 70:30) relieved the damage to the ruminal epithelium. Thiamine supplementation improves the ruminal epithelial barrier function by regulating Nrf2-NFκB signaling pathways during high-concentrate-diet feeding.

Under normal conditions, intake from dietary thiamine and ruminal synthesis is sufficient. However, there are situations where the thiamine finally available to the animal can be a limiting factor (INRA, 1988, 2018; Zinn, 1992; NRC, 1996, 2016). For example, when rations contain high levels of concentrate or are rich in quickly fermentable carbohydrates, typical of intensive feeding systems, abrupt drops in the ruminal pH can occur, releasing thiaminases (exogenous enzymes), which destroy thiamine.

Also, in acidosis situations, thiamine destruction by thiaminase has been linked to the appearance of polioencephalomalacia (PEM) or cerebro-cortical necrosis. A similar situation may occur in rations or water with excessive sulfur levels (Zinn, 1992; NRC, 1996, 2016; Patterson et al., 2003; Pritchard, 2007). Conditions of low ruminal pH also favor the reduction of sulfur to its gaseous form of hydrogen sulfide (H_2S), increasing its concentration in the rumen. H_2S, when eructed, can be inhaled by the animal and trigger PEM. This fact, coupled with the blood levels of thiamine, is considered responsible for the appearance of PEM in cattle (McAllister et al., 1997; Loneragan et al., 1998). The positive effect of supplementation by thiamine, independent of the clinical diagnosis of PEM syndrome, may be because this precedes the subclinical apparition of PEM or because supplementary thiamine may prevent the deficiency (Ward and Patterson, 2004). Under these conditions, thiamine supplementation may alleviate symptoms and improve animal performance (Ward and Patterson, 2004), although parenteral administration is more advisable.

Another vital aspect to consider is the meat's thiamine content since this, together with the presence of the sulfurous components, principally cysteine is involved in the production of certain intermediary compounds responsible for the development and boosting of certain aromas characteristic of meat while it is being cooked (Jooh et al., 2002).

Riboflavin (vitamin B$_2$)

Riboflavin is a constituent of many enzymes which participate in intermediary metabolism. Ruminal microorganisms synthesize abundant quantities of this vitamin, some 15.2 mg/kg organic matter digested. This synthesis and the flow of riboflavin in the rumen appear to be independent of the level of concentrate in the ration (Zinn et al., 1987). Furthermore, ruminal degradation is almost complete (Zinn et al., 1987), and intestinal digestibility is approximately 25% (Miller et al., 1986; Zinn et al., 1987). Therefore, it is quite improbable that riboflavin deficiencies can occur in ruminants. Riboflavin deficiencies have only been observed in young pre-ruminant animals (NRC, 1996, 2016). Supplementation should be only considered in animals under stress and with a low feed intake when bacterial supplies are diminished (Zinn, 1992).

Neither the NRC (1996, 2016) nor INRA (1988, 2018) and dsm-firmenich (2022b) has established specific recommendations for riboflavin for beef cattle or feedlot calves. In milk replacers for veal calves NRC (2001) and NASEM (2021) proposed a supplementation of 6.5 mg/kg DM, and dsm-firmenich (2022b) recommended 2.5–4.5 mg/kg DM. (Table 5.1a). Zinn (1992) calculated, using data collected from pigs (NRC, 1979), that the requirements for feedlot or finisher cattle were 0.32 mg/kg BW$^{0.75}$.

Recently, Ren et al. (2023) evaluated the influences of riboflavin supply (0, 15, 30, and 45 mg/kg DM) on growth performance, nutrient digestibility, and ruminal fermentation in lambs. Increasing riboflavin supply did not affect the DMI but quadratically increased the average daily gain and linearly decreased the FCR. Total-tract DM, neutral-detergent fiber, acid detergent fiber, and crude protein digestibility increased quadratically. Rumen pH and propionate molar percentage decreased linearly, total volatile fatty acids concentration, acetate proportion, and the ratio of acetate to propionate increased linearly. However, ammonia nitrogen concentration was unchanged with increasing riboflavin supply. Linear increases were observed in the activities of carboxymethyl-cellulase, xylanase, pectinase, and protease, and the populations of bacteria, fungi, protozoa, dominant cellulolytic bacteria, *Ruminobacter amylophilus,* and *Prevotella ruminicola*. Methanogen population was not affected by riboflavin supplementation. The microbial protein amount and urinary total purine derivatives excretion increased quadratically. The results indicated that 30 mg/kg DM riboflavin supply improved growth performance, rumen fermentation, and nutrient digestion in lambs.

Niacin (vitamin B$_3$)

Niacin is an active component of 2 coenzymes (NAD and NADP), which are fundamental in metabolizing carbohydrates, lipids, and amino acids. Niacin is found in high concentrations in by-products of animal origin and cereals. Ruminal bacteria synthesize abundant quantities of niacin (Zinn et al., 1987). Zinn (1992) calculated that niacin synthesis in the rumen occurs at a rate of 107.02 mg/kg of organic matter. However, when added to the ration, the quantity of niacin that reaches the intestine may be even less than that provided in the ration due to the inhibition of bacterial synthesis in the presence of exogenous niacin (Abdouli and Schaefer, 1986). Moreover, between 94 and 99% of niacin present in the diet is degraded in the rumen (Zinn, 1992), although other studies have estimated that between 17 and 30% of dietary niacin reaches the small intestine (Harmeyer and Kollenkirchen, 1989; Campbell et al., 1994).

Niacin stimulates microbial protein synthesis (Mizwicki, 1976; Bartley et al., 1979; Ridell et al., 1981; Arambell et al., 1982), the production of propionic acid (Ridell et al., 1981, 1989; Arambell et al., 1982; Hannah and Stern, 1985), and digestion of cellulose (Hannah and Stern, 1985). On the metabolic level, niacin participates in lipid and energy metabolism. Supplementation with niacin increases glucose concentration in the blood and decreases the concentration of β-hydroxybutyric acid and free fatty acids in plasma, indicating its activity as a gluconeogenesis stimulator.

Niacin is required in rations for calves before weaning due to the scant microbial synthesis in the rumen. Hopper and Johnson (1955) observed that calves fed synthetic milk deficient in niacin presented with diarrhea within 48 hours. There was an immediate improvement the day after administering an oral dose of 6 mg/day or an IM dose of 10 mg/day nicotinic acid. The NRC (2001) recommends the incorporation of 10 mg/kg DM of niacin in milk replacer. There is no evidence that niacin supplementation improves the growth rate of calves. Ridell et al. (1981) supplemented calves between 110 and 370 kg with 1.3 g/day niacin and observed no benefit, which suggests that a functional rumen provides enough niacin for the growth and normal development of the calves.

No recommendations have been established for niacin in feedlot cattle (NRC, 1996, 2016; INRA, 1988, 2018; dsm-firmenich, 2022b) due to its sufficient synthesis in the rumen.

Only in the case of veal calf production is recommended the inclusion in milk replacers of niacin. NRC (2001) and NASEM (2021) indicated 10 mg /kg DM and dsm-firmenich (2022b) suggested 9–18 mg/kg DM (Table 5.1a).

By extrapolating from the requirements for pigs (NRC, 1979), Zinn (1992) calculated that the requirements for growing and finishing calves were 1.75 mg/kg $LW^{0.75}$. Since microbial synthesis is 107.02 mg/kg of organic matter (Zinn, 1992), the supply by ruminal bacteria would be sufficient to meet these requirements. However, when animals are fed rations with an imbalance in amino acids, an inadequate supply of energy, or containing rancid ingredients, niacin requirements are altered (NRC, 1996).

Specifically, an excess of leucine, arginine, or glycine, an excess of energy, or the incorrect use of antibiotics increases niacin requirements. In experiments on production, niacin supplementation at up to 10 times the theoretical requirements up to entry to the feedlot improved effective yield (Cole et al., 1982; Zinn et al., 1987). However, Overfield and Hatfield (1976) observed improvements in growth when supplementing with niacin (250–500 mg/kg). Hutcheson (1990) also observed an improvement of 20% in weight gain when supplementing starter rations for healthy calves with 125 ppm niacin. However, a positive response was only observed in sick calves with a higher dosage (250 ppm).

Pyridoxine (vitamin B$_6$)

As with other B group vitamins, neither INRA (1988, 2018) nor the NRC (1996, 2001, 2016) and dsm-firmenich (2022b) have established recommendations for adult bovines.

Regarding veal calves, NRC (2001) and NASEM (2021) recommended incorporating 6.5 mg/kg DM in milk replacers and dsm-firmenich (2022b) suggested supplementing milk replacers with 2.5–4.5 mg/kg DM (Table 5.1a).

Zinn (1992), extrapolating the data collected from pigs (NRC, 1979), proposed a supply of 0.14 mg/kg $BW^{0.75}$ for feedlot and finishing calves. Pyridoxine is not degraded in the rumen but is synthesized abundantly, so a deficit is very unlikely (Zinn, 1992).

Cobalamin (vitamin B$_{12}$)

Vitamin B$_{12}$ is the cofactor of methylmalonyl-CoA mutase (necessary for converting from propionate to succinate) and tetrahydrofolate methyl transferase (which participates in methionine metabolism).

Up to 90% of vitamin B$_{12}$ of dietary origin is degraded in the rumen (Zinn, 1992). Bacteria are the only natural source of vitamin B$_{12}$.

The NRC (2001, 2016) considered that the requirements of milk cows are between 0.34 and 0.68 μg/kg BW. However, using the requirements for fattening pigs (NRC, 1979), Zinn (1992) calculated the requirements for growing and finishing cattle as 1.42 g/kg $BW^{0.75}$.

Owing to the high ruminal degradability of dietary vitamin B_{12}, the supply by the rumen is of fundamental importance. Microbial synthesis of B_{12} depends on the presence of cobalt and increases in a linear fashion when cobalt is administered (in chloride form) up to levels of 0.2–0.25 mg/kg (Stangl *et al.*, 2000; Tiffany *et al.*, 2003; Tiffany and Spears, 2005). Under normal conditions, ruminal bacteria synthesize at a rate of 4.1 mg/kg of organic matter, and synthesis increases in rations high in forage (Sutton and Elliot, 1972; Walker and Elliot, 1972). It is unlikely that a vitamin B_{12} deficiency would occur in beef cattle, considering both its requirements and the capacity for ruminal synthesis, except when there is a cobalt deficiency (Zinn *et al.*, 1987).

The NRC (2001) and NASEM (2021) recommended supplementing 0.07 mg/kg DM in milk replacers, whereas in its last OVN™ recommendations, dsm-firmenich (2022b) proposed for milk replacers a supplementation level of 0.04–0.08 mg/kg DM (Table 5.1a).

Other than this exception, there is no evidence in the literature to suggest a need for vitamin B_{12} supplementation of rations for beef cattle, provided that the ration contains, as said above, enough cobalt.

Fast-growing beef cattle may need more mineral and vitamin intake (Celi, 2011). Lopes *et al.* (2021) evaluated the effects of supplementing finishing beef cattle with inorganic trace minerals and non-protected B vitamin blend or organic trace minerals and rumen-protected B vitamin blend during the finishing phase on liver metabolism. The results indicated that the supplementation with organic trace minerals and protected B vitamins alters the abundance of proteins associated with the electron transport chain and other oxidation-reduction pathways, boosting the production of reactive oxygen species, which appear to modulate proteins linked to oxidative-damage responses to maintain cellular homeostasis.

Biotin (vitamin B_7)

Biotin is a cofactor of enzymes that catalyze carboxylation reactions and intervene in the tricarboxylic acid cycle, gluconeogenesis, and fat synthesis (Campbell *et al.*, 2000). It is also involved in the control and production of keratin, so supplementation with biotin at 10 mg of biotin/animal/day is recommended to reduce laminitis in beef cattle (Tomlinson *et al.*, 2004; Schwab and Shaver, 2005) and exerts a positive effect in the prevention of foot problems in beef cattle (Campbell *et al.*, 2000). Hoof health improved when cattle were supplemented with 10–20 mg of biotin/day (Spears and Weiss, 2014).

Chiquette *et al.* (1993) observed no differences in the digestibility or ruminal fermentation of growing calves supplemented with 2 mg/kg BW of biotin in diets based on forage or concentrate.

Ruminal bacteria synthesize large quantities of biotin depending on the availability of energy and are estimated to be 0.79 mg/kg of organic matter by Briggs *et al.* (1964). However, this synthesis is reduced with an increase in the amount of concentrate in the ration (>50% of the ration).

In milk replacers, NASEM (2021) recommended 0.1 mg/kg DM, which was already recommended in its previous book (NRC, 2001). In the last OVN™ dsm-firmenich (2022b) recommended a supplementation level of 0.2–0.3 mg/kg (Table 5.1a).

Folic acid (vitamin B_9)

Folic acid participates in the metabolism as a methyl group donor. Methionine is also used as a methyl group donor, so supplementation with folic acid increases the availability of methionine for productive functions.

Zinn (1992) used data collected from pigs (NRC, 1987) to extrapolate folic acid requirements for feedlot and finisher cattle and concluded that the requirements were 0.75 mg/kg of $LW^{0.75}$.

A significant amount of folic acid is synthesized in the rumen (0.42 mg/kg of organic matter) depending on the availability of energy (Zinn, 1992). By comparing the estimated requirements with the microbial synthesis of folic acid Zinn (1992) concluded that this vitamin could be of limited use in cattle.

In pre-ruminant calves, poor bacterial synthesis may lead to deficiency. Daily injection of 40 mg of folic acid between weeks 1 and 16 of life increased average weight gain by 8% between weeks 7 and 12 (Dumoulin et al., 1991).

No recommendation has been established for beef cattle. As for other B vitamins, recommendations are given for milk replacer for veal calves (Table 5.1a): NRC (2001) and NASEM (2021) suggested adding 0.5 mg/kg DM and recently dsm-firmenich (2022b) suggested in its OVN™ guidelines a supplementation of 0.2–0.3 mg/kg DM.

Owing to the high level of ruminal degradation (97%, Zinn, 1992), oral supplementation in adult animals would only be justified if a protection system against ruminal degradation were developed.

Recently, Wang et al. (2023) examined the influences of coated folic acid (CFA), 0 or 6 mg of folic acid/kg DM, and coated riboflavin (CRF), 0 or 60 mg riboflavin/kg DM on bull performance, nutrients digestion, and ruminal fermentation. Supplementation of CRF in diets with CFA had a greater increase in daily weight gain and feed efficiency than in diets without CFA. Supplementation with CFA or CRF enhanced the digestibility of DM, organic matter, crude protein, neutral-detergent fiber, and non-fiber carbohydrates. Ruminal pH and ammonia-N content decreased, and the total volatile fatty acids concentration and acetate to propionate ratio elevated for CFA or CRF addition. Supplementation with CFA or CRF increased the activities of fibrolytic enzymes and the numbers of total bacteria, protozoa, fungi, dominant fibrolytic bacteria and P. ruminicola. The activities of α-amylase, protease, and pectinase and the numbers of Butyrivibrio fibrisolvens and R. amylophilus were increased by CFA but were unaffected by CRF. The blood concentration of folate increased, and homocysteine decreased for CFA addition. The CRF supplementation elevated blood concentrations of folate and RF. These findings suggested that CFA or CRF inclusion had facilitating effects on performance and ruminal fermentation, and combined addition of CFA and CRF had a greater increase in performance than CFA or CRF addition alone in bulls.

Pantothenic acid

Pantothenic acid is a constituent of coenzyme A, and it is essential in many reactions, including fatty acid oxidation metabolism, amino acid catabolism, and acetylcholine synthesis.

As with other B group vitamins, there are no recommendations on the requirements of pantothenic acid in beef cattle but only for veal calves: both NRC (2001) and NASEM (2021) recommended 13 mg/kg, and dsm-firmenich (2022b) indicated a range of 7–9 mg/kg DM (Table 5.1a).

Zinn (1992) estimated, from the requirements of growing pigs (NRC, 1979), that the requirements of fattening calves were 1.42 mg/kg $BW^{0.75}$. Considering that synthesis by ruminal bacteria is 2.2 mg/kg DM, and ruminal degradation of dietary pantothenic acid is 78%, it appears that supplementation may be necessary (Zinn et al., 1987; Zinn, 1992), especially in the case of animals under stress or with low feed intake. Developing less degradable forms in the rumen may provide an opportunity to improve the dietary supply and obtain possible production responses.

Vitamin C (ascorbic acid)

Vitamin C is synthesized fundamentally as ascorbic acid within the cells of adult ruminants. It is provided depending on the synthesis of vitamin C in the liver since most of the vitamin C delivered in the diet is degraded in the rumen. It is generally accepted that adult cattle synthesize sufficient ascorbic acid to cover their vitamin C requirement (Toutain *et al.*, 1997). Thus, there is no data on the effects of oral vitamin C supplementation in adult animals. However, ruminants are considered the domestic species least likely to present vitamin C deficiencies when in some cases, the synthesis of ascorbic acid is insufficient. Calves cannot synthesize it until 3 weeks old, so it is considered an essential nutrient only for young calves.

Vitamin C is an antioxidant and participates in regulating steroid synthesis. Roth and Kaeberle (1985) suggested it is implicated in the immune response. Under stress conditions, the plasma concentration of vitamin C diminishes as much in young as in growing calves (Cummins and Brunner, 1991; Hidiroglou *et al.*, 1977).

Oral supplementation of 1–2 g of vitamin C in pre-ruminant calves increased the plasma concentration of vitamin C (Hidiroglou *et al.*, 1995), which might be related to improving the immune response (Eicher-Pruiett *et al.*, 1992). In sheep, supplementation of the ration with 4 g/day of vitamin C resulted in a rise in the plasma concentration of vitamin C (Hidiroglou *et al.*, 1995). In no case did supplementation with vitamin C improve production. However, parenteral administration of vitamin C is indeed recommended in cases of stress since its provision in the diet for a prolonged period might cause adverse effects on the immune response due to the potential of vitamin C for acting as a pro-oxidant in high concentrations (Rose and Bode, 1993). The vitamin C content in the tissues also varies according to the nutritional system of the calves.

For example, the concentration of ascorbic acid (µg/g of muscle) in the psoas major muscle (selected for its high susceptibility to deterioration during storage) ranged from 15.92 µg/g of muscle in grain-based diets to 25.30 µg/g of muscle in pastured calves (Descalzo *et al.*, 2005). Although neither the NRC (1996, 2016) nor the INRA (1988, 2018) and dsm-firmenich (2022b) set recommendations for beef cattle, it is necessary to monitor the requirements and supplies of this vitamin, above all in feedlot cattle fed diets which include high quantities of concentrate, because of its effects on the quality of the carcass and the meat, such as its capacity to reduce the oxidative capacity of lipids, and the improvement and persistence of its color when treated post mortem (Descalzo and Sancho, 2008).

On the opposite, for the production of veal calves, both the NRC (2001) and NASEM (2021) did not indicate a supplementation and dsm-firmenich (2022b) suggested a level of 250–500 mg/kg DM in milk replacers.

In a literature review, Ranjan *et al.* (2012) reported that although cattle can synthesize vitamin C from D-Glucose or D-Galactose, several reports suggest decreased tissue concentrations during various diseases and stress and beneficial effects of their supplementation in the maintenance of health and fertility. In addition, Ranjan *et al.* (2012) indicated that supplementation with the appropriate dose of vitamin C may be necessary for heat stress management, the management of the diarrhea of the calves, mastitis, infertility, and fattening, as was discussed by Matsui (2012).

Takahashi *et al.* (1999) reported that plasma vitamin C concentrations decreased during fattening in cattle. Matsui (2012) mentioned that this research group sampled Japanese Black cattle to measure plasma vitamin C. They used 135 calves, 238 fattening heifers, 524 fattening steers, 127 replacement heifers, and breeding but not lactating cows. Their results (Figure 5.4) indicated that the individual variations in plasma vitamin C concentrations were substantial, and that sex did not affect plasma vitamin C concentrations in growing and fattening cattle. The plasma vitamin C concentrations were stable by 13.4 months of age 22.5±3.3 µM (mean ±

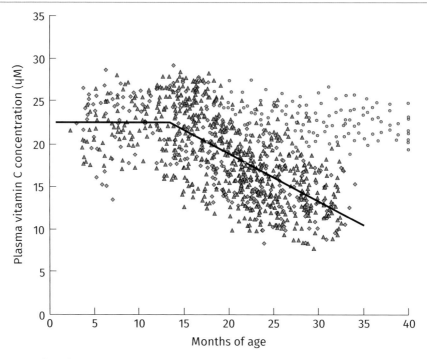

Figure 5.4 Relationship between plasma vitamin C concentrations and age in beef cattle. Female calves and heifers (♦) castrated male calves and steers (▲), and replacement heifers and dry cows. The regression lines were evaluated using the non-linear regression procedure of SAS in all cattle except for replacement heifers and dry cows; Y (µM) = 22.5 when X (month) ≤13.4; Y (µM) = −0.556X (month) +29.9 when X (month) ≥13.4, (P < 0.0001). (Source: Matsui, 2012)

SD) but gradually decreased after that. On the other hand, plasma vitamin C concentrations did not change with aging in replacement heifers and dry cows (22.7±2.1 µM), similar to growing cattle. These results show that plasma vitamin C concentration decreases as cattle gain weight and fat but not by chronological age. Obesity is well recognized to induce oxidative stress (Styskal *et al.*, 2012), and plasma vitamin C concentration is inversely related to human body fat percentage (Johnston, 2006). Thus, fattening *per se* can be considered an oxidative stressor that decreases plasma vitamin C concentration by enhancing vitamin C metabolic use (Matsui, 2012).

Vitamin C supplementation can reduce the environmental stress in lactating cows and improve implantation of embryos (Li *et al.*, 2014). Padilla *et al.* (2006) observed that heat stress could decrease plasma vitamin C concentration in lactating cows from 18 µM (ambient temperature 18°C) to 9 µM (28°C constant ambient temperature).

Supplemental vitamin C can probably improve marbling in feedlot cattle consuming high-sulfur diets. Several studies reported that vitamin C supplementation in beef cattle might increase marbling, metabolizable energy, and meat percentage in Angus crossbred steers (Maciel *et al.*, 2022). Vitamin C supplementation in fattening cattle was reported to improve the firmness and texture of the beef (Oohashi *et al.*, 2000; Mori *et al.*, 2006). However, the mechanisms that indicate how vitamin C supplementation affects the firmness and texture of beef remain unclear.

Pogge and Hansen (2013) fed 120 Angus steers in an experiment with 3 diets: T1: 0.22% of sulfur + 10.3 g of vitamin C per steer per day; T2: 0.34% of sulfur + 10.3 g of vitamin C per steer per day; T3: 0.55% of sulfur + 10.3 g of vitamin C per steer per day. These authors concluded that the supplementation of 10.3 g of vitamin C per day in Angus steers and feeding a diet high in sulfur (0.55%) could improve marbled scores. Plasma vitamin C levels in cattle fall below the normal range of 2.4 to 4.7 mg/l during the late finishing phase, demonstrating that vitamin C may play an essential role in adipogenesis (Kawachi, 2006; Pogge and Hansen, 2013). The increase in lipogenesis is related to the result of the positive effect of vitamin C on the differentiation of adipocytes (Gregoire *et al.*, 1998; Kawachi, 2006; Pogge and Hansen, 2013).

Doğan *et al.* (2021) evaluated the effect of vitamin C on oxidizing and antioxidant parameters in cattle vaccinated against anthrax. Forty healthy cattle aged 6–8 months were classified into 4 treatments: T1: control; T2: 1 ml of anthrax vaccine; T3: 1 ml of anthrax vaccine + 5 mg/kg of vitamin C; T4: 5 mg/kg of vitamin C. The results indicated that nitric oxide and malondialde levels decreased significantly in vaccinated bovines with 1 ml of anthrax vaccine + 5 mg/kg of vitamin C. Vitamin C could be beneficial in terms of reducing oxidative stress (Doğan *et al.*, 2021; Doğan 2023).

Beenken *et al.* (2021) examined the effects of injectable vitamin C on feedlot performance, inflammation, and muscle fatigue in beef cattle as a result of the antioxidant properties of ascorbate. One hundred thirty-two Angus crossbred steers (393±4 kg) were stratified by BW to a 2 × 2 factorial of intramuscular injection (INJ; 20 ml/steer): vitamin C (250 mg sodium ascorbate/ml) or saline (SAL) and road traffic duration (DUR): 18 hours (18-hour; 1,770 km) or 8 hours (8-hour; 727 km). On day 0, steers were weighed and given either vitamin C or SAL INJ immediately before transport. Upon return (day 1), body weight and blood were collected before steers were returned to pens equipped with GrowSafe bunk beds. Steers were weighed on days 0, 1, 7, 15, 30, 31, 54, and 55. The results indicated that vitamin C application before long-haul transit positively influenced antioxidant capacity; however, vitamin C did not improve overall post-transit performance. Matsui (2012) concluded that vitamin C supplementation may not help fatten cattle with relatively high plasma ascorbic acid concentrations and hypothesized that the efficacy of vitamin C supplementation on beef marbling is conditional.

Injectable vitamin C for stress due to transportation seems to have positive effects. Deters and Hansen (2020) determined that pre-transit intramuscular injection of vitamin C (5 g sodium ascorbate/steer) to 90 newly weaned calves mitigated the decline in plasma ascorbate concentrations and resulted in superior feedlot performance compared to post-transit administration. A pre-transit vitamin C injection improved steer average daily gain from day 7 to 31 ($P = 0.05$) and overall (day 1 to 57; $P = 0.02$), resulting in greater BW on day 30/31 ($P = 0.03$) and a tendency for greater final BW (day 56/57; $P = 0.07$). Steers that received vitamin C pre- or post-transit had greater DM intake from day 31 to 57 ($P = 0.01$) and overall ($P = 0.02$) compared to control steers.

Choline

Choline is not a vitamin in the traditional sense as it is not part of an enzyme system, and it is required in grams and not in milligrams like true vitamins.

Phosphatidylcholine is the leading natural form of choline present in food, although a small quantity of free choline may also exist in vegetable matter. As a phospholipid and acetylcholine component, it fulfills an essential role in the metabolism, serving as a methyl group donor. Biologically active methyl groups may also be obtained from methionine, so one of the advantages of supplementing choline is an increase in the availability of methionine for protein synthesis.

It has been demonstrated that both choline naturally present in feedstuffs and synthetic supplements of choline degrade by between 80 and 99% in the rumen, depending on the source (Sharma and Erdman, 1989a). The flow of choline of microbial origin to the duodenum is slight, and the little available comes from protozoal synthesis (Sharma and Erdman, 1988). Choline is an essential nutrient in lipid transport and metabolism. Supplementation should, therefore, come from sources that guarantee it is protected from ruminal degradability.

NRC (2001) and NASEM (2021) recommended incorporating in milk replacers 1,000 mg/kg DM. dsm-firmenich (2022b) suggested a 500–700 mg/kg supplementation of milk replacer DM.

In calves, signs of deficiency include muscular weakness, fatty liver infiltration, and renal hemorrhage, as is observed in other species. Johnson et al. (1951) observed a choline deficiency in 1-week-old calves when milk replacers contained 15% casein. The choline requirements calculated in this experiment were 260 mg/l milk replacer (1,733 mg/kg of DM).

Rumsey (1989) showed that supplementing choline in rations for calves fed with concentrates did not alter the effective yields, ruminal fermentation characteristics, or carcass quality. Protected choline has improved the productive behavior of fatted calves with no adverse effects on the characteristics of the carcass (Bryant et al., 1999; Bindel et al., 2000, 2005). While Bindel et al. (2005), who carried out choline infusions in the abomasum (5 g/day), with and without supplementary fat supply in the fatting calf ration, did not observe changes in the digestion of nutrients nor the concentrations of metabolites in plasma.

Several feed materials used in animal nutrition contain choline, but this naturally occurring choline is rapidly degraded in the rumen, therefore, it should be offered as RPC in ruminant animal species. Kawas et al. (2020) studied the effect of RPC on growth, carcass, and some blood metabolites in feedlot lambs. RPC supplementation did not significantly affect DM intake, weight gain, gain:feed ratio, or carcass weights. However, RPC supplementation was associated with lower blood triglycerides and increased backfat thickness and yield grade, thus suggesting an effect of RPC on lipid metabolism. The RPC supplementation was also associated with a reduced height to the shoulder and *longissimus* muscle area, suggesting an inhibitory effect of RPC on growth. Consequently, the results of this study do not support the use of RPC supplementation to improve animal performance or carcass characteristics in feedlot lambs.

Supply of vitamins and nutritional value of beef cattle for human consumption

Beef cattle are seen as an essential source of nutrition for the human population (Table 5.4). Various factors such as breed, the ingredients used in the feeding of livestock, the kind of cut you might consider, the post mortem handling of the carcass, and other factors will have a substantial effect on its composition and nutritional value (MacRae et al., 2005; Williams, 2007).

The lean component of beef meat is a well-known excellent source of human nourishment. Beef meat has a high protein content of great biological value with the makeup and proportion of amino acids they can provide, with vitamins – like niacin, riboflavin iron, B_6, B_{12}, pantothenic acid, folic acid, and sometimes even vitamin D, minerals – like iron, zinc, P, selenium and copper – endogenous antioxidants and other bioactive substances (MacRae et al., 2005; Williams, 2007). The content of these macro- and micronutrients, with their organoleptic properties of tenderness, texture, juiciness, and savor (MacRae et al., 2005; Dhiman et al., 2006), make beef an essential ingredient in the human diet.

Numerous studies indicate that supplementation with vitamins A, D, E, and C, and those from the B complex, can positively affect different parameters of beef quality. Thus, for example, some data indicate that vitamin D has a positive influence on improving the tenderness of the meat and increasing the levels of Ca in muscle (Swanek *et al.*, 1999; Montgomery *et al.*, 2002; Foote *et al.*, 2004), even though the positive effects have not always been evident (Wertz *et al.*, 2004). Nevertheless, this management practice has little acceptance as a commercial strategy because, due to the high supplementation levels required, it reduces voluntary ingestion and animal productivity (Dikeman, 2007). In addition, excessive vitamin D supplementation (in doses of 2×10^6 IU/day of vitamin D_3) can cause toxicity in beef cattle, and its harmlessness to human health has not been demonstrated (Dikeman, 2007). Moreover, vitamin D supplementation levels are restricted to a maximum by local regulations.

Vitamins A, C, and E intervene in lipids' metabolism and IMF deposition. This characteristic, in turn, is related to an improvement in the flavor of meat and a change in the profile and provision of mono and PUFAs (Siebert *et al.*, 2003; Kawachi, 2006; Dhiman *et al.*, 2006; Dikeman, 2007; Gorocica-Buenfil *et al.*, 2007a,b, 2008). Another aspect related to the quality of meat is the preservation of its color and its resistance to oxidation in post mortem treatment, in which this group of vitamins also plays a vital role with its antioxidant effect.

Beef also provides an integral part of other bioactive substances (e.g., ubiquinones, glutathione, carnosine, anserine, L-carnitine, taurine, creatinine, etc.), which act as endogenous antioxidants and contribute to an improvement in the human immune system (Arihara, 2006; Williams, 2007).

Conclusion

Vitamins play a fundamental role in numerous vital functions. In productive conditions, vitamin deficiencies should not only be considered from the perspective of maintaining physiological functions. Vitamins should also permit optimum production and reduced incidence of clinical or subclinical pathologies.

In the last few years, vitamin recommendations established by ration formulation systems and those applied in field conditions by the industry have been increased. This is true, especially in intensive systems that aim to improve productivity and reduce pathologies. The most critical increases in recommended levels affect vitamins A and E. Other vitamins, especially of the B group, which have not until now been considered necessary in formulations for adult ruminants, are necessary in the case of pre-ruminants and may be necessary in adults under conditions of stress or high production, but for this application, systems must be developed to protect vitamins to avoid or reduce their ruminal degradability.

The establishment of requirements and provision of vitamins for the nutrition and feeding of beef cattle should be seen not only from the animal's point of view but also from the implications on the final product in the production system, i.e., the meat and the importance this has in the human diet.

Chapter 6

Optimum vitamin nutrition in dairy cattle

The development of vitamin recommendations for dairy cattle has been limited by analytical difficulties and by the lack of sufficiently precise response criteria with which to determine specific values for recommendations. However, the increase in productive yield of the dairy cow has revealed a series of production problems which, in recent years, have enabled deficiencies of some vitamins to be identified, and recommended amounts of these vitamins for commercial conditions are being modified.

Vitamins are generally classified as fat-soluble and water-soluble. Due to microbial synthesis in the rumen, water-soluble vitamins have traditionally been considered non-essential for ruminants. However, recent data suggest several benefits from their supplementation in dairy cows. We have summarized in some tables the vitamin supplementation levels recommended by various research committees and feed industry organizations (NRC, 2001; NASEM, 2021; dsm-firmenich, 2022b).

Vitamin supplementation for calves in milk replacers and starter and grower feed is given in Tables 6.1a and 6.1b. Table 6.2 provides an overview of the adequate intake (AI) levels of vitamins A, D, and E, as proposed by NASEM (2021). The suggested AI intakes expressed in units/kg BW have been multiplied by an average weight of heifers of 550 kg and cows of 700 kg for dry and lactating cows to give an average suggested supplementation per animal/day.

In Table 6.3, we have summarized the more detailed indications of adequate intake given by NASEM (2021) for Holstein growing calves and heifers for dairy replacement and dry cows according to age, BW growth rate, and feed intake.

Table 6.4 gives the adequate intake for primiparous and pluriparous Holstein lactating cows according to milk yield. In both cases, we have calculated an average adequate intake per animal per day based on the dry matter (DM) intake and suggested adequate intake per kg of DM.

Finally, Tables 6.5, 6.6, and 6.7 give an overview of the recommendations for heifers, dry cows, and lactating cows as proposed by NRC (2001), NASEM (2021), and dsm-firmenich (2022b). In most cases, the recommended levels were increased considerably from previous reports. This chapter discusses these new recommendations and their justification and critically evaluates the available scientific literature.

Table 6.1a Vitamin level in natural milk and vitamin inclusion level in milk replacers for calves according to research committees and feed industry organizations (units/kg DM)

Vitamin	Units	NRC (2001)[1]	NASEM (2021)[2]	OVN™ 2022 (dsm-firmenich, 2022b)[3]
Vitamin A	IU	9,000	11,000	20,000–32,000
Vitamin D$_3$	IU	600	3,200	2,000–4,000
Vitamin E	mg	50	200	150–200
Vitamin K	mg	–[4]	–[4]	1–1.5
Vitamin B$_1$	mg	6.5	6.5	2.5–5
Vitamin B$_2$	mg	6.5	6.5	2.5–4.5
Vitamin B$_6$	mg	6.5	6.5	2.5–4.5
Vitamin B$_{12}$	mg	0.07	0.07	0.04–0.08
Niacin	mg	10	10	9–18
d-pantothenic acid	mg	13	13	7–9
Folic acid	mg	0.5	0.5	0.2–0.3
Biotin	mg	0.1	0.1	0.05–0.1
Vitamin C	mg	–	–	250–500
Choline	mg	1,000	1,000	500–750
β-carotene	mg	–	–	100

Notes: [1]These values assume a 45 kg calf consuming 0.53 kg of milk replacer solids (DM)/day. Concentrations should be reduced if calves are fed substantially more significant amounts of milk replacer (e.g., ≥1 kg/day of solids).
[2]These values assume a 60 kg calf consuming 0.6 kg of milk replacer solids. Concentrations should be reduced if calves are fed substantially more significant amounts of milk replacer (e.g., ≥1 kg/day of solids).
[3]OVN™, 2022 was based on current industry practices.
[4]Microbial synthesis of vitamin K within the intestines appears adequate, and supplemental vitamin K is usually unnecessary (Nestor and Conrad, 1990).

Table 6.1b Vitamin inclusion level for calves during starter and grower phases[1] according to research committees and feed industry organizations (units/kg DM)

Vitamin	Units	NRC (2001)	NASEM (2021)	OVN™ 2022 (dsm-firmenich, 2022b)
Vitamin A	IU	4,000	3,700	7,500–10,000
Vitamin D$_3$	IU	600	1,100	2,200–3,000
Vitamin E	mg	25	67	135–200

Note: [1]These values assume during starter phase an 80-kg calf consuming 2.4 kg of starter DM and during grower phase a 110 kg calf consuming 3.3 kg of grower DM.

Table 6.2 Adequate intake of vitamins A, D, and E (adapted from NASEM, 2021)

Vitamin	Units	Heifers[1]	Dry cows[2]	Lactating cows[2]	Pre-fresh cows[2] (2–5 weeks pre)
Vitamin A	IU/kg BW	110	110	110	110
	IU/head/day	60,500	77,000	77,000	77000[3]
Vitamin D	IU/kg BW	30	30	40	40
	IU/head/day	16,500	21,000	28,000	28,000
Vitamin E	IU/kg BW	0.8	1.6	0.8	3
	IU/head/day	440	1,120	560	2,100

Notes: [1] Heifers 550 kg BW.
[2] Dry and lactating cows 700 kg BW.
[3] If milk production is >35 kg/day adequate intake must be corrected with this formula: 110 IU* BW + [1,000*(Milk production kg - 35)]; e.g. if milk production is 55 kg/day adequate intake will be 97,000 IU/head day.

Table 6.3 Recommendations for growing calves, heifers for dairy replacement and dry cows (source: adapted from NASEM, 2021)

Holstein		Growing calves and heifers						Dry cows	
								Days prepartum	
								60–21 days	<21 days
Age, days		30	100	225	350	475	600		
BW, kg		65	120	230	330	420	530	740	740
Growth rate, kg/day		0.7	0.7	0.9	0.8	0.7	0.9	0.1	0.1
DM intake, kg/day		1.4	3.9	6.6	8.5	9.8	11	13.9	13
Vitamin A	IU/kg DM	5,218	3,390	3,829	4,265	4,698	5,288	5,850	6,272
Vitamin D	IU/kg DM	1,518	924	1,044	1,163	1,281	1,442	1,595	1,710
Vitamin E	IU/kg DM	86	49	56	62	68	77	85	171
Vitamin A[1]	IU/head/day	7,300	13,000	25,000	36,000	46,000	58,000	81,000	81,500
Vitamin D[1]	IU/head/day	2,100	3,600	7,000	10,000	12,500	16,000	22,000	22,000
Vitamin E[1]	IU/head/day	120	190	370	525	660	850	1,200	2,400

Note: [1]Recommendations in IU/head/day are calculated from DM intake kg/d and IU/kg DM; figures are rounded.

Table 6.4 Recommendations of vitamins (IU/kg) for lactating cows by parity (BW) and days-in milk (source: adapted from NASEM, 2021)

Holstein		First (570 kg)			Mature (700 kg)	
Days in Milk		15	150	20	100	200
Milk, kg		33	39	53	55	43
Fat, %		3.9	3.6	3.7	3.5	3.8
Protein, %		3.1	3	2.8	2.8	3.3
Dry matter intake, kg/day		20.8	23.9	25.8	29.4	27.4
ME, Mcal/kg		2.39	2.61	2.58	2.73	2.6
NE $_{Lactation}$, Mcal/kg		1.51	1.72	1.61	1.8	1.73
Vitamin A	IU/kg DM	3,021	2,796	3,687	3,303	3,103
Vitamin D	IU/kg DM	1,099	954	1,085	952	1,02˙
Vitamin E	IU/kg DM	22	19	22	19	20
Vitamin A[1]	IU/head/day	62,800	66,800	95,000	97,100	85,000
Vitamin D[1]	IU/head/day	23,000	22,800	28,000	28,000	28,00˙
Vitamin E[1]	IU/head/day	460	455	570	560	550

Note: [1]Recommendations in IU/head/day are calculated from DM intake kg/day and IU/kg DM; figures are rounded.

Table 6.5 Vitamin inclusion level (units per head per day) for heifers according to research committees or feed industry organizations

Heifers: dairy replacement, Growing

Vitamin	Units	NRC, 2001	NASEM, 2021[1]	OVN™ (dsm-firmenich, 2022b)	References
Vitamin A	IU	22,000-60,000	25,000-58,000	20,000-60,000	NASEM, 2021
Vitamin D$_3$	IU	6,000-16,350	7,000-16,000	6,000-16,350	NASEM, 2021
Vitamin E	mg	160-436	370-850	300-500	NASEM, 2021; Industry practice
Biotin	mg	–	–	10-20[2]	Chen et al., 2011; Industry practice
β-carotene	mg	–	–	300-500[3]	Madureira et al., 2020; Industry practice

Heifers: dairy replacement, 4–6 weeks pre-calving

Vitamin	Units	NRC, 2001	NASEM, 2021[2]	OVN™ (dsm-firmenich, 2022b)	References
Vitamin A	IU	75,000	81,000	80,000-100,000	NASEM, 2021; Industry practice
Vitamin D$_3$	IU	20,000	22,000	20,000-25,000	NASEM, 2021; Industry practice
25(OH)D$_3$ (HyD®)	mg	–	–	3[4]	Martinez et al, 2018
Vitamin E	mg	1,200	1200-2,400	2,000-3,000	NASEM, 2021; Industry practice
Niacin	mg	–	–	6,000-12,000[5]	Schwab et al., 2005; Aragona et al., 2020
Biotin	mg	–	–	20[2]	Chen et al., 2011; Industry practice
β-carotene	mg	–	–	500-1,000[6]	Madureira et al., 2020; Industry practice

Notes: [1] Ranges are taken from Tab. 6.3 considering heifers from 230 to 530 kg BW.
[2] For optimum hoof health.
[3] 6–8 weeks before 1st insemination/mating when intake of green forage is low.
[4] 3 weeks before calving.
[5] From 2 week befoew parturition until peak lactation.
[6] Lower level 8 weeks before 1st calving, upper level 4 weeks before 1st calving when intake of green forage is low.

Table 6.6 Vitamin inclusion level (units per head per day) for dry cows according to research committees or feed industry organizations

			Dairy cows, Dry cows, far-off		
Vitamin	**Units**	**NRC (2001)**	**NASEM (2021)[1]**	**OVN™ (dsm-firmenich, 2022b)**	**References**
Vitamin A	IU	80,300	81,000	80,000–120,000	NASEM (2021); Industry practice
Vitamin D$_3$	IU	21,900	22,000	25,000–30,000	Industry practice
Vitamin E	mg	1,168	1,200	1,100–4,000[2]	NASEM (2021); Industry practice
Niacin	mg	–	–	6,000–12,000[3]	Schwab et al. (2005); Aragona et al. (2020)
Biotin	mg	–	–	20–40[4]	Lischer et al. (2002)
β-carotene	mg	–	–	500–1,000[5]	Madureira et al. (2020); Industry practice

			Dairy cows, Dry cows, close-up		
Vitamin	**Units**	**NRC (2001)**	**NASEM (2021)[1]**	**OVN™ (dsm-firmenich, 2022b)**	**References**
Vitamin A	IU	83,270	81,500	80,000–120,000	NASEM (2021)
Vitamin D$_3$	IU	22,700	22,000	25,000–30,000	Industry practice
25OHD$_3$ (HyD®)	mg	–	–	3[6]	Martinez et al. (2018)
Vitamin E	mg	1,211	2,400	2,000–4,000[2]	NASEM (2021)
Niacin	mg	–	–	6,000–12,000[3]	
Biotin	mg	–	–	20–40[4]	Lischer et al. (2002)
β-carotene	mg	–	–	500–1,000[5]	Madureira et al. (2020); Industry practice

Notes: [1] See Table 6.3 for detail about the ranges.
[2] Upper level from 3 weeks pre-partum until 4 weeks post-partum.
[3] From 2 weeks before calving until peak of lactation.
[4] For optimum hoof health and milk yield.
[5] Lower level during entire dry period (Far-off and Close-up); upper level 3–4 weeks before calving (Close-up only).
[6] 3 weeks before calving.

Table 6.7 Vitamin inclusion level (units per head per day) for lactating cows according to research committees or feed industry organizations

Vitamin	Units	NRC (2001)[1]	NASEM (2021)[1]	OVN™ (dsm-firmenich, 2022b)[3]	References
Vitamin A	IU	75,000	85,000–95,000	100,000–150,000	NASEM (2021); Jin et al. (2014); Industry practice
Vitamin D$_3$	IU	21,000	28,000	25,000–40,000	Industry practice
25OHD$_3$ (HyD®)	mg	–	–	1	Poindexter et al. (2020, 2023a,b)
Vitamin E	mg	545	550–570[4]	600–1,000[5]	Industry practice
Niacin	mg	–	–	6,000–12,000[6]	Schwab et al. (2005); Aragona et al. (2020)
Biotin	mg	–	–	20–40[7]	Lischer et al. (2002); Majee et al. (2003); Chen et al. (2011)
β-carotene	mg	–	–	300–500[8]	Madureira et al. (2020); Industry practice

Notes: [1]Mature Holstein cows 680 kg BW.
[2]Mature Holstein cows 700 kg BW; see Table 6.4 for details about the ranges.
[3]Mature Holstein cows 700 kg BW.
[4]Increase the level up to 1,200 mg/head/day in pre-fresh cows (2–5 weeks pre).
[5]Upper level for optimum udder health.
[6]From 2 weeks before calving until peak lactation.
[7]For optimum hoof health and milk yield.
[8]Start during dry period until pregnancy is confirmed.

FAT-SOLUBLE VITAMINS

Vitamin A and the ß-carotenes

Introduction

Vitamin A activity is defined in retinol equivalent units. All-trans-retinol is the isomer of the greatest potency and activity and the only important one for practical purposes (Ullrey, 1972). One international unit (IU) of vitamin A corresponds to 0.3 µg of all-trans-retinol (equivalent to 0.344 µg all-trans-retinyl acetate). Retinol is not found in plants but is obtained from the β-carotenes (or provitamin A). One milligram of β-carotene has an activity equivalent to 400 IU of vitamin A (equivalent to 120 µg of retinol).

In plants, most of the β-carotenes are found in the vegetative material. Therefore, forage is the primary source of this vitamin. β-carotenes are transferred from the plant to the animal and can modify the color of milk and its derivatives and the fat deposited in muscle tissues (Priolo *et al.*, 2002; Havemose *et al.*, 2004; Nozière *et al.*, 2006). The β-carotene in milk gives a creamy, off-white appearance to most dairy products and seems to directly influence consumer's color perception (Faulkner *et al.*, 2018).

Various factors affect the β-carotene content of plants and thus the supply of vitamin A. Among the factors indicated are their physical state, the pH value (significant in silage), the temperature, and the presence of oxygen. These factors modify the availability of the animals that consume them. Their content diminishes with maturity, and they rapidly oxidize once the plant is cut, so the concentration in hay and silage is much lower than that in fresh plants (Chauveau-Duriot *et al.*, 2005), even though most domestic species convert β-carotenes to vitamin A. Still, conversion in dairy cattle is low (24%), and their storage capacity varies according to breed, as some (e.g., Guernsey, Jersey) have a greater capacity than others like Holstein. In breeds such as Holsteins, supplementation may be beneficial. Rosendo *et al.* (2010) observed that multiparous cows with mild fatty liver may have issues regulating blood retinol concentrations.

The most common commercial forms of vitamin A are all-*trans*-retinyl acetate, palmitate, or propionate. They are more stable than natural sources, losing around 1% per month under correct storage conditions. However, when stored with other minerals or feedstuffs, losses increase to 5–9% monthly (Coelho, 1991).

Calves

The NASEM (2021) recommendations remained like the NRC 2001 report. The vitamin A requirement for suckling calves is 110 IU/kg of BW (NASEM, 2021). However, the calculation in NRC (2001) was based on a 45 kg calf consuming 0.53 kg DM/day, whereas NASEM (2021) considered a 60 kg calf with a daily intake of 0.6 kg DM/day. Therefore, the units/kg DM increased from 9,000 to 11,000 IU/kg DM. The suggested supplementation by dsm-firmenich (2022b) is significantly higher, 20,000 to 32,000 IU/kg DM, primarily based on industry practice (Table 6.1a).

In the starter and grower phases, the recommendation was to supplement 4,000 IU/kg DM (NRC, 2001), and it remained at 3,700 IU/kg DM, according to NASEM (2021). Also, in this case, industry practice is the primary driver of the recommendation given by dsm-firmenich (2022b) OVN™, from 7,500 to 10,000 IU/kg DM (Table 6.1b).

The recommendation provided by NASEM (2021) is still based on studies by Eaton *et al.* (1972), who, using the dose that permits maintenance of appropriate cerebrospinal fluid pressure as a selection criterion, established a recommendation of 97 IU/kg LW. However, the build-up or loss of vitamin A in the liver is a more precise measure of the vitamin A status of the animal. Swanson *et al.* (2000) used this criterion. They observed that supplementation with 134 IU/kg LW led to the accumulation of vitamin A in the liver, while supplementation with 93 IU/kg led to a reduction in hepatic reserves of vitamin A. These results suggest appropriate supplementation is between 93 and 134 IU/kg. However, where there are doubts about the intake or the quality of the colostrum administered to calves, or when stressful conditions are detected, often due to intensive production systems, the recommendation may be increased to 134–200 IU/kg LW without risk of toxicosis.

The vitamin A status of calves depends significantly on the intake of vitamin A through the colostrum. Calves are born with low vitamin A levels because transfer through the placenta is very low. Waldner and Uehlinger (2016) identified that drought conditions, dam peripartum health problems, and inadequate colostrum intake contribute to low vitamin A and E concentrations and adverse health outcomes in beef calves. Transferring vitamins from the colostrum to the calf is vital to health (Seymour, 2004; Puvogel *et al.*, 2008). A delay in the supply from colostrum of more than 12 hours after parturition affects plasma levels of β-carotenes, vitamin A, and vitamin E during the first month of the calf's life (Zanker *et al.*, 2000; Debier *et al.*, 2005; Puvogel *et al.*, 2008; Jin *et al.*, 2014). If the vitamin A levels remain low after parturition, the calf's health and subsequent growth may be negatively affected (Debier and Larondelle, 2005).

Additional supplementation is needed if there are insufficient quantities of vitamin A rich colostrum. McGill *et al.* (2019) demonstrated the importance of vitamin A in colostrum for immunity in dairy heifers vaccinated and challenged with bovine respiratory syncytial virus (BRSV). They used 43 Holstein calves that did not receive colostrum from their dams and split them into 2 treatments: sufficient (VAS) and deficient vitamin A (VAD). All calves received colostrum replacer within 4 hours of birth. The 2 colostrum replacers contained 150 g of bovine globulin protein concentrated from colostral whey. Colostrum was essentially devoid of all fat-soluble vitamins A, D_3, and E. Vitamins D_3 (150,000 IU of cholecalciferol/dose) and E (1,500 IU α-tocopherol/dose) were added back to the colostrum replacer for all calves. Only the VAS replacer had 150,000 IU retinyl palmitate. Each animal received 375 g of fractionated colostrum replacer reconstituted in 1.9 l of water at approximately 40°C. Later, the milk replacers had either 45,000 IU of vitamin A (retinyl palmitate) for VAS or no vitamin A for VAD. At 2 weeks, calves were offered starter pellets without (VAD) or 4,000 IU/kg (VAS). These calves were vaccinated at 6 weeks of age and later challenged with BRSV. The results demonstrated that the VAD calves could not respond to the mucosal BRSV vaccine and did not have protection during the challenge, causing significant lung abnormalities due to the inflammatory response.

Cows fed with rations rich in vitamin A during the dry period produce more colostrum with a greater vitamin A concentration. On the other hand, underfeeding with vitamin A during the dry period generates colostrum with a low vitamin A concentration, which affects the vitamin status of the calf (Debier *et al.*, 2005). Supplementation to the cow should be achieved with sources of vitamin A and not just replacing it with β-carotenes due to its reduced intestinal absorption (Yonekura and Nagao, 2007) or low capacity for converting β-carotenes into retinol by the young calf (Nonnecke *et al.*, 2001). These considerations demand the administration of a minimum of 165 to 200 IU/kg LW for the first months of life to achieve normal hepatic reserves.

Erdman (1992) and Krueger *et al.* (2016) reported that supplying vitamin A concentrations above recommended levels in milk replacers is standard practice. Supplementation at much higher levels – 87,000 IU/kg of milk replacer and 44,000 IU/kg DM in milk replacer – according to Swanson *et al.*, (2000) had neither positive nor negative effects. Therefore, increasing such high dosages does not appear to be justified. On the other hand, Nonnecke *et al.* (1999) observed the harmful effects of overdosage of vitamin A in young calves. Franklin *et al.* (1998) observed a deterioration in the health of calves supplemented with 30,000 IU/day of vitamin A during the first 6 weeks of life. In both cases, the deterioration in health was attributed to the interference of vitamin A with the vitamin E status of the animals. Therefore, where large amounts of vitamin A are supplemented, the vitamin E levels in the milk replacer should also be raised (Badman *et al.*, 2019).

Heifers

NASEM (2021) indicated an AI of vitamin A of 110 IU/kg BW (Table 6.2). Supplementation level during the growing phase up to mating (Table 6.3), i.e., from 65 to 530 kg BW increases from 7,300 to 58,000 IU/head/day, providing the indicated AI. This level must be increased in pre-partum up to 81,000 IU/day. Comparing the different sources of information (Table 6.5), we can see that the supplementation proposed by NRC (2001), NASEM (2021), and dsm-firmenich (2022b) were very similar both during the growing phase and pre-calving. In the latter case, dsm-firmenich (2022b) indicates some higher levels because of industry practice.

Lactating cows

The NASEM (2021) confirmed the AI for dairy cattle indicated in the previous report (NRC, 2001) of 110 IU/day of vitamin A per kg BW (Table 6.2), but introduced a correction factor according to milk production using the following formulas:

- If milk production ≤35 kg/day vitamin A AI = BW × 110 IU
- If milk production ≥35 kg/day vitamin A AI = BW × 110 IU + 1,000 × (milk yield − 35)

Therefore, for a 700 kg BW Holstein cow producing 35 kg of milk/day, the AI of vitamin A is 77,000 IU/head per day. However, if milk yield is 45 kg/day or 55 kg/day the AI increases respectively to 87,000 and 97,000 IU/head per day.

It is now accepted that milk production requires retinol. The concentration in milk is between 3 and 11 mg/kg of milk fat. This means 0.1 to 0.4 mg/kg of milk when the fat milk content is 3.7% or 1,000 IU of vitamin A/kg of milk.

A cow producing 35 kg of milk per day (3.7% fat) with a BW of 625 kg secretes 10 mg of retinol daily, equivalent to 30,000 IU and consuming about 69,000 IU. But, when milk production is higher, cows are typically fed higher-concentrate diets and less forage with lower vitamin A intake. Consequently, the new NASEM (2021) (Table 6.4) recommendations were established based on milk production above 35 kg milk/day.

The previous recommendations from NRC (1989, 2001) were based on long-term reproduction studies of relatively low-yielding animals fed rations containing a high proportion of forage (Swanson *et al.*, 1968). However, in current production systems, many animals are fed with rations containing a higher proportion of concentrate, even at lower production rates. A confrontation of recommendation (Table 6.7) shows that NASEM (2021) has increased compared to NRC (2001) for the reasons mentioned above. In its OVN™ tables, dsm-firmenich (2022b) is proposing higher levels 100,000 to 150,00 IU/head day mainly because of the industry practice as well as the beneficial effect of higher dosages on immune function (Jin *et al.*, 2014).

Rode *et al.* (1990) and Weiss *et al.* (1995) demonstrated that the bioavailability of vitamin A was reduced during the first months of life to achieve normal hepatic reserves. Some experimental studies suggested that increasing the vitamin supplement above these recommended levels may be beneficial. Oldham *et al.* (1991) observed an increase in milk production from 35 to 40 kg/day when the ration was supplemented with 250 IU of vitamin A per kg BW, compared with rations supplemented with 75 IU/kg BW. Michal *et al.* (1994) did not observe production responses when rations were supplemented with 200 IU of vitamin A/kg BW. Still, the incidence of retained placentas and milk fever was reduced by 33%.

Supplementing vitamin A in amounts much higher than recommended (166 vs. 1,660 IU/kg BW) increased heat detection from 26 to 60%, reducing the somatic cell count in weeks 2–8 postpartum (Chew and Johnston, 1985). These results suggest that, under commercial conditions, in which animals are subjected to more significant productive stress and in which rations contain a higher proportion of concentrate, the current recommendations (110 IU/kg BW) may be increased by 50 to 100%. It must be remembered that the current recommendations were established for rations based on forage and that ruminal degradability of vitamin A increases from 40 to 80% as the forage content of the ration decreases (Ullrey, 1972; Rode, 1990). Jin *et al.* (2014) concluded that dietary supplementation with 220 IU of vitamin A/kg LW for Holstein cows might enhance the antioxidant and immune functions (Table 6.8). These cows had an intake of 17.30 ± 0.50 kg DM intake (DMI) per day, lactated for 150 ± 10 days, and produced 20.75 ± 0.50 kg of milk/day.

The wide safety margin of vitamin A permits the increase without risk of toxicity. However, in some cases, there have been indications that supplying very high concentrations of vitamin A in the diet to approximately 8 times the NASEM's (2021) recommendations, can provoke reductions in the production of milk and its fat content (Puvogel *et al.*, 2005). These levels should serve as a reference for maximum levels.

Dry and prepartum cows
A confrontation of the different sources is given in Table 6.6. NRC (2001) and NASEM (2021) indicate supplementation of 81,000 IU/day. In contrast, the last OVN recommendations (dsm-firmenich, 2022b) propose a range of 80,000–120,000 IU/day considering an industry practice which is most probably due to the observed responses in different conditions, including stress and safety margin. The NASEM (2021) decided on the same recommendations for dry cows as for growing heifers (110 IU/kg BW), and consequently, levels vary according to breed, growth rate, and body weight (Table 6.2 and 6.3).

Weiss (1998) endorsed this recommendation based on improved immune competence and fewer problems with MG health and postpartum reproduction. Many research studies have confirmed a reduction in vitamin A concentration peripartum (Tjoelker *et al.*, 1988; Heirman *et al.*, 1990; Michal *et al.*, 1994; Akar and Gazioglu, 2006; Strickland *et al.*, 2020; Figure 6.1). This reduction is partially due to the loss of vitamin A in colostrum (Goff *et al.*, 2002).

However, in current production systems, animals are fed with rations containing a higher proportion of concentrate. Rode *et al.* (1990), Oldham *et al.* (1991), and Weiss *et al.* (1995) demonstrated that the bioavailability of vitamin A was reduced by 30 to 60% in rations containing more than 50% of concentrate. Hence, several studies show that supplementation with vitamin A during the dry period reduces the incidence of mastitis in the dry and productive periods (Dahlquist and Chew, 1985; Chew and Johnston, 1985; LeBlanc *et al.*, 2004).

Tjoelker *et al.* (1988) compared the 80 versus 350 IU/kg LW supply with 300–400 mg of β-carotenes, but they did not observe improvements in the function of neutrophils and lymphocytes. Supplementation of 170,000 IU of vitamin A/day during the dry and early lactation periods stimulated more milk production with lower fat content (Oldham *et al.*, 1991).

Michal *et al.* (1994) observed that supplementing prepartum rations with 120,000 IU/day of vitamin A improved polymorphonuclear neutrophil function and a 28% reduction in retained placentas (Figure 6.2). Weiss (1998) suggested that higher recommendations for vitamin A (150 IU/kg LW) should also be applied to dry cows. LeBlanc *et al.* (2004) reported that in the last week prepartum, a 100 ng/ml increase in serum retinol was associated with a 60% decrease in the risk of early lactation clinical mastitis. There were significant positive associations of peripartum serum concentrations among α-tocopherol, β-carotene, and retinol. Supplementation

Table 6.8 Effect of vitamin A supplementation level on antioxidant and immune function of dairy cows after 60 days of supplementation (source: Jin et al., 2014)

Antioxidant function parameters	Levels of vitamin A (IU/kg BW[a])		SEM[b]	P-value
	110	220		
Glutathione peroxidase, U/ml	155.1	248.03	32.5	0.01
Selenoprotein P, mg/l	3.11	3.97	0.23	0.007
Thioredoxin reductase, U/l	29.59	34.2	3.2	0.27
Superoxide dismutase, U/ml	108.05	137.9	12.18	0.04
Catalase, U/ml	4.08	5.03	0.6	0.02
OH[c] U/ml	338.1	436.15	18.39	0.001
Total antioxidant capacity, U/ml	4.09	6.05	0.69	0.02
ROS[d] fluorescence intensity/ml	593.5	591.25	0.39	0.01
Malonaldehyde, nmol/ml	4.14	2.31	0.6	0.01

Immunological parameters	Levels of vitamin A (IU/kg BW[a])		SEM[b]	P-value
	110	220		
Immunoglobulin M, g/l	1.23	1.71	0.13	0.01
Immunoglobulin G, g/l	14.04	16.52	0.88	0.01
Immunoglobulin A, g/l	0.79	0.98	0.07	0.02
Interleukin-1, ng/ml	0.25	0.41	0.04	0.001
Interleukin-2, ng/ml	4.27	4.76	0.34	0.3
Interleukin-4, ng/ml	0.88	1	0.15	0.43
Interleukin-6, pg/ml	118.4	105.07	8.69	0.48
Tumor necrosis factor-α, ng/ml	0.75	0.91	0.05	0.03
Soluble CD4, U/ml	74.85	93.44	4.14	0
Soluble CD8, U/ml	48.16	42.42	2.44	0.03
sCD4/sCD8	1.8	2.04	0.07	0.02
Vitamin A, µg/ml	0.43	0.48	0.02	0.003
Somatic cell count, ×10[3]/ml	192.75	139.84	21.3	0.03

Note: [a]BW, Body weight; [b]SEM, standard error of the mean; [c]OH, hydroxyl radical inhibition capability; [d]ROS, reactive oxygen species.

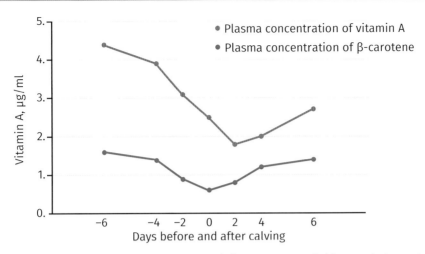

Figure 6.1 Average plasma concentration of vitamin A (●) and β-carotene (●) in cows during peripartum (source: adapted from Akar and Gazioglu, 2006)

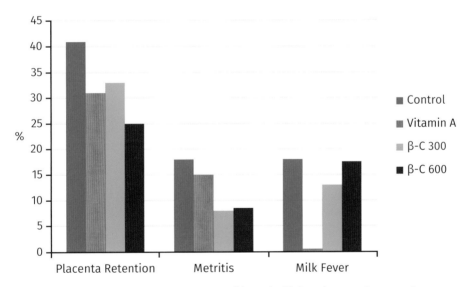

Figure 6.2 The incidence of retained placentas, metritis, and milk fever in control cows and cows supplemented with 120,000 IU/day of vitamin A or 300 or 600 mg/day of β-carotenes (source: adapted from Michal *et al.*, 1994)

at levels 50% greater than current recommendations (NASEM, 2021) may be advisable, given the reduction in problems peripartum and maintaining retinol concentrations in plasma and the colostrum postpartum (Puvogel *et al.*, 2005).

Recently, Rodriguez *et al.* (2023) investigated the effects of supplementing vitamin A (0, 75,000, 187,500 IU/day) during the transition period on plasma metabolites, the prevalence of ketosis, and early milk production. The results indicated that supplementation of vitamin A did not affect production, mobilization of body fat, and risk of ketosis. However, the highest level of vitamin A may have negatively affected the immune response, partly contributing to increased milk somatic cell counts during early lactation.

Recommendations for β-carotene

The NASEM (2021) and the NRC (2001) considered that data was very inconsistent to justify specific recommendations for β-carotene whereas dsm-firmenich (2022b) recommends 500–1,000 mg/day for dry cows: the lower level is suggested when the administration occurs during the whole dry period, whereas the highest dose is recommended when administered during close-up only (Table 6.6).

However, there is evidence that β-carotene has functions other than serving as a precursor for retinol and its concentration decreases peripartum (Tjoelker et al., 1988; Michal et al., 1994; Chawla and Kaur, 2004; Calderón et al., 2007; Kawashima et al., 2009a,b) and the benefits observed in some experimental studies suggest that, under some conditions, β-carotene supplementation may be beneficial. The consumption of low-quality forage during the dry period and the increase in immunological requirements around the peripartum may explain the reduction in the plasma concentration of β-carotenes peripartum and the possible need to supplement the ration.

Several studies have shown that supplementing rations with between 300 and 600 mg/day of β-carotene results in an increase in the proliferation of polymorphonuclear neutrophils and their phagocytic capacity (Michal et al., 1994; Tjoelker et al., 1990; Chew, 1993), as well as an increase in the plasma concentration of both β-carotenes and retinol (Michal et al., 1994; Chawla and Kaur, 2004). The improved response capacity of the immune system may explain the improvements observed in MG health, reduced somatic cell count, reduction in the number of new mammary infections, and mastitis during the dry period (Dahlquist and Chew, 1985) as well as during lactation (Chew and Johnston, 1985; Meyer et al., 2005; Koutsoumpas et al., 2013). Chew (1993) observed a negative correlation between the level of β-carotene in plasma and the somatic cell count because β-carotene protects cells against oxidation, optimizing cellular function. Jukola et al. (1996) reported increased mastitis in cows with low plasma β-carotene. However, the action of carotenoid compounds on the immune response is variable and depends not only on its type and concentration but also on the cell and animal species (Chew and Park, 2004).

Dietary supplements of 300 and 600 mg/day of β-carotene reduced the incidence of mastitis and intramammary infections during the dry period and peripartum (Chew, 1987; Wang et al., 1988a,b; Chawla and Kaur, 2004; Meyer et al., 2005; Akar and Gazioglu, 2006; Koutsoumpas et al., 2013). Other authors did not observe effects on udder health (Oldham et al., 1991; LeBlanc et al., 2004), although discrepancies may be due to the presence of β-carotene in the basal ration.

Hurley and Doane (1989) observed an improvement in reproductive function following the administration of β-carotene (300–400 mg/day). In their review, reproductive parameters improved in 12 of the 22 studies in which vitamin A was supplemented in quantities that met or exceeded those recommended by the NRC (1989). Cows supplemented with β-carotene experienced more rapid uterine recovery (Wang et al., 1988b; Rakes et al., 1985; Kawashima et al., 2009a,b), a shorter interval from parturition to first estrus (Rakes et al., 1985; Bremel et al., 1982; Kawashima et al., 2006), a more intense estrus, a shorter interval from parturition to conception (Lotthammer et al., 1979), a higher conception rate, or fewer inseminations per cow, and lower incidence of follicular cysts (Bremel et al., 1982; Larson et al., 1983; Iwańska et al., 1985).

Michal et al. (1994) observed that the incidence of retained placentas fell from 41% in unsupplemented cows to 31% in those supplemented with 300 mg/day of β-carotene and to 25% with supplementation of 600 mg/day of β-carotene and the incidence of metritis was reduced by 25% (Figure 6.2). However, some authors observed no positive effects, most probably because these studies were either carried out on Jersey cows that accumulate β-carotene (Bremel et al.,

1982) or because β-carotene was only supplemented during lactation and not during the dry period (Bindas *et al.*, 1984a). Furthermore, Aréchiga *et al.* (1998) observed that supplementation with 400 mg/day of β-carotene 15 days before insemination increased milk production by 6–11%. Chawla and Kaur (2004) observed a 28% increase in milk production when supplementing with 1,000 mg/day of β-carotene prepartum. These numbers suggest that the benefits may be derived from reduced incidence of pathologies, reproductive improvements, and increased milk production.

Akar and Gazioglu (2006) concluded that poor fertility parameters in cows with retained placenta, compared to the control group, could relate to the low content of vitamin A and especially β-carotene. Kaewlamun *et al.* (2011) observed no effect of β-carotene on ovarian activity. Still, they suggested that uterine involution was lower and reduced inflammation in cows supplemented with 1,000 mg β-carotene/day. De Bie *et al.* (2016) indicated that daily supplementation of β-carotene (2,000 mg/d) can substantially improve β-carotene and retinol availability in the oocyte's micro-environment, irrespective of the energy balance, which may affect follicular development and oocyte quality in the presence of maternal metabolic stress.

Halik *et al.* (2016) demonstrated the positive effects of dietary supplementation with 400 mg/day β-carotene during the last drying-off period and in the initial stage of lactation. β-carotene reduced milk somatic cell count, days to first estrus after calving, the inter-gestation period, and increased progesterone levels in milk on day 23 after insemination. Ježek *et al.* (2020), in an extensive survey of 176 farms and 604 cows sampled, concluded that β-carotene deficiency may have affected fertility in some of the farms investigated. The median value of β-carotene was 5.02 mg/l (minimum 0.63 mg/l, maximum 16.10 mg/l). Values below 4.0 mg/l could be related to infertility. On the other hand, in pregnant cows already receiving adequate vitamin A but with low serum β-carotene concentration, supplementation of β-carotene (800 mg/day) increased concentrations of β-carotene and vitamin A in blood serum but did not affect production, reproduction, or health (Prom *et al.*, 2022).

Mary *et al.* (2021) also assessed the status of vitamin E and β-carotene in commercial dairy cows in Europe. Blood concentrations of these vitamins were measured in 2,467 dairy cows from 127 farms in Belgium, Germany, Spain, Portugal, and the Netherlands. More than 75% and 44% were deficient in vitamin E and β-carotene, with blood concentrations below 3.0 and 3.5 mg/l, respectively. Blood concentrations were positively related to the total estimated daily vitamin intake. Consequently, dietary supplementation could contribute to providing adequate amounts of these vitamins during lactation, to ensure their lifetime performance and improve their fertility.

Madureira *et al.* (2020) also observed that cows with greater concentrations of β-carotene at the moment of artificial insemination were more likely to have greater concentrations of pregnancy-associated glycoproteins (PAG) at 31-day post-artificial insemination (Table 6.9). The concentration of β-carotene at artificial insemination was affected by the body condition score, which indicates better feed intake and parity. Cows with higher concentrations of plasma β-carotene at AI had greater pregnancy/artificial insemination (Figure 6.3), lower pregnancy losses, and greater concentrations of PAG at day 31 post-artificial insemination, suggesting it may be associated with placental function in lactating dairy cows (Table 6.9).

The available information suggests that supplementation with between 300 and 1,000 mg/day of β-carotenes during the critical dry period and the 2 or 3 months postpartum may improve MG health and reproductive function.

Table 6.9 Association between β-carotenes in plasma and pregnancy loss[†] (source: Madureira et al., 2020)

b-carotene (µg/mL)	All cows			Only cows that ovulated[4]		
	Ovulation failure[1] (%/ [n*])	P/AI[2] (%/[n])	PAG at 31 days[3] (ng/mL)	P/AI (%/[n])	PAG at 31 days (ng/mL)	Pregnancy loss[5] (%/[n])
≤ 3.30	19.7 ± 3.2[a] [98]*	19.2 ± 4.5[a] [109]	2.6 ± 0.3[a]	29.8 ± 5.3[a] [80]	2.6 ± 0.9[a]	41.9 ± 4.8[a] [28]
3.31–4.02	20.5 ± 3.1[a] [98]	33.7 ± 4.7[a] [100]	3.5 ± 0.3[a]	44.6 ± 5.4[a] [87]	3.7 ± 0.9[a]	20.4 ± 3.7[b] [41]
4.03–5.04	10.3 ± 3.1[b] [96]	36.9 ± 5.0[b] [96]	3.7 ± 0.3[bc]	45.1 ± 5.4[b] [87]	4.1 ± 0.8[a]	22.1 ± 4.1[b] [41]
≥5.05	4.5 ± 2.7[b] [94]	39.8 ± 5.4[b] [94]	4.1 ± 0.3[c]	41.7 ± 5.5[b] [92]	6.0 ± 0.8[b]	15.7 ± 4.2[b] [41]

Notes: [†]Mean ± SE for ovulation failure, pregnancy/AI (P/AI), pregnancy loss, and concentration of pregnancy-associated glycoproteins (PAG) at 31 d ays post-AI according to beta-carotene concentration classified in quartiles, considering all cows and only cows that ovulated.
[a-c]Different letters indicate the difference between variables within columns (P < 0.05).
[1]Cows that did not have a CL on 7 days post-AI.
[2]Number of cows pregnant/number of cows inseminated.
[3]Concentration of PAG at 31 days post-AI.
[4]Only cows that had a CL on 7 days post-AI.
[5]Number of cows pregnant at 60 days/number of cows pregnant at 31 days.
[*]Number of cows in each quartile [n].

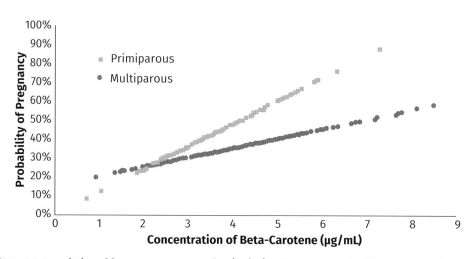

Figure 6.3 Association of β-carotene concentration (µg/ml) at the moment of artificial insemination on pregnancy per artificial insemination according to parity (primiparous (n = 143) P < 0.01, multiparous (n = 221) P < 0.05 (source: Madureira et al., 2020)

Vitamin D

Introduction

Vitamin D, also known as antirachitic, is a prohormone required to regulate Ca metabolism and maintain correct Ca levels in the blood (Nelson and Merriman, 2014; Eder and Grundmann, 2022). Much vitamin D is produced within the skin through the photoconversion of 7-dehydrocholesterol to vitamin D_3 (Figure 6.4). The plasma concentration of $25OHD_3$ (Horst et al.,

1994) is generally recommended to evaluate the animal's vitamin D status. The usual range of plasma 25OHD$_3$ in cattle is 20–50 ng/ml. However, as already mentioned in Chapter 4, the recommended 25OHD$_3$ plasma level in dairy cattle is around 100 ng/ml (Nelson *et al.*, 2018) to support, besides Ca and P metabolism, performance improvement (milk yield) and the modulation of the immune system.

Vitamin D is involved in the active transport of Ca and P across the intestinal epithelial cells and boosts the action of parathyroid hormone in reabsorbing bone Ca. It has also been demonstrated that vitamin D maintains immune function by stimulating humoral immunity and inhibiting cell-mediated immunity (Reinhardt and Hustmyer, 1987; Daynes *et al.*, 1995; Nelson *et al.*, 2012; Corripio-Miyar *et al.*, 2017; Ahmadi and Mohri, 2021; Ahmadi *et al.*, 2022; Eder and Grundmann, 2022; Flores-Villalva, 2022). McGrath *et al.* (2018) and Celi *et al.* (2020) discussed the interactions between the antioxidant system, vitamin D metabolism, and the rumen microbiome that affect skeletal health, redox balance, and gastrointestinal functionality of modern dairy cows. Vitamin D status is also related to reproductive physiology in cattle (Panda *et al.*, 2001; Nelson and Merriman, 2014).

Plants generally contain vitamin D$_2$, while animal-origin feedstuffs contain vitamin D$_3$. Horst and Littledike (1982) demonstrated that ruminants obtain little biological activity from vitamin D$_2$ due to its reduced ability to bind to the transport protein, which leads to faster metabolic degradation and a shorter average lifetime. Hymøller and Jensen (2010a) demonstrated that Vitamin D$_3$ was about twice as effective at elevating the concentration of 25OHD$_3$ in the plasma of dairy cows as vitamin D$_2$ (Eder and Grundmann, 2022).

The NASEM (2021) considered vitamin D$_3$ to be the predominant source of supplemental vitamin D used for livestock and assumes the adequate intake to be based on this source (1 µg equals 40 IU). As with other fat-soluble vitamins, oxidized fats in the ration can destroy the vitamin D present and limit its absorption (McDowell, 2006).

As explained in Chapter 4, the assessment of the vitamin D nutritional status is done using the first metabolite 25OHD$_3$ as a marker. According to Horst *et al.* (1994) and Nelson and

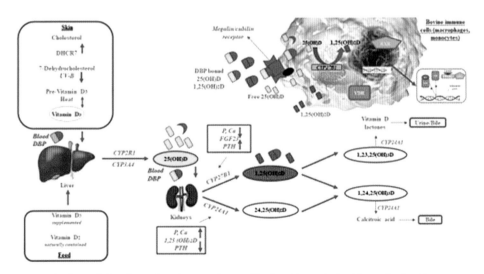

Figure 6.4 Metabolism of vitamin D. Vitamin D synthesized in the skin or derived from the feed is absorbed in the small intestine and delivered to the liver, where it is hydroxylated to 25-hydroxyvitamin D [25(OH)D] by various 25-hydroxylases (source: adapted from Eder and Grundmann, 2022)

Merriman (2014) blood concentrations below 30 ng/ml are considered insufficient, impairing immune function, and below 5 ng/ml indicate vitamin D deficiency and, leading to rickets in young animals and osteomalacia in adults. Levels above 200–300 ng/ml indicate toxicosis.

The optimal $25OHD_3$ range for humans is considered to be 30–50 ng/ml. For ruminants adequate levels are considered 40–80 ng/ml – for Ca and P metabolism and modulation of the immune function (Nelson *et al.*, 2016a, b; NASEM, 2021) and optimal levels are above 100 ng/ml providing positive effects on colostrum and milk production and quality and immunity (Poindexter et al., 2020; Silva *et al.*, 2022; Xu *et al.*, 2021). Nelson *et al.* (2016) did a survey in the United States to check the $25OHD_3$ in plasma in dairy and beef cows. They collected 702 blood samples from 12 different dairy herds from cows receiving 30,000–50,000 IU of vitamin D_3 daily. The majority of the cows showed levels below 100 ng/ml with average around 60 ng/ml. Similar results were obtained in beef cows on pasture in northern and southern regions of the US. In Ireland, 842 blood samples collected from 12 spring calving farms – at calving, 7 days post-partum and 21 days post-partum – and all cows in all phases had $25OHD_3$ below 60 ng/ml. The $25OHD_3$ concentrations are correlated positively with immune cell populations and based on the survey, the current supplementation strategies may not equip cows for optimal immune function.

Vinet *et al.* (1985) observed that the plasma concentrations of vitamin D in housed dry cows fed on maize silage were 19 ng/ml 2 weeks prepartum and only 10 ng/ml 35 days postpartum. Supplementing the ration with 7.5 or 15 IU of vitamin D/kg BW was sufficient to maintain the plasma concentration between 25 and 31 ng/ml.

Hodnik *et al.* (2020) and Eder and Grundmann (2022) reviewed the importance of vitamin D in dairy cattle. Hodnik *et al.* (2020) described the variability observed in a commercial farm in the vitamin D status of high-producing Holstein-Friesian cows housed in closed barns throughout the year without access to sunshine. The content of vitamin D_3 in the diet was less than 400 IU/kg DM, which is very low. Under these conditions, most cows had low vitamin D values in all tests. The average plasma level of all cows was 22.26 ng/ml. The range was 17.2 to 23.9 ng/ml, except for one cow, which was above 30 ng/ml in October and November but only 18.9 ng/ml in December. Supplementation of 10,000 to 50,000 IU/day of vitamin D (15 to 75 IU/kg BW) usually maintains plasma concentrations of $25OHD_3$ greater than 30 ng/ml (NASEM, 2021). Interest in vitamin D has centered on its roles in anionic-cationic balance and Ca metabolism (Seymour, 2004). The average concentration of $1,25(OH)_2D_3$ is between 20–80 pg/ml at the end of gestation and 70–200 pg/ml at parturition. Levels can increase to 200–300 pg/ml in recurrent cases of milk fever (Horst *et al.*, 1997, 2005). The increase in the plasma levels of $1,25(OH)_2D_3$ is a response to the fall in ionized Ca concentration in blood. There is an inverse relationship between the plasma levels of $1,25(OH)_2D_3$ and the presence of hypocalcemia in dairy cattle (Joyce *et al.*, 1997). However, sufficient vitamin D or its precursors are not the only factors maintaining Ca homeostasis peripartum (Taylor *et al.*, 2008).

Recommendations for vitamin D

The *in vivo* synthesis of vitamin D_3 depends on the duration and intensity of exposure to solar radiation. The solar intensity will depend on latitude, season, and cloud cover. Animals exposed to sunlight or animals fed with sun-dried hay may not, in theory, need supplementary vitamin D. Nevertheless, vitamin D supplements may improve intake, production, and some immune and reproductive parameters.

However, an excess of vitamin D may be toxic. The NRC (1987) suggested that toxic levels are reached with concentrations of 2,200 IU/kg DM over long periods or short-term at 25,000 IU/kg DM in the ration. Littledike and Horst (1982) suggested that vitamin D toxicity in dairy cows begins to occur as 25OHD$_3$ concentrations exceed 200 ng/ml and levels above 200 ng/ml for long periods can result in calcification of soft tissues. There are plants synthesizing 1,25(OH)$_2$D$_3$ glycosides. Machado *et al.* (2020) reviewed the calcinogenic principles, clinical and pathological findings observed when cattle consume *Solanum glaucophyllum* (waxyleaf nightshade), *Trisetum flavescens* (yellow oatgrass or golden oat grass). *Cestrum diurnum* (day-blooming cestrum or day-blooming jasmine), and *Stenotaphrum secundatum* (St. Augustine grass). Other plant species involved in enzootic calcinosis are: *Nierembergia rivularis* (whitecup or water nierembergia), *Nierembergia veitchii* (trailing cup plant), *Solanum torvum* (turkey berry or devil's fig) and *Solanum stuckertii*.

Calves

Even though the optimum plasmatic 25OHD$_3$ level is still unknown, the NASEM (2021) set up the AI at 32 IU/kg, which will be 2,100 IU/day for the 65 kg calf. Considering an intake of 0.6 kg/day, the milk replacer must contain 3,200 IU of vitamin D$_3$/kg DM to meet this AI (Table 6.1a). These values are higher than the NRC (2001) which recommended 600 IU/kg DM. The recommendation given by dsm-firmenich (2022b) is a range of 2,000–4,000 IU/kg DM, considering the beneficial effects of this vitamin on immune competence (as discussed below).

During the starter and grower phases, NASEM (2021) recommends 1,100 IU/kg DM, almost double the level compared to NRC (2001) of 600 IU/kg. dsm-firmenich (2022b) suggested a higher supplementation of 2,200–3,000 IU/kg DM, also driven by the effects on immune response (Table 6.1b).

The average serum 25OHD$_3$ concentration of newborn calves under 4 days of age was 15 ± 11 ng/ml, ranging from 0 to 39 ng/ml (Nelson *et al.*, 2016b). These concentrations in the calves correlated with the concentrations in their dams. In this survey, Nelson *et al.* (2016b) observed that 25% of the calves may have serum 25OHD$_3$ concentrations below 10 ng/ml. These low levels can indicate a great risk for impaired health and development if they are not supplemented.

Infection with the bovine diarrhea virus decreases 25OHD$_3$ plasma concentrations (Nonnecke *et al.*, 2014). López-Constantino *et al.* (2022) showed that reduced serum 25OHD$_3$ levels below 30 ng/ml are associated with diminished mycobactericidal capacity. In contrast, increased 25OHD$_3$ in culture media enhances phagocytosis and nitric oxide production, improving immunological response to combat *Mycobacterium bovis*. In this study, tuberculin-positive cattle had average serum concentrations of 48.86 ng/ml 25(OH)D$_3$, while tuberculin-negative had a serum concentration of 87.12 ng/ml. This indicates the importance of this vitamin during infection. Krueger *et al.* (2016) demonstrated that young calves fed colostrum replacers supplemented with 5,000 IU/day of vitamin D$_3$ tended to have fewer health issues than calves fed no supplemental vitamin D. This effect could be related to the changes in the intestinal microbiota due to milk replacer composition described by Badman *et al.* (2019).

The responses of dairy calves to supplemental vitamin D$_3$ are presented in Figure 6.5 (Nelson *et al.*, 2016b). Data represent the outcome of 2 experiments in which Holstein bull calves were fed milk replacers containing increasing amounts of supplemental vitamin D$_3$. In Experiment 1, calves were fed milk replacers containing 1,700 (*n* = 16) or 17,900 IU (*n* = 8) of vitamin D$_3$/kg DM. In Experiment 2, calves were fed 400 (*n* = 12) or 11,000 (*n* = 12) IU of vitamin D$_3$/kg DM. To obtain a 25(OH)D$_3$ serum concentration of 30 ng/ml, calves must consume approximately 2,100 IU of vitamin D$_3$/day (Nelson *et al.*, 2016b).

The 25OHD$_3$ can be fed as a feed additive to calves to increase the 25OHD$_3$ plasmatic concentrations. Celi *et al.* (2018) confirmed that 25OHD$_3$ can be fed to calves at 1.7, 5.1, and 8.5 μg/kg feed without adverse effects. Feeding high doses of 25OHD$_3$ (12,000 IU per calf per day) could effectively improve growth performance, plasma minerals, and hormones concentration and

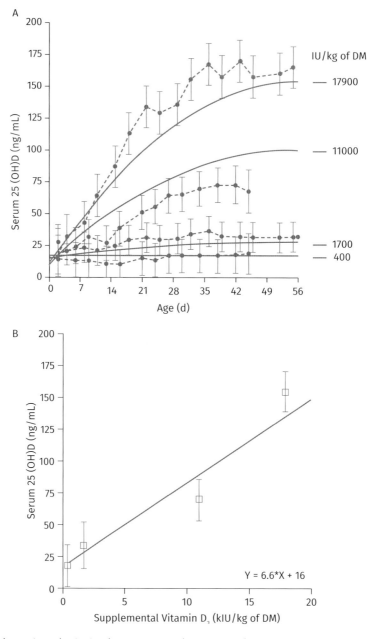

Figure 6.5 (A). Predicted (solid lines) and observed (dashed lines) serum 25-hydroxyvitamin D [25(OH)D] concentrations of experimental calves in response to the rate of supplemental vitamin D_3 and day of age. Data points and error bars represent the mean and 95% CI for each group according to day of age. The equation of the predicted response was [25(OH)D] = 16.02 ng/ml + (−0.00031 × IU of vitamin D_3) + (−0.024 × d) + (0.00029 × IU of vitamin D_3 × d) + (−2.59 × 10-6 × IU of vitamin D_3 × d2). (B) The solid line represents the slope and intercept of the regression analysis of serum 25(OH)D concentrations of samples collected at 30 d of age and older as a function of supplemental vitamin D_3. The slope (6.6 ng/ml per 1,000 IU of vitamin D_3) and intercept (16.1 ng/ml) were significant (P < 0.001). The symbols and error bars represent the observed means with 95% CI of samples from calves in each group at 30 d of age and older. (Source: Nelson et al., 2016b).

enhance the antioxidant capacity and immunoglobulin of pre-weaning Holstein calves (Wang L.H. *et al.*, 2022). The 25OHD$_3$ supplementation improved growth, feed efficiency, plasma total Ca and P levels, growth hormone, insulin-like growth factor I, plasma catalase, superoxide dismutase, and immunoglobulin G.

Heifers
The latest recommendation by the NASEM (2021) upholds the previous recommendations by the NRC (2001) of an AI of 30 IU/kg BW (Table 6.2). From growing to the mating phase (from 65 to 530 kg BW), this AI means to provide from 2,100 to 16,000 IU/head day. Supplementation must be increased to some 22,000 IU/day approaching parturition (Table 6.3). The confrontation of different sources indicates a good agreement, reflected by industry practice (Table 6.5).

Nelson *et al.* (2016b) reported the results of a survey of heifers carried out in April with an estimated daily dietary supplementation between 11,000 and 12,000 IU/day. These heifers had serum 25OHD$_3$ concentrations between 69±8 and 82±18 ng/ml, respectively, which can be considered adequate.

Lactating cows
The NASEM (2021) recommended an AI of supplemental vitamin D for lactating cows of 40 IU/kg BW (Table 6.2). Suggested supplementation is some 23,000 IU/day for primiparous Holstein cows and 28,000 IU/day for mature cows (Table 6.4). This suggested AI shows an increase compared to the previous recommendation given by NRC (2001). The recommendation provided by dsm-firmenich (2022b) in its OVN™ guidelines ranged from 25,000 to 40,000 IU/day. This industry source also recommends the administration of 1 mg/day of the metabolite 25OHD$_3$ (commercial name HyD®) (Table 6.7).

In a review of several studies carried out at Ohio State University, Hibbs and Conrad (1983) concluded that cows supplemented with 50–70 IU of vitamin D/kg BW produced more milk and generally consumed more DM than those animals that were not supplemented or which were supplemented with 100–140 IU of vitamin D/kg BW.

Holcombe *et al.* (2018) determined that healthy lactating cows reduce serum vitamin D concentrations at calving and postpartum. This indicates the need for enhanced vitamin D supplementation during this period. Guo *et al.* (2018) observed that supplemental 6 mg 25OHD$_3$ enhances dairy cow plasma 25OHD$_3$ concentrations but does not necessarily milk concentrations.

Poindexter *et al.* (2020) confirmed that 25OHD$_3$ is a more effective feed additive than supplemental vitamin D$_3$, resulting in increased serum mineral concentrations (Ca, mg, and P), increased expression of vitamin D-responsive genes, and altered immune responses to inframammary bacterial challenge. New studies recently confirmed these results (Flores-Villalva, 2022; Poindexter *et al.*, 2023a,b).

Recently, Ahmadi and Mohri (2021), Eder and Grundmann (2022), and Flores-Villalva (2022) reviewed the functions of vitamin D and highlighted the cellular mechanisms where vitamin D and its metabolite 25OHD$_3$ could enhance the immune function in dairy cows and be helpful for the prevention and therapy of mastitis. However, they indicated that the number of studies reported on this topic is limited. Previous studies like Yue *et al.* (2018) have failed to demonstrate that repletion to physiologically normal plasma 25OHD$_3$ levels of vitamin D-depleted healthy dairy cows did not influence immune parameters. In contrast, Corripio-Miyar *et al.* (2017) and Wherry *et al.* (2022) have reported positive effects of 1,25(OH)$_2$D$_3$ on immune responses against *Mycobacterium*, causing tuberculosis and paratuberculosis. Vieira-Neto *et al.* (2021b) observed that feeding additional vitamin D as cholecalciferol in the last 3 weeks of gestation of dairy cows changed the profile of blood leukocytes and attenuated granulocyte phagocytosis during the transition period, whereas supplementing 25OHD$_3$ prepartum increased mRNA expression of genes involved in immune cell function, including genes related to pathogen recognition and antimicrobial effects of leukocytes.

Dry cows
Recommended AI by NASEM (2021) is 40 IU/kg BW (Table 6.2), which means a supplementation of 22,000 IU/day during both far-off and close-up (Table 6.3). Both levels are similar to what was proposed by NRC (2001) and dsm-firmenich (2022b), which indicates a larger range of 25,000–30,000 IU/day. During close-up, they also recommend the supplementation of 3 mg/day of 25OHD$_3$ (commercial name HyD®) (Table 6.6).

Ward *et al.* (1972) reduced the interval between calving and first estrus interval by 16 days when supplementing cows with 43,000 IU/day of vitamin D. Wisnieski *et al.* (2019) determined that serum concentrations of 25OHD$_3$ at dry-off and close-up for lower risk of increased urine ketone concentrations during early lactation were below 103.4 and 91.1 ng/ml, respectively. Increased urine ketone concentrations are not necessarily harmful or diagnostic for ketosis but do indicate the development of negative energy balance, metabolic stress, and an increased risk of early lactation disease.

Nutritional interventions applied in the pre-calving period can have a prolonged positive effect on dairy cow production and health well into lactation, particularly prepartum dietary interventions that prevent mineral-related disorders like hypocalcemia in early lactation (Nelson *et al.*, 2016b). Ca and mineral metabolism are of particular interest during this period. Rodney *et al.* (2018) evaluated the effect of modifications on the dietary cation-anion difference (DCAD) and the sources of vitamin D in the antepartum diet of pregnant Holstein cows, 28 nulliparous and 51 parous. Treatments were arranged as a factorial with 2 levels of DCAD, positive (+130 mEq/kg) or negative (–130 mEq/kg), and 2 sources of vitamin D, calcidiol (25OHD$_3$) or cholecalciferol, fed at 3 mg for each 11 kg of diet DM. The experiment followed a randomized complete block design with the cow as the experimental unit. Supplementing with calcidiol increased plasma concentrations of 25OHD$_3$, 3-epi 25OHD$_3$, 25OHD$_2$, 1,25(OH)D$_3$, and 24,25(OH)$_2$D$_3$ compared with supplementing with cholecalciferol. Cows fed the diet with negative DCAD had lesser concentrations of vitamin D metabolites before and after calving than cows fed the diet with positive DCAD, except for 25OHD$_2$. Feeding the diet with negative DCAD induced a compensated metabolic acidosis that attenuated the decline in blood ionized Ca (iCa) and serum total Ca (tCa) around calving, particularly in parous cows. In contrast, cows fed the diet with positive DCAD and supplemented with calcidiol had the greatest 1,25(OH)$_2$D$_3$ concentrations and the lowest iCa and tCa concentrations on day 1 and 2 postpartum. The acidogenic diet or calcidiol markedly increased urinary losses of tCa and tMg, and feeding calcidiol tended to increase colostrum yield and losses of tCa and tMg in colostrum. Cows fed the diet with negative DCAD had increased concentrations of serotonin and C-terminal telopeptide of type 1 collagen prepartum compared with cows fed the diet with positive DCAD. Concentrations of undercarboxylated and carboxylated osteocalcin and those of adiponectin did not differ with treatment. These results provide evidence that dietary manipulations can induce metabolic adaptations that improve mineral homeostasis with the onset of lactation. This might explain some of the improvements observed in health and production when cows are fed diets with negative DCAD or supplemented with 25OHD$_3$.

Martinez *et al.* (2018a, b) supplemented 1 mg/head day of 25OHD$_3$ to dairy cows during transition period with or without anionic diets (–130 mEq/kg DCAD or +130 mEq/kg DCAD). Milk yield as 3.5% FCM (fat-corrected milk) were increased in both cases, with and without negative

DCAD diets supplemented with 25OHD$_3$. ECM (energy-corrected milk), protein and fat yield were higher when negative DCAD diet was fed.

In a new study Poindexter *et al.* (2023a) tested 25OHD$_3$ and regular vitamin D$_3$ given at 1 and 3 mg/cow/day of each source before and after calving. The cows receiving 3 mg of 25OHD$_3$ before calving increased milk yield in the first 42 days in-milk, tended to increase percentage of milk fat and increase the milk fat content.

Serum vitamin D is believed to be associated with antioxidant potential in periparturient cows. Strickland *et al.* (2021) determined the association between serum vitamins and bio-markers of oxidative stress in healthy cows. Results indicated that serum vitamin D concentrations are positively associated with antioxidant potential (AOP) in peripartum cattle. Still, common antioxidant vitamins, including vitamins A, E, and β-carotene, are not associated with AOP. Supplementary vitamin D could significantly impact oxidative stress and disease prevention in periparturient cows. Golder *et al.* (2021) evaluated the supplementation of 2 mg/day of 25OHD$_3$ from approximately 21 day prepartum to parturition and 1 mg/day in lactation in dairy cows. The supplemented cows had 0.2 lower log somatic cell count than control cows (4.21 ± 0.045 versus 4.01 ± 0.050, respectively). Multiparous supplemented cows had a 41±23% higher probability of pregnancy/day than multiparous control cows, resulting in a 22-day median decrease in time to pregnancy.

Vieira-Neto *et al.* (2021a) injecting subcutaneously 200 or 300 µg of 1α,25(OH)$_2$D$_3$ (calcitriol) within 6 hours of calving observed improving concentrations of iCa, tCa, and tP, which reduced the risk of hypocalcemia. Calcitriol treatment reduced the pregnancy rate, and health performance benefits were limited to over-conditioned cows. Thus, treatment of all cows is not supported, and proper identification of cohorts of cows that benefit from postpartum interventions that increase blood calcitriol or Ca is needed.

However, dietary supplementation of 3 mg/day of 25OHD$_3$ during the prepartum period had diverse positive effects in dairy cows. Silva *et al.* (2022) supplemented dairy cows with 3 mg/day of 25OHD$_3$ compared to supplementing vitamin D$_3$ at 0.625 mg/day and reported improved energy metabolism and lactation performance. Feeding 25OHD$_3$ increased colostrum yield. The 25OHD$_3$ plasmatic concentration was increased with dietary 25OHD$_3$ supplementation. 25OHD$_3$ supplementation increased plasma glucose concentration at parturition. Treatments did not influence the postpartum DMI. Cows fed 25OHD$_3$ produced 2.8 kg/day more milk than those fed the control diets. The 25OHD$_3$ supplementation increased 3.5% fat-corrected milk and energy-corrected milk and improved milk yield components in early lactation.

Recently, Nisar *et al.* (2024) concluded that 25OHD$_3$ significantly influences redox balance and energy profile in pregnant ewes. The 25OHD$_3$ blood status can be a predictor for subclinical pregnancy toxemia. Correlation analysis revealed a positive association of 25OHD$_3$ with fructosamine, Ca, and total antioxidant capacity and a negative correlation with non-esterified fatty acid and total oxidant status.

Vitamin E
Introduction
The vitamin E content of feed for dairy cattle is very variable. Consequently, obtaining accurate estimates of vitamin E concentration in the diet is difficult. The adequate daily intake of this vitamin is expressed as supplemental vitamin E and not total dietary vitamin E. To keep track of the units of supplementation, it is essential to remember that one IU vitamin E equals 1 mg of all-*rac*-α-tocopherol acetate, which is also the most common commercial form. Therefore, IU and mg are both used, indicating the same dose. Depending on their maturity state, forages contain between 80 and 200 IU of vitamin E/kg DM (Tramontano *et al.*, 1993; Jukola *et al.*,

1996). As with other fat-soluble vitamins, the plant concentration and quantity available to the animal depend on various environmental and agricultural management factors. The α-to-copherol concentration decreases rapidly once the plant is cut. Prolonged exposure to oxygen or sunlight increases the rate of degradation (Thafvelin and Oksanen, 1966). Silage and hay contain between 20 and 80% less tocopherol than fresh forage. Concentrate feeds are low in vitamin E except for whole soybeans and cottonseed.

The main focus of the studies undertaken to evaluate the role of vitamin E in ruminants arises from its potential as an antioxidant, as it can prevent the damage caused by free radicals at the tissue level and prevent or retard the development of certain degenerative inflammatory diseases. Vitamin E also appears to play a fundamental role in immune function (Ndiweni and Finch, 1995; Politis *et al.*, 1996; Baldi, 2005) and MG health (Weiss *et al.*, 1990a, 1997; Njeru *et al.*, 1994a; Morgante *et al.*, 1999; Baldi *et al.*, 2008; McGrath *et al.*, 2018; Kuhn and Sordillo, 2021).

Recommendations for vitamin E
Calves

The NASEM (2021) recommended an adequate intake of 2 IU/kg BW, 120 IU/day for a 60 kg calve, or 200 IU/kg of milk replacer DM if the intake will be 0.6 kg of milk replacer daily. Accordingly, dsm-firmenich (2002b) indicated a supplementation of 150–200 mg/kg DM of milk replacer. These values are higher than the NRC (2001) recommendation, which was 50 IU/kg of milk replacer solids or 30 IU/d. This change is based on the increased requirement by animals in stressful situations typical of current production systems, where an extra vitamin E supplement may boost the immune system (Table 6.1a).

However, the recommendations depend significantly on the colostrum intake and its vitamin E content since the transfer of vitamin E through the placental membrane is low (Van Saun *et al.*, 1989). It is, therefore, essential to ensure the supply of colostrum in the first hours of the calf's life, since from 24 hours after parturition, the efficiency of its intestinal absorption is reduced. Weiss *et al.* (1992) observed that the vitamin E concentration in colostrum increased by 40% when the ration for dry cows was supplemented with 70 IU/day during the dry period. Quigley and Bernard (1995) evaluated the effects of adding vitamin E (0, 100, or 1,000 IU) to colostrum on the absorption of α-tocopherol and immunoglobulin in neonatal calves. In this study, adding vitamin E increased the absorption of α-tocopherol but did not affect the absorption of immunoglobulins. Lacetera *et al.* (1996) observed increased colostrum production and vitamin E content when dry cow rations were supplemented with 25 IU/day of vitamin E during the 3 weeks of prepartum.

Stobo (1983) suggested that the vitamin E concentration in the milk replacer should depend on the ration's unsaturated fatty acid content and recommended a 1.5–2.5 IU ratio of vitamin E per gram of linoleic acid. In standard milk replacers, this ratio is achieved with daily intakes of between 25 and 63 IU/kg of DM. The NRC (2001) indicated that vitamin E intake needs to be 30 IU/day to prevent oxidative stress caused by polyunsaturated fatty acids (PUFA).

Hidiroglou *et al.* (1995) supplemented the ration of newborn calves with 1,000 IU/day vitamin E. They observed an increase in the plasma concentration in the first week, and this concentration remained constant afterward. Immunoglobulin levels and average weight gain (0.34 kg/day *vs.* 0.42 kg/d) tended to increase in the group treated with vitamin E. Reddy *et al.* (1986 and 1987) observed that young calves supplemented with 125 or 250 IU vitamin E per day had faster growth rate, more leukocyte activity, higher concentrations of immunoglobulins and serum cholesterol, and reduced indicators of cellular membrane lesions. However, they only obtained a growth rate of <150 g/day.

Animals with low growth rates tend to have higher needs for vitamin E. For example, Nonnecke *et al.* (2010) observed that after feeding calves with approximately 300 IU/day, calves gaining 0.55 kg/day had higher serum α-tocopherol than those gaining 1.2 kg/day. Similarly, calves supplemented with 500 IU of vitamin per day gained more weight when fed diets varying in energy and protein, targeting 0.5 kg/day, but did not affect calves with diets set for a growth rate of 0.25 kg/day (Krueger *et al.*, 2014).

Nevertheless, sometimes, higher supplementation to fast-growing calves does not have an effect. Sehested *et al.* (2004) did not observe significant differences in growth rate between Holstein calves fed 0 or 500 IU of supplemental vitamin E. In another study, Mohri *et al.* (2005) evaluated the effect of pre-weaning supplementation of suckling calves with 300 IU vitamin E and 6 mg selenium per 45 kg BW (corresponding to 6,7 IU/kg and 0.13 mg/kg respectively) administered parenterally at 24 and 48 hours and 7, 14, 21 and 28 days after parturition. The extra supplies did not improve the calves' immune response or post-weaning growth, except for a significant increase in the hematocrit and the concentration of β-globulins (Ballou, 2012).

Although there is no solid evidence to justify an increase in these recommendations, the NASEM (2021) recognizes that these recommendations may not be adequate for fast-growing calves. Despite the limited information available, there are situations in which higher levels merit consideration. First, frequent digestive disorders in young calves reduce vitamin E absorption. Second, supplementation with high quantities of vitamin A interferes with vitamin E absorption. Third, infections can deplete vitamin E stores. For these reasons, and because of the comprehensive safety margin of vitamin E, it may be justified to increase the recommendations, at least in some situations.

During both the starter and grower phases, NASEM (2021) recommends supplementation of 67 IU/kg DM, which is much higher than the 25 mg/kg feed proposed by NRC (2001). dsm-firmenich (2022b) indicated a supplementation of 135 to 200 IU/kg DM feed, which considers the important effects of this vitamin in modulating the antioxidant system and the immune response (Table 6.1b).

Calves often have lower plasma vitamin E concentration than the recommended level (3 mg/l) after weaning, which seems to be a challenge for a good immune response. Lashkari *et al.* (2021) conducted 2 studies evaluating the effects of natural vitamin E supplementation in the starter concentrate to increase the plasma vitamin E concentration of calves around weaning. In the first study, the standard concentrate used at the farm was fed either unsupplemented (CON) or supplemented with 490±24 (Means ± SD) mg of RRR-α-tocopherol (RRR-α-T)/kg of diet by mixing a vitamin E-enriched pellet with the standard concentrate pellet in the ratio of 1:10. In the second study, calves were fed either a common concentrate pellet with 48±8 mg/kg all-rac-α-tocopheryl acetate (CON) or a common concentrate pellet with 245±30 (Means ± SD) mg/kg RRR-α-T with a similar dietary composition. The results indicated that regardless of the approach used for preparing the concentrate pellets, supplementation with a high amount of natural vitamin E (RRR-α-T) significantly increased the plasma vitamin E concentration above 3 mg/l at weaning and post-weaning and decreased the plasma cortisol and serum amyloid A concentration in calves post-weaning.

Heifers
NASEM (2021) recommendation for growing heifers was 0.8 IU/kg BW (Table 6.2). This recommendation did not increase compared to the NRC (2001). Recommendations given by NASEM (2021) for heifers at different weights are given in Table 6.3. Confrontation of different sources (Table 6.5) shows that there is a good agreement between the levels suggested by NRC (2001), NASEM (2021), and dsm-firmenich (2022b).

Lactating cows

NASEM (2021) confirmed an AI of vitamin E of 0.8 IU/kg BW for lactating cows, which means 560 IU/day for a 700 kg Holstein lactating cow (Tables 6.2 and 6.4). NASEM (2021) recommendation is substantially aligned with what was proposed by NRC (2001) but they also recommended increasing the supplementation to 1,200 mg/day in pre-fresh cows. dsm-firmenich (2022b) finally proposed a range of 600–1,000 IU/day, indicating that the upper level optimizes udder health (Table 6.7).

It is important to consider that grazing cattle consume fresh forage that may supply 35 mg/kg of α-tocopherol (50 IU/kg) more than hay and silage. Consequently, the requirement for supplemental vitamin E should be reduced theoretically by 50 IU/day for every kilogram of fresh pasture DM consumed by a cow.

Recommendations are higher than those established by INRA (1988) or previously by the NRC (1989; 15 IU/kg DM, or 300 IU/d). This increase was based on the review by Weiss (1998), who established a clear inverse relationship between vitamin E intake and the incidence of mastitis. Weiss *et al.* (1990a) observed that supplementing vitamin E in the lactation ration reduced the incidence of clinical mastitis. Clinical mastitis cases increased in over half the herds when the supply was below 23 IU/kg of diet, suggesting that supplementation above the recommended levels could benefit MG health. On the other hand, many researchers have observed that the plasma concentration of vitamin E in herds with a high somatic cell count or with a high incidence of mastitis was lower than in those herds with a lower somatic cell count (Weiss *et al.* 1990a), which suggests that low vitamin E plasma levels increase the risk of mastitis (Weiss, 1998). Weiss *et al.* (1994 and 1997) suggested that the plasma concentration of vitamin E should be greater than or equal to 3 µg/ml to reduce the risk of reproductive or MG problems.

Therefore, a vitamin E supplementation for lactating animals in the range of 500 IU/day appears adequate for most normal production situations (Weiss, 2005). In general, the quantity of ingested vitamin E is considered appropriate when the plasma levels of α-tocopherol are higher than 3.0–3.5 µg/ml or higher than 2.0 µg/ml when expressed concerning cholesterol concentration in plasma. No additional benefits have been observed with higher plasma levels (Baldi, 2005). An increase in vitamin E supplies could be considered when there is an excess of vitamin A or a deficit of selenium.

Bourne *et al.* (2007b) evaluated the effect of the supplementation method in dairy cows at peak or mid-lactation (610, 1,864, and 737 mg of vitamin E per day for the control, oral, and parenteral treatments, respectively). Oral supplementation above the recommendations (1,864 mg/day) did not translate into an increase in the concentration of vitamin E in plasma compared with the control dose (610 mg/day). The vitamin E level was higher in cows that received additional supplementation parenterally (737 mg/day in the food + 2,100 mg parenteral per week), which suggests that injection is more effective if the objective is a higher supplementation of this vitamin in lactating dairy cattle. Stowe *et al.* (1988), after supplementing the lactation ration with vitamin E (500 IU/day) during 2 consecutive production cycles, observed an increase in the plasma concentration of vitamin E and a tendency to fewer services per conception. Weiss *et al.* (1997) observed increased DM intake when vitamin E supplements increased from 100 to 1,000 IU/day.

It is difficult to discuss the requirements of vitamin E in dairy cattle without considering the requirements or supplies of selenium because the effects of both micronutrients on animal health and productivity are closely related. In some cases, although not always, vitamin E can be substituted to a certain extent by selenium or vice versa. Although selenium cannot replace vitamin E completely, it reduces its requirements and delays the appearance of symptoms of vitamin E deficiency in the animal (Spears, 2000; Hemingway, 2003). The NASEM (2021) has recommended a maximum of 0.3 ppm selenium, which is limited because of its toxicity. If the rations have a selenium content lower than the requirements, an additional supply of vitamin E is recommended (Grasso et al., 1990).

Recently, Jung et al. (2023) investigated the effects of road transportation and administration of vitamin E and selenium on circulating cortisol, haptoglobin, blood metabolites, oxidative biomarkers, white blood cell profiles, and behaviors in pregnant dairy heifers. The supplemented group received 70 IU/kg DM feed of dl-α-tocopheryl acetate and 0.3 mg/kg DM feed of sodium selenite once daily from 7 days before transportation to 3 days after transportation. Their results indicated that transported heifers supplemented with vitamin E and selenium had greater total antioxidative status levels at 48 hours after transportation than those non-supplemented. Supplementation did not affect white blood cell numbers, neutrophil and lymphocyte percentages, and lying time. Road transportation caused temporal oxidative stress in pregnant heifers. Vitamin E and selenium supplementation partially alleviated the stress, suggesting that this could be a viable strategy to reduce stress in transporting pregnant heifers and improving animal welfare.

Another important aspect when evaluating the requirements and practical recommendations for vitamin E supplementation in dairy cattle relates to the quality of the milk and its vitamin E content (Haug et al., 2007; Krol et al., 2020). The concentration of vitamin E in milk depends on various factors, among them the type, quantity, and method of administering the vitamin E to the animal. Bourne et al. (2007a) observed that the vitamin E concentration in milk was higher in cows supplemented parenterally with vitamin E (4,200 mg parenteral per day for 3 weeks). The same authors showed a significant relationship between the vitamin E content in the plasma and cows' milk. However, the correlation was significant only when cows were supplemented parenterally ($r = 0.44$; $P < 0.001$). A similar tendency was observed by Calderón et al. (2007), who observed the effect of supplying, over 6 weeks, increasing levels of vitamin E (73.9; 510.2; 942.6 and 1384.9 mg/day) in the ration of dairy cattle during mid-lactation. The concentration of vitamin E in plasma increased similarly to the supply of vitamin E in the ration.

Dry cows

NASEM (2021) indicated an AI of vitamin E of 1.6 IU/kg BW for dry cows, approximately 85 IU/kg DM, or 1,200 IU/day for a 700 kg BW Holstein cow. The recommendation is increased to 2,400 IU/day or 3 mg/kg BW 3 weeks before expected calving. dsm-firmenich (2022b) suggested higher levels with a range of 1,100–4,000 during far-off and 2,000–4,000 during close-up. The proposed upper level of 4,000 mg/day is recommended from 3 weeks pre-partum until 4 weeks postpartum (Tables 6.2, 6.3 and 6.6). The benefits of higher levels of vitamin E during this period are discussed in this paragraph.

The AI proposed by NASEM (2021) is the same as recommended 20 years ago (NRC, 2001) and higher than the 15 IU/ kg DM (or 150 IU/day) established by INRA (1988) or the previous recommendation by the NRC (1989). The increase was based on the immune system's response improvements, translating into better mg and reproductive health. However, mastitis and other health issues are still common. Stowe et al. (1988) demonstrated that supplementing the lactation ration with vitamin E (500 IU/day) during 2 consecutive productive cycles did not allow the storage of enough vitamin E to maintain an unsupplemented dry period, indicating the need for specific supplementation during this period.

In their meta-analysis, Bourne et al. (2007a) concluded that supplementation with vitamin E during the dry period is associated with a reduction in the risks of the occurrence of retained placentas in dairy cattle since out of 44 studies analyzed, 20 showed a positive effect, 21 showed no effect, and only in 3 was an increase in the incidence of retained placentas

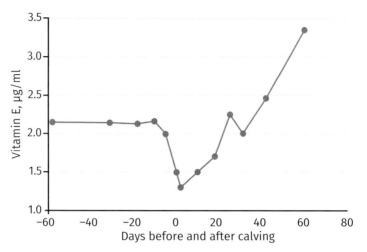

Figure 6.6 Evolution of plasma concentration of vitamin E in the peripartum (source: adapted from Weiss *et al.*, 1990b)

observed in the treated cows. Bourne *et al.* (2008) came to a similar conclusion, as supplementation with vitamin E and selenium was related to a decrease in the culling of cows from the herd because of reproductive problems, as well as a lower incidence of mastitis (8%) and retained placentas (dropping from 6.5 to 3%). Furthermore, Bourne *et al.* (2007b) also compared the use of natural sources of vitamin E against synthetic forms. They recommended the latter, which was more effective than their natural equivalents.

The plasma concentration of vitamin E falls in the peripartum period, especially 2 weeks from calving (Smith *et al.*, 1985; Weiss *et al.*, 1990a, b; 1992; Goff *et al.*, 2002; Calderón *et al.*, 2007; Figure 6.6). The reduction in the plasma concentration of vitamin E in this period is partially due to increased immune system activity, reduced intake, and the excretion of vitamin E in colostrum. This reduction coincides with the most critical time concerning immunocompetence and an increase in the incidence of diseases (Smith *et al.*, 1985; Weiss *et al.*, 1990b).

The NASEM (2021) recommendation for late gestation within 2–5 weeks pre-calving is 3.0 IU/kg BW (Table 6.2). The parenteral supply of vitamin E during this peripartum period has proven positive effects (Bourne *et al.*, 2007a). Oral or parenteral administration of vitamin E (1,000 or 3,000 IU/day) during the peripartum period improved macrophage and neutrophil function (Hogan *et al.*, 1990, 1992; Politis *et al.*, 1995, 1996; Ndiweni and Finch, 1996; Mohri *et al.*, 2005; Meydani and Han, 2006; Figure 6.7). However, oral administration of up to 1,000 IU/day of vitamin E did not prevent a reduction in plasma concentration of vitamin E during the peripartum period. Only a parenteral injection of 3,000 IU on days 10 and 5 prepartum successfully increased the plasma concentration of vitamin E during the critical peripartum days (Hogan *et al.*, 1992; Weiss *et al.*, 1992). It has also been suggested that the additional supply of vitamin E by this method could help to reduce the risk of oxidative stress, which occurs peripartum (Castillo *et al.*, 2005) derived from a reduction in feed intake (Grummer *et al.*, 2004).

Improved immune function translates into a greater capacity to fight mammary infections. Smith *et al.* (1984) reduced the incidence (–37%) and duration (-62%) of mammary infections and the number of cases of clinical mastitis by supplementing vitamin E at 1,000 IU/day during the 60 days of the dry period. Smith *et al.* (1985) also observed a reduction in the incidence of mastitis. Supplemental selenium and vitamin E during the prepartum period resulted in a reduction of 42% in the rate of mammary infections, 32% in clinical mastitis cases, and 59% in

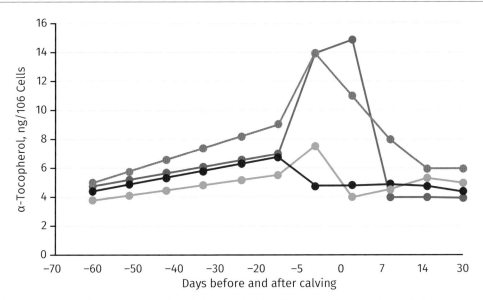

Figure 6.7 Changes in the concentration of vitamin E in blood leukocytes in control cows (●), or cows supplemented with 1000 IU/day of vitamin E orally (●), injected vitamin E (●), or the combination of 1000 IU/day of oral and injected vitamin E (●) (source: adapted from Weiss et al., 1992)

the total number of infected days of lactation (Erskine et al., 1989). Hogan et al. (1993) obtained similar results. Smith et al. (1985) observed that first lactation heifers, supplemented with 1,000 IU/day during the 60 days prepartum, had fewer mammary infections, other infections throughout lactation, and clinical cases and the duration of the infections and somatic cell counts were reduced. Batra et al. (1992) also observed a reduction in the incidence of clinical cases and their duration after supplementing vitamin E during the dry period (1,000 IU/day). On the other hand, Bourne et al. (2008) did not observe any effect on the somatic cell count with a supplementary supply of vitamin E and selenium (2 injections: 2,100 mg vitamin E + 7 mg of sodium selenite per injection, 2 weeks before parturition and one day after parturition) in 3 herds of dairy cattle (n = 594 cows).

These results demonstrate that the increase in the vitamin E recommendations from 1,200 IU/day established in the NRC's 2001 report to 2,400 IU/day in NASEM (2021), while not resolving the reduction in the plasma concentration of vitamin E during the peripartum period, does improve immune competence and MG health.

The summary presented by Weiss (2005) shows that, based on the data in the literature, the supply of high doses of vitamin E (above 1,000 IU/day) peripartum can be beneficial for a general improvement in the health of dairy cattle. Politis et al. (1995) observed that supplementation of 3,000 IU/day of vitamin E from 4 weeks prepartum to 8 weeks postpartum prevented the reduction in the immune response by polymorphonuclear neutrophils and macrophages typical of the peripartum period, suggesting that supplementation above current recommendations could be beneficial. The results obtained by Weiss et al. (1997), who supplemented 100, 1,000, and 4,000 IU/day of vitamin E during the 2 weeks before parturition, found that the highest level reduced the incidence of clinical mastitis by 80%, and intramammary infections by 60%. Still, supplementation of 100 and 1,000 IU/day did not prevent the reduction of plasma concentration of vitamin E peripartum. Supplementation with 4,000 IU/day of vitamin E maintained the plasma level throughout the peripartum period (Figure 6.8). Compared with supplementation with 100 and 1000 IU/day, supplementation with 4,000 IU/day of vitamin E increased the concentration of vitamin E in polymorphonuclear neutrophils by 200%. The incidence of intramammary infections was reduced compared with the control group by 11.8, 31.8, and 32.1% with 100, 1000, and 4000 IU/day, respectively. Prevalence was 26, 14, and 9% in Staphylococcal infections with 100, 1000, and 4000 IU/d, respectively. The prevalence of clinical mastitis was 25, 17, and 3% of udders when supplemented with 100, 1,000, and 4,000 IU/day, respectively (Figure 6.9). The effect of supplementation with vitamin E on the prevalence of clinical mastitis was greatest in primiparous (37, 14, and 0% of udders when supplemented with 100, 1,000, and 4,000 IU/day, respectively). The results demonstrated, furthermore, that the reduction in the plasma concentration of vitamin E peripartum is an important mastitis risk factor because if the plasma concentration was below 3 µg/ml, the risk of mastitis was 9.4 times higher.

Vitamin E not only affects MG health, but there is considerable evidence of its effects on reproductive function (Aoki et al., 2014). Harrison et al. (1984) demonstrated that supplementation, during the 3 prepartum weeks, of a combination of oral vitamin E (740 IU/day) and parenteral selenium (0.1 mg/kg BW) 21 days before projected calving completely prevented the incidence of retained placenta in a herd with a previous incidence of 20% and resulted in a quicker return to estrus. However, the incidence of mastitis and ovarian cysts remained unchanged. Lacetera et al. (1996) also observed a reduction in the incidence of retained placenta from 33 to 8% following parenteral supplementation of selenium (5 mg per 100 kg) and vitamin E (25 IU per 100 kg) 3 and 1.5 weeks prepartum, and an increase of 10% in milk production. However, the increase in milk production is an effect that is not always evident (Kay et al., 2005; Pottier et al., 2006). In a recent study, Kadek et al. (2021) also concluded that parenteral application of vitamins A, E, and β-carotene to pregnant cows affected the blood concentrations of these vitamins, total antioxidant status, and hematologic indices in their calves. This project confirmed the transgenerational effect of vitamin supplementation.

Moghimi-Kandelousi et al. (2020) summarized the effects of vitamin E supplementation on dairy cows during the transition phase in a meta-analysis and meta-regression. The effects of vitamin E supplementation on serum and colostrum enrichment, milk yield, somatic cell counts (SCC), and various reproductive variables of transition cows were evaluated. This analysis showed that supplementing vitamin E did not affect SCC or colostrum quality but improved the reproductive performance of transition cows, an effect consistent with increased levels of serum vitamin E and, for some variables, being modulated by Se supplementation. Cows receiving additional vitamin E had, on average, 6.1% fewer cases of retained placenta, whereby Se supplementation and breed were key factors improving the effect of vitamin E to reduce retained placenta. In this regard, breeds other than Holstein responded better, and these cows showed a lower incidence of retained placenta. The supplemented cows showed fewer days open (effect size: –0.31), and this improvement was affected linearly by increasing the dosage administered. Also, cows showed fewer services per conception with increasing dosages of vitamin E.

Campbell and Miller (1998) reported a quicker return to estrus (from 60 to 42 days) and a reduction in the days to conception (from 71 to 62 days) when supplementing the ration for dry cows with 1,000 IU/day for 42 days (Figure 6.10). Because vitamin E was not supplemented in the postpartum ration, the effects on reproduction were attributed to the residual effects of prepartum supplementation. Other authors (Harrison et al., 1984; Miller et al., 1993; Segerson et al., 1981; Brzezinska-Slebodzinska et al., 1994) obtained similar results which link supplementing the prepartum ration with vitamin E and improved reproductive activity.

Focant et al. (1998) studied the effect of supplementing vitamin E in rations rich in canola and flax seeds. Including these ingredients reduced the protein and fat concentrations in the milk and increased the C:18 content and the proportion of unsaturated fatty acids

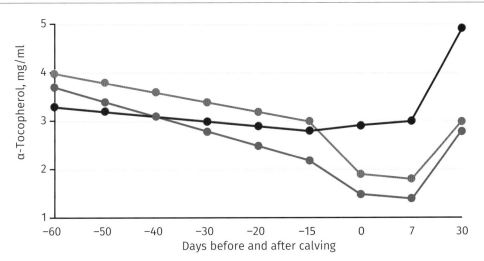

Figure 6.8 Plasma concentration of vitamin E in cows supplemented with 100 IU/day of vitamin E (●), 1,000 IU/day of vitamin E prepartum, and 500 IU/day of vitamin E postpartum (●) or 1,000 IU/day of vitamin E in dry period, 4,000 IU/day of vitamin E over 2 weeks prepartum, and 2,000 IU/day of vitamin E postpartum (●) (source: adapted from Weiss *et al.*, 1997)

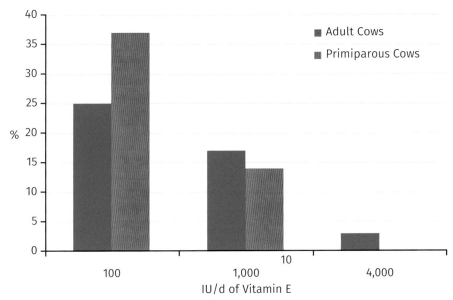

Figure 6.9 Prevalence of clinical mammary infections in adult and primiparous cows supplemented with 100, 1,000, and 4,000 IU/day of vitamin E (source: adapted from Weiss *et al.*, 1997)

(from 2.7 to 10.8%). This increase in unsaturation in milk fat enhances the risk of rancidity. Supplementing 9,600 IU vitamin E/day increased the vitamin E concentration in the milk by 45%. It prevented both the drop in milk fat and the oxidation of the unsaturated fatty acids. These results are similar to those obtained by Charmley and Nicholson (1994), who supplemented the ration with 8,000 IU/day. Kay *et al.* (2005) observed that the addition of 10,000 IU/day of α-tocopherol resulted in an increase of 6% in the fat content of the milk.

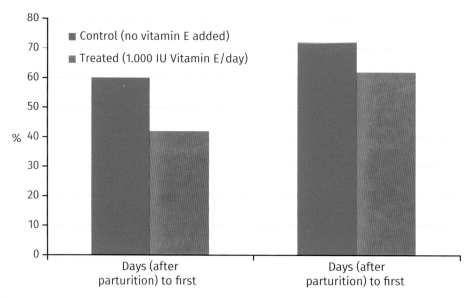

Figure 6.10 Effect of supplementation of 1,000 IU/day of vitamin E on the occurrence of the first estrus and days to first insemination (source: adapted from Campbell and Miller, 1998)

The difference was even more significant in the study conducted by Pottier *et al.* (2006), where the addition of 12,000 IU of α-tocopherol in the diet containing flax (extruded seed, 10%, and oil, 1% of DM) increased the fat content in milk by 18% compared with the same diet without supplemental vitamin E. These results suggest that the current recommendations for dry cows (1,000 IU/day) could be increased to 3,000–4,000 IU/day to boost the immune function and to 9,000 IU/day for milk quality when selenium levels in the ration are marginal, the polyunsaturated fatty acid content of the ration is high, the incidence of mammary or reproductive disorders is high, or to reduce the risk of milk fat oxidation, without risk of reaching toxicity levels.

Effective supplementation of minerals and vitamins during the transition period is very important to cope with the increased requirement due to the loss of nutrients during this phase of life. The deficiency of vitamins and minerals leads to most of the periparturient disorders in dairy cattle and buffaloes. Likewise, Khan *et al.* (2014) reviewed the literature available and concluded that vitamins and minerals are essential to dairy animal production and reproduction. The bioavailability of the minerals to the animals needs to address the issues of the soil-plant-animal relationship for scientific supplementation of the critical components related to periparturient disorders. Therefore, the region-specific, more concisely area-specific mineral mixture must be developed to improve periparturient disorders (Khan *et al.*, 2014, 2022).

Similarly, vitamin E can decrease oxidative stress by scavenging free radicals (Celi, 2011). Typically, vitamin E radicals formed when vitamin E reacts with free radicals are regenerated by a network of other antioxidants, termed the "vitamin E regeneration system" (VERS). In the case of vitamin E supplementation, the VERS should be sufficient to regenerate formed vitamin E radicals; if not, oxidative stress might increase instead of decrease (Bouwstra *et al.*, 2010). Additionally, oxidative stress and vitamin E levels might be critical physiological states to evaluate before supplementation (Celi, 2011). In a clinical trial, Bouwstra *et al.* (2010) evaluated retrospectively which physiological states influenced the effect of vitamin E supplements. The oxidative stress reaches the highest levels during the dry period of 2 weeks of antepartum.

High oxidative stress in this period was related to a higher risk of clinical mastitis, and not all cows responded well to high (3,000 IU/day) vitamin E supplementation. However, the results of this study are not consistent with most of the literature as reviewed by Politis (2012), who concluded that supplementation of 3,000 IU vitamin E/cow per day in the late dry period is still recommended because it is generally associated with decreased risk of mastitis. Conditional or opposite effects have not been repeated and require further research before changing recommendations for vitamin E supplementation.

Dairy cattle are routinely supplemented with the vitamin E analog α-tocopherol to mitigate the severity of oxidative stress. Nonetheless, oxidative stress remains a disease-predisposing condition for many dairy cattle. A better method of optimizing the antioxidant functions of vitamin E is needed. α-tocopherol is only one of 8 analogs of vitamin E, all of which have varying antioxidant properties in other mammals, albeit a shorter physiological half-life compared with α-tocopherol. Kuhn and Sordillo (2021) used a primary bovine mammary endothelial cell oxidant challenge model to determine the functions of vitamin E analogs: γ-tocopherol or γ-tocotrienol. The results suggested that γ-tocopherol has antioxidant activities that reduce cellular damage and loss of function due to oxidant challenge as effectively as α-tocopherol. These data set the foundation for further investigation into the antioxidant properties of vitamin E analogs in other bovine cell types or whole animal models.

Haga *et al.* (2021) discussed at least 6 physiological phenomena that occur during the transition period and may be candidate factors predisposing to a decreased blood α-tocopherol level and hypovitaminosis E with changes in α-tocopherol-related gene expression. Based on recent literature, the 6 physiological factors are:

● the decline in α-tocopherol intake from the close-up period
● the changes in the digestive and absorptive functions of α-tocopherol
● the decline in plasma high-density lipoprotein as an α-tocopherol carrier
● the increasing oxidative stress and consumption of α-tocopherol
● the decreasing hepatic α-tocopherol transfer to circulation
● the increasing mammary α-tocopherol transfer from blood to colostrum may be involved in α-tocopherol deficiency during the transition period.

However, the mechanisms and pathways are poorly understood, and further studies are needed to understand the physiological role of α-tocopherol-related molecules in cattle.

In summary, the continuous overproduction of reactive oxygen species during the transition from late gestation to peak lactation leads to the development of oxidative stress. Oxidative stress is usually the main contributor to diseases such as retained placenta, fatty liver, ketosis, mastitis, and metritis in periparturient dairy cattle. The oxidative stress is generally balanced by the naturally available antioxidant system in the body of dairy cattle. However, in some special conditions, such as the peri-periparturient period, a body's natural antioxidant system cannot balance the reactive oxygen species production. The antioxidants are supplied to the dairy cattle from external sources to cope with this situation.

Natural antioxidants such as selenium and vitamin E have been found to restore normal health by minimizing the harmful effects of excessive reactive oxygen species production. Se and vitamin E deficiencies have been reported to be associated with various diseases in periparturient dairy cattle including mastitis (Abd Ellah, 2013). Omur *et al.* (2016) administered antioxidant vitamins (A, D, E) and trace elements (Cu, Mn, Se, Zn) to dairy cows. They concluded that it is possible to control blood concentrations of negative energy balance, non-esterified fatty acids, and β-hydroxybutyric acid around the transition period. Xiao *et al.* (2021)

highlighted new insights into supplementing Se and vitamin E as antioxidant agents in the health regulation of periparturient dairy cattle.

To sum up, redox balance is essential in regulating several biological processes. However, an imbalance between the production of oxidants and the animal body's natural antioxidant system may lead to serious health issues in periparturient dairy cattle. Therefore, the external antioxidant source may contribute to balancing the situation of oxidative stress. Vitamin E and Se are well studied for their antioxidant and immune-regulating properties. Thus, properly supplementing Se and vitamin E during the periparturient period could be an excellent choice to relieve oxidative stress and the resulting consequences on dairy cattle's health.

It has been discussed that synthetic vitamin supplementation is not consistent with organic production. Consequently, Johansson et al. (2014) investigated whether dairy cows can maintain their health and production without adding synthetic vitamins to their diet. In basic dairy cow diets, provitamin A (β-carotene) and vitamin E are mainly found in pasture, grass, and legume silages, but the concentrations are highly variable. In this study, the vitamin status and health of cows without synthetic vitamin supplementation (NSV group) with control cows (CON group) fed synthetic vitamins according to Swedish recommendations (600 IU of vitamin E and 80,000 IU of vitamin A per cow per day) were investigated. Vitamin concentrations in blood plasma and milk, health, fertility, milk yield, and milk composition were measured. All cows were fed a 100% organic diet containing grass-legume silage, cold-pressed rapeseed cake, peas, cereal grains, and minerals. Blood samples were collected from each cow 3 weeks before expected calving, at calving, 3 weeks, 3 to 5 months, and 7 to 9 months after calving. Colostrum and milk samples 4 days after calving were collected, and simultaneously, 3 blood samplings after calving.

The only difference in vitamin status between these groups was found in colostrum in year 1, when CON cows tended to have a higher concentration of α-tocopherol, and their β-carotene concentration was higher than NSV cows. The NSV cows tended to have more cases of mastitis than CON cows in year 2. Within the NSV group, fewer cows were healthy, and more cases of mastitis were observed in year 2 than in year 1. The groups did not differ in production parameters. In conclusion, the vitamin status in the blood and milk of the studied cows indicated that cows in organic dairy production can fulfill their requirements of vitamins A and E without any supplementation of synthetic vitamins, except at the time around calving, when the requirements are high. However, the impaired health of NSV cows in year 2 may indicate a long-term negative health effect in cows fed no synthetic vitamins (Johansson et al., 2014).

Vitamin K

Vitamin K includes a group of quinones that have antihemorrhagic effects. The most common isomers are polyquinones (K_1), menaquinones (K_2), and menadione (K_3). Plant chloroplasts are an essential source of vitamin K_1, bacteria provide a substantial amount of vitamin K_2, and vitamin K_3 is a synthetic isomer used as a feed additive. Cows need vitamin K to synthesize a series of coagulation factors and to activate thrombin in the coagulation process (Combs, 2022). Under normal production conditions, good health, and functional rumen, vitamin K deficiency seldom occurs, as the ruminal bacteria synthesize enough vitamin K to cover requirements (McDowell, 2006). Deficiency is only described in situations where anticoagulant substances have been consumed, as may occur with the consumption of forage contaminated with dicumarol of fungal origin. The toxicity of vitamin K has not been studied in cattle.

For suckling calves, recently dsm-firmenich (2022b) suggested supplementation of 1–1.5 mg/kg DM. Both NRC (2001) and NASEM (2021) did not provide any supplementation considering adequate the intestinal microbial synthesis (Nestor and Conrad, 1990) (Table 6.1a).

There are no recommendations for vitamin K for heifers and dry and lactating cows. Lastly, it is essential to remember that, as with other fat-soluble vitamins, ruminal synthesis, and consequently, the intestinal availability of vitamin K can be negatively affected by the presence of oxidized fats in the ration or when there are problems with fat absorption (McDowell, 2006).

Recently, vitamin K supplementation has received more attention. Bai et al. (2021) evaluated the effects of supplementing vitamin K_3 (50 or 200 mg/day) to Holstein dairy cows. Results indicated that the molar ratio of propionate in ruminal fluid was significantly increased on feeding 200 mg/day vitamin K_3. Additionally, menaquinone 4 (MK-4) concentrations significantly increased in plasma and milk after vitamin K_3 feeding. In ruminal fluid, MK-4 concentrations increased after 200 mg/day of vitamin K_3 feeding. These results suggest that vitamin K_3 may be a good source of MK-4, the biologically active form of vitamin K, in Holstein dairy cows during their late lactation periods. This study provides a basis for understanding the physiological role of vitamin K in dairy cows.

Kuroiwa et al. (2022) examined the effects of dietary vitamin K_3 supplementation on immune-related substances in milk, oxidative stress indices in plasma and Vitamin K_1, and MK-4 in plasma and milk in periparturient dairy cows. Forty healthy perinatal Holstein-Friesian dairy cows were used in this study. Twenty-one animals were randomly selected and categorized into the vitamin K_3 supplemented (50 mg/day/head as vitamin K_3) group; the remaining 19 were categorized into the control group. Blood and milk were sampled on day 3 after calving, and their chemical components were determined. The vitamin K_3-supplemented group had significantly higher MK-4 levels in plasma and milk on day 3 postpartum than the control group. In addition, there was a significant increase in the immunoglobulin G (IgG) level in milk. Vitamin K_3 may be absorbed from the gastrointestinal tract and converted to MK-4, the biologically active form of vitamin K_3, in the MG and other tissues. It was thought that the increase in MK-4 level in plasma and milk induced an increase in the concentration of IgG in milk. Vitamin K_3 supplementation to periparturient dairy cows may contribute to the production of colostrum with high concentrations of IgG and MK-4 (Kuroiwa et al., 2022).

WATER-SOLUBLE VITAMINS

In ruminants, the B vitamin supply not only depends on vitamin intake, but also on microbial synthesis in the rumen and intestines, the ruminal degradation due to fermentation, and final amounts available in the duodenum. Therefore they have been traditionally considered non-essential for cattle mostly because of the contribution of synthesis by ruminal microorganisms. Erdman (1992) produced some estimates using published data that correlated animal requirements with live weight (estimated using data collected from pigs; NRC, 1987), milk production (according to the concentration of the vitamins in milk), vitamin synthesis in the rumen, and food supplements and their ruminal degradability. Recently Girard and Graulet (2021) reevaluated these calculations using modeling techniques and their estimations are presented in Tables 6.10 and 6.11.

Vitamin intake of B vitamins is very variable since vitamin concentration in forages varies due to many factors (Table 6.12). The ruminal microbes play an important role in destroying dietary sources and synthesis. The final duodenal flow of B vitamins is the amount available to the cow (Table 6.10). Currently, many efforts have been made to estimate these values, but it is still under development (Robinson, 2019; Girard and Graulet, 2021).

Table 6.10 Daily intake, duodenal flow, and apparent ruminal synthesis (ARS) or degradation of B vitamins in lactating dairy cows (minimum and maximum) (source: Girard and Graulet, 2021)

Vitamin	Intake (mg)	Duodenal flow (mg)	Apparent ruminal synthesis or degradation (mg)
B_1	25 to 72	15–75	−35–39
B_2[a]	476–2,350	547–1,729	−1,110–578
Niacin[b]	373–4,434	1,002–3,866	−3,166–2,831
B_6[c]	61–368	18–88	−294–−29
Folic acid	4–24	19–106	9–92
B_{12}	−[d]	3–24	3–24

Notes: [a]Sum of riboflavin and flavin adenine dinucleotide.
[b]Sum of nicotinic acid and nicotinamide.
[c]Sum of pyridoxal/pyridoxal-5-phosphate, pyridoxine, and pyridoxamine.
[d]Under the limit of detection.

Table 6.11 B vitamin concentrations (mg/kg DM) in some feed ingredients of dairy cow diets (source: Girard and Graulet, 2021)

Ingredients	Vitamin B_1	Vitamin B_1[a]	Niacin[b]	Vitamin B_6[c]	Folic acid
Alfalfa silage (*n* = 8)					
Mean	1.6	90	119	11	0.38
Range	0.4–2.8	50–148	21–291	4–24	0.21–0.57
Orchard grass silage (*n* = 6)					
Mean	1.5	99	75	12	0.55
Range	1.0–2.4	43–172	52–93	3–19	0.21–1.45
Corn silage (*n* = 4)					
Mean	1	52	98	11	0.08
Range	0.6–1.4	33–73	8–204	7–17	0.05–0.1
Corn (*n* = 9)					
Mean	3.5	10	22	2.9	0.14
Range	2.8–4.1	5–16	13–30	2.3–3.9	0.08–0.25
Soybean meal[d] (*n* = 10)					
Mean	2.3	26	45	3.4	1.9
Range	1.2–4.7	11–43	31–58	2.1–5.7	1.2–3.3
Soy Pluse (*n* = 8)					
Mean	1.1	34	90	3.1	2.3
Range	0.5–1.8	19–43	25–173	1.4–5.7	1.0–4.7

Notes: [a]Sum of riboflavin and flavin adenine dinucleotide.
[b]Sum of nicotinic acid and nicotinamide.
[c]Sum of pyridoxal/pyridoxal-5-phosphate, pyridoxine, and pyridoxamine.
[d]Solvent extracted.
[e]Mechanical expeller process.

Table 6.12 The concentration of B complex vitamins in cattle diets and typical vitamin intake in dairy cattle[1] (source: adapted from Weiss, 2007, who in turn used data supplied by Santschi *et al.*, 2005a,b; Schwab *et al.*, 2006)

Vitamins	Average concentration (mg/kg DM)	Range of variation in concentration (mg/kg MS)	Average intake (mg/day)
Thiamine	2	1.5–2.6	45
Riboflavin	5.4	4.3–6.7	123
Niacin total	46	22.6–94.8	1,045
Vitamin B$_6$	5.2	3.2–8.5	118
Total folates	0.5	0.4–0.7	11
Biotin	6.9	6.3–7.8	157
Biotin	0.4	0.33–0.41	8

[1] Based on average ingestion of 22.7 kg/day.

Erdman (1992) information suggested that the intake of most vitamins is sufficient to meet requirements. However, the calculations indicated that folic acid, pantothenic acid, and choline supplies may not cover requirements, so supplementation is recommended. On the other hand, when the rumen is not functioning fully, as in the case of pre-ruminant calves and abnormal ruminal situations (acidosis, indigestion, reduced intake, etc.), the intake of water-soluble vitamins may be a limiting factor. Girard and Graulet (2021) concluded that the positive production and metabolic responses to B vitamin supplements given to dairy cows, especially during the transition period and in early lactation, are indicative of subclinical deficiency. However, there is a need to build a substantial database to predict B vitamin supply including numerous feed ingredients and forages. There is also a need to identification and validation of biomarkers to rapidly assess B vitamin status of dairy cows. There are very few data on concentrations of pantothenic acid and inositol concentrations in feed ingredients and digesta.

There is a growing interest in knowing the actual requirements and how these vitamins affect the production and health of cows. There is also interest in the development of a method of improving the supply of these vitamins in milk and dairy products (Cooke *et al.*, 2007; Ferreira and Weiss, 2007; Enjalbert *et al.*, 2008; Girard and Matte, 2005a,b; Drackley *et al.*, 2006; Swensson and Lindmark-Månsson, 2007; Baldi *et al.*, 2008; Ashwin *et al.*, 2018).

The NASEM (2021) recognized that biotin, niacin, and vitamin B$_{12}$ could be considered in diet formulation for dairy cows. Additionally, high-yield dairy cows may benefit from B vitamin supplementation. Increasing their concentrations in colostrum and milk may benefit calf health and human consumers of dairy products.

Data were obtained from bibliographical sources, with analytical methods different from the rest (Zinn *et al.*, 1987; Frigg *et al.*, 1993; Midla *et al.*, 1998).

Biotin (vitamin B$_7$)

Biotin is a vitamin of the B complex considered essential for ruminants. Biotin acts as a cofactor of various enzymes that catalyze carboxylation reactions and other metabolic routes directly related to milk synthesis in the MG so that its supplementation can improve the adequate response in high-production dairy cattle (Weiss, 2005, 2007; Chen *et al.*, 2011). Ruminal bacteria synthesize substantial amounts of biotin depending on the availability of energy

(0.79 mg/kg digestible organic material; Zinn, 1992), although other data suggest that this synthesis is reduced when the amount of concentrate in the ration increases (Da Costa Gomez et al., 1998), and it has been suggested that this effect is associated with the fall in the cellulolytic microbial population which occurs when ruminal pH falls. Biotin does not degrade largely in the rumen, and oral supplementation almost always increases the biotin flow to the duodenum and its concentration in plasma and milk (Frigg et al., 1993; Midla et al., 1998).

Recommendations for biotin

Suckling calves

NRC (2001) and NASEM (2021) recommended supplementing milk replacers with 0.1 mg of biotin/kg DM. The recent OVN™ (dsm-firmenich, 2022b) recommends 0.05–0.1 mg/kg DM (Table 6.1a).

Growing calves and heifers

Both NRC (2001) and NASEM (2021) did not recommend supplementing the diet of these ruminant categories with biotin. Only dsm-firmenich (2022b) in its OVN™ suggested supplementation with 10–20 mg/head day in growing heifers and 20 mg/head day in pre-calving heifers (Table 6.5).

Dry and lactating cows

Estimates of requirements and supplies carried out by Erdman (1992) indicate that, under normal conditions, the supplies are sufficient to cover the requirements of cows in production. NRC (2001), NASEM (2021), and INRA (1988; 2018) did not indicate any supplementation, whereas OVN™ (dsm-firmenich, 2022b) suggests a supplementation of 20–40 mg/kg feed (Tables 6.6 and 6.7).

Some studies indicate that biotin deficiency is related to the development of laminitis in dairy cattle (Distl and Schmid, 1994; Bergsten et al., 1999; Campbell et al., 2000; Fitzgerald et al., 2000; Seymour, 2000; Hedges et al., 2001; Pötzsch et al., 2003; Margerison et al., 2003; Tomlinson et al., 2004; Franco da Silva et al., 2010) because there appears to be a relationship between high levels of biotin in the plasma and the hardness of hooves and an increase in milk production (McDowell, 2004). Thus, many studies indicated that supplementing 20 mg/day of biotin improves hoof health (Midla et al., 1998; Bergsten et al., 1999, 2003; Fitzgerald et al., 2000). Figure 6.11 shows the difference in cows with and without supplementation observed with lameness for 2 years. Hedges et al. (2001) supplemented 20 mg/day of biotin for 18 months in 5 commercial herds in which the average incidence of laminitis was 69%. In 2 herds, biotin supplements reduced the incidence of laminitis by half. Lischer et al. (2002) supplemented 40 mg/day of biotin for only 50 days and in the biotin-treated animals, the newly formed epidermis covering the sole ulcers was found to be of significantly better histological quality after 50 days than at the start of the study. The significant improvement in histological horn quality found in the biotin-treated animals suggests that biotin exerts a positive influence on the healing of sole ulcers. However the study period of 50 days appears to have been too short to permit macroscopic detection of the improvement in horn quality. Pötzsch et al. (2003), using 20 mg/day, also obtained similar results in reducing lameness and recommended supplementing cows over long periods (>6 months) to achieve an effective reduction in the risk of the occurrence of these problems.

Some authors have observed that milk production increased by between 1.0 kg/day (Midla et al., 1998) and 2.9 kg/day (Bergsten et al., 1999) in response to biotin supplementation. Zimmerly and Weiss (2001) supplemented the cows' rations in production with biotin (10 or 20 mg/day) from 2 weeks prepartum to 100 days of lactation. Milk production increased from 36.9 kg/day in the control group to 37.8 and 39.7 kg/day, respectively, with biotin supplements.

Concentration in plasma, milk, and colostrum also increased with the supplement. Several studies confirm the importance of the supplementary supply of biotin for dairy cattle. The production of milk or its main components is not always improved by supplementary biotin because the response may be affected by various factors such as the composition of the diet, the state of lactation, and the status of biotin in the cow (Ferreira *et al.*, 2007).

Other results suggest that supplementation with biotin reduces the occurrence of fatty liver syndrome in high-producing dairy cattle. This effect has been associated with reduced non-esterified fatty acids in the blood, the concentration of lipids in the liver, and increased blood glucose levels (Rosendo *et al.*, 2004, 2010; Ferreira and Weiss, 2007). This effect may be because supplementation with biotin favors gluconeogenesis (Rosendo *et al.*, 2004) and lipolysis (Enjalbert *et al.*, 2008) in the liver. However, biotin supplementation did not affect fiber digestibility (Rosendo *et al.*, 2003).

Lean and Rabiee (2011) reviewed 9 publications describing randomized controlled trials to evaluate the effectiveness of biotin supplementation on milk yield and its composition and hoof health in lactating dairy cows, explored sources of heterogeneity among studies, and evaluated publication bias. Biotin increased milk production by 1.29 kg/head/day (95% confidence interval = 0.35 to 2.18 kg) with no evidence of heterogeneity (I2 = 0.0%). Treatment did not affect milk fat or protein percentages, and a trend to increase fat and protein yields was observed. The duration of treatment before calving, parity, or diet type did not affect milk production and composition results. Assessment of biotin supplementation on hoof health indicated that more studies had improved rather than negative or neutral outcomes.

Ferreira *et al.* (2015) hypothesized that pantothenic acid reduces the absorption of biotin in lactating dairy cows. Therefore, they conducted a study to evaluate the plausible interaction between biotin and pantothenic acid on production performance and concentration of

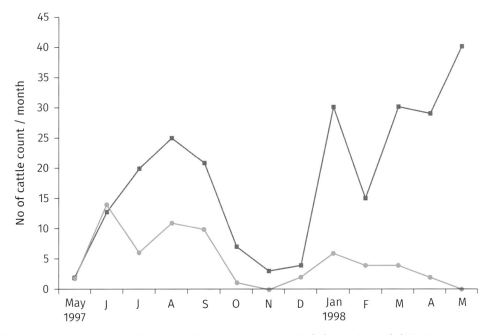

Figure 6.11 Reported monthly incidence of lameness in cattle with (●) and without (■) biotin supplementation (source: Fitzgerald *et al.*, 2000)

avidin-binding substances (ABS), an indicator of biotin concentration, in the blood and milk of lactating dairy cows. Eight primiparous and 16 multiparous Holstein cows were assigned to 1 of 4 diet sequences in a replicated 4 × 4 Latin square design with 18 day periods. Treatments consisted of a control diet that contained no B vitamins, a biotin diet that contained 0.87 mg of biotin per kg DM, a pantothenic acid diet that contained 21 mg of pantothenic acid per kg DM, and a biotin plus pantothenic acid diet that contained 0.87 mg of biotin and 21 mg of calcium pantothenic acid per kg DM. The supplementation of pantothenic acid did not affect the concentration of ABS in plasma when either supplemented alone or in combination with biotin. Biotin supplementation increased the concentration of ABS in milk relative to control. When cows were supplemented with biotin and pantothenic acid, the concentration of ABS in milk was like that of cows supplemented with biotin alone.

Folic acid (vitamin B$_9$)

Folic acid is essential in synthesizing purines and pyrimidines and forms part of the enzymes involved in transferring methyl groups (Girard and Matte, 2005b). Methionine may also act as a methyl group donor, so folic acid reduces the need to use methionine for this purpose. A folic acid deficiency can be critical for cell division and protein metabolism (Mason, 2003; Girard and Matte, 2005a). Several studies have been conducted to evaluate the effect of folic acid supplementation together with vitamin B$_{12}$ on dairy cattle's productive responses, especially during early lactation (Weiss and Fereira, 2006a, b; Girard and Duplessis, 2022). However, there is insufficient evidence to date to determine the exact requirements and make recommendations for its use in practical conditions.

Most dietary folic acid (approximately 97%) is degraded in the rumen (Zinn, 1992; Santschi *et al.*, 2005a). On the other hand, a significant amount of folic acid is synthesized in the rumen depending on the availability of energy (0.42 mg/kg of digestible organic material; Zinn, 1992). The synthesis and degradation of folic acid in the rumen, in turn, determines the quantity available to be absorbed in the small intestine of the ruminant. Few studies have estimated this vitamin's synthesis and degradation, so there are no bioavailability values for the folic acid in ruminant feed ingredients (Ragaller *et al.*, 2008). The apparent intestinal absorption of folic acid seems very low, probably due to interaction with bile secretions (Santschi *et al.*, 2005a).

Recommendations for folic acid

Suckling calves

NRC (2001) and NASEM (2021) recommended supplementing milk replacers with 0.5 mg of folic acid/kg DM and in the recent OVN™ dsm-firmenich (2022b) recommended 0.2–0.3 mg/kg DM (Table 6.1a).

Growing calves and heifers

None of the academic and industrial sources recommended supplementing the diet of these ruminant categories with folic acid.

Dry and lactating cows

There are no recommendations for supplementing cow's diets with folic acid. Until recently, the published data indicated that the amount of folic acid provided in the basal ration and synthesized in the rumen was sufficient to prevent deficiency symptoms in cows (Girard *et al.*, 1995). However, this estimate is different from that of Erdman (1992), which suggests that supplementing this vitamin could increase productive efficiency. Other studies support this hypothesis (Girard and Matte, 2005b; Drackley *et al.*, 2006; Graulet *et al.*, 2007). Nevertheless, due to the high ruminal degradation, oral supplementation would only be justified if protection against ruminal degradation were developed.

In pre-ruminant calves, poor bacterial synthesis may lead to deficiency. Daily injection of 40 mg of folic acid between weeks 1 and 16 of life increased average weight gain by 8%. In adult cows, parenteral supplementation of 160 mg folic acid each week from 45 days of gestation to 6 weeks postpartum tended to increase milk yield and milk protein production during the second half of lactation in primiparous and in multiparous cows (Girard et al., 1995). In the postpartum period, the protein content of milk increased during the first 6 weeks in multiparous animals. Girard and Matte (1998) observed a linear increase in milk production when supplementing rations with 0.2 and 4 mg of folic acid/kg LW. The plasma concentration of folic acid also showed a linear increase, which suggests that at least a part of the folic acid escapes rumen degradation. The observed responses may be a direct effect of folic acid or an indirect effect due to the reduction in the use of methionine as a methyl donor.

Supplementation with folic acid (dose between 2 and 3 g/day) results in variable responses in milk production and composition and DMI. Girard and coworkers have explored the effects of vitamin B_{12}, folic acid, and methionine metabolism in lactating dairy cows for several years and multiple experiments (Girard and Matte, 1998; Girard and Matte, 2005a; Preynat et al., 2009; 2010; Girard et al., 2009). After observing an inverse relationship between serum vitamin B_{12} and folate concentrations during lactation, Girard and Matte (1998) conducted an experiment in which primiparous heifers were fed a diet supplemented with both folic acid and methionine and injected with either vitamin B_{12} or a placebo. In this preliminary trial, vitamin B_{12} supplementation tended to increase milk production (8.8%), milk solids production (12%), and milk fat yield (16%), suggesting that vitamin B_{12} status may affect the response of lactating cows to folic acid and methionine supplementation.

Separate previous findings (Girard and Matte, 1998; 2005a; Girard et al., 2005) showed that, in early lactation, a positive response of milk production and milk component yields to supplementary folic acid was observed in cows with higher plasma concentrations of vitamin B_{12}. Graulet et al. (2007) evaluated the effect of folic acid (0 vs. 2.6 g/day) and vitamin B_{12} (0 vs. 0.5 g/day) from the third prepartum week to 8 weeks postpartum. In this case, supplementation with folic acid increased the production of milk (+5.8%), fat (+16.2%), and protein (+3.3%).

When folic acid was given in combination with vitamin B_{12}, metabolic efficiency was improved, as suggested by similar lactational performance and DMI over cows fed folic acid supplements alone. The effects of folic acid and vitamin B_{12} on lactation performance were not mainly explained by methionine economy because of a more efficient methyl neogenesis but were rather related to increased glucose availability and changes in methionine metabolism (Preynat et al., 2009; 2010). These findings support the hypothesis that, in early lactation, the supply of vitamin B_{12} was not optimal and limited the lactation performance of the cows. Girard et al. (2019) demonstrated that the supplementation of both folic acid (320 mg) and vitamin B_{12} (10 mg) improved insulin sensitivity in feed-restricted lactating dairy cows.

In recent studies, Liu et al. (2021) investigated the effect of cobalt and folic acid on growth performance and rumen fermentation in Holstein male calves. Forty animals were randomly assigned to 4 groups according to their BW. Cobalt sulfate at 0 or 0.11 mg Co/kg DM and folic acid at 0 or 7.2 mg/kg DM were used in a 2 × 2 factorial design. The average daily gain was improved with folic acid or cobalt supplementation, but the effect was more significant for supplementing cobalt in diets without folic acid than with folic acid. Supplementing folic acid or cobalt increased DM intake and total-tract nutrient digestibility. Rumen pH was unaltered with folic acid but reduced with cobalt supplementation. The rumen's total volatile fatty acids concentration was increased with folic acid or cobalt inclusion. Acetate percentage and acetate to propionate ratio were augmented with folic acid inclusion. Supplementing cobalt decreased the acetate percentage and increased the propionate percentage. Activities of xylanase and α-amylase and total bacteria, fungi, protozoa, *Ruminococcus albus*, *Fibrobacter succinogenes,* and *Prevotella ruminicola* increased with folic acid or cobalt inclusion. Activities of carboxymethyl-cellulase and pectinase increased with folic acid inclusion, and the population of methanogens decreased with cobalt addition. Blood folates increased, and homocysteine decreased with folic acid inclusion. Blood glucose and vitamin B_{12} increased with cobalt addition. The data suggested that supplementing 0.11 mg cobalt/kg DM in diets containing 0.09 mg cobalt/kg DM increased growth performance and nutrient digestibility but did not improve the effects of folic acid addition in calves.

Li *et al.* (2016) evaluated the effects of rumen-protected folic acid (RPFA) dietary supplements on lactation performance, energy balance, reproductive performance, and blood parameters of dairy cows. Ninety-six multiparous Holstein cows were assigned to 4 groups of 24 each according to their previous 305 day milk production. The treatments were: control (0), low (1) RPFA (LRPFA), medium (2) RPFA (MRPFA), and high (3) RPFA (HRPFA) with 0–3 g RPFA/cow per day, respectively. Supplements of RPFA were top-dressed and manually mixed into the upper one-third of the ration during the morning feeding from 3 weeks before the expected calving date to 15 weeks after parturition. The results indicated (Table 6.13) that supplementary RPFA in cow diets positively affected feed intake and milk production, increased plasma glucose and serum folate concentrations, decreased plasma concentrations of non-esterified fatty acids, β-hydroxybutyrate, and serum concentration of homocysteine, and improved energy balance and reproductive performance. These data suggest that RPFA improved lactation, energy balance, and reproductive performance in a dose-dependent manner.

The perinatal period is critical in dairy cattle due to negative energy balance and high milk production stress. Folic acid could play a critical role in milk production in the biosynthesis and methylation cycle, as it was reviewed by Khan *et al.* (2020a). Khan *et al.* (2020b) conducted a study to evaluate the effect of folic acid supplementation on milk production in periparturient cows. In this study, 123 cows having similar parity, weight, and expected date of calving were randomly selected and divided into 3 groups: A (n = 41, folic acid 240 mg/500 kg cow BW/day), B (n = 40, FA 120 mg/500 kg cow BW/day) and C (control, n = 42). Folic acid was supplemented for 21 days (14 days pre- and 7 days post-calving), and 3 samples of blood lymphocytes were taken on day 7 post-calving from each folic acid-treated and control group. In addition,

Table 6.13 Effects of rumen-protected folic acid supplementation on dry matter intake, milk yield, and milk components (source: Li *et al.*, 2016)

Item	Rumen-protected folic acid (g)				SEM	P-value
	0	1	2	3		
Intake						
Dry matter (kg/day	18.7	19.3	20	20.3	0.57	0.045
NE (MJ/day)	127	131	135	137	0.96	0.036
Milk production (kg/day)						
Actual	30.6	31.3	31.9	32.1	1.47	0.019
4% FCM	27.8	28.5	29.2	29.5	1.35	0.021
Milk protein	0.99	1.02	1.07	1.09	0.036	0.037

the milk samples for each folic acid-treated group were collected during the 2nd, 3rd, and 4th months of lactation. The transcriptomic analysis revealed that folic acid treatment regulated many essential metabolic-related genes (DGAT2, ALOX5, LAP3, GPAT3, GGH, ALDOA, TKT) and pathways (glycolysis, folate biosynthesis, glutathione metabolism, etc.) in periparturient dairy cattle. It was concluded that 120 mg/500 kg cow BW of folic acid could be considered a standard during the periparturient period to enhance the milk production performance of dairy cows. The transcriptomic profile revealed several metabolic and milk production-associated genes, which could be a helpful addition to the marker selection for enhancing the metabolism and milk production of periparturient dairy cows.

Khan *et al.* (2020c) reported the transcriptomic profile of blood lymphocytes of Chinese Holstein cows supplemented orally with coated folic acid during the periparturient period. The data suggested that the low folic acid supplementation (120 mg/500 kg cow BW) could be an excellent choice to boost appropriate immunity and anti-inflammation and might be applied to the health improvement of perinatal dairy cows. The analysis revealed that more genes and pathways were regulated in response to high and low folic acid supplementation than controls. Khan *et al.* (2022) also reviewed the combined effects of folic acid with vitamin E and selenium on alleviating bovine mastitis during the periparturient period.

Niacin (vitamin B$_3$)
Introduction
Niacin is an active component of 2 coenzymes (NAD and NADP), which are fundamental in metabolizing carbohydrates, lipids, and amino acids (Pires and Grummer, 2007). This water-soluble vitamin may be formed in the liver from tryptophan and is found in 2 forms: nicotinic acid and nicotinamide. Both compounds have similar nutritional properties and can be used interchangeably to synthesize NAD. Still, they are metabolized by different routes and have different properties when administered at supra-physiological levels (Carlson, 2005). As a vitamin from the B complex, niacin is widely available in products and by-products of animal origin and cereals.

Bioavailability
The flow of niacin to the duodenum is generally greater than niacin intake when rations are not supplemented, indicating that ruminal bacteria synthesize it abundantly (Zinn *et al.*, 1987). Zinn (1992) estimated that niacin synthesis in the rumen was 107.02 mg/kg of digestible organic material. However, when niacin is added to the ration, the quantity that reaches the intestine may be even less than that provided in the ration due to the inhibition of bacterial synthesis in the presence of exogenous niacin (Abdouli and Schaefer, 1986). While one review estimated that between 94 and 99% of niacin present in the diet is degraded in the rumen (Zinn, 1992), other studies have found that between 17 and 30% of dietary niacin reaches the small intestine (Bartley *et al.*, 1979; Harmeyer and Kollenkirchen, 1989; Campbell *et al.*, 1994).

The study of the nutritional effects on the animal of supplying niacin is complicated, given the capacity of ruminants to synthesize niacin from tryptophan (with adequate levels of vitamin B$_6$ and riboflavin) and its high ruminal degradation, which determines the necessity of using protected sources (Seymour, 2004).

Recommendations for niacin
Suckling calves
Niacin is required in calf rations before weaning because microbial synthesis in the rumen is limited. Hopper and Johnson (1955) observed that calves fed with milk replacers deficient in niacin presented with diarrhea within 48 hours. There was an immediate improvement the

day after administering an oral dose of 6 mg/day or an intramuscular dose of 10 mg/day of nicotinic acid. Both the NRC (2001) and the NASEM (2021) recommended the incorporation of 10 mg of niacin per kg DM in milk replacers, whereas the supplementation proposed by dsm-firmenich (2022b) is 9 to 18 mg/kg (Table 6.1a).

Growing calves and heifers

The NRC (2001) and the NASEM (2021) did not recommend any supplementation with niacin during these phases. On the other hand, dsm-firmenich (2022b) proposed including 6 to 12 g/head per day in heifers' diet during the period 4 to 6 weeks pre-calving (Table 6.5).

Dry and lactating cows

The NRC (1989; 2001), NASEM (2021), and INRA (1988; 2018) have not established recommendations for niacin. However, they recognize that supplementing adult cows with 6–12 g/day from prepartum to the peak of lactation has resulted in some positive effects. This supplementation results in increased milk production, often also raising the fat and protein content. It has also been found to prevent ketosis and fatty liver (Schwab et al., 2005). In this line, dsm-firmenich (2022b) proposed supplementing cow's diet both during dry and lactation phases with 6–12 g/head/day (Tables 6.6 and 6.7).

Ridell et al. (1981, 1989) reported improved microbial protein synthesis and milk production during early lactation. Niacin increased the rumen bacterial protein, ammonia, and propionic acid concentrations. It reduced the concentration of urea nitrogen, but there were no differences in the amino acid composition of rumen bacteria. In contrast, Kung et al. (1980) and Horner et al. (1986, 1988) observed that including niacin (3, 6, or 12 g in 20.5 kg DM) accompanied by whole cottonseed in the ration of Holstein cows in lactation affected neither the ruminal pH nor the ammonia-N concentration. Fat and protein content in milk tended to fall, although total fat and milk production was more outstanding with the addition of 12 g of niacin/head/day.

Drackley (1992) summarized a set of 23 studies and concluded that supplementation of niacin resulted in a slight increase in average milk production (+0.62 kg/day) and in fat content (+0.033 g/l) and protein content (+0.002 g/l). Most negative responses occurred when the basal ration contained supplemental fat (Drackley, 1992). Erdman (1992) compared 29 published studies and calculated an average rise in milk production of 0.3 kg/day without effects on fat and protein composition. However, when the results were broken down according to lactational status, the average increase in animal production in early lactation was 0.4 kg/day, a value close to that obtained by Drackley (1992). In 3 studies carried out on commercial farms in which supplements of 6 g/day of niacin were given, the responses were inconsistent, from an absence of improvements (Jaster et al., 1983) to an increase in 1 kg/day during the first 70 days of lactation (Bartlett et al., 1983) or 0.9 kg/day during the first 90 days postpartum (Muller et al., 1986). The response observed in high-yielding cows was more significant than the production response in less productive animals.

More recently, Schwab et al. (2005) analyzed the published data from 27 studies related to the effect of supplementation with nicotinic acid in dairy cattle. The authors conclude that a response to the supplementation is achieved with 6–12 g/day, with small positive changes in milk production (0.4 kg/day) and moderate fat and protein content increases.

However, it is not clear that the response justifies the cost entailed by supplementation throughout lactation, and in any case, its use is recommended during the peripartum period. In other cases, high doses of nicotinic acid (48 g/day) over 30 days prepartum reduced the levels of non-esterified fatty acids in plasma and the fall in DMI the week before parturition

(French, 2004). However, a subsequent study conducted by the same group of investigators could not replicate these effects (Chamberlain and French, 2006). Pires and Grummer (2007) infused nicotinic acid post-ruminally (between 0 and 60 mg/kg BW). They observed a fall in the concentration of non-esterified fatty acids in the blood, which coincided with an increase in insulin concentration and a slight effect on glucose concentration in the blood. The authors concluded that supplementation with nicotinic acid could be beneficial in regulating non-esterified fatty acids and preventing problems related to lipid metabolism during the transition stage in high-yielding dairy cows. Driver *et al.* (1990) observed with high-yielding cows in early lactation that the percentage of milk protein was more significant when heat-treated soy was supplemented with niacin (6 g/day), suggesting that niacin ameliorated the drop in milk protein, which is frequently associated with the supply of large quantities of fat in the ration. Furthermore, niacin tended to reduce the blood plasma concentration of non-esterified fatty acids. Zimmerman *et al.* (1992) also reported that supplementation with 12 g/day of niacin interacted with dietary crude protein in multiparous cows, increasing blood glucose, decreasing blood β-hydroxybutyrate, and non-esterified fatty acid concentration with the high crude protein and normal fiber diet. However, Campbell *et al.* (1994) observed no benefits when supplementing rations with niacin or nicotinamide, although the apparent digestibility of most of the nutrients increased.

Kung *et al.* (1980) obtained favorable results when supplementing niacin (6 g/day) in early lactation. As well as the production responses, niacin has been used to prevent ketosis and fatty liver through its antilipolytic action (Fronk and Schultz, 1979; Waterman *et al.*, 1972; Jaster *et al.*, 1983). Erickson *et al.* (1992) observed in cows in early lactation that supplementing with 12 g of niacin/head day increased the levels of methionine and phenylalanine produced in the MG content and the total protein production in milk. These results agree with Lanham *et al.* (1992), who observed an increase in casein synthesis following supplementation of the ration with niacin at the beginning of lactation. In 14 experimental studies in which niacin was supplemented (NRC, 2001), non-esterified fatty acids in plasma were reduced in only 1 study, increased in 2, and did not change in the others.

The results from these experiments are contradictory. While the NASEM (2021) concludes that no evidence supports clear recommendations on niacin requirements, the production response has sometimes been significant. In these cases, the best responses are produced by supplementing 6 g of niacin per animal per day from the period just before parturition and during early lactation (up to 12 weeks) based on improved production and composition of milk and a reduced risk of ketosis. When symptoms of ketosis are apparent, supplementation with between 20 and 50 g of niacin per cow every 2 hours reduces the likelihood of a sudden fall in yield. It improves normal plasma levels of free fatty acids, β-hydroxy-butyrate, glucose, and insulin.

In a literature review, Mishra *et al.* (2018) reported that niacin supplementation during heat stress in dairy animals leads to inconsistent results as observed by Rungruang *et al.* (2014), who concluded that encapsulated niacin did not improve thermotolerance of winter-acclimated lactating dairy cows exposed to moderate thermal stress in Arizona. The doses Mishra *et al.*(2018) reviewed were between 6 to 36 g/day. Therefore, it is still impossible to define the dose and effect of niacin during the heat stress period. However, it was evident that supplementation of niacin is beneficial in postpartum dairy animals under heat stress and negative energy balance, but economics need to be taken into consideration. Specific knowledge gaps need to be resolved by conducting more trials with this vitamin during hot weather regarding production and digestibility. Khan *et al.* (2018) investigated the effect of different levels of niacin supplementation (0, 600, and 800 mg/kg) on physiological

Table 6.14 Effect of niacin supplementation on levels of plasma cortisol, SOD, catalase, glucose, urea, and NEFA in lactating crossbred cows (source: adapted from Khan *et al.*, 2018). Different superscript letters on the line indicate significant difference (*P* < 0.05)

	Niacin supplementation (mg/kg)		
	0	600	800
Cortisol (ng/ml)	$4.83^x \pm 0.17$	$4.59^{xy} \pm 0.18$	$4.34^y \pm 0.13$
SOD (U/ml)	$3.28^y \pm 0.05$	$3.08^x \pm 0.05$	$3.05^x \pm 0.06$
Catalase (nmol/min/ml)	$51.27^y \pm 1.15$	$48.97^x \pm 0.85$	$48.93^x \pm 0.89$
Glucose (mg/dl)	46.74 ± 0.70	47.00 ± 0.72	48.07 ± 0.69
Urea (mg/dl)	$24.90^x \pm 0.42$	$25.37^x \pm 0.49$	$26.59^y \pm 0.40$
NEFA (µmol/l)	$365.98^y \pm 9.07$	$345.63^x \pm 8.38$	$345.17^x \pm 9.21$

Note: [x,y]Different superscript letters on the line indicate significant difference (*P* < 0.05).

and blood biochemical parameters during the heat stress period (April to August; 120 days), 18 crossbred early lactating cows (2nd to 4th lactation; 11.56 ± 1.74 days-in milk). They concluded that 800 mg/kg niacin supplementation to lactating crossbred cows resulted in better stress alleviation, as the improved biomarker values indicated. SOD, catalase, cortisol, and skin temperature (Table 6.14).

Recently, Petrović *et al.* (2020) conducted a study to determine the influence of niacin application on inflammatory response and functional status of the liver (expressed with liver functional index, LFI) in cows in early lactation. Thirty Holstein-Friesian cows were included in the experiment. Niacin was applied to 15 cows 2 weeks before and 2 weeks after calving, and 15 cows were included in the negative control group. Fine granular powder of

Table 6.15 Influence of niacin application on inflammatory parameters on the liver of dairy cows during early lactation (source: Petrović *et al.*, 2020)

	Week	Niacin	Control	SEM	*P*-value
TNF-α (ng/ml)	0	0.24	0.39	0.004	0.01
	1	0.28	0.52		
	2	0.27	0.61		
Haptoglobin (mg/dl)	0	0.39	0.76	0.012	0.01
	1	0.44	0.82		
	2	0.47	0.89		
Albumin (g/l)	0	39.1	32.2	0.42	0.01
	1	37.82	31.5		
	2	38.9	33.6		
Total bilirubin (mol/l)	0	6.8	8.1	0.21	0.01
	1	7.2	9.5		
	2	8.1	10.2		

nicotinic acid was used at a dosage that allows 6–12 g in the gastrointestinal tract. Dosage was applied daily (60–120 g/day in total mixed ration meal). In recent studies, that dosage was suggested as the optimal biologic concentration. Niacin was applied for 2 weeks before and after calving. In this study, the antilipolytic and anti-inflammatory action of niacin was noted. That is the vital mechanism in liver hepatocyte protection in early lactation. A significant influence of niacin on TNF-α concentration was detected (Table 6.15). This cytokine is correlated with the functional status of liver hepatocytes, lipolysis parameters, and inflammatory response.

Pantothenic acid (vitamin B$_5$)

Pantothenic acid is a constituent of coenzyme A, and it is essential in many reactions, including fatty acid oxidation metabolism, amino acid catabolism, and acetylcholine synthesis. Ruminal microorganisms synthesize between 20 and 30 times more pantothenic acid than the cow requires; hence, supplementation is unnecessary. The rumen degraded 78% of dietary pantothenic acid (Zinn *et al.*, 1987). Erdman (1992) determined, based on maintenance and production requirements calculations and microbial and dietary supplies, that pantothenic acid might be limited under some conditions. Although the estimates of vitamin requirements made in the latest version of the NRC report for dairy cattle do not recommend its supplementation due to a lack of supporting scientific data, it mentions that pantothenic acid could become a limiting factor in high-yielding cows and some supplementation studies have shown positive effects (NASEM, 2021).

Recommendations for pantothenic acid

Suckling calves
Both the NRC (2001) and NASEM (2021) recommended 10 mg/kg, and dsm-firmenich (2022b) proposed a range of 7 to 9 mg/kg (Table 6.1a).

Growing calves, heifers, dry and lactating cows
NASEM (2021) suggested to incorporate 13.0 mg/kg DM in milk replacers. As with other B group vitamins, there are no recommendations on pantothenic acid requirements for adult bovines (INRA, 1988, 2018; NRC, 2001 NASEM, 2021; dsm-firmenich, 2022b). The study conducted by Majee *et al.* (2003) compared the effect of supplementing dairy cattle with biotin (20 *vs.* 40 mg/day) and a mixture of B complex vitamins (thiamine, riboflavin, pyridoxine, niacin, biotin, folic acid, B$_{12}$), which included 475 or 950 mg/day of pantothenic acid, they observed no additional benefit in response to the inclusion of the mixture of B complex vitamins in the diet. As a final recommendation, they noted the need to use vitamin B sources resistant to ruminal degradation. Sacadura *et al.* (2008) conducted 2 experiments to evaluate the effect of a mixture of protected B complex vitamins on dairy cattle production (at the start and mid-point of lactation). The mixture contained biotin, folic acid, and pantothenic acid. The results indicated that supplementation increased production (kg/day) of milk, fat, and protein at the start of lactation. It also improved the general state of the herd (physical condition and locomotion problems) without effects on the DMI. The positive effects of the supplementation were less evident in the case of dairy cattle in mid-lactation. As the supplementation was done with a mixture of vitamins, the beneficial effect cannot be attributed to any one vitamin. The authors suggested that the active mechanism in supplementing the mixture of B complex vitamins contributes to greater efficiency in metabolic function.

Ragaller *et al.* (2011) studied the effect of pantothenic acid on duodenal nutrient flows, blood, and milk variables. In the first experiment of the study, 2 dry and 6 lactating cows received a diet with a forage-to-concentrate (F:C) ratio of 34:66 (high concentrate, HC), whereas in the second experiment, a diet with a F:C ratio of 66:34 (high forage, HF) was fed to 4 dry and 5 lactating cows. The cows received both rations with or without 1 g pantothenic acid/day. By supplementing pantothenic acid to the HC ration, the molar percentage of acetic acid increased, whereas the concentration of total short-chain fatty acids, the efficiency of microbial protein synthesis in the rumen, and the serum glucose levels decreased. With the HF ration, the pantothenic acid decreased the molar percentage of propionic acid and increased the amount of ruminally fermented organic matter. Based on these results, the supplementation with pantothenic acid does not provide any benefits. Ferreira *et al.* (2015) also did not observe the effect of pantothenic acid (21 mg/kg DM) fed alone or in combination with biotin (0.87 mg/kg DM) for 18 days on DM intake and yields of milk or milk components.

Riboflavin (vitamin B$_2$)
Riboflavin is one of the numerous vitamins that participate in intermediary metabolism, especially energy metabolism (Weiss, 2007) and oxidation-reduction reactions (Zempleni *et al.*, 2007). In dairy cattle, no requirements have been established since ruminal microorganisms are presumed to synthesize abundant quantities of this vitamin (15.2 mg/kg of digestible organic material; Zinn, 1992). Furthermore, ruminal degradation is almost total (Zinn *et al.*, 1987; Santschi *et al.*, 2005a), so extra supplies should resist ruminal degradation (Majee *et al.*, 2003; Santschi *et al.*, 2005a). On the other hand, it is estimated that intestinal digestibility is approximately 25% (Miller *et al.*, 1986; Zinn *et al.*, 1987).

Recommendations for riboflavin
Suckling calves
The NRC (2001) and NASEM (2021) recommended the inclusion of 6.5 mg/kg DM in milk replacers whereas dsm-firmenich (2022b), suggested a supplementation of 2.5–4.5 mg/kg DM (Table 6.1a).

Growing calves, heifers, dry and lactating cows
Although the requirements and practical recommendations for the incorporation of riboflavin in the ration of adult cattle have not been established, the data provided by the analyses of Santschi *et al.* (2005a,b) and Schwab *et al.* (2006) indicated that the average intake of riboflavin in dairy cattle fed with a regular diet was 123 mg/day (Table 6.12).

As with the other vitamins of the B complex, the increase in dairy cattle production indicates that the requirements for riboflavin have increased in the same proportion. Furthermore, the only experimental work (Majee *et al.*, 2003) evaluated the effect of incorporating biotin with or without a mixture of B complex vitamins, which supplied 150 or 300 mg/day of riboflavin. Although the supplementation improved animal production in one of the experiments, the benefit cannot be attributed to any one vitamin. Given the limited number of studies and inconsistent results, no practical recommendations for supplementing this vitamin can be made for these phases.

Poulsen *et al.* (2015) realized a study aimed to quantify milk riboflavin content using reverse-phase HPLC in 2 major Danish dairy breeds. Milk from Danish Jersey cows contained significantly higher levels of riboflavin (1.93 mg/l of milk) than Danish Holstein cows (1.40 mg/l of milk). The results showed substantial interbreed differences in milk riboflavin content. They concluded that variation in riboflavin content in milk is mainly related to genetic factors, and SLC52A3, a riboflavin transporter gene, is thought to play a significant role in milk riboflavin regulation. However, more directed studies still need to explore the underlying mechanism.

Thiamine (vitamin B$_1$)

Thiamine is a coenzyme that acts as a cofactor in many reactions of oxidative metabolism of carbohydrates and proteins and as an intermediary in the synthesis of fatty acids (Harmeyer and Kollenkirchen, 1989; Weiss and Fereira, 2006b; Zempleni et al., 2007; EFSA, 2010). The quantity of thiamine synthesized in the rumen (between 28 and 72 mg/day) is the same as or higher than that ingested in the ration (Breves et al., 1981). No requirements have been established for ruminants in good health and with a functional rumen. Supplies from microbial synthesis and dietary thiamine are sufficient to meet the requirements of cows, even considering a ruminal degradation of dietary thiamine of 48% (Zinn et al., 1987). Santschi et al. (2005a) indicated that 66% of dietary thiamine degrades in the rumen, although Weiss (2007) suggested a lower value (53.1%). For ruminants, thiamine is not toxic (NRC, 1987), and deficiencies only occur in abnormal situations, such as consumption of feed rich in thiaminases or high in sulfates or situations in which the ruminal pH drops suddenly (Zinn et al., 1987; Harmeyer and Kollenkirchen, 1989; Gould et al., 1991; Zempleni et al., 2007). Pan et al. (2018) reviewed thiamine metabolism, its application in dairy cow production (Figure 6.12), and its impact on the rumen.

Thiamine supplementation can balance the bacterial community by increasing the abundance of cellulolytic bacteria, including Bacteroides, Ruminococcus, Pyramidobacter, Succinivibrio, and Ruminobacter. Such increases enhance fiber degradation and ruminal acetate production; increased acetate concentrations are transported to the MG to increase milk fat synthesis. On the other hand, thiamine supplementation suppresses the ruminal epithelium inflammatory response by decreasing ruminal lipopolysaccharide (LPS) production and repressing NFκB protein activation. TPP, thiamine pyrophosphate; LBP, LPS-binding protein (Wang et al., 2014; Pan et al., 2018).

Recommendations for thiamine

Suckling calves

The NRC (2001) and NASEM (2021) recommended incorporating 6.5 mg of thiamine per kg DM in milk replacers. Recently dsm-firmenich (2022b) proposed a supplementation with 2.5–5.0 mg/kg DM (Table 6.1a).

Growing calves, heifers, dry and lactating cows

No specific recommendations of thiamine for cows have been established. However, under certain specific conditions, such as in the case of animals subjected to stressful situations and in high-yielding dairy cattle at the start of lactation, some investigators recommend increasing dietary supplies of thiamine (McDowell, 2006). Because a significant proportion is degraded in the rumen, supplementary sources should resist ruminal degradation (Majee et al., 2003). The average supply of thiamine is considered less variable than other vitamins in the B complex, with an average intake of 45 mg/day in diets typically formulated for high-yielding dairy cattle. As with most vitamins in the B complex, the scant data available (Shaver and Bal, 2000; Majee et al., 2003) do not allow a clear conclusion on the benefits of a supplementary supply of thiamine for dairy cattle.

Pan et al. (2016) detected relationships between thiamine concentrations and pH (favorable), acetate (positive), and lactate (negative), indicating that thiamine affects rumen fermentation and carbohydrate metabolism (Figure 6.13). They also found thiamine deficiency in

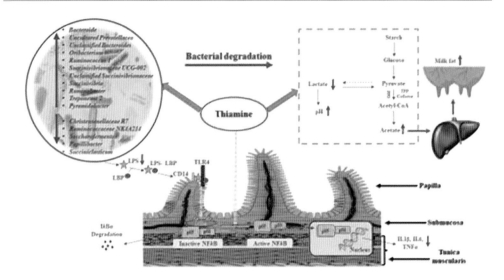

Figure 6.12 The potential mechanisms by which thiamine supplementation attenuates high-grain-induced subacute ruminal acidosis in dairy cows (source adapted from: Pan *et al.*, 2018)

dairy cows with subacute rumen acidosis (SARA). Ruminal infusion of thiamine (180 mg/kg of DMI) could help attenuate the ruminal pH depression of SARA by improving the proportions of volatile fatty acids (VFA) and reducing lactate concentrations in rumen fluid and blood. Moreover, exogenous thiamine might enhance thiamine absorption by improving ruminal fermentation and alleviating inflammatory response.

In 2017, Pan *et al.* studied 3 treatments: control (20% dietary starch, DM basis), high-grain diet (HG, 33.2% dietary starch, DM basis), and HG diet supplemented with 180 mg of thiamine/kg of DMI. This study concluded that thiamine could attenuate epithelial inflammation during high grain feeding. Thiamine supplementation decreased ruminal LPS (49,361 *vs.* 134,380 endotoxin units/ml) and attenuated the HG-induced inflammation response as indicated by a reduction in plasma cytokine IL6 and decreasing gene and protein expression of pro-inflammatory cytokines in rumen epithelium. The protective effects may be due to its ability to suppress toll-like receptor 4 (TLR4-mediated), the phosphorylation of nuclear factor kappa B (NFκB) unit p65 and signaling pathways.

Thiamine also has been suggested as a cofactor to avoid ketogenesis in cows postpartum. However, the contribution of thiamine in the diet of dairy cows, if not protected from the action of microorganisms of the rumen, may not have the desired effect. Therefore, Melendez *et al.* (2021) conducted a study on a dairy herd with 650 cows, randomly assigned to a treatment group receiving orally 60 g rumen-protected thiamine daily for 10 days postpartum and a control group. On days 3 and 10, postpartum β-hydroxyl butyrate (BHB) levels were similar between groups; however, on day 7, BHB concentrations were different (0.57 and 0.83 mmol/L for treated and control groups, respectively, *P* ≤ 0.05). It was concluded that a rumen-protected thiamine oral product decreased the blood concentrations of BHB during the first 10 days postpartum. Based on this pilot study, this additive deserves further investigation to elucidate its potential mechanism of physiological action to prevent ketosis and improve milk production in lactating dairy cows.

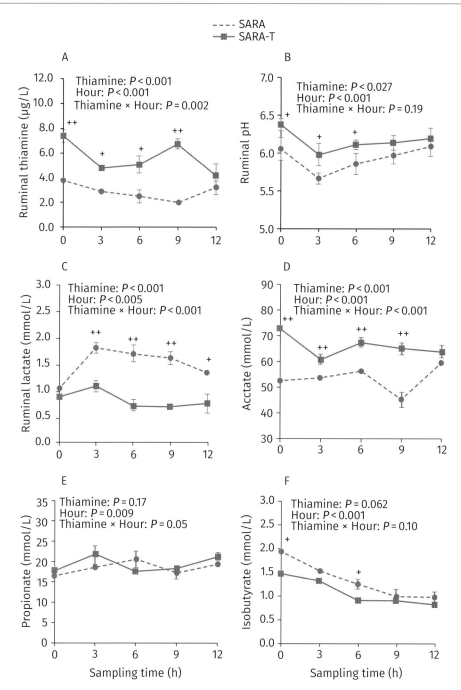

Figure 6.13 Effects of thiamine supplementation on ruminal pH, concentrations of thiamine, lactate, acetate, propionate, isobutyrate, butyrate, isovalerate, valerate, and total VFA (TVFA) in the rumen fluid of dairy cows. SARA represents Subacute Ruminal Acidosis cows without thiamine supplement. SARA + T represents SARA cows supplemented with thiamine. (source: Pan et al., 2016) Data are presented as means ± SE. *indicates differences between treatments at $P \leq 0.05$; **indicates differences between treatments at $P \leq 0.01$.

Vitamin B$_{12}$ (cobalamin)

Vitamin B$_{12}$ is a cofactor in 2 crucial enzyme reactions in animal metabolism. The first is with methylmalonyl-CoA mutase, which is necessary for converting from propionate to succinate during the oxidation of branched-chain fatty acids and the catabolism of ketogenic amino acids. The second is with tetrahydrofolate methyl transferase, which participates in methionine metabolism and is crucial for protein synthesis (NRC, 2001; Zempleni *et al.*, 2007). The ruminal degradation of dietary vitamin B$_{12}$ ranges between 90% and 100% (Zinn, 1992; Schwab *et al.*, 2006). Bacteria are the only natural source of vitamin B$_{12}$, for which an adequate cobalt supply is required (McDowell, 2000a).

Recommendations for vitamin B$_{12}$

Suckling calves

In milk replacers for calves, both the NRC (2001) and NASEM (2021) indicated to supplement 0.07 mg/kg DM, and similarly, dsm-firmenich (2022b) recommended 0.04–0.08 mg/kg DM of milk replacer (Table 6.1a). Supplementing weaned calves may be strictly necessary under some conditions like stress (Duncan and Webster, 1953; Lassiter *et al.*, 1953).

Growing calves, heifers, dry and lactating cows

No recommendations are given for other categories of adult ruminants. The NRC (2001) considered that the requirements of dairy cows range between 0.34 and 0.68 µg/kg BW. Due to the high degradation of vitamin B$_{12}$ in the rumen, the microbial synthesis of vitamin B$_{12}$ is fundamental. It depends on the presence of cobalt, the rate increasing linearly up to levels of 0.2 mg/kg (Andrews *et al.*, 1960). A supplementary supply of cobalt in the diet (0.17 *vs.* 0.29 mg of cobalt per kg DM) higher than the NRC's 2001 recommendations (0.11 mg/kg) stimulates the synthesis of vitamin B$_{12}$, which suggests that these recommendations should also be set higher (Stemme *et al.*, 2008).

   Under normal conditions, ruminal bacteria synthesize at a rate of 4.1 mg of vitamin B$_{12}$ per kg of digestible organic matter, and synthesis is higher in rations rich in forage (Sutton and Elliot, 1972; Walker and Elliot, 1972; Croom *et al.*, 1981). However, these data contradict the results Schwab *et al.* (2006) obtained in dairy cattle, who estimated an average synthesis of 7.8 mg/kg of digestible organic material (6.4–9.4 mg/kg). The total dietary supply is estimated to be between 60 and 130 mg/day (Santschi *et al.*, 2005b; Schwab *et al.*, 2006; Weiss, 2007). Considering the requirements and the capacity for ruminal synthesis of vitamin B$_{12}$, a deficiency in dairy cattle is unlikely, except where there is a cobalt deficiency (Erdman, 1992).

   The results of other studies (Girard and Matte, 2005b) suggest that supplementation with vitamin B$_{12}$ in high-yielding dairy cattle in early lactation may interfere with other B complex vitamins, such as folic acid, and become a limiting nutrient. Graulet *et al.* (2007) evaluated the effect of supplementation with folic acid and vitamin B$_{12}$. They only demonstrated an additive effect of both vitamins for milk fat content, while a supply of vitamin B$_{12}$ alone had no effects. Nevertheless, Girard and Matte (2005b) suggested the need to evaluate the possible deficiencies of folic acid and vitamin B$_{12}$ in dairy cattle since supplementation with vitamin B$_{12}$ considerably increased the content of the vitamin in milk, improving its nutritional quality for human consumption. This research group has provided important information about factors that affect the variability of vitamin B$_{12}$ in milk (Duplessis *et al.*, 2015, 2018, 2019, 2020a, b, 2021).

   A 250 ml glass of milk contains about 46% of the daily recommended dietary allowance of B$_{12}$ for individuals over 13 years old. However, the concentration of vitamin B$_{12}$ in cows' milk is highly variable (Franco-Lopez *et al.*, 2020; Duplessis *et al.*, 2021). There is interest in determining what causes the variability of vitamin B_{12}. Currently, some research studies report the possibility of a correlation between the ruminal microbiota and the concentration of vitamins in cattle (Franco-Lopez *et al.*, 2020; Duplessis *et al.*, 2020a, b, 2021, 2023).

Franco-Lopez *et al.* (2020) evaluated 92 sets of rumen, feces, blood, and milk samples from Holstein cows equipped with rumen cannulas collected at various stages of lactation. The cows studied were classified into 4 treatments: dry group (cows between 51 and 33 days before the calving date); close-up group (cows between 12 and 0 days before the calving date); group 1 (lactating cows; average 125 days of lactation); group 2 (lactating cows; average 320 days of lactation). The results found that the interaction between the composition of the rumen microbiota and other factors, such as the cows' lactation status, can significantly affect the final concentration of vitamin B_{12} in the rumen, feces, and milk. A high ruminal concentration of vitamin B_{12} was found to be correlated with a higher abundance of *Prevotella*, while a low ruminal concentration of vitamin B_{12} was correlated with a higher abundance of *Bacteroidetes*, *Ruminiclostridium*, and *Butyrivibrio* (Franco-Lopez *et al.*, 2020).

Vitamin B_{12} is firmly bound to several specific carrier proteins, predominantly transcobalamin (TC) and haptocorrin (HC) (Fedosov *et al.*, 2019). Since the type of vitamin B_{12} binder can influence cobalamin bioavailability, Fedosov *et al.* (2019) examined vitamin B_{12} carriers in combined milk samples derived from European and Indian herds of cows and buffaloes. In that study, more than 3,000 milk samples were collected. All samples had similar concentrations of cobalamin (Cbl) (≈3 nM) but differed in their sets of cobalamin-binding proteins: transcobalamin, haptocorrin, and caseins. The samples were classified into 4 treatments: T1: Milk samples from Danish cows (*Bos taurus* × Holstein-Friesian breed) × Transcobalamins + Caseins; T2: Milk samples from Indian cows (*B. indicus* × local Friesians) × Transcobalamins + Haptocorrins; T3: Milk samples from Indian buffaloes (*Bubalus bubalis*, local animals × Murrah breed) × Transcobalamins + Haptocorrins; T4: Milk samples from Italian buffaloes (*B. bubalis*, Italian Mediterranean breed) × Haptocorrhinas.

The results showed that the milk of Italian buffaloes was characterized by a high content of haptocorrins, which exceeded endogenous cobalamin. This could result in impaired B_{12} assimilation by humans drinking the milk because buffalo haptocorrin is resistant to both acid treatment (similar to stomach conditions) and proteolytic degradation by trypsin and chymotrypsin (similar to haptocorrin intestinal conditions). On the contrary, the authors identified that the milk of cows and buffaloes from India showed a lower amount of haptocorrins and a higher presence of B_{12}-transporting transcobalamins susceptible to low pH and the process of oxidation and proteolysis. Additionally, Danish cows produced milk without a significant amount of haptocorrins, and the number of transcobalamin was insufficient to bind all the endogenous cobalamin. Similar results had been reported by Mahalle *et al.* (2018).

In a literature review, González-Montaña *et al.* (2020) studied the relationship between vitamin B_{12} and cobalt metabolism in domestic ruminants. Cobalt functions as a component of vitamin B_{12} and participates as a coenzyme in 2 enzyme systems: methylmalonyl-CoA mutase, which requires adenosylcobalamin, and methionine synthetase, which requires methylcobalamin, both necessary to obtain energy through ruminal metabolism. According to González-Montaña *et al.* (2020), cobalt needs are around 0.11 mg/kg, with the possibility of supplementing by increasing the amount to 0.20 mg/kg. However, in the study carried out by Hackbart *et al.* (2010), cobalt supplementation of 2.1 mg/kg during the dry period and 1.1 mg/kg during lactation can stimulate milk production in cows. Similarly, Weiss (2007) stated that increasing cobalt supplementation from 0 to 1 mg/kg can increase milk production in multiparous cows. Still, it is not possible to show effects in primiparous cows. Likewise, Stemme *et al.* (2006) reported that oral extra-supplementation of cobalt 0.13 mg/kg *vs.* 0.27 mg/kg in dairy cows during pregnancy could increase serum cobalamin levels. Finally, a study by Kincaid and Socha (2007) reported that cobalt supplementation of 0.15, 0.89, or 1.71 mg/kg in prepartum cows could increase the ruminal synthesis of vitamin B_{12} in colostrum and milk.

Vitamin B_{12} synthesized in the rumen from cobalt can majorly affect metabolism in the peri-parturient period. Thus, Weerathilake et al. (2019) evaluated the effect of dietary inclusion of cobalt, vitamin B_{12} or injecting vitamin B_{12} on the metabolism, health, and performance of high-yielding dairy cows. Fifty-six Holstein-Friesian dairy cows (12 primiparous and 44 multiparous) were classified into 4 treatments: C, no added Co; DC, additional 0.2 mg Co/kg DM; DB, additional 0.68 mg vitamin B_{12}/kg DM; IB, intramuscular injection of vitamin B_{12} to supply 0.71 mg/cow per day prepartum and 1.42 mg/cow per day postpartum. The basal and lactation rations both contained 0.21 mg Co/kg DM. Results indicated that the dietary supplementation of cobalt at a concentration of 0.21 mg/kg provides enough cobalt for the correct synthesis of vitamin B_{12}, which would be necessary to develop metabolic functions and improve the performance and digestibility of the diet of the high-yielding dairy cows.

Duplessis et al. (2014a) determined the effect of a combined folic acid + vitamin B_{12} supplement administered at the beginning of lactation on the slaughter rate, metabolic disorders, and reproduction of commercial dairy cows. A total of 805 cows were studied: (271 primiparous and 534 multiparous) in 15 dairy herds. Every 2 months from February to December 2010 and within each herd, cows were assigned according to the parity number, previous 305 day milk production, and calving interval to 5 ml of (1) saline solution at 0.9% NaCl (control group) or (2) 320 mg folic acid + 10 mg vitamin B_{12} (vitamin group). Treatments were administered weekly by intramuscular injections. As a result of this experiment, multiparous cows receiving the vitamin supplement experienced less difficulty at calving than multiparous control cows.

Pyridoxine (vitamin B_6)

Pyridoxine, or vitamin B_6, is a coenzyme that actively participates in the metabolism of amino acids, and requirements are established according to the quantity of protein intake (Zempleni et al., 2007). Most published data indicate that the ruminal degradability of pyridoxine is very low, and it is synthesized abundantly in the rumen, so a deficiency is unlikely (Zinn, 1992; Schwab et al., 2006). However, Santschi et al. (2005a,b) and Schwab et al. (2006) indicated that the intestinal flow of vitamin B_6 could be between 50–70 mg lower than the estimates of the NASEM (2021).

Vitamin B_6 is also necessary during the transition period, as it is a strategic donor of methyl groups (Mason, 2003). This role links it directly with the metabolism of lipids and the development of ketosis and fatty liver (Seymour, 2004; Zempleni et al., 2007). The importance of this productive period in cows should drive revision of the recommendations.

Recommendations for vitamin B_6
Suckling calves
NRC (2001) and NASEM (2021) suggested a supplementation of 6.5 mg/kg and dsm-firmenich (2022b) proposed 2.5–4.5 mg/kg DM (Table 6.1a).

Growing calves, heifers, dry and lactating cows
As with other B group vitamins, there are no established recommendations for adult cattle. Beaudet et al. (2016) quantified an apparent ruminal synthesis (ARS) of riboflavin, folates, and vitamin B_{12} but degradation of thiamine, niacin, and vitamin B_6. The high-starch diets increased the synthesis of riboflavin and folates and reduced apparent ruminal degradation of vitamin

B_6, whereas vitamin B_{12} synthesis was more significant with the high-fiber diets. The low-N diets decreased the ruminal synthesis of riboflavin and folates. Overall, riboflavin, niacin, and folate ARS was negatively correlated with NDF and ADF intakes. In contrast, vitamin B_{12} followed the opposite pattern in the range of the studied diets, which all had the same forage-to-concentrate ratio. The intake of nutrients did not influence thiamine and vitamin B_6. Moreover, only vitamin B_6 ARS was correlated with its intake. This study confirmed that diet characteristics influence B vitamin supply for dairy cows, probably by affecting microbial population and activity.

Collective B vitamin supplementation

Many researchers have evaluated the supplementation of B vitamin combinations in dairy cows. However, not all results have been consistent. Morrison et al. (2018) evaluated the supplementation of a complex of rumen-protected B vitamins and choline to transition cows in a large multi-herd trial under field conditions and observed no effect on hyperketonemia incidence, clinical health disorders, milk production, or reproductive performance. In contrast, Watanabe and Bito (2018) reported that vitamin B_{12} modulates intestinal microbial ecology. The genes involved in the uptake or transport of cobalamin were not found, which implies that there are associations related to genes involved in unknown processes, such as the production of B_{12} in ruminants or the secretion of B_{12} by the MG. Kaur et al. (2019) also evaluated the supplementation of rumen-protected B vitamins during the transition and early lactation periods, respectively. Vitamin B supplementation upregulated several genes related to embryo development, immune system, and adhesion. Vitamin B supplementation did not affect embryo size and ovulatory follicle or corpus luteum diameter at embryo collection. In conclusion of this study, the benefits of strategic dietary vitamin B supplementation during the transition and early lactation might be directly linked to endometrial functions required for embryo survival during the peri-implantation period.

Duplessis and Girard (2019) evaluated the effect of maternal supplementation of biotin (20 mg/day), folic acid (2.6 g/day), and vitamin B_{12} (10 mg intramuscular injection) 26 days before calving on colostral and calf plasma concentrations of these B vitamins. In this experiment, no treatment effect was noted on colostral or calf plasma concentration of IgG ($P > 0.54$). However, biotin, folic acid, and vitamin B_{12} supplementation given to the dam before calving increased the concentrations of these vitamins in the colostrum. The colostral levels increased from 26.8 to 253.7, 673 to 1,094 (SE: 52), and 28.6 to 57.9 (SE: 3.3) ng/ml by their respective vitamin supplementation. In the same way, calf plasma concentrations of these vitamins were increased. This is important since newborn calves rely on an external supply of these B vitamins to fulfill their requirements before developing their functional rumen.

The impact of the management and composition of the diet on the concentration of vitamin B_{12} in the milk of Holstein cows was evaluated. Duplessis et al. (2019) studied milk samples from 100 commercial dairy herds in Québec province, Canada. Information was collected on 1,484 first, 1,093 second, and 1,763 third and highest parity Holstein cows in 100 herds during 3 consecutive milkings. The cows were milked twice daily: in the morning and the afternoon. The cows evaluated in the treatments were housed in fixed stables ($n = 98$) and free stables ($n = 2$). Herd size ranged from 16 to 113 lactating dairy cows. Total mixed ration (TMR) was used in 31 herds, while the automatic component feeding system (AFS) was used in 49 herds, and manual component feeding (MCF) in 20 herds. The results showed that the average concentration of vitamin B_{12} in milk ranged from 2,861 to 5,892 pg/ml. Cows that have calved more than 3 times had a higher concentration of vitamin B_{12} in their milk than cows in their first and second calving. Additionally, concentrations of dietary fiber, such as acid detergent fiber (ADF) and neutral-detergent fiber (NDF), and energy-related compounds, such as non-fiber carbo-hydrates (NFC) and starch, were associated, respectively, positively and negatively with the concentration of vitamin B_{12} in milk.

Khan *et al.* (2020a) identified that folic acid and vitamin B_{12} are essential nutrients, which must be supplemented in dairy cattle during the peripartum period to overcome metabolic and immunological stress and improve peripartum milk production. Additionally, vitamin B_{12} is essential in metabolism since it acts as a coenzyme of the enzyme methionine synthase, necessary for transferring a methyl group from folic acid to homocysteine, thus promoting methionine generation.

The supplementation with B vitamins may be related to improvements in milk production, health, and reproductive efficiency of dairy cows. Therefore, Kaur *et al.* (2019) evaluated the effects of rumen-protected vitamin B complex supplementation in the transition and the lac-tation period, compared with a control diet containing no supplements on endometrial out-comes on day 14 of pregnancy. The study was completely randomized, 42 multiparous Holstein cows were used in the study 3 weeks before calving. Cows were supplemented with 100 g/cow per day of rumen-protected B vitamins and choline for transition cows, containing choline, riboflavin, folic acid, and vitamin B_{12} from 3 weeks prepartum to 14 days-in milk (DIM) and with 4 g of rumen-protected B vitamins for lactating cows, containing folic acid, vitamin B_{12}, biotin, pyridoxine, and pantothenic acid, diluted with 36 g of a palmitic fat source, from 15 DIM until endometrial biopsy (around 72 DIM). Supplementation with rumen-protected B vitamins improved the marking of some critical genes necessary for establishing pregnancy in Holstein dairy cows. For this reason, it can be concluded that the upregulation of essential genes in the endometrium before implantation may be related to the action of vitamin B molecules in the endometrium (Kaur *et al.*, 2019).

Suboptimal B vitamin supply may affect metabolic efficiency in dairy cows (Brisson *et al.*, 2022). At the same time, B vitamin supply cannot be adequately estimated by dietary intake. The rumen microbiota has been shown to play a significant role in synthesizing and utilizing B vitamins. Brisson *et al.* (2022) developed a meta-analysis to describe the actual B vitamin supply to the cow: post-ruminal flow (PRF) and ARS. This meta-analysis used data from 340 individual cow observations, representing 36 treatment means and 16 experiments from 15 studies conducted by 3 research groups (Michigan State University (MSU), the National Institute for Agriculture, Food and Environment (INRAe), and Agriculture and Agri-Food Canada (AAFC)). Post-ruminal digesta samples were analyzed for the content of B vitamins (B_1, B_2, B_3, B_6, B_9, B_{12}), and univariate and multivariate linear form equations were considered. Models describing ARS considered DMI (kg/day), B vitamin dietary concentration (mg/kg of DM), and rumen-level variables such as rumen digestible NDF and starch (g/kg of DM), total volatile fatty acids (VFA, mM), acetate, propionate, butyrate, and valerate molar proportions (% of VFA), mean pH, and fractional rates of degradation of NDF and starch (%/hour). Models describing PRF considered dietary-level driving variables such as DMI, B vitamin dietary concentration (mg/kg DM), starch and crude protein (g/kg DM), and forage NDF (g/kg DM). The results obtained from both the ARS and PRF models suggested that diet composition and rumen dynamics correlate with the synthesis and resulting variations in post-ruminal flow and PRF of each B vitamin differently. Additionally, this paper emphasized that B vitamin intake is not the primary factor controlling B vitamin (post-ruminal flow, PRF).

Changes in the composition of the diet can affect the microbial population in the rumen, and its metabolism of vitamin B. Diets based on alfalfa silage may have greater thiamine and vitamin B_6 degradation in the rumen (Castagnino *et al.*, 2017). Castagnino *et al.* (2016) offered diets containing either alfalfa or orchard grass (OG) silages as the sole forage to ruminally and duodenally cannulated lactating Holstein cows in crossover design experiments. Experiment 1 compared diets containing alfalfa and OG (~23% forage neutral NDF and ~27% total NDF) offered to 8 cows in 2 15-day treatment periods. Experiment 2 compared diets containing alfalfa and OG (~25% forage NDF and ~30% total NDF) offered to 13 cows in 2 18-day treatment periods. Thiamine, riboflavin, niacin, vitamin B_6, folates, and vitamin B_{12} were analyzed in feeds and duodenal digesta. The ARS was calculated as the duodenal flow of each vitamin minus its intake. Herd sizes ranged from 150 to 450 lactating cows. A randomized controlled trial in 3 commercial dairy herds (n = 1,346 cows with a group as an experimental unit; Experiment 1) and a university research herd (n = 50 cows with the cow as an experimental unit; Experiment 2) evaluated the use of 100 g/cow per day of a commercially available proprietary rumen-protected blend of B vitamins and choline (RPBC) supplement or a placebo, fed 3 weeks before to 3 weeks after calving. In Experiment 2, liver biopsies were taken at 4 and 14±1 DIM to measure triacylglycerol concentrations and the expression of 28 genes selected to represent relevant aspects of hepatic metabolism.

In both experiments, alfalfa diets increased vitamin B_6 and decreased folate intakes. In experiment 1, riboflavin and niacin intakes were greater with the OG diet, whereas in experiment 2, thiamine intake was greater, but riboflavin intake was smaller with the OG diet. Despite the low contribution of either silage to the dietary folate content, folate intake was greater with OG diets than with alfalfa due to the difference in soybean meal contribution between diets. Niacin and folate ARS were not affected by the forage family. Duodenal microbial nitrogen flow was positively correlated with ARS of riboflavin, niacin, vitamin B_6, folates, and vitamin B_{12} but tended to be negatively correlated with thiamine ARS. The ARS of folates and vitamin B_{12} appears to be related to microbial biomass activity. Changes in the nutrient composition of the diets likely affected the microbial population in the rumen and their B vitamin metabolism.

Castagnino et al. (2018) also evaluated the effect of endosperm type (floury vs. vitreous, vitreousness of 25 and 66%, respectively) and particle size (fine 2 mm screen vs. medium 6 mm screen) of dry corn grain on ARS and duodenal flow of B vitamins in lactating dairy cows. These factors are known to affect starch digestibility in the rumen. Results indicated that the duodenal flow of thiamine, riboflavin, niacin, folates, and vitamin B_{12}, expressed per unit of DMI, decreased with an increase in particle size. Similarly, the apparent degradation of thiamine and riboflavin was greater, and the ARS of niacin, folates, and vitamin B_{12} was reduced when cows were fed coarser dry corn grain particles. Neither endosperm type nor particle size affected the duodenal flow and ARS of vitamin B_6. The ARS, expressed per unit of DMI, of all studied B vitamins, but thiamine was negatively correlated with apparent ruminal digestibility of NDF. The duodenal flow of microbial N was positively correlated with ARS of riboflavin, niacin, vitamin B_6, and folates.

Beaudet et al. (2016) evaluated the effects of nitrogen level and carbohydrate source on ARS of thiamine, riboflavin, niacin, vitamin B_6, folates, and vitamin B_{12}. This experiment used 4 lactating Holstein cows distributed in a 4 × 4 Latin square design with treatments following a 2 × 2 factorial arrangement. Cows were fitted with cannulas in the rumen and proximal duodenum. The treatments were 2 N levels and 2 carbohydrate sources. The diet with the high N level provided 14% crude protein, calculated to meet 110% of the protein requirements, and an adequate supply of rumen-degradable protein. In contrast, the diet with the low N level contained 11% crude protein, calculated to meet 80% of the protein requirements with a shortage in rumen-degradable protein. Carbohydrate source treatments differed by nature (i.e., high in starch from barley, corn, and wheat or high in fiber from soybean hulls and dehydrated beet pulp). Results indicated that diet characteristics influence B vitamin supply for dairy cows, probably by affecting microbial population and activity. For example, vitamin B_{12} was positively correlated with NDF and ADF intakes.

Seck et al. (2017) evaluated the effects of the forage-concentrate ratio on the ARS of thiamine, riboflavin, niacin, vitamin B_6, folates, and vitamin B_{12}. Fourteen Holstein cows were evaluated, and the cows had duodenal and ruminal cannulas. The experiment was a crossover design with 2 15-d treatment periods and a 14-d preliminary period in which cows were fed a diet intermediate in composition between the treatment diets. Two treatments were established, T1: a diet containing low forage (44.8% forage, 32.8% starch, 24.4% NDF); T2: a diet containing high-forage (61.4% forage, 22.5% starch, 30.7% NDF) concentrations. The 2 nutritional diets were formulated with different proportions of the same ingredients. Consequently, ARS of riboflavin, niacin, folates, and vitamin B_{12} correlated positively with the amount of starch digested in the rumen and duodenal flow of microbial N, whereas these correlations were negative for thiamine.

According to Castagnino et al. (2018), factors affecting the digestibility of dry corn kernel starch in the rumen can change the B vitamin values available in dairy cows. In that study, 8 multiparous lactating Holstein cows were evaluated. The studied cows were equipped with ruminal and duodenal cannulas. The evaluated cows were randomly assigned to a treatment sequence according to a 2 × 2 factorial arrangement in a 4 × 4 Latin square design experiment in duplicate. At the beginning of the experiment, the cows had 132 (SD = 42.1) DIM. The duration of each experimental period was 21 days. The factors studied were T1: type of endosperm (floury vs. vitreous) and T2: particle size (fine vs. medium) of the dry corn grain. The vitreous proportion was 25% for the floury endosperm group and 66% for the vitreous group in dry corn grain endosperm. As demonstrated by these authors, except for thiamine or vitamin B_1, the effects of factors that increase the digestibility of dry corn grain starch in the rumen on the amounts of B vitamins available for dairy cow absorption may be significantly related to differences in rumen digestibility of neutral vitamins, detergent fiber, and on duodenal microbial nitrogen flux.

Duplessis et al. (2020b) evaluated plasma folate and vitamin B_{12} concentrations and their relationship to dietary composition in Holstein dairy cows in the United States and Canada. Twenty-two and 24 US and Canadian dairy herds were examined, totaling 427 and 476 cows at 10–197 DIM (Table 6.16). Parity and DIM described the variation in plasma concentrations of those 2 vitamins. Among the evaluated dietary nutrient composition variables, plasma folate concentrations were negatively correlated with fiber concentrations and positively with NFC concentrations. In comparison, plasma vitamin B_{12} concentrations were positively correlated with fiber. In 2021, Duplessis et al. concluded that B_{12} concentration increases when the rumen conditions are optimal, such as with elevated pH. These authors also indicated that bedding type (recycled manure solid bedding or straw) does not correlate with milk B_{12} concentration.

The literature review published by McFadden et al. (2020) concluded that an inadequate supply of methyl donors might contribute to oxidative stress, inflammation, hepatic triglyceride accumulation, and compromised milk production in the transition of dairy cows from gestation to lactation. For this reason, to address potential methyl donor deficiencies in the peripartum cow, supplementation with dietary folic acid, B vitamins, methionine, choline, and betaine is a nutritional practice that deserves consideration.

Duplessis et al. (2022) evaluated the effects on lactation performance, energy, protein metabolism, and hormones by combining biotin (B_7), folic acid (B_9), and vitamin B_{12} supplementation during the transition period to dairy cows. Thirty-two multiparous Holstein cows were evaluated and classified into 4 treatments: T1: Intramuscular injection of 2 ml of saline solution (0.9% NaCl; B_7-/B_9B_{12}-) x week; T2: Intramuscular injection of 2 ml of saline solution

Table 6.16 Plasma folate and vitamin B_{12} concentrations in different US and Canadian regions (source: Duplessis et al., 2020b)

Region	Cows, n	Folates[1] (ng/ml)		Vitamin B_{12}[2,3] (pg/ml)	
		Mean	95% CI	Mean	95% CI
United States					
Northwest	58	16.6[a]	15.1–18.2	249[a]	210–296
California	119	11.4[c]	10.3–12.5	213[ab]	189–241
Southwest	59	14.1[ab]	12.6–15.6	211[ab]	178–251
Upper Midwest	100	13.2[bc]	11.8–14.5	186[abc]	160–216
Southeast	71	14.1[ab]	12.7–15.4	183[abc]	157–213
Canada					
British Columbia	97	14.1[ab]	12.9–15.3	170[bc]	148–194
Alberta	79	15.2[ab]	13.8–16.7	191[abc]	163–224
Ontario	100	13.3[bc]	12.1–14.5	179[bc]	156–204
Québec and New York[4]	120	15.7[ab]	14.6–16.8	155[c]	137–176
Nova Scotia	100	14.1[ab]	12.9–15.3	166[bc]	145–189

Notes: [a-c]Means in the same row with different superscripts differ (P < 0.10).
[1]Region effect, P < 0.0001.
[2]Geometric means and 95% CI for log-transformed data computed as ex.
[3]Region effect, P = 0.002.
[4]Because only one herd was enrolled in New York State, it was included in the closest region, Québec, Canada (103 km from Montreal, QC, Canada).

(0.9% NaCl; $B_7+/B_9B_{12}-$) × week + 20 mg/day of B_7 in the diet (without protection against ruminal degradation); T3: Intramuscular injection of 2 ml of 10 mg of B_{12} ($B_7-/B_9B_{12}+$) × week + 2.6 g/day of B_9 in the diet (without protection against ruminal degradation); T4: Intramuscular injection of 2 ml of 10 mg of B_{12} ($B_7+/B_9B_{12}+$) × week + 20 mg/day of B_7 in the diet + 2.6 g/day of B_9 in the diet. The combined supplementation of biotin, folic acid, and vitamin B_{12} can positively affect lactation in Holstein cows in the peripartum. Additionally, B_9 and B_{12} supplementation can improve the efficiency of energy metabolism in cows in early lactation. Similarly, folic acid and cobalamin supplementation increased plasma concentrations of cysteine and homocysteine postpartum but did not affect the plasma concentration of methionine. The results indicate plasma glucose concentration during infusions at 43 days of lactation for cows supplemented with B_7 was higher when given in combination with B_9 and B_{12}. Accordingly, a combination of biotin, folic acid, and vitamin B_{12} supplementation during the transition period to dairy cows significantly affects plasma glucose concentration. In conclusion, results indicated that the combination of biotin, folic acid, and vitamin B_{12} supplementation during the transition period to dairy cows significantly affects body weight, milk production, and the concentration of fatty acids in milk.

Vitamin C

Vitamin C is a cofactor in many biochemical and oxidation-reduction reactions and processes (NRC, 2001; Zempleni et al., 2007). It acts as an antioxidant, protecting cells against damage from free radicals (McDowell, 2004) and regulating steroid synthesis. Vitamin C is synthesized inside the cells of adult ruminants, principally in the liver and kidneys (Weiss, 2007), except for young calves, which cannot synthesize it until 3 weeks of age (Cummins and Brunner, 1991), so it is considered an essential nutrient only for this type of animal. Vitamin C requirements also increase in conditions of stress (Padilla *et al.*, 2006; McDowell, 2006) when the plasma concentration falls rations rich in non-fibrous carbohydrates (Schwab *et al.*, 2006; Cummins and Brunner, 1991; Hidiroglou *et al.* (1977).

Recommendations for vitamin C

Suckling calves
Vitamin C recommendation for this category is only given by dsm-firmenich (2022b) recommending 250–500 mg/kg DM of milk replacers (Table 6.1a).

Oral supplementation of 1–2 g of vitamin C in pre-ruminant calves increased vitamin C plasma concentration (Hidiroglou *et al.*, 1995) and prevented diarrhea (Seifi *et al.*, 1996). The positive effects attributed to vitamin C refer to the immune response, as it stimulates the neutrophils and, in some cases, reduces mastitis indicators (Chaiyotwittayakun *et al.*, 2002; Naresh *et al.*, 2002; Weiss *et al.*, 2004; Kleczkowski *et al.*, 2005; Ranjan *et al.*, 2005; Weiss and Hogan, 2007).

Growing calves, heifers, dry and lactating cows
No recommendation is given for adult ruminants. Data on the effects of oral vitamin C supplementation in adult animals show no solid evidence which would permit practical recommendations to be made (Weiss, 2007). Vitamin C plasma concentration decreases due to heat stress, liver injuries, fattening, and infectious diseases such as mastitis in production cows (Weiss *et al.*, 2004; Weiss and Hogan, 2007).

It has been proposed that vitamin C improves fertility in dairy cattle (Gonzáles-Maldonado *et al.*, 2019a,b). However, the optimal dose and time of vitamin C supplementation needs to be determined. Mittal *et al.* (2014) evaluated the antioxidant capacity of vitamins E, C, and their combination in cryopreserved bull semen. The results indicated that the combination of vitamin E + C has the most profound effect in protecting sperms against reactive oxygen species production and cold shock when compared to vitamin E and vitamin C supplemented alone in the extender for semen dilution utilized for cryopreservation. Vitamin C also improves oocyst (Yassen *et al.*, 2020) and embryo development for embryo transfer (Zhang *et al.*, 2020).

With the same objective, Afiati *et al.* (2016) evaluated the effect of vitamin C administration in diluent media on the quality of dairy cattle thawed spermatozoa. Semen samples were from a 4-year-old Friesian Holstein bull. The sperm isolation factors were sexed and un-sexed sperm (x and y) and were classified into 4 treatments: T1: control. 0% vitamin C in the diluent; T2: 0.25% vitamin C in the diluent; T3: 0.50% vitamin C in the diluent; T4: 0.75% vitamin C in the diluent. It was determined that the optimal concentration of vitamin C in diluent media to improve the quality of defrosted sperm of dairy cattle (*B. taurus*) was 0.25%. The optimal concentration of vitamin C in a diluent medium to improve the quality of defrosting sperm of dairy cattle (*B. taurus*) was 0.50%.

It has been proposed that vitamin C, in combination with vitamin E, could improve fertility in cows (Li *et al.*, 2014; Maldonado *et al.*, 2017; González-Maldonado *et al.*, 2019b; Zhou *et al.*, 2019; Yassen *et al.*, 2020). However, when combined injections of vitamin C (3,000 mg) and E (3,000 IU) were evaluated, no significant effects were detected on reproductive parameters in dairy cattle. The lowest dose of vitamins sustained similar pregnancy rates among treatments, even though they had lower progesterone concentrations.

Kirdeci *et al.* (2021) evaluated the effect of vitamin C on the pregnancy rate and hydroxy deoxyguanosine (8-OHDG) levels during heat stress in postpartum dairy cattle. Eighty multiparous Holstein dairy cows were evaluated and classified into 2 treatments: T1: Control, (*n* = 40) received 10 ml of isotonic standard saline solution; T2: (*n* = 40) They received vitamin C (4 mg/kg) on the day of artificial insemination (day 0) and days 4, 8, and 12 after insemination. Kirdeci *et al.* (2021) showed that vitamin C supplementation during the postpartum period increases the pregnancy rate after insemination and reduces the oxidative stress metabolite 8-OHDG levels.

Choline
Choline is not a vitamin in the traditional sense as it is not part of an enzyme system, and it is required in grams and not in milligrams like most vitamins. Choline can be formed from serine and methionine (Zempleni *et al.*, 2007). Phosphatidylcholine is the leading natural form of choline in food, although a small quantity of free choline may also exist in plant material. Choline is necessary for the biosynthesis of phospholipids and acetylcholine (Zempleni *et al.*, 2007), and it plays a fundamental role in the metabolism as a methyl group donor. Biologically active methyl groups may also be obtained from methionine, so one of the advantages of supplementing choline is an increase in the availability of methionine for protein synthesis. Harper *et al.* (1977) considered that choline deficiencies only occur when the ration is deficient in protein. Most rations contain enough choline to cover the minimum requirements of ruminants. Due to the high degradation of dietary choline, it is probable that in high-producing dairy cattle, methionine, betaine (derived from the degradation of choline), and *de novo* synthesis play an essential role as methyl group donors (Aliev and Burkova, 1987; NASEM, 2021). However, the supplementation with RPC positively affects DMI. This effect has been associated with increased milk yield without improving the energy balance and metabolic profile of the cows (Humer *et al.*, 2019). Consequently, improved health status and reproduction have not been consistent findings.

Recommendations for choline
Suckling calves
Johnson *et al.* (1951) found choline deficiency in one-week-old calves given milk replacer rations containing 15% casein. The choline requirements estimated in this experiment were 260 mg/l of milk replacer (1,733 mg/ kg DM).

NRC (2001), and NASEM (2021) recommended incorporating 1,000 mg of biotin/kg DM in the milk replacement. dsm-firmenich (2022b) recently suggested adding 500–750 mg/kg DM (Table 6.1a).

Growing calves, heifers, dry and lactating cows
No recommendation is provided for adult ruminants. Despite its essential role in metabolism, the quantity of choline available for absorption in the small intestine is small, and the use of sources protected against ruminal degradation is recommended. Post-ruminal supplementation or supplementation in the protected form of 15–90 g of choline per day increased milk production of between 0 and 3 kg/day. Grummer *et al.* (1987) obtained an increase in milk production (from 29.5 to 31.6 kg of milk per day) by infusing 22 g of choline per day. Erdman and Sharma (1991) supplemented 0.24% protected choline chloride between weeks 5 and 21 postpartum and obtained an increase in milk yield of 2.6 kg/day compared with the control group.

Sharma and Erdman (1988) observed that while the oral dosage of choline (0, 10, and 20 g/kg DM) resulted in low recovery of choline in the duodenum and brought no production response, abomasal infusion of 30 g/day resulted in an increase of 0.45 and 0.14% fat and protein, respectively, in milk. Atkins *et al.* (1988) also observed no positive results on administering an oral choline supplement. The NASEM (2021) indicates that establishing recommendations for the transition and production cow would require more experimental studies.

However, since the recommendations of the NRC (2001), interest in the supplementary supply of choline has increased, as demonstrated by the growing number of studies published subsequently (Pinotti *et al.*, 2002, 2003, 2020; Piepenbrink and Overton, 2003; Brusemeister and Sudekum, 2006; Cooke *et al.*, 2007; Elek *et al.*, 2008; De Veth *et al.*, 2016; Humer *et al.*, 2019). However, the NASEM (2021) committee did not indicate a recommendation for choline except for milk replacers. Some of the data suggest that supplementing choline as RPC may effectively improve the yield and composition of milk, especially in rations low in protein or with limited availability of methionine (Eastridge, 2006). Weiss (2007) summarized the results of 12 experimental studies and concluded that the median increase in milk production when RPC was fed was about 2.3 kg/day during the first 2 months of lactation. With this level of response, the additional supply of RPC in the diet is considered profitable. The effects on the incidence of fatty liver are less clear. Concerning the recommended dose, Pinotti *et al.* (2005) concluded that, although the data are insufficient to establish the fundamental requirements of choline in dairy cattle, supplementation of between 12 and 20 g/day would be appropriate for dairy cattle in transition.

Bollatti *et al.* (2019a, b, 2020) supplementing 12.9 g/day of an RPC form as a top dress to parous Holstein cows from 21 days prepartum to 21 days postpartum observed greater hepatic triacylglycerol content and plasma BHB concentration in the first 21 days postpartum. Still, concentrations of inflammatory markers and liposoluble vitamins in plasma were unaffected. Treatment did not affect the incidence of clinical diseases; however, RPC increased the plasma triacylglycerol concentration but reduced the incidence of subclinical hypocalcemia. It is suggested that the increase in hepatic triacylglycerol in cows fed RPC is partly mediated by the improvements in lactation performance not followed by concurrent changes in DMI, which resulted in a more negative energy balance. Based on the current findings, the improved lactation performance and feed efficiency observed in the companion manuscript with supplementing 12.9 g/day of choline ion cannot be explained by the reduced fatty liver or improved peripartum health or inflammatory status. Other mechanisms are suggested, and they might be related to the potential effects of choline on mammary epithelial cell proliferation or enhanced uptake of nutrients.

Potts *et al.* (2020) also evaluated RPC or rumen-protected methionine (RPM), or both, during the periparturient period. Fifty-four Holstein cows (25 primiparous, 29 multiparous) were used in a randomized block design experiment with a 2 × 2 factorial treatment structure. Cows were blocked by expected calving date and parity and assigned to 1 of 4 treatments: (1) no supplemental choline or methionine (control, CON); (2) 60 g/day of RPC (13.0 g/day of choline ion); (3) 12 g/day of RPM prepartum and 18 g/day of RPM postpartum (9 g/day or 13.5 g/day of dl-Met, respectively); and (4) a combination of RPC and RPM treatments (RPC + RPM; 60 g/day of RPC plus 12 g/day of RPM prepartum and 18 g/day of RPM postpartum). Treatments were applied once daily as a top dress from 3 weeks before through 5 weeks after calving. Results indicated that primiparous and multiparous cows have different requirements for choline and methionine. Supplemental methionine as RPM during the periparturient period positively affected milk fat concentration for multiparous cows. Feeding choline as RPC to multiparous cows increased milk yield only in the absence of RPM. In contrast, RPC positively affected milk yield for primiparous cows, irrespective of RPM supplementation. During the periparturient period, feeding RPC could decrease hepatic triacylglycerol concentration and probably increase milk yield.

Also, Zenobi et al. (2020) evaluated the supplementation of RPC. Ninety-three multiparous Holstein cows were randomly assigned to 1 of 4 dietary treatments in a 2 × 2 factorial arrangement at 47±6 days before the expected calving date. Cows were fed energy to excess (EXE; 1.63 Mcal of net energy for lactation (NEL)/kg of dietary DM) or maintenance (MNE; 1.40 Mcal of NEL/kg of dietary DM) ad libitum throughout the nonlactating period. The RPC was fed at 0 or 60 g/day to supply 0 or 12.9 g/day of choline ions top-dressed for 17±4.6 days prepartum through 21 days postpartum. After calving, cows were fed the same methionine-supplemented diet, apart from RPC supplementation. Supplementation with RPC modulated several parameters of immune status in the postpartum period, contributing to increased milk production in prepartum cows.

NUTRITIONAL VALUE OF COW'S MILK IN HUMAN NUTRITION

The ultimate objective of producing foodstuffs of animal origin is to obtain nutritional, quality products for human consumption (Hartman and Dryden, 1974; MacRae et al., 2005; Zempleni et al., 2007; Haug et al., 2007; Krol et al., 2020). The vitamin requirements for humans are described in Table 6.17. Milk makes an important, although variable, contribution to providing the daily requirement of vitamins for human nutrition (Figure 6.14). Table 6.18 provides the composition of cows' milk from different countries and the average daily allowance. The composition and proportion of nutrients supplied by cow's milk depend on various factors intrinsic and extrinsic to the animal. Among the factors related to the animal are the lactation phase, age, breed, the energy balance of the animal, health of the udder and the cow, etc. (Lucas et al., 2006; Nozière et al., 2006; Haug et al., 2007; Swensson and Lindmark-Månsson, 2007; Kailasapathy, 2016; Krol et al., 2020; Shetty et al., 2020; Conboy Stephenson et al., 2021).

Even more critical, the milk's composition can be modified through different management and feeding strategies (forage-to-concentrate ratio, type, and proportion of ingredients used, vitamin-mineral supplementation, incorporating specific feed additives, etc.). Thus, for example, one can achieve considerable changes (>100% of change) in the content of conjugated

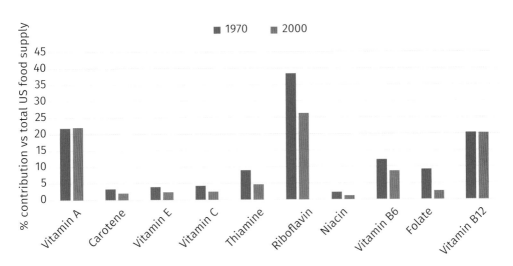

Figure 6.14 Contribution of milk and milk products to human daily vitamin requirements (source: adapted from Swensson and Lindmark-Månsson, 2007)

Table 6.17 Vitamin reference dietary requirements for humans in the United States (source: Price and Preedy, 2020)

	0–6 months	6–12 months	1–3 years	4–8 years	9–13 years	14–18 years	19–50 years	51–70 years	>70 years
Fat-soluble									
Vitamin A (µg/day)	400	500	300	400	600	900 M – 700 F	900 M – 700 F	900 M – 700 F	900 M – 700 F
Vitamin D (µg/day)	10	10	15	15	15	15	15	15	20
Vitamin E (mg/day)	4	5	6	11	15	15	15	15	15
Vitamin K (µg/day)	2	2.5	30	55	60	75	120 M – 90 F	120 M – 90 F	120 M – 90 F
Water-soluble									
B_1 thiamine (mg/day)	0.2	0.3	0.5	0.6	0.9	1.2 M – 1.0 F	1.2 M – 1.1 F	1.2 M – 1.1 F	1.2 M – 1.1 F
B_2 riboflavin (mg/day)	0.3	0.4	0.5	0.6	0.9	1.3 M – 1.0 F	1.3 M – 1.1 F	1.3 M – 1.1 F	1.3 M – 1.1 F
B_3 niacin (mg/day)	2	4	6	8	12	16 M – 14 F	16 M – 14 F	16 M – 14 F	16 M – 14 F
B_6 pyridoxine (mg/day)	0.1	0.3	0.5	0.6	1	1.3 M – 1.2 F	1.3	1.7 M – 1.5 F	1.7 M – 1.5 F
B_9 folate (µg/day)	65	80	150	200	300	400	400	400	400
Pantothenic acid (mg/day)	1.7	1.8	2	3	4	5	5	5	5
Biotin (µg/day)	5	6	8	12	20	25	30	30	30
B_{12} cobalamin (µg/day)	0.4	0.5	0.9	1.2	1.8	2.4	2.4	2.4	2.4
Vitamin C (mg/day)	40	50	15	25	45	75 M – 65 F	90 M – 75 F	90 M – 75 F	90 M – 75 F

Table 6.18 Variation in the vitamin content of milk and comparison with the recommended daily supplies in different countries

Content[1] (per 100 g of milk)	Unit	Spain[2]	Sweden[3]	Denmark[4]	USA[5]	Australia /New Zealand[6]	Averages[7]	
							Intake	% of RDI
Water	g	88.6	86.8	87.7	88.1	90.6	87.8	–
Protein	g	3.2	3.37	3.4	3.27	3.4	3.3	–
Lipids	g	3.6	4.34	3.5	3.2	3.5	3.7	–
Energy	kJ	260	NI	261	256	279	259.3	–
Cholesterol	mg	13	13.9	14	13.5	13	13.6	–
Vitamin A	mg RE	42	39.6	32.3	32	43	35.9	8.5
β-carotene	mg	22	20	16	7	18	19.3	–
Vitamin D	mg	0.03	0.03	0.1	0.96*	0.1	0.04	0.5
Vitamin E	mg	100	101	90	50	100	87.8	0.6
Vitamin K	mg	NI	0.41	–	0.2	–	0.2	0.2
Vitamin B_1 (thiamine)	mg	40	40	42	56	23	40.5	3.7
Vitamin B_2 (riboflavin)	mg	180	141	173	138	188	162.8	13.6
Niacin	mg	80	64	92	105	86	81	0.5
Vitamin B_6 (pyridoxine)	mg	40	42	47	61	20	42.3	3.3
Vitamin B_{12} (cobalamine)	mg	0.3	0.41	0.45	0.54	0.4	0.4	17.2
Pantothenic acid	mg	NI	340	340	362	360	340	6.8
Folic acid	mg	5	5.6	11	NI	5	7.2	1.8
Vitamin C	mg	1.8	1.16	1.2	0.82	0	0.9	2.1

Notes: [1]–, no content; NI, not indicated; vitamin A: μg of retinol equivalents.
[2]Adapted from Moreira et al. (2013); whole pasteurized milk.
[3]Adapted from Lindmark-Månsson et al. (2003); raw milk.
[4]Adapted from FRIDA Foodata.dk (consulted online 28/11/2023); whole milk, 3.5% fat.
[5]Adapted from: USDA, Food Data Central (consulted online 28/11/2023); whole milk, 3.25% fat, *with added vitamin D.
[6]Adapted from Food Standards Australia /New Zealand Food Composition Database (consulted online 28/11/2023) Milk, cow, fluid, regular fat (3.5% fat).
[7]% RDI, % of recommended daily intake. The approximate mean value, estimated from data available in the table, data appearing as – and Tr were computed as zero (0). RDI, recommended daily intake for an adult (19–65 years).

linoleic acid and vitamins A and E, moderate changes (between 25 and 100% of change) in the fat and unsaturated fatty acid content, and minor changes (<25% of change) in the folate, riboflavin, and vitamin B_{12} content (Haug et al., 2007).

Fat-soluble micronutrients, including fat-soluble vitamins, are embedded in the milk fat fraction, which has important implications for their bioaccessibility and bioavailability from milk (Baldi and Pinotti, 2008). A study conducted in Sweden by Lindmark-Månsson et al. (2003) compared the changes in the composition of cow's milk between 1970 and 1996, observing a significant increase in the content of total solids, fat, casein, calcium, and phosphorous, which is evidence that there is a real possibility of modifying the nutritional composition of milk. Another study (Swensson and Lindmark-Månsson, 2007) compared the changes in the vitamin supply of milk products per capita between 1970 and 2000 (Figure 6.14). The supply has decreased for most of them, except for vitamin A, which increased by 1.3%, and vitamin B_{12}, the supply of which remains constant. The most significant decreases have been in folic acid (71.4%), thiamine (47.2%), niacin (45.5%), and vitamin C (40.5%). More recently, Weir et al. (2020) concluded that vitamin D_3 fortification of cows' milk with 1, 1.5, and 2.0 µg/100 g theoretically increased median vitamin D intakes from 2.0 to 4.2, 5.1, and 5.9 µg/day, respectively. Higher vitamin D_3 in milk from this study than in food composition tables suggests further analysis is warranted. This model suggests that vitamin D_3 fortification of cows' milk is an effective strategy to help more of the population achieve recently revised reference nutrient intakes (RNIs) for vitamin D_3. Considering that the consumption of milk and dairy products is vital in the human diet, it is necessary to reconsider some of the recommendations for feeding dairy cattle, considering the contribution of milk to human nutrition (Graulet et al., 2013; Graulet and Girard, 2017; Krol et al., 2020). Baldi and Pinotti (2008) indicated that an advantage of augmenting milk microconstituents by animal nutrition rather than milk fortification is that it helps safeguard animal health, which is a primary factor in determining the quality, safety, and wholesomeness of animal-origin foods for human consumption.

CONCLUSION

Vitamins play a fundamental role in numerous vital functions. Under commercial conditions, vitamin deficiencies should not only be considered from the perspective of maintaining physiological functions. They are also required to allow optimum production and to prevent clinical or subclinical pathologies. In the last decades, vitamin recommendations established by ration formulation systems and those applied in field conditions by the industry have substantially increased, taking improved productivity, health, and welfare as evaluation criteria. The increases have been significant in vitamin E and moderate in vitamin A. Other vitamins previously considered unnecessary in the diet of adult ruminants, such as some of the water-soluble vitamins, may be beneficial under stress or high productivity conditions. However, their use under commercial conditions might require developing new forms less susceptible to degradation in the rumen. Finally, the vitamin supply in dairy cattle is essential not only from the perspective of animal production and its profitability. The ultimate objective is the production of quality milk that supplies all the nutrients and vitamins to meet the requirements of consumers.

Bibliography

Abaker, J. A., Xu, T. L., Jin, D., Chang, G. J., Zhang, K., & Shen, X. Z. (2017). Lipopolysaccharide derived from the digestive tract provokes oxidative stress in the liver of dairy cows fed a high-grain diet. *Journal of Dairy Science*, 100(1), 666–678. https://doi.org/10.3168/jds.2016-10871

Abd Ellah, M. R. (2013). Role of free radicals and antioxidants in mastitis. *Journal of Advanced Veterinary Research*, 3(1), 1–7. https://advetresearch.com/index.php/AVR/article/download/103/101

Abdouli, H., & Schaefer, D. M. (1986). Impact of niacin and length of incubation on protein synthesis, soluble to total protein ratio and fermentative activity of ruminal microorganisms. *Journal of Animal Science*, 62(1), 244–253. https://doi.org/10.2527/jas1986.621244x

Abrams, J. T. (1952). Livestock and their environments: Sunlight and vitamin D. *Veterinary Record*, 64, 151–157.

Abrams, J. T. (1978). Nutrient deficiencies in animals: Vitamin D. In *Handbook series in nutrition and food, 2* p. 179. CRC Press. Section E: Nutritional Disorders" (M. Rechcigl, Jr., ed).

Acedo, T. S., de Gouvea, V. N., de Vasconcellos, G. F., Arrigoni, M., Martins, C. L., Millen, D., Muller, L. R., de Melo, G. F., Rizzieri, R. A., da Costa, C. F., & Sartor, A. B. D. (2018). Effect of 25-hydroxyvitamin-D3 on feedlot cattle. *Journal of Animal Science*, 96(Suppl. 3) [Abstract].

Adams, C. R. (1973). Effect of environmental conditions on the stability of vitamins in feeds. In *Effect of processing on the nutritional value of feeds*. National Academy of Sciences, National Research Council.

Adams, C. R. (1978). Vitamin product forms for animal feeds. In *Vitamin nutrition update-seminar series 2* p. 5483/1078. Hoffman-La Roche, Inc.. RCD

Adams, C. R., Eoff, H. J., & Zimmerman, C. R. (1975). Protecting feeds from vitamin E and A deficits in lightweight moldy and blighted corn. *Feedstuffs*, 47(36), 24.

Adams, R. S., Sautter, J. H., Gullickson, T. W., & Gander, J. E. (1959). Some effects of feeding various filled milks to dairy calves. IV. Necropsy findings, electrocardiographic studies, and creatinuria ratios. *Journal of Dairy Science*, 42(9), 1580–1591. https://doi.org/10.3168/jds.S0022-0302(59)90770-2

Adil, M., Iqbal, M., Kanwal, S., & Abbas, G. (2024). Toxicity and adverse effects of veterinary pharmaceuticals in animals. In *Pharmaceuticals in aquatic environments* (pp. 141–159). CRC Press.

Afiati, F., Lestari, D. A., & Malini, D. M. (2016). Effect of vitamin C administration in diluent media to quality of dairy cattle thawed spermatozoa. *Jurnal Ilmu Ternak dan Veteriner*, 21(2), 124–134. https://doi.org/10.14334/jitv.v21i2.1360

Ahmadi, S., & Mohri, M. (2021). New outlook to vitamin D functions in dairy cows: Nonclassical roles. Iran. *Journal of Veterinary Science and Technology*, 13(2), 1–11. https://doi.org/10.22067/IJVST.2021.70605.1044

Ahmadi, S., Farzaneh, N., & Mohri, M. (2022). Changes and relations of 25(OH) vitamin D and some inflammatory and oxidative stress indicators in healthy dairy cows during transition period. *Comparative Clinical Pathology*, 31(6), 917–924. https://doi.org/10.1007/s00580-022-03392-8

Ahmed, F., Jones, D. B., & Jackson, A. A. (1990). The interaction of vitamin A deficiency and rotavirus infection in the mouse. *The British Journal of Nutrition*, 63(2), 363–373. https://doi.org/10.1079/bjn19900122

Airado-Rodríguez, D., Intawiwat, N., Skaret, J., & Wold, J. P. (2011). Effect of naturally occurring tetrapyrroles on photooxidation in cow's milk. *Journal of Agricultural and Food Chemistry*, 59(8), 3905–3914. https://doi.org/10.1021/jf104259p

Aitkin, F. C., & Hankin, R. G. (1970). *Vitamins in feed for livestock*. CAB.

Akar, Y., & Gazioglu, A. (2006). Relationship between vitamin A and β-carotene levels during the postpartum period and fertility parameters in cows with and without retained placenta. *Bulletin of the Veterinary Institute in Pulawy*, 50, 93–96.

Akordor, F. Y., Stone, J. B., Walton, J. S., Leslie, K. E., & Buchanan-Smith, J. G. (1986). Reproductive per-formance of lactating Holstein cows fed supplemental beta-carotene. *Journal of Dairy Science, 69*(8), 2173–2178. https://doi.org/10.3168/jds.S0022-0302(86)80650-6

Al-Attar, A. M. (2011). Vitamin E attenuates liver injury induced by exposure to lead, mercury, cadmium and copper in albino mice. *Saudi Journal of Biological Sciences, 18*(4), 395–401. https://doi.org/10.1016/j.sjbs.2011.07.004

Albonico, F., & Fabris, A. (1958). Fattori influenzanti il contenuto vitaminico e clorofillico di alcune foraggere leguminose. *Agrochimica, 2*, 147–176 (in Italian).

Alderson, N. E., Mitchell, G. E., Little, C. O., Warner, R. E., & Tucker, R. E. (1971). Preintestinal disappearance of vitamin E in ruminants. *The Journal of Nutrition, 101*(5), 655–659. https://doi.org/10.1093/jn/101.5.655

Ali, A., Morrical, D. G., Hoffman, M. P., & Al-Essa, M. F. (2004). Evaluation of vitamin E and selenium supple-mentation in late gestation on lamb survival and preweaning growth. *The Professional Animal Scientist, 20*(6), 506–511. https://doi.org/10.15232/S1080-7446(15)31355-3

Aliev, A. A., & Burkova, L. M. (1987). Effect of choline chloride on the metabolism of nitrogen and choline in the stomach and intestines of lactating cows. *Skh. Biol., 4*, 80.

Allahdad, Z., Varidi, M., Zadmard, R., & Saboury, A. A. (2018). Spectroscopic and docking studies on the interaction between caseins and β-carotene. *Food Chemistry, 255*, 187–196. https://doi.org/10.1016/j.foodchem.2018.01.143

Allen, W. M., Bradley, R., Berrett, S., Parr, W. H., Swannack, K., Barton, C. R. Q., & Macphee, A. (1975). Degenerative myopathy with myoglobinuria in yearling cattle. *The British Veterinary Journal, 131*(3), 292–308. https://doi.org/10.1016/S0007-1935(17)35286-7

Alonso, N., Meinitzer, A., Fritz-Petrin, E., Enko, D., & Herrmann, M. (2023). Role of vitamin K in bone and muscle metabolism. *Calcified Tissue International, 112*(2), 178–196. https://doi.org/10.1007/s00223-022-00955-3

Alosilla, C. E., McDowell, L. R., Wilkinson, N. S., Staples, C. R., Thatcher, W. W., Martin, F. G., & Blair, M. (2007). Bioavailability of vitamin A sources for cattle. *Journal of Animal Science, 85*(5), 1235–1238. https://doi.org/10.2527/jas.2006-251

Alstad, A. D., Casper, H. H., & Johnson, L. J. (1985). Vitamin K treatment of sweet clover poisoning in calves. *Journal of the American Veterinary Medical Association, 187*(7), 729–731. PubMed: 2414258

Álvarez, R., Meléndez-Martínez, A. J., Vicario, I. M., & Alcalde, M. J. (2015). Carotenoid and vitamin A contents in biological fluids and tissues of animals as an effect of the diet: A review. *Food Reviews International, 31*(4), 319–340. https://doi.org/10.1080/87559129.2015.1015139

Alves de Oliveira, L., Jean-Blain, C., Komisarczuk-Bony, S., Durix, A., & Durier, C. (1997). Microbial thiamine metabolism in the rumen simulating ferementer (RUSITEC): The effect of acidogenic conditions, a high súlfur level and added thiamine. *The British Journal of Nutrition, 78*(4), 599–613. https://doi.org/10.1079/bjn19970177

Amat, S., Olkowski, A. A., Atila, M., & O'Neill, T. J. (2013). A review of polioencephalomalacia in ruminants: Is the development of malacic lesions associated with excess sulfur intake independent of thiamine deficiency. Vet. Med. *Animal Science, 1*(1), 1. https://doi.org/10.7243/2054-3425-1-1

Amin, M. R., & Onodera, R. (1998). Effects of salinomycin and vitamin B_6 on *in vitro* metabolism of pheny-lalanine and its related compounds by ruminal bacteria, protozoa and their mixture. *The Journal of General and Applied Microbiology, 44*(1), 1–9. https://doi.org/10.2323/jgam.44.1

Aminifard, Z., & Kiani, A. (2023). Determination of fermentation and digestibility parameters of tomato pomace in comparison with wheat bran under *in vitro* conditions. *J. Anim. Sci. Res., 33*(2), 93–105. https://doi.org/10.22034/as.2022.41844.1583

Aminifard, Z., Kiani, A., & Azarfar, A. (2022). Determination of nutritional value and digestibility of tomato pomace before and after oil extraction *in vitro* and evaluation of ruminal disappearance of lycopene *in situ*. *J. Animal Production, 24*(4), 441–452. https://doi.org/10.22059/jap.2022.338142.623673

Anderson, P. H., Berrett, S., & Patterson, D. S. P. (1976). The significance of elevated plasma creatine phos-phokinase activity in muscle disease of cattle. *Journal of Comparative Pathology, 86*(4), 531–538. https://doi.org/10.1016/0021-9975(76)90062-1

Andrews, E. D., Hart, L. I., & Stephenson, B. J. (1960). Vitamin B$_{12}$ and cobalt in livers from grazing cobalt-deficient lambs and from others given various cobalt supplements. *New Zealand Journal of Agricultural Research*, *3*(2), 364–376. https://doi.org/10.1080/00288233.1960.10418091

Andrews, E. D., Hartley, W. J., & Grant, A. B. (1968). Selenium-responsive diseases of animals in New Zealand. *New Zealand Veterinary Journal*, *16*(1–2), 3–17. https://doi.org/10.1080/00480169.1968.33738

Aoki, M., Ohshita, T., Aoki, Y., & Sakaguchi, M. (2014). Plasma thiobarbituric acid reactive substances, vitamin A and vitamin E levels and resumption of postpartum ovarian activity in dairy cows. *Animal Science Journal*, *85*(5), 532–541. https://doi.org/10.1111/asj.12181

Aragona, K. M., Rice, E. M., Engstrom, M., & Erickson, P. S. (2020). Supplementation of nicotinic acid to pre-partum Holstein cows increases colostral immunoglobulin G, excretion of urinary purine derivatives, and feed efficiency in calves. *Journal of Dairy Science*, *103*(3), 2287–2302. https://doi.org/10.3168/jds.2019-17058

Arambell, M. J., Dennis, S. M., Riddel, D. O., Bartley, E. E., Camac, J. L., & Dayton, A. D. (1982). Effect of heat-treated soybean meal with and without niacin on rumen fermentation. *Journal of Animal Science*, *55*(1), 405.

Ardalan, M., Rezayazdi, K., & Dehghan-Banadaky, M. (2010). Effect of rumen-protected choline and methionine on physiological and metabolic disorders and reproductive indices of dairy cows. *Journal of Animal Physiology and Animal Nutrition*, *94*(6), e259–e265. https://doi.org/10.1111/j.1439-0396.2009.00966.x

Aréchiga, C. F., Ortíz, O., & Hansen, P. J. (1994). Effect of prepartum injection of vitamin E and selenium on postpartum reproductive function of dairy cattle. *Theriogenology*, *41*(6), 1251–1258. https://doi.org/10.1016/0093-691X(94)90482-X

Aréchiga, C. F., Staples, C. R., McDowell, L. R., & Hansen, P. J. (1998). Effects of timed insemination and supplemental beta-carotene on reproduction and milk yield of dairy cows under heat stress. *Journal of Dairy Science*, *81*(2), 390–402. https://doi.org/10.3168/jds.S0022-0302(98)75589-4

Arellano-Rodriguez, G., Meza-Herrera, C. A., Rodriguez-Martinez, R., Dionisio-Tapia, R., Hallford, D. M., Mellado, M., & Gonzalez-Bulnes, A. (2009). Short-term intake of β-carotene-supplemented diets enhances ovarian function and progesterone synthesis in goats. *Journal of Animal Physiology and Animal Nutrition*, *93*(6), 710–715. https://doi.org/10.1111/j.1439-0396.2008.00859.x

Arihara, K. (2006). Strategies for designing novel functional meat products. *Meat Science*, *74*(1), 219–229. https://doi.org/10.1016/j.meatsci.2006.04.028

Arikan, S., & Rodway, R. G. (2000). Effects of high-density lipoprotein containing high or low beta-carotene concentrations on progesterone production and beta-carotene uptake and depletion by bovine luteal cells. *Animal Reproduction Science*, *62*(4), 253–263. https://doi.org/10.1016/S0378-4320(00)00122-6

Arikan, S., Sands, H. S., Rodway, R. G., & Batchelder, D. N. (2002). Raman spectroscopy and imaging of β-carotene in live *corpus luteum* cells. *Animal Reproduction Science*, *71*(3–4), 249–266. https://doi.org/10.1016/S0378-4320(02)00020-9

Arizmendi-Maldonado, D., McDowell, L. R., Sinclair, T. R., Mislevy, P., Martin, F. G., & Wilkinson, N. S. (2003). α-tocopherol and β-carotene concentrations in tropical grasses as affected by increasing daylength. *Communications in Soil Science and Plant Analysis*, *34*(3–4), 519–530. https://doi.org/10.1081/CSS-120017836

Arnold, R. N., Scheller, K. K., Arp, S. C., Williams, S. N., Buege, D. R., & Schaefer, D. M. (1992). Effect of long- or short-term feeding of α-tocopheryl acetate to Holstein and Crossbred beef steers on performance, carcass characteristics, and beef color stability. *Journal of Animal Science*, *70*(10), 3055–3065. https://doi.org/10.2527/1992.70103055x

Ascarelli, I., Edelman, Z., Rosenberg, M., & Folman, S. (1985). Effect of dietary carotene on fertility of high yielding dairy cows. *Animal Production*, *40*, 195–207. https://doi.org/10.1017/S0003356100025307

Ashwin, K., Paladan, V., Uniyal, S., Sahoo, J. K., Perween, S., Gupta, M., & Singh, A. (2018). An update on B vitamin nutrition for cattle. *International Journal of Current Microbiology and Applied Sciences*, *7*(7), 188–192. https://doi.org/10.20546/ijcmas.2018.707.023

Asson-Batres, M. A., Smith, W. B., & Clark, G. (2009). Retinoic acid is present in the postnatal rat olfactory organ and persists in vitamin A–depleted neural tissue. *The Journal of Nutrition*, *139*(6), 1067–1072. https://doi.org/10.3945/jn.108.096040

Astrup, H. N., & Nedkvitne, J. J. (1987). Effect of vitamin D supplement on cows and sheep. *Norwegian Journal of Agricultural Sciences*, *1*, 87.

Atef, S. H. (2018). Vitamin D assays in clinical laboratory: Past, present and future challenges. *The Journal of Steroid Biochemistry and Molecular Biology*, 175, 136–137. https://doi.org/10.1016/j.jsbmb.2017.02.011

Atkins, K. B., Erdman, R. A., & Vandersall, J. H. (1988). Dietary choline effects on milk and duodenal choline flow in dairy cattle. *Journal of Dairy Science*, 71(1), 109–116. https://doi.org/10.3168/jds.S0022-0302(88)79531-4

Axelrod, A. E. (1971). Immune processes in vitamin deficiency states. *The American Journal of Clinical Nutrition*, 24(2), 265–271. https://doi.org/10.1093/ajcn/24.2.265

Axelsson, S. (1991). Origin and significance of acetylcholine and choline in plasma and serum from normal and paretic cows. *Zentralblatt Fur Veterinarmedizin. Reihe A*, 38(10), 737–748. https://doi.org/10.1111/j.1439-0442.1991.tb01073.x

Azzi, A., Breyer, I., Feher, M., Pastori, M., Ricciarelli, R., Spycher, S., Staffieri, M., Stocker, A., Zimmer, S., & Zingg, J. M. (2000). Specific cellular responses to α-tocopherol. *The Journal of Nutrition*, 130(7), 1649–1652. https://doi.org/10.1093/jn/130.7.1649

Bâ, A. (2008). Metabolic and structural role of thiamine in nervous tissues. *Cellular and Molecular Neurobiology*, 28(7), 923–931. https://doi.org/10.1007/s10571-008-9297-7

Babior, B. M. (1984). The respiratory burst of phagocytes. *The Journal of Clinical Investigation*, 73(3), 599–601. https://doi.org/10.1172/JCI111249

Babu, S., & Srikantia, S. G. (1976). Availability of folates from some foods. *The American Journal of Clinical Nutrition*, 29(4), 376–379. https://doi.org/10.1093/ajcn/29.4.376

Bachmann, H., Offord-Cavin, E., Phothirath, P., Horcajada, M. N., Romeis, P., & Mathis, G. A. (2013). 1, 25-dihydroxyvitamin D_3-glycoside of herbal origin exhibits delayed release pharmacokinetics when compared to its synthetic counterpart. *The Journal of Steroid Biochemistry and Molecular Biology*, 136, 333–336. https://doi.org/10.1016/j.jsbmb.2012.09.016

Badman, J., Daly, K., Kelly, J., Moran, A. W., Cameron, J., Watson, I., Newbold, J., & Shirazi-Beechey, S. P. (2019). The effect of milk replacer composition on the intestinal microbiota of pre-ruminant dairy calves. In *Frontiers in Veterinary Science*, 6, 371. https://doi.org/10.3389/fvets.2019.00371

Badwey, J. A., & Karnovsky, M. L. (1980). Active oxygen species and the functions of phagocytic leukocytes. *Annual Review of Biochemistry*, 49, 695–726. https://doi.org/10.1146/annurev.bi.49.070180.003403

Bai, H., Arai, H., Ikuta, K., Ishikawa, S., Ohtani, Y., Iwashita, K., Okada, N., Shirakawa, H., Komai, M., Terada, F., & Obara, Y. (2021). Effects of dietary vitamin K3 supplementation on vitamin K1 and K2 (menaquinone) dynamics in dairy cows. *Journal of Animal Science*, 93, e13680. https://doi.org/10.1111/asj.13680

Bailey, L. B., & Gregory, J. F. (1999). Folate metabolism and requirements. *The Journal of Nutrition*, 129(4), 779–782. https://doi.org/10.1093/jn/129.4.779

Bailey, L. B., & Gregory, J. F. (2006). Folate. In B. Bowman & R. Russell (Eds.), *Present knowledge in nutrition* (pp. 278–301). International Life Sciences Institute.

Bailey, L. B., Da Silva, V., West, A. A., & Caudill, M. A. (2013). Folate. In J. Zempleni, J. Suttie, J. Gregory, & P. J. Stover (Eds.), *Handbook of vitamins* (5th ed.) (pp. 421–446). CRC Press, Taylor & Francis Group, LLC ISBN 9781466515567.

Baker, D. H., Allen, N. K., & Kleiss, A. J. (1973). Efficiency of tryptophan as a niacin precursor in young chicks. *Journal of Animal Science*, 36(2), 299–302. https://doi.org/10.2527/jas1973.362299x

Baker, S. S., & Cohen, H. J. (1983). Altered oxidative metabolism in selenium-deficient rat granulocytes. *Journal of Immunology*, 130(6), 2856–2860. https://doi.org/10.4049/jimmunol.130.6.2856, PubMed: 6304192

Baldi, A. (2005). Vitamin E in dairy cows. *Livestock Production Science*, 98(1–2), 117–122. https://doi.org/10.1016/j.livprodsci.2005.10.004

Baldi, A., & Pinotti, L. (2008). Lipophilic microconstituents of milk. *Advances in Experimental Medicine and Biology*, 606, 109–125. https://doi.org/10.1007/978-0-387-74087-4_3

Baldi, A., Bontempo, V., Cheli, F., Carli, S., Sgoifo Rossi, C. S., & Dell'orto, V. (1997). Relative bioavailability of vitamin E in dairy cows following intraruminal administration of three different preparations of DL-α-tocopheryl acetate. *Veterinary Research*, 28(6), 517–524. PubMed: 9428145

Baldi, A., Cheli, F., Pinotti, L., & Pecorini, C. (2008). Nutrition in mammary gland health and lactation: Advances over eight Biology of Lactation in Farm Animals meetings. *Journal of Animal Science*, 86(13) (Suppl.), 3–9. https://doi.org/10.2527/jas.2007-0286

Baldwin, R. L., & Allison, M. J. (1983). Rumen metabolism. *Journal of Animal Science, 57*(2)(Suppl. 2), 461–477. PubMed: 6352592

Ballet, N., Robert, J. C., & Williams, P. E. V. (2000). 19 vitamins in forages. In D. I. Givens, E. Owen, R. F. E. Axford, & H. M. Omed (Eds.). ISBN-0-85199-344-3, *Forage evaluation in ruminant nutrition* (pp. 399–431In).

Ballou, M. A. (2012). Immune responses of Holstein and Jersey calves during the preweaning and immediate post weaned periods when fed varying planes of milk replacer. *Journal of Dairy Science, 95*(12), 7319–7330. https://doi.org/10.3168/jds.2012-5970

Barash, P. G. (1978). Nutrient toxicities of vitamin K. In M. Rechcigl, Jr. (Ed.), *CRC Handbook series in nutrition and food, section E: Nutrition Disorders* (p. 97). CRC Press.

Bargai, U., & Levin, D. (1993). Lameness in the Israeli dairy herd: A national survey of incidence, types, distribution and estimated cost. *Israel Journal of Veterinary Medicine, 48*(2), 88–90.

Barouh, N., Bourlieu-Lacanal, C., Figueroa-Espinoza, M. C., Durand, E., & Villeneuve, P. (2022). Tocopherols as antioxidants in lipid-based systems: The combination of chemical and physicochemical interactions determines their efficiency. *Comprehensive Reviews in Food Science and Food Safety, 21*(1), 642–688. https://doi.org/10.1111/1541-4337.12867

Bartlett, C. A., Schwab, C. G., Smith, J. W., & Holter, J. B. (1983). Supplemental niacin for dairy cows under field conditions. II. Effects on production. *Journal of Dairy Science, 66*(1), 176 [Abstr.].

Bartley, E. E., Herod, E. L., Bechtle, R. M., Sapienza, D. A., Brent, B. E., & Davidovich, A. (1979). Effect of monensin or lasalocid, with and without niacin or amicloral, on rumen fermentation and feed efficiency. *Journal of Animal Science, 49*(4), 1066–1075. https://doi.org/10.2527/jas1979.4941066x

Barton, C. R., & Allen, W. M. (1973). Possible paralytic myoglobinuria of unknown actiology in young cattle. *The Veterinary Record, 92*(11), 288–290. https://doi.org/10.1136/vr.92.11.288

Bates, C. J. (2006). Thiamine. In B. A. Bowman & R. M. Russell (Eds.), *Present knowledge in nutrition* (9th ed.) (pp. 242–249). International Life Sciences Institute.

Batra, T. R., Hidiroglou, M., & Smith, M. W. (1992). Effect of vitamin E on incidence of mastitis in dairy cattle. *Canadian Journal of Animal Science, 72*(2), 287–297. https://doi.org/10.4141/cjas92-036

Bauernfeind, J. C. (1981). Carotenoids as colorants and vitamin A precursors. Technological and nutritional applications. *Food science and technology* [Monographs]. Academic Press.

Baugh, C. M., & Krumdieck, C. L. (1971). Naturally occurring folates. *Annals of the New York Academy of Sciences, 186*, 7–28. https://doi.org/10.1111/j.1749-6632.1971.tb46952.x

Beaudet, V., Gervais, R., Graulet, B., Nozière, P., Doreau, M., Fanchone, A., Castagnino, D. D. S., & Girard, C. L. (2016). Effects of dietary nitrogen levels and carbohydrate sources on apparent ruminal synthesis of some B vitamins in dairy cows. *Journal of Dairy Science, 99*(4), 2730–2739. https://doi.org/10.3168/jds.2015-10521

Beck, M. A. (1997). Increased virulence of coxsackievirus B$_3$ in mice due to vitamin E or selenium deficiency. *The Journal of Nutrition, 127*(5)(Suppl.), 966S–970S. https://doi.org/10.1093/jn/127.5.966S

Beck, M. A. (2007). Selenium and vitamin E status: Impact on viral pathogenicity. *The Journal of Nutrition, 137*(5), 1338–1340. https://doi.org/10.1093/jn/137.5.1338

Beck, M. A., Kolbeck, P. C., Rohr, L. H., Shi, Q., Morris, V. C., & Levander, O. A. (1994). Vitamin E deficiency intensifies the myocardial injury of Cosxackievirus B$_3$ infection of mice. *The Journal of Nutrition, 124*(3), 345–358. https://doi.org/10.1093/jn/124.3.345

Becker, D. E., & Smith, S. E. (1951). The level of cobalt tolerance in yearling sheep. *Journal of Animal Science, 10*(1), 266–271. https://doi.org/10.2527/jas1951.101266x

Beeckman, A., Vicca, J., Van Ranst, G., Janssens, G. P. J., & Fievez, V. (2010). Monitoring of vitamin E status of dry, early and mid-late lactating organic dairy cows fed conserved roughages during the indoor period and factors influencing forage vitamin E levels. *Journal of Animal Physiology and Animal Nutrition, 94*(6), 736–746. https://doi.org/10.1111/j.1439-0396.2009.00956.x

Beenken, A. M., Deters, E. L., & Hansen, S. L. (2021). The effect of injectable vitamin C and road transit duration on inflammation, muscle fatigue, and performance in pre-conditioned beef steer calves. Journal of Animal Science, 99(12). https://doi.org/10.1093/jas/skab312

Beharka, A., Redican, S., Leka, L., & Meydani, S. N. (1997). Vitamin E status and immune function. *Methods in Enzymology, 282*, 247–263. https://doi.org/10.1016/S0076-6879(97)82112-X

Beisel, W. R. (1982). Single nutrients and immunity. *The American Journal of Clinical Nutrition, 35*(2)(Suppl.), 417–468. https://doi.org/10.1093/ajcn/35.2.417

Bell, A. W., & Bauman, D. E. (1997). Adaptations of glucose metabolism during pregnancy and lactation. *Journal of Mammary Gland Biology and Neoplasia, 2*(3), 265–278. https://doi.org/10.1023/A:1026336505343

Bender, D. A. (1992). *Nutritional biochemistry of the vitamins.* Cambridge University Press. https://doi.org/10.1017/CBO9780511615191

Bendich, A. (1987). Role of antioxidant vitamins on immune function. In "Proc. Roche Technical Symp.: "The role of vitamins on animal performance and immune response." RCD 7442. Hoffmann–La Roche, Inc.

Bendich, A. (1989). Carotenoids and immune response. *The Journal of Nutrition, 119*(1), 112–115. https://doi.org/10.1093/jn/119.1.112

Bendich, A. (1993). Physiological role of antioxidants in the immune system. *Journal of Dairy Science, 76*(9), 2789–2794. https://doi.org/10.3168/jds.S0022-0302(93)77617-1

Benevenga, N. J., Baldwin, R. L., & Ronning, M. (1966). Alterations in liver enzyme activities and blood and urine metabolite levels during the onset of thiamine deficiency in the dairy calf. *The Journal of Nutrition, 90*(2), 131–140. https://doi.org/10.1093/jn/90.2.131

Benito, E., & Bosch, M. A. (1997). Impaired phosphatidylcholine biosynthesis and ascorbic acid depletion in lung during lipopolysaccharide-induced endotoxemia in guinea pigs. *Molecular and Cellular Biochemistry, 175*(1–2), 117–123. https://doi.org/10.1023/a:1006883628365

Benoit, S. L. A., Bequett, B. J., & Erdman, R. A. (2010). Rumen-protected choline affects methionine methyl group metabolism in lactating dairy cows. *Journal of Dairy Science, 93*(1), 473 [Abstr.].

Bergsten, C., Greenough, P. R., Gay, J. M., Dobson, R. C., & Gay, C. C. (1999). A controlled field trial of the effects of biotin supplementation on milk production and hoof lesions. *Journal of Dairy Science, 82*(1), 34 [Abstr.].

Bergsten, C., Greenough, P. R., Gay, J. M., Seymour, W. M., & Gay, C. C. (2003). Effects of biotin supplementation on performance and claw lesions on a commercial dairy farm. *Journal of Dairy Science, 86*(12), 3953–3962. https://doi.org/10.3168/jds.S0022-0302(03)74005-3

Bettendorff, L. (2013). Vitamin B₁. In J. Zempleni, J. Suttie, J. Gregory, & P. J. Stover (Eds.), *Handbook of vitamins* (5th ed.) (pp. 267–324). CRC Press, Taylor & Francis Group.

Bhandari, S. D., & Gregory, J. F. (1992). Folic acid, 5-methyl-tetrahydrofolate and 5-formyl-tetrahydrofolate exhibit equivalent intestinal absorption, metabolism and *in vivo* kinetics in rats. *The Journal of Nutrition, 122*(9), 1847–1854. https://doi.org/10.1093/jn/122.9.1847

Bhat, M. K., & Cama, H. R. (1978). Thyroidal control of hepatic release and metabolism of vitamin A. *Biochimica et Biophysica Acta, 541*(2), 211–222. https://doi.org/10.1016/0304-4165(78)90394-X

Bierer, T. L., Merchen, N. R., & Erdman, J. W. (1995). Comparative absorption and transport of five common carotenoids in preruminant calves. *The Journal of Nutrition, 125*(6), 1569–1577. https://doi.org/10.1093/jn/125.6.1569

Bindas, E. M., Gwazdauskas, F. C., Aiello, R. J., Herbein, J. H., McGilliard, M. L., & Polan, C. E. (1984a). Reproductive and metabolic characteristics of dairy cattle supplemented with β-carotene. *Journal of Dairy Science, 67*(6), 1249–1255. https://doi.org/10.3168/jds.S0022-0302(84)81431-9

Bindas, E. M., Gwazdauskas, F. C., McGilliard, M. L., & Polan, C. E. (1984b). Progesterone responses to human chorionic gonadotropin in dairy cattle supplemented with β-carotene. *Journal of Dairy Science, 67*(12), 2978–2985. https://doi.org/10.3168/jds.S0022-0302(84)81663-X

Bindel, D. J., Drouillard, J. S., Titgemeyer, E. C., Ives, S. E., & Wessels, R. H. (1998). Effects of ruminally protected choline and dietary fat on blood metabolites of finishing heifers. *Journal of Animal Science, 76*(1), 52. https://doi.org/10.2527/2000.78102497x

Bindel, D. J., Drouillard, J. S., Titgemeyer, E. C., Wessels, R. H., & Löest, C. A. (2000). Effects of ruminally protected choline and dietary fat on performance and blood metabolites of finishing heifers. *Journal of Animal Science, 78*(10), 2497–2503. https://doi.org/10.2527/2000.78102497x

Bindel, D. J., Titgemeyer, E. C., Drouillard, J. S., & Ives, S. E. (2005). Effects of choline on blood metabolites associated with lipid metabolism and digestion by steers fed corn-based diets. *Journal of Animal Science, 83*(7), 1625–1632. https://doi.org/10.2527/2005.8371625x

Binkley, N. C., & Suttie, J. W. (1995). Vitamin K nutrition and osteoporosis. *The Journal of Nutrition, 125*(7), 1812–1821. https://doi.org/10.1093/jn/125.7.1812

Birdsall, J. J. (1975). Technology of fortification of foods. *Proceedings of the National Academy of Sciences of the United States of America, 126*. https://doi.org/10.17226/20201

Bito, T., & Watanabe, F. (2022). *Seaweeds as a source of vitamin B_{12}. Sustainable global resources of seaweeds volume 2: Food, pharmaceutical and health applications* p. 339. https://doi.org/10.1007/978-3-030-92174-3_18

Bjørneboe, A., Bjørneboe, G. E. A., & Drevon, C. A. (1990). Absorption, transport and distribution of vitamin E. *The Journal of Nutrition, 120*(3), 233–242. https://doi.org/10.1093/jn/120.3.233

Black, W. D., & Hidiroglou, M. (1996). Pharmacokinetic study of ascorbic acid in sheep. *CJVR, 60*(3), 216–221. http://www.ncbi.nlm.nih.gov/pmc/articles/pmc1263836/

Blair, L., & Cummins, K. A. (1984). Effect of dietary ascorbic acid on blood immunoglobulin concentration in dairy calves. *Journal of Dairy Science, 67*(Suppl. 1), 138.

Blaxter, K. L. (1962). The significance of selenium and vitamin E in nutrition. Muscular dystrophy in farm animals: Its cause and prevention. *The Proceedings of the Nutrition Society, 21*(2), 211–216. https://doi.org/10.1079/PNS19620034

Blaylock, L. G., & Richardson, L. R. (1950). Peanut meal, mixtures of soybean and cottonseed and mixtures of soybean and peanut meals as sources of protein for baby chicks. *Poultry Science, 29*(5), 656–660. https://doi.org/10.3382/ps.0290656

Block, E. (1984). Manipulating dietary anions and cations for prepartum dairy cows to reduce incidence of milk fever. *Journal of Dairy Science, 67*(12), 2939–2948. https://doi.org/10.3168/jds.S0022-0302(84)81657-4

Block, E., & Farmer, B. (1987). The status of beta-carotene and vitamin A in Quebec dairy herds: Factors affecting their status in cows and their effects on reproductive performance. *Canadian Journal of Animal Science, 67*(3), 775–788. https://doi.org/10.4141/cjas87-080

Blomhoff, R. (1994). *Vitamin A in health and disease.* Marcel Dekker, Inc.

Blomhoff, R., Green, M. H., Green, J. B., Berg, T., & Norum, K. R. (1991). Vitamin A metabolism: New perspectives on absorption, transport and storage. *Physiological Reviews, 71*(4), 951–990. https://doi.org/10.1152/physrev.1991.71.4.951

Blum, J. W., & Baumrucker, C. R. (2002). Colostral and milk insulin-like growth factors and related substances. Mammary gland and neonatal (intestinal and systemic) targets. *Domestic Animal Endocrinology, 23*(1–2), 101–110. https://doi.org/10.1016/S0739-7240(02)00149-2

Bobe, G., Young, J. W., & Beitz, D. C. (2004). Invited review: Pathology, etiology, prevention, and treatment of fatty liver in dairy cows. *Journal of Dairy Science, 87*(10), 3105–3124. https://doi.org/10.3168/jds.S0022-0302(04)73446-3

Bollatti, J. M., Zenobi, M. G., Artusso, N. A., Lopez, A. M., Barton, B. A., Staples, C. R., & Santos, J. E. P. (2019a). Effects of rumen-protected choline on the inflammatory and metabolic status and health of dairy cows during the transition period. *Journal of Dairy Science, 103*, 4192–4205. https://doi.org/10.3168/jds.2019-17294

Bollatti, J. M., Zenobi, M. G., Barton, B. A., Staples, C. R., & Santos, J. E. P. (2019b). Responses to rumen-protected choline in transition cows do not depend on prepartum body condition. *Journal of Dairy Science, 103*(3), 2272–2286. https://doi.org/10.3168/jds.2019-17302

Bollatti, J. M., Zenobi, M. G., Artusso, N. A., Alfaro, G. F., Lopez, A. M., Barton, B. A., Nelson, C. D., Staples, C. R., & Santos, J. E. P. (2020). Timing of initiation and duration of feeding rumen-protected choline affects performance of lactating Holstein cows. *Journal of Dairy Science, 103*(5), 4174–4191. https://doi.org/10.3168/jds.2019-17293

Bonjour, J. P. (1991). Biotin. In L. J. Machlin (Ed.), *Handbook of vitamins* (2nd ed.). Marcel Dekker, Inc.

Bonsembiante, M., Bittante, G., & Andrighetto, I. (1986). *Beta-carotene effect on fertility of beef heifers and cows.* F. Hoffmann-La Roche, and Co., Ltd.

Booth, A., Reid, M., & Clark, T. (1987). Hypovitaminosis A in feedlot cattle. *Journal of the American Veterinary Medical Association, 190*(10), 1305–1308. PubMed: 3583885

Booth, S. L., & Mayer, J. (1997). Skeletal functions of vitamin K-dependent proteins: Not just for clotting anymore. *Nutrition Research Reviews, 55*(7), 282–284. https://doi.org/10.1111/j.1753-4887.1997.tb01619.x

Bourne, N., Laven, R., Wathes, D. C., Martinez, T., & McGowan, M. (2007a). A meta-analysis of the effects of vitamin-E supplementation on the incidence of retained fetal membranes in dairy cows. *Theriogenology*, *67*(3), 494–501. https://doi.org/10.1016/j.theriogenology.2006.08.015

Bourne, N., Wathes, D. C., McGowan, M., & Laven, R. A. (2007b). A comparison of the effects of parenteral and oral administration of supplementary vitamin E on plasma vitamin E concentrations in dairy cows at different stages of lactation. *Livestock Science*, *106*(1), 57–64. https://doi.org/10.1016/j.livsci.2006.07.001

Bourne, N., Wathes, D. C., Lawrence, K. E., McGowan, M., & Laven, R. A. (2008). The effect of parenteral supplementation of vitamin E with selenium on the health and productivity of dairy cattle in the UK. *Veterinary Journal*, *177*(3), 381–387 [Abstract]. https://doi.org/10.1016/j.tvjl.2007.06.006

Bouwstra, R. J., Nielen, M., Newbold, J. R., Jansen, E. H. J. M., Jelinek, H. F., & Van Werven, T. (2010). Vitamin E supplementation during the dry period in dairy cattle. Part II: Oxidative stress following vitamin E supplementation may increase clinical mastitis incidence postpartum. *Journal of Dairy Science*, *93*(12), 5696–5706. https://doi.org/10.3168/jds.2010-3161

Bowland, J. P., & Owen, B. D. (1952). Supplemental pantothenic acid in small grain rations for swine. *Journal of Animal Science*, *1*, 757 [Abstr.].

BR Corte (2023) Exigências Nutricionais de Zebuínos Puros e Cruzados (Nutritional Requirements of Purebred and Crossbred Zebu). de Campos Valadares Filho, S., Saraiva, D. T., Benedeti, P., de Sales Silva, F.A. and Chizotti, M.L. editors. 4th edition Produção Independente. ISBN: 9788581791920

Bradfield, D. & Behrens, W. C. (1968). Effects of injectable vitamins on productive performance of beef cattle. Proc. West. Sec. Am. Soc. Anim. Sci. 19:361.

Bramley, P. M., Elmadfa, I., Kafatos, A., Kelly, F. J., Manios, Y., Roxborough, H. E., Schuch, W., Sheehy, P. J. A., & Wagner, K. H. (2000). Vitamin E. *Journal of the Science of Food and Agriculture*, *80*(7), 913–938. https://doi.org/10.1002/(SICI)1097-0010(20000515)80:7<913::AID-JSFA600>3.0.CO;2-3

Brass, E. P. (1993). Hydroxycobalamin [c-lactam] increases total coenzyme A content in primary culture hepatocytes by accelerating coenzyme A biosynthesis secondary to acyl-CoA accumulation. *The Journal of Nutrition*, *123*(11), 1801–1807. https://doi.org/10.1093/jn/123.11.1801

Braun, F. (1986). The effect of bile on intestinal absorption of calcium and vitamin D. *Wiener Klinische Wochenschrift*, *98*(166), 23. PubMed: 3008448

Bräunlich, K. (1974). *Vitamin B$_6$*, *1451*. F. Hoffmann-La Roche, and Co., Ltd.

Bräunlich, K., & Zintzen, H. (1976). *Vitamin B$_1$*, *1593*. F. Hoffmann-La Roche, and Co. Ltd.

Bray, D. L., & Briggs, G. M. (1984). Decrease in bone density in young male guinea pigs fed high levels of ascorbic acid. *The Journal of Nutrition*, *114*(5), 920–928. https://doi.org/10.1093/jn/114.5.920

Bremel, D. H., Hemken, R. W., Heersche, Jr., G., Edgerton, L. A., & Olds, D. (1982). Effects of β-carotene on metabolic and reproductive parameters in lactating dairy cows. *Journal of Dairy Science*, *65*(1), 178 [Abstr.].

Brent, B. E., & Bartley, E. E. (1984). Thiamin and niacin in the rumen. *Journal of Animal Science*, *59*(3), 813–822. https://doi.org/10.2527/jas1984.593813x

Breves, G., Brandt, M., Hoeller, H., & Rohr, K. (1981). Flow of thiamin to the duodenum in dairy cows fed different rations. *The Journal of Agricultural Science*, *96*(3), 587–591. https://doi.org/10.1017/S0021859600034559

Brigelius-Flohé, R. (2021). Vitamin E research: Past, now and future. *Free Radical Biology and Medicine*, *177*, 381–390. https://doi.org/10.1016/j.freeradbiomed.2021.10.029

Brigelius-Flohé, R., Kelly, F. J., Salonen, J. T., Neuzil, J., Zingg, J. M., & Azzi, A. (2002). The European perspective on vitamin E: Current knowledge and future research. *The American Journal of Clinical Nutrition*, *76*(4), 703–716. https://doi.org/10.1093/ajcn/76.4.703

Briggs, M. H., Heard, T. W., Whitcroft, A., & Hogg, M. L. (1964). Studies of urea fed cattle: Rumen levels of B vitamins and related coenzymes. *Life Sciences*, *3*, 11–14. https://doi.org/10.1016/0024-3205(64)90219-X

Brin, M. (1969). The effects of cell age and thiamine on erythrocyte transketolase activity. *Journal of Nutritional Science and Vitaminology*, *15*(4), 338–339.

Brisson, V., Girard, C. L., Metcalf, J. A., Castagnino, D. S., Dijkstra, J., & Ellis, J. L. (2022). Meta-analysis of apparent ruminal synthesis and post ruminal flow of B vitamins in dairy cows. *Journal of Dairy Science*, *105*(9), 7399–7415. https://doi.org/10.3168/jds.2021-21656

Bronner, F., & Stein, W. D. (1995). Calcium homeostasis-An old problem revisited. *The Journal of Nutrition*, *125*(7)(Suppl.), 1987S–1995S. https://doi.org/10.1093/jn/125.suppl_7.1987S

Bronzo, V., Lopreiato, V., Riva, F., Amadori, M., Curone, G., Addis, M. F., Cremonesi, P., Moroni, P., Trevisi, E., & Castiglioni, B. (2020). The role of innate immune response and microbiome in resilience of dairy cattle to disease: The mastitis model. *Animals: An Open Access Journal from MDPI*, *10*(8), 1397. https://doi.org/10.3390/ani10081397

Brosnan, J. T., Brosnan, M. E., Bertolo, R. F. P., & Brunton, J. A. (2007). Methionine: A metabolically unique amino acid. *Livestock Science*, *112*(1–2), 2–7. https://doi.org/10.1016/j.livsci.2007.07.005

Brouwer, D. A., van Beek, J., Ferwerda, H., Brugman, A. M., van der Klis, F. R., van der Heiden, H. J., & Muskiet, F. A. (1998). Rat adipose tissue rapidly accumulates and slowly releases an orally administered high vitamin D dose. *The British Journal of Nutrition*, *79*(6), 527–532. https://doi.org/10.1079/BJN19980091

Brown, E. S. (1964). Isolation and assay of dipalmityl lecithin in lung extracts. *The American Journal of Physiology*, *207*, 402–406. https://doi.org/10.1152/ajplegacy.1964.207.2.402

Brown, F. (1953). The tocopherol content of farm feedingstuffs. *Journal of the Science of Food and Agriculture*, *4*(4), 161–165. https://doi.org/10.1002/jsfa.2740040401

Brown, G. M. (1962). The biosynthesis of folic acid. *Journal of Biological Chemistry*, *237*(2), 536–540. https://doi.org/10.1016/S0021-9258(18)93957-8

Brownlee, N. R., Huttner, J. J., Panganamala, R. V., & Cornwell, D. G. (1977). Role of vitamin E in glutathione-induced oxidant stress: Methemoglobin, lipid peroxidation, and hemolysis. *Journal of Lipid Research*, *18*(5), 635–644. https://doi.org/10.1016/S0022-2275(20)41605-0

Bruhn, J. C., & Oliver, J. C. (1978). Effect of storage on tocopherol and carotene concentration in alfalfa hay. *Journal of Dairy Science*, *61*(7), 980–982. https://doi.org/10.3168/jds.S0022-0302(78)83677-7

Bruns, N. J., & Webb, Jr., K. E. (1990). Vitamin A deficiency: Serum cortisol and humoral immunity in lambs. *Journal of Animal Science*, *68*(2), 454–459. https://doi.org/10.2527/1990.682454x

Brusemeister, F., & Sudekum, K. (2006). Rumen- protected choline for dairy cows: The *in-situ* evaluation of a commercial source and literature evaluation of effects on performance and interactions between methionine and choline metabolism. *Animal Research*, *55*(2), 93–104. https://doi.org/10.1051/animres:2006002

Bryant, T. C., Rivera, J. D., Galyean, M. L., Duff, G. C., Hallford, D. M., & Montgomery, T. H. (1999). Effects of dietary level of ruminally protected choline on performance and carcass characteristics of finishing beef steers and on growth and serum metabolites in lambs. *Journal of Animal Science*, *77*(11), 2893–2903. https://doi.org/10.2527/1999.77112893x

Bryant, T. C., Wagner, J. J., Tatum, J. D., Galyean, M. L., Anthony, R. V., & Engle, T. E. (2010). Effect of dietary supplemental vitamin A concentration on performance, carcass merit, serum metabolites, and lipogenic enzyme activity in yearling beef steers. *Journal of Animal Science*, *88*(4), 1463–1478. https://doi.org/10.2527/jas.2009-2313

Brzezinska-Slebodzinska, E., Miller, J. K., Quigley, J. D., Moore, J. R., & Madsen, F. C. (1994). Antioxidant status of dairy cows supplemented prepartum with vitamin E and selenium. *Journal of Dairy Science*, *77*(10), 3087–3095. https://doi.org/10.3168/jds.S0022-0302(94)77251-9

Bunnell, R. H., Keating, J. P., & Quaresimo, A. J. (1968). Alpha-tocopherol content of feeds. *Journal of Agricultural and Food Chemistry*, *16*(4), 659–664. https://doi.org/10.1021/jf60158a008

Cabrera, M. C., & Saadoun, A. (2014). An overview of the nutritional value of beef and lamb meat from South America. *Meat Science*, *98*(3), 435–444. https://doi.org/10.1016/j.meatsci.2014.06.033

Cadenas, S., Rojas, C., & Barja, G. (1998). Endotoxin increases oxidative injury to proteins in guinea pig liver: Protection by dietary vitamin C. *Pharmacology and Toxicology*, *82*(1), 11–18. https://doi.org/10.1111/j.1600-0773.1998.tb01391.x

Calderón, F., Chauveau-Duriot, B., Pradel, P., Martin, B., Graulet, B., Doreau, M., & Nozière, P. (2007). Variations in carotenoids, vitamins A and E, and color in cow's plasma and milk following a shift from hay diet to diets containing increasing levels of carotenoids and vitamin E. *Journal of Dairy Science*, *90*(12), 5651–5664. https://doi.org/10.3168/jds.2007-0264

Calderón-Ospina, C. A., & Nava-Mesa, M. O. (2020). B Vitamins in the nervous system: Current knowledge of the biochemical modes of action and synergies of thiamine, pyridoxine, and cobalamin. *CNS Neuroscience and Therapeutics*, *26*(1), 5–13. https://doi.org/10.1111/cns.13207

Camarena, V., & Wang, G. (2016). The epigenetic role of vitamin C in health and disease. *Cellular and Molecular Life Sciences*, *73*(8), 1645–1658. https://doi.org/10.1007/s00018-016-2145-x

Campbell, M. H., & Miller, J. K. (1998). Effect of supplemental dietary vitamin E and zinc on reproductive performance of dairy cows and heifers fed excess iron. *Journal of Dairy Science*, *81*(10), 2693–2699. https://doi.org/10.3168/jds.S0022-0302(98)75826-6

Campbell, J. M., Murphy, M. R., Christensen, R. A., & Overton, T. R. (1994). Kinetics of niacin supplements in lactating dairy cows. *Journal of Dairy Science*, *77*(2), 566–575. https://doi.org/10.3168/jds.S0022-0302(94)76985-X

Campbell, J. R., Greenough, P. R., & Petrie, L. (2000). The effects of dietary biotin supplementation on vertical fissures of the claw wall in beef cattle. *Canadian Veterinary Journal*, *41*(9), 690–694. PubMed Central: PMC1476396

Camporeale, G., & Zempleni, J. (2006). Biotin. In B. A. Bowman & R. M. Russell (Eds.), *Present knowledge in nutrition* (9th ed.). International. Life. *Sciences. Institute*, 250–259.

Campos, C. F., Costa, T. C., Rodrigues, R. T. S., Guimarães, S. E. F., Moura, F. H., Silva, W., Chizzotti, M. L., Paulino, P. V. R., Benedeti, P. D. B., Silva, F. F., & Duarte, M. S. (2020). Proteomic analysis reveals changes in energy metabolism of skeletal muscle in beef cattle supplemented with vitamin A. *Journal of the Science of Food and Agriculture*, *100*(8), 3536–3543. https://doi.org/10.1002/jsfa.10401

Cantatore, F. P., Loperfido, M. C., Magli, D. M., Mancini, L., & Carrozzo, M. (1991). The importance of vitamin C for hydroxylation of vitamin D_3 to $1,25(OH)_2D_3$ in man. *Clinical Rheumatology*, *10*(2), 162–167. https://doi.org/10.1007/BF02207657

Cappa, C. (1958). Le metabolisme de la vitamine C chez les ruminants. *Rivista. Zoot*, *31*, 299.

Capuco, A. V., Ellis, S. E., Hale, S. A., Long, E., Erdman, R. A., Zhao, X., & Paape, M. J. (2003). Lactation persistency: Insights from mammary cell proliferation studies. *Journal of Animal Science*, *81*(3)(Suppl. 3), 18–31. https://doi.org/10.2527/2003.81suppl_318x

Cardinault, N., Doreau, M., Poncet, C., & Nozière, P. (2006). Digestion and absorption of carotenoids in sheep given fresh red clover. *Animal Science*, *82*(1), 49–55. https://doi.org/10.1079/ASC200514

Carlson, L. A. (2005). Nicotinic acid: The broad- spectrum lipid drug. A 50th anniversary review. *Journal of Internal Medicine*, *258*(2), 94–114. https://doi.org/10.1111/j.1365-2796.2005.01528.x

Carmel, R. (1994). *In vitro* studies of gastric juice in patients with food-cobalamin malabsorption. *Digestive Diseases and Sciences*, *39*(12), 2516–2522. https://doi.org/10.1007/BF02087684

Carnagey, K. M., Huff-Lonergan, E. J., Lonergan, S. M., Trenkle, A., Horst, R. L., & Beitz, D. C. (2008a). Use of 25-hydroxyvitamin D_3 and dietary calcium to improve tenderness of beef from the round of beef cows. *Journal of Animal Science*, *86*(7), 1637–1648. https://doi.org/10.2527/jas.2007-0406

Carnagey, K. M., Huff-Lonergan, E. J., Trenkle, A., Wertz-Lutz, A. E., Horst, R. L., & Beitz, D. C. (2008b). Use of 25-hydroxyvitamin D_3 and vitamin E to improve tenderness of beef from the *longissimus* dorsi of heifers. *Journal of Animal Science*, *86*(7), 1649–1657. https://doi.org/10.2527/jas.2007-0502

Carpenter, K.J. (1981) *"Pellagra"*. Hutchinson Ross, Stroudsburg, PA.

Carpenter, K. J., Schelstraete, M., Vilicich, V. C., & Wall, J. S. (1988). Immature corn as a source of niacin for rats. *The Journal of Nutrition*, *118*(2), 165–169. https://doi.org/10.1093/jn/118.2.165

Carrica, J. M., Brandt, R. T., & Lee, R. W. (1986). Influence of vitamin E on feedlot performance and carcass traits of beef steers fed either lasalocid or monensin. *Journal of Animal Science*, *63*(Suppl. 1), 432–437.

Carrillo, B. J. (1973). *Effecto de la intoxicacíon de Solanum malacoxylon en sistema óseo*. Rev. Invest. Agropecu. Patol. Anim. 10:65, 4.

Carson, D. A., Seto, S., & Wasson, D. B. (1987). Pyridine nucleotide cycling and poly(ADP-ribose) synthesis in resting human lymphocytes. *Journal of Immunology*, *138*(6), 1904–1907. https://doi.org/10.4049/jimmunol.138.6.1904

Carter, E. G. A., & Carpenter, K. J. (1982). The available niacin values of foods for rats and their relation to analytical values. *The Journal of Nutrition*, *112*(11), 2091–2103. https://doi.org/10.1093/jn/112.11.2091

Carter, J. N., Gill, D. R., Krehbiel, C. R., Confer, A. W., Smith, R. A., Lalman, D. L., Claypool, P. L., & McDowell, L. R. (2005). Vitamin E supplementation of newly arrived feedlot calves. *Journal of Animal Science*, *83*(8), 1924–1932. https://doi.org/10.2527/2005.8381924x

Carvalho, V. V., & Perdigão, A. (2019). Supplementation of 25-hydroxyvitamin-D3 and increased vitamin E as a strategy to increase carcass weight of feedlot beef cattle. *Journal of Animal Science, 97*(Suppl. S3). https://doi.org/10.1093/jas/skz258.871

Casas, E., Leach, R. J., Reinhardt, T. A., Thallman, R. M., Lippolis, J. D., Bennett, G. L., & Kuehn, L. A. (2013). A genome wide association study identified CYP2J2 as a gene controlling serum vitamin D status in beef cattle. *Journal of Animal Science, 91*(8), 3549–3556. https://doi.org/10.2527/jas.2012-6020

Casas, E., Lippolis, J. D., Kuehn, L. A., & Reinhardt, T. A. (2015). Seasonal variation in vitamin D status of beef cattle reared in the central United States. *Domestic Animal Endocrinology, 52*, 71–74. https://doi.org/10.1016/j.domaniend.2015.03.003

Cashman, K. D. (2018). Vitamin D requirements for the future—Lessons learned and charting a path forward. *Nutrients, 10*(5), 533–545. https://doi.org/10.3390/nu10050533

Cashman, K. D., & O'Connor, E. (2008). Does high vitamin K, intake protect against bone loss in later life? *Nutrition Reviews, 66*(9), 532–538. https://doi.org/10.1111/j.1753-4887.2008.00086.x

Casper, H. H., Alstad, A. D., Tacke, D. B., Johnson, L. J., & Lloyd, W. E. (1989). Evaluation of vitamin K$_3$ feed additive for prevention of sweet clover disease. *Journal of Veterinary Diagnostic Investigation, 1*(2), 116–119. https://doi.org/10.1177/104063878900100204

Castagnino, D. S., Seck, M., Beaudet, V., Kammes, K. L., Linton, J. A. V., Allen, M. S., Gervais, R., Chouinard, P. Y., & Girard, C. L. (2016). Effects of forage family on apparent ruminal synthesis of B vitamins in lactating dairy cows. *Journal of Dairy Science, 99*(3), 1884–1894. https://doi.org/10.3168/jds.2015-10319

Castagnino, D. S., Harvatine, K. J., Allen, M. S., Gervais, R., Chouinard, P. Y., & Girard, C. L. (2017). Short communication: Effect of fatty acid supplements on apparent ruminal synthesis of B vitamins in lactating dairy cows. *Journal of Dairy Science, 100*(10), 8165–8169. https://doi.org/10.3168/jds.2017-13087

Castagnino, D. S., Seck, M., Longuski, R. A., Ying, Y., Allen, M. S., Gervais, R., Chouinard, P. Y., & Girard, C. L. (2018). Particle size and endosperm type of dry corn grain altered duodenal flow of B vitamins in lactating dairy cows. *Journal of Dairy Science, 101*(11), 9841–9846. https://doi.org/10.3168/jds.2018-15131

Castillo, C., Hernandez, J., Bravo, A., Lopez-Alonso, M., Pereira, V., & Benedito, J. L. (2005). Oxidative status during late pregnancy and early lactation in dairy cows. *Veterinary Journal, 169*(2), 286–292. https://doi.org/10.1016/j.tvjl.2004.02.001

Catani, M. V., Savini, I., Rossi, A., Melino, G., & Avigliano, L. (2005). Biological role of vitamin C in keratinocytes. *Nutrition Reviews, 63*(3), 81–90. https://doi.org/10.1111/j.1753-4887.2005.tb00125.x

Celi, P. (2011). Oxidative stress in ruminants. In S. C. Bondy & A. Campbell (Eds.). ISSN 2197-7224, *Studies on veterinary medicine* (pp. 191–231). https://doi.org/10.1007/978-1-61779-071-3_13

Celi, P., Williams, S., Engstrom, M., McGrath, J., & La Marta, J. (2018). Safety evaluation of dietary levels of 25-hydroxyvitamin D3 in growing calves. *Food and Chemical Toxicology, 111*, 641–649. https://doi.org/10.1016/j.fct.2017.11.053

Celi, P., Kindermann, M., Tamassia, L. F. M., & Walker, N. (2020). Skeletal health, redox balance and gastrointestinal functionality in dairy cows: Connecting bugs and bones. *The Journal of Dairy Research, 87*(4), 410–415. https://doi.org/10.1017/S0022029920001090

Cetinkaya, N., & Ozcan, H. (1991). Investigation of seasonal variations in cow serum retinol and beta-carotene by high performance liquid chromatographic method. *Comparative Biochemistry and Physiology. A, Comparative Physiology, 100*(4), 1003–1008. https://doi.org/10.1016/0300-9629(91)90328-a

Chaiyotwittayakun, A., Erskine, R. J., Bartlett, P. C., Herdt, T. H., Sears, P. M., & Harmon, R. J. (2002). The effect of ascorbic acid and L-histidine therapy on acute mammary inflammation in dairy cattle. *Journal of Dairy Science, 85*(1), 60–67. https://doi.org/10.3168/jds.S0022-0302(02)74053-8

Chamberlain, J. L., & French, P. D. (2006). The effects of nicotinic acid supplementation during late gestation on lipolysis and feed intake during the transition period. *Journal of Animal Science, 89*, 232. https://ir.library.oregonstate.edu/concern/graduate_thesis_or_dissertations/c821gn84n

Chan, M. M. (1991). Choline and carnitine. In L. J. Machlin (Ed.), *Handbook of vitamins* (2nd ed.) (pp. 537–556). Marcel Dekker.

Chao, M. D., Domenech-Pérez, K. I., & Calkins, C. R. (2017). Feeding vitamin E may reverse sarcoplasmic reticulum membrane instability caused by feeding wet distillers grains plus solubles to cattle. *The Professional Animal Scientist, 33*(1), 12–23. https://doi.org/10.15232/pas.2016-01569

Charmley, E., & Nicholson, J. W. G. (1994). Influence of dietary fat source on oxidative stability and fatty acid composition of milk from cows receiving a low or high level of dietary vitamin E. *Canadian Journal of Animal Science*, 74(4), 657–664. https://doi.org/10.4141/cjas94-095

Chatterjee, G. C. (1967). Effects of ascorbic acid deficiency in animals. In *The enzymes* Vol. I Sebrell, W.H. and Harris, R.S. (Eds.) Academic Press, Inc. New. York.

Chauveau-Duriot, B., Thomas, D., Portelli, J., & Doreau, M. (2005). Carotenoids content in forages: Variation during conservation. *Renc. Rech. Ruminants*, 12, 117.

Chawla, R., & Kaur, H. (2004). Plasma antioxidant vitamin status of periparturient cows supplemented with α-tocopherol and β-carotene. *Animal Feed Science and Technology*, 114(1–4), 279–285. https://doi.org/10.1016/j.anifeedsci.2003.11.002

Chawla, J., & Kvarnberg, D. (2014). Hydrosoluble vitamins. *Handbook of Clinical Neurology*, 120, 891–914. https://doi.org/10.1016/B978-0-7020-4087-0.00059-0

Cheli, F., Politis, I., Rossi, L., Fusi, E., & Baldi, A. (2003). Effects of retinoids on proliferation and plasminogen activator expression in a bovine mammary epithelial cell line. *The Journal of Dairy Research*, 70(4), 367–372. https://doi.org/10.1017/S0022029903006496

Chen, B., Wang, C., Wang, Y. M., & Liu, J. X. (2011). Effect of biotin on milk performance of dairy cattle: A meta-analysis. *Journal of Dairy Science*, 94(7), 3537–3546. https://doi.org/10.3168/jds.2010-3764

Chen, C., Wang, Z., Li, J., Li, Y., Huang, P., Ding, X., Yin, J., He, S., Yang, H., & Yin, Y. (2019). Dietary vitamin E affects small intestinal histomorphology, digestive enzyme activity, and the expression of nutrient transporters by inhibiting proliferation of intestinal epithelial cells within jejunum in weaned piglets1. *Journal of Animal Science*, 97(3), 1212–1221. https://doi.org/10.1093/jas/skz023

Chen, J. (1990). *Technical service internal reports*. BASF, Corp.

Chen, Y. F., Huang, C. F., Liu, L., Lai, C. H., & Wang, F. L. (2019). Concentration of vitamins in the 13 feed ingredients commonly used in pig diets. *Animal Feed Science and Technology*, 247, 1–8. https://doi.org/10.1016/j.anifeedsci.2018.10.011

Chew, B. P. (1987). Vitamin A and carotene on host defense. *Journal of Dairy Science*, 70(12), 2732–2743. https://doi.org/10.3168/jds.S0022-0302(87)80346-6

Chew, B. P. (1993). Role of carotenoids in the immune response. *Journal of Dairy Science*, 76(9), 2804–2811. https://doi.org/10.3168/jds.S0022-0302(93)77619-5

Chew, B. P. (1995). Antioxidant vitamins affect food animal immunity and health. *The Journal of Nutrition*, 125(6)(Suppl.), 1804S–1808S. https://doi.org/10.1093/jn/125.suppl_6.1804S

Chew, B. P., & Johnston, L. A. (1985). Effects of supplemental vitamin A and β-carotene on mastitis in dairy cows. *Journal of Dairy Science*, 68(1), 191.

Chew, B. P., & Park, J. S. (2004). Carotenoid action on the immune response. *The Journal of Nutrition*, 134(1), 257S–261S. https://doi.org/10.1093/jn/134.1.257S

Chew, B. P., Holpuch, D. M., & O'Fallon, J. V. (1984). Vitamin A and beta-carotene in bovine and porcine plasma, liver, corpora lutea and follicular fluid. *Journal of Dairy Science*, 67(6), 1316–1322. https://doi.org/10.3168/jds.S0022-0302(84)81439-3

Chew, B. P., Hollen, L. L., Hillers, J. K., & Herlugson, M. L. (1982). Relationship between vitamin A and β-carotene in blood plasma and milk and mastitis in Holsteins. *Journal of Dairy Science*, 65(11), 2111–2118. https://doi.org/10.3168/jds.S0022-0302(82)82469-7

Chhabra, A., & Arora, S. P. (1987). Effect of dietary zinc on the conversion of beta-carotene to vitamin A in crossbred calves. *Indian Journal of Dairy Science*, 40, 322.

Chhabra, A., Arora, S. P., & Kishan, J. (1980). Note on the effect of dietary zinc on β-carotene conversion to vitamin A. *Indian Journal of Animal Sciences*, 50, 879.

Chien, C. T., Chang, W. T., Chen, H. W., Wang, T. D., Liou, S. Y., Chen, T. J., Chang, Y. L., Lee, Y. T., & Hsu, S. M. (2004). Ascorbate supplement reduces oxidative stress in dyslipidemic patients undergoing apheresis. *Arteriosclerosis, Thrombosis, and Vascular Biology*, 24(6), 1111–1117. https://doi.org/10.1161/01.ATV.0000127620.12310.89

Chilliard, Y., & Ottou, J. F. (1995). Duodenal infusion of oil in midlactation cows. 7. Interaction with niacin on response to glucose, insulin and B-agonist challenges. *Journal of Dairy Science*, 78(11), 2452–2463. https://doi.org/10.3168/jds.S0022-0302(95)76873-4

Chiquette, J., Girard, C. L., & Matte, J. J. (1993). Effect of diet and folic acid addition on digestibility and ruminal fermentation in growing steers. *Journal of Animal Science*, *71*(10), 2793–2798. https://doi.org/10.2527/1993.71102793x

Chow, C. K. (1979). Nutritional influence on cellular antioxidant defense systems. *The American Journal of Clinical Nutrition*, *32*(5), 1066–1081. https://doi.org/10.1093/ajcn/32.5.1066

Christensen, K. (1983). Pools of cellular nutrients. In P. M. Riis (Ed.), *Dynamic biochemistry of animal production* Elsevier. Sci. Pub.

Christensen, S. (1973). The biological fate of riboflavin in mammals. A survey of literature and own investigations. *Acta Pharmacologica et Toxicologica*, *32*, 3–72. https://doi.org/10.1111/j.1600-0773.1973.tb03313.x

Church, D. C., & Pond, W. G. (1974). *Basic animal nutrition and feeding*. Albany printing, Albany, New York.

Cipriano, J. E., Morrill, J. L., & Anderson, N. V. (1982). Effect of dietary vitamin E on immune responses of calves. *Journal of Dairy Science*, *65*(12), 2357–2365. https://doi.org/10.3168/jds.S0022-0302(82)82509-5

Clifford, A. J., Jones, A. D., & Bills, N. D. (1990). Bioavailability of folates in selected foods incorporated into amino acid-based diets fed to rats. *The Journal of Nutrition*, *120*(12), 1640–1647. https://doi.org/10.1093/jn/120.12.1640

Coburn, S. P., Mahuren, J. D., Kennedy, M. S., Schaltenbrand, W. E., & Townsend, D. W. (1992). Metabolism of 14C and 32P pyridoxal 5′-phosphate and 3H pyridoxal administered intravenously to pigs and goats. *The Journal of Nutrition*, *122*(2), 393–401. https://doi.org/10.1093/jn/122.2.393

Coelho, M. B. (1991). Vitamin stability in premixes and feeds: A practical approach. *BASF Tech., Symp. Bloomington, MN*, 56–71.

Coen, G., Ballanti, P., Silvestrini, G., Mantella, D., Manni, M., Di Giulio, S., Pisanò, S., Leopizzi, M., Di Lullo, G., & Bonucci, E. (2009). Immunohistochemical localization and mRNA expression of matrix gla protein and fetuin-A in bone biopsies of hemodialysis patients. *Virchows Archiv*, *454*(3), 263–271. https://doi.org/10.1007/s00428-008-0724-4

Cohen, N., Scott, C. G., Neukon, C., Lopresti, R. L., Weber, G., & Saucy, G. (1981). Total synthesis of all 8 stereoisomers of alpha-tocopheryl acetate. Analysis of their diastereomeric and enantiomeric purity by gas chromatography. *Helvetica Chimica Acta*, *64*, 1158–1173. https://doi.org/10.1002/hlca.19810640422

Cole, C. L., Rasmussen, R. A., & Thorp, F. (1944). Ascorbic acid deficiency in cow. *Veterinary Medicine*, *39*, 204.

Cole, N. A., McLaren, J. B., & Hutcheson, D. P. (1982). Influence of preweaning and B-vitamin supplementation of the feedlot receiving diet on calves subjected to marketing and transit stress. *Journal of Animal Science*, *54*(5), 911–917. https://doi.org/10.2527/jas1982.545911x

Combs, Jr., G. F., & McClung, J. P. (2022). *The vitamins. Fundamental aspects in nutrition and health* (6th ed.). Elsevier. ISBN: 978032390473.

Comitato, R., Ambra, R., & Virgili, F. (2017). Tocotrienols: A family of molecules with specific biological activities. *Antioxidants*, *6*(4), 93. https://doi.org/10.3390/antiox6040093

Conboy Stephenson, R., Ross, R. P., & Stanton, C. (2021). Carotenoids in milk and the potential for dairy based functional foods. *Foods*, *10*(6), 1263. https://doi.org/10.3390/foods10061263

Cooke, R. F., Silva del Río, N., Caraviello, D. Z., Bertics, S. J., Ramos, M. H., & Grummer, R. R. (2007). Supplemental choline for prevention and alleviation of fatty liver in dairy cattle. *Journal of Dairy Science*, *90*(5), 2413–2418. https://doi.org/10.3168/jds.2006-028

Collick, D. W., Ward, W. R., & Dobson, H. (1989). Associations between types of lameness and fertility. *The Veterinary Record*, *125*(5), 103–106. https://doi.org/10.1136/vr.125.5.103

Commonwealth Scientific and Industrial Research Organization. (2007). Nutrient requirements of domesticated ruminants. *Primary Industries Standing Committee*. https://doi.org/10.1071/9780643095106

Cooper, J. R., Roth, R. H., & Kini, M. M. (1963). Biochemical and physiological function of thiamine in nervous tissue. *Nature*, *199*, 609–610. https://doi.org/10.1038/199609a0

Correa, R. (1957). Deficiency of cobalt in cattle. 1. Clinical study and experimental demonstration of the existence of the disorder in Brazil. Inst. Biol., *24*, 199–228.

Corripio-Miyar, Y., Mellanby, R. J., Morrison, K., & McNeilly, T. N. (2017). 1,25-dihydroxyvitamin D3 modulates the phenotype and function of monocyte derived dendritic cells in cattle. *BMC Veterinary Research*, *13*(1), 390. https://doi.org/10.1186/s12917-017-1309-8

Coya, R., Carro, E., Mallo, F., & Diéguez, C. (1997). Retinoic acid inhibits *in vivo* thyroid-stimulating hormone secretion. *Life Sciences*, *60*(16), PL 247–PL 250. https://doi.org/10.1016/S0024-3205(97)00091-X

Craven, N., & Williams, M. R. (1985). Defenses of the bovine mammary gland against infection and prospects for their enhancement. *Veterinary Immunology and Immunopathology*, *10*(1), 71–127. https://doi.org/10.1016/0165-2427(85)90039-X

Croom, W. J., Rakes, A. H., Linnerud, A. C., Ducharme, G. A., & Elliot, J. M. (1981). Vitamin B$_{12}$ administration for milk fat synthesis in lactating dairy cows fed a low fiber diet. *Journal of Dairy Science*, *64*(7), 1555–1560. https://doi.org/10.3168/jds.S0022-0302(81)82725-7

Cummins, K. A., Bush, L. J., & White, T. W. (1992). Ascorbate in cattle: A review. *The Professional Animal Scientist*, *8*(1), 22–29. https://doi.org/10.15232/S1080-7446(15)32101-X

Cummins, K. A., & Brunner, C. J. (1989). Dietary ascorbic acid and immune response in dairy calves. *Journal of Dairy Science*, *72*(1), 129–134. https://doi.org/10.3168/jds.S0022-0302(89)79088-3

Cummins, K. A., & Brunner, C. J. (1991). Effect of calf housing on plasma ascorbate and endocrine and immune function. *Journal of Dairy Science*, *74*(5), 1582–1588. https://doi.org/10.3168/jds.S0022-0302(91)78320-3

Cunha, T. J. (1985). Nutrition and disease interaction. *Feedstuffs*, *57*(41), 37.

Cushnie, G. H., Richardson, A. J., Lawson, W. J., & Sharman, G. A. (1979). Cerebrocortical necrosis in ruminants: Effect of thiaminase type 1-producing Clostridium sporogenes in lambs. *The Veterinary Record*, *105*(21), 480–482. https://doi.org/10.1136/vr.105.21.480

CVB Tabellenboek Voeding Herkauwers. (2022) Voedernormen Rundvee, Schapen, Geiten en voederwaarden voedermiddelen voor Herkauwers CVB-reeks nr. 65 November 2022.

Da Costa-Gomez, C., Al Masri, M., Steinberg, W., & Abel, H. (1998). *Effect of varying hay/barley proportions on microbial biotin metabolism in the rumen simulating fermenter (RUSITEC)*. Proc. Soc. Nutr. Physiol., *7* [Abstr.].

Dabrowski, K. (1990). Gastro-intestinal circulation of ascorbic acid. Comparative Biochemistry and Physiology Part A, 95(4), 481–486. https://doi.org/10.1016/0300-9629(90)90727-A.

Dagnelie, P. C., van Staveren, W. A., & Van Den Berg, H. (1991). Vitamin B$_{12}$ from algae appears not to be bioavailable. *The American Journal of Clinical Nutrition*, *53*(3), 695–697. https://doi.org/10.1093/ajcn/53.3.695

Dahlquist, S. P., & Chew, B. P. (1985). Effect of vitamin A and β-carotene on mastitis in dairy cows during the early dry period. *Journal of Dairy Science*, *68*(1), 191.

Daily, J. W., & Sachan, D. S. (1995). Choline supplementation alters carnitine homeostasis in humans and guinea pigs. *The Journal of Nutrition*, *125*(7), 1938–1944. https://doi.org/10.1093/jn/125.7.1938

Dakshinamurti, S., & Dakshinamurti, K. (2013). Vitamin B$_6$. In J. Zempleni, J. Suttie, J. Gregory, & P. J. Stover (Eds.), *Handbook of vitamins* (5th ed.) (pp. 351–396). CRC Press, Taylor & Francis Group.

Dalto, D. B., & Matte, J. J. (2017). Pyridoxine (vitamin B$_6$) and the glutathione peroxidase system; a link between one-carbon metabolism and antioxidation. *Nutrients*, *9*(3), 189. https://doi.org/10.3390/nu9030189

Daniel, L. R., Chew, B. P., Tanaka, T. S., & Tjoelker, L. W. (1991a). β-carotene and vitamin A effects on bovine phagocyte function *in vitro* during the peripartum period. *Journal of Dairy Science*, *74*(1), 124–131. https://doi.org/10.3168/jds.S0022-0302(91)78152-6

Daniel, L. R., Chew, B. P., Tanaka, T. S., & Tjoelker, L. W. (1991b). *In vitro* effects of β-carotene and vitamin A on peripartum bovine peripheral blood mononuclear cell proliferation. *Journal of Dairy Science*, *74*(3), 911–915. https://doi.org/10.3168/jds.S0022-0302(91)78240-4

Daniel, M. J., Arnett, A. M., & Dikeman, M. E. (2008). Vitamin A restriction during finishing benefits beef retail color display life. *Kansas Agricultural Experiment Station Research Reports*, *95*(1), 28–30. https://doi.org/10.4148/2378-5977.1509

Darby, W. J., McNutt, K. W., & Todhunter, E. N. (1975). Niacin. *Nutrition Reviews*, *33*(10), 289–297. https://doi.org/10.1111/j.1753-4887.1975.tb05075.x

Dash, S. K., & Mitchell, D. J. (1976). Storage, processing reduce vitamin A. Anim. *Nutrition and Health*, *31*(7), 16.

David, C. W., Norrman, J., Hammon, H. M., Davis, W. C., & Blum, J. W. (2003). Cell proliferation, apoptosis, and B- and T-lymphocytes in Peyer's patches of the ileum, in thymus and in lymphnodes of preterm calves and in full-term calves at birth and on day 5 of life. *Journal of Dairy Science*, *86*(10), 3321–3329. https://doi.org/10.3168/jds.S0022-0302(03)73934-4

David, V., Dai, B., Martin, A., Huang, J., Han, X., & Quarles, L. D. (2013). Calcium regulates FGF-23 expression in bone. *Endocrinology*, *154*(12), 4469–4482. https://doi.org/10.1210/en.2013-1627

Davidson, S., Hopkins, B. A., Odle, J., Brownie, C., Fellner, V., & Whitlow, L. W. (2008). Supplementing limited methionine diets with rumen-protected methionine, betaine, and choline in early lactation Holstein cows. *Journal of Dairy Science*, *91*(4), 1552–1559. https://doi.org/10.3168/jds.2007-0721

Davies, E. T., Pill, A. H., & Austwick, P. K. (1968). Possible involvement of thiamine in aetiology of cerebro-cortical necrosis. *Veterinary Record Open*, *83*(26), 681.

Daynes, R. A., Araneo, B. A., Hennebold, J., Enioutina, E., & Mu, H. H. (1995). Steroids as regulators of the mammalian immune response. *The Journal of Investigative Dermatology*, *105*(1) (Suppl.), 14S–19S. https://doi.org/10.1111/1523-1747.ep12315187

De Bie, J., Langbeen, A., Verlaet, A. A. J., Florizoone, F., Immig, I., Hermans, N., Fransen, E., Bols, P. E. J., & Leroy, J. L. M. R. (2016). The effect of a negative energy balance status on β-carotene availability in serum and follicular fluid of nonlactating dairy cows. *Journal of Dairy Science*, *99*(7), 5808–5819. https://doi.org/10.3168/jds.2016-10870

De Boer-van den Berg, M. A., Verstijnen, C. P., & Vermeer, C. (1986). Vitamin K-dependent carboxylase in skin. *The Journal of Investigative Dermatology*, *87*(3), 377–380. https://doi.org/10.1111/1523-1747.ep12524848

De la Huerga, J., & Popper, H. (1952). Factors influencing choline absorption in the intestinal tract. *The Journal of Clinical Investigation*, *31*(6), 598–603. https://doi.org/10.1172/JCI102646

De Ondarza, M. B., Emanuele, S., & Putnam, D. (2007). Effect of rumen protected choline (Reashure®) supplemented to high-producing cows on milk production, milk components, and intake. *Journal of Dairy Science*, *90* (Suppl. 1), 353 [Abstr.].

De Ondarza, M. B., Wilson, J. W., & Engstrom, M. (2009). Case study: Effect of supplemental β-carotene on yield of milk and milk components and on reproduction of dairy cows. *The Professional Animal Scientist*, *25*(4), 510–516. https://doi.org/10.15232/S1080-7446(15)30742-7

De Ondarza, M. B., Sniffen, C. J., Dussert, L., Chevaux, E., & Sullivan, J. (2011). *Live yeast aids rumen function, milk yield. Feedstuffs. Reprinted with permission from 83:24.*

De Veth, M. J., Artegoitia, V. M., Campagna, S. R., Lapierre, H., Harte, F., & Girard, C. L. (2016). Choline absorption and evaluation of bioavailability markers when supplementing choline to lactating dairy cows. *Journal of Dairy Science*, *99*(12), 9732–9744. https://doi.org/10.3168/jds.2016-11382

Debier, C., & Larondelle, Y. (2005). Vitamins A and E: Metabolism, roles and transfer to offspring. *The British Journal of Nutrition*, *93*(2), 153–174. https://doi.org/10.1079/BJN20041308

Debier, C., Pottier, J., Goffe, C., & Larondelle, Y. (2005). Present knowledge and unexpected behaviors of vitamins A and E in colostrum and milk. *Livestock Production Science*, *98*(1–2), 135–147. https://doi.org/10.1016/j.livprodsci.2005.10.008

DeHoogh, W. (1989). Dicumarol toxicity in a herd of Ayrshire cattle fed moldy sweet clover. *Bov. Pract*, 173–175. https://doi.org/10.21423/bovine-vol0no24p173-175

DeLuca, H. F. (1979). The vitamin D system in the regulation of calcium and phosphorus metabolism. *Nutrition Reviews*, *37*(6), 161–193. https://doi.org/10.1111/j.1753-4887.1979.tb06660.x

DeLuca, H. F. (1992). New concepts of vitamin D functions. *Annals of the New York Academy of Sciences*, *669*, 59–68; discussion 68. https://doi.org/10.1111/j.1749-6632.1992.tb17089.x

DeLuca, H. F. (2008). Evolution of our understanding of vitamin D. *Nutrition Reviews*, *66*(10) (Suppl. 2), S73–S87. https://doi.org/10.1111/j.1753-4887.2008.00105.x

DeLuca, H. F. (2014). History of the discovery of vitamin D and its active metabolites. *BoneKEy Reports*, *3*, 479. https://doi.org/10.1038/bonekey.2013.213

Deming, D. M., Teixeira, S. R., & Erdman, Jr., J. W. (2002). All-trans β-carotene appears to be more bioavailable than 9-cis or 13-cis β-carotene in gerbils given single oral doses of each isomer. *The Journal of Nutrition*, *132*(9), 2700–2708. https://doi.org/10.1093/jn/132.9.2700

Denisova, N. A., & Booth, S. L. (2005). Vitamin K and sphingolipid metabolism: Evidence to date. *Nutrition Reviews*, *63*(4), 111–121. https://doi.org/10.1111/j.1753-4887.2005.tb00129.x

Dersjant-Li, Y., Jensen, S. K., Bos, L. W., & Peisker, M. R. (2009). Bio-discrimination of α-tocopherol Stereoisomers in rearing and veal calves fed milk replacer supplemented with all-rac-α-tocopheryl acetate. *International Journal for Vitamin and Nutrition Research. Internationale Zeitschrift Fur*

Vitamin- und Ernahrungsforschung. Journal International de Vitaminologie et de Nutrition, 79(4), 199–211. https://doi.org/10.1024/0300-9831.79.4.199

Descalzo, A. M., Insani, E. M., Biolatto, A., Sancho, A. M., García, P. T., Pensel, N. A., & Josifovich, J. A. (2005). Influence of pasture or grain-based diets supplemented with vitamin E on antioxidant/oxidative balance of Argentine beef. *Meat Science, 70*(1), 35–44. https://doi.org/10.1016/j.meatsci.2004.11.018

Descalzo, A. M., & Sancho, A. M. (2008). A review of natural antioxidants and their effects on oxidative status, odor and quality of fresh beef produced in Argentina. *Meat Science, 79*(3), 423–436. https://doi.org/10.1016/j.meatsci.2007.12.006

Deters, E. L., & Hansen, S. L. (2020). Pre-transit vitamin C injection improves post-transit performance of beef steers. *Animal, 14*(10), 2083–2090. https://doi.org/10.1017/S1751731120000968

Deuchler, K. N., Piperova, L. S., & Erdman, R. A. (1998). Milk choline secretion as an indirect indicator of post-ruminal choline supply. *Journal of Dairy Science, 81*(1), 238–242. https://doi.org/10.3168/jds.S0022-0302(98)75571-7

Dewett, D., Lam-Kamath, K., Poupault, C., Khurana, H., & Rister, J. (2021). Mechanisms of vitamin A metabolism and deficiency in the mammalian and fly visual system. *Developmental Biology, 476*, 68–78. https://doi.org/10.1016/j.ydbio.2021.03.013

Dhiman, T. R., & Poulson, C. S. (2006). Cornforth, D. and ZoBell, D.R. (2006) conjugated linoleic acid (CLA) and vitamin E levels in pasture forages for beef cattle. Utah State. *Univ. Cooperative Extension. AG/Beef, 03.* http://doi.org/10.1016%2Fj.livprodsci.2004.07.012

Dhur, A., Galan, P., & Hercberg, S. (1991). Folate status and the immune system. *Progress in Food and Nutrition Science, 15*(1–2), 43–60. PubMed: 1887065

Di Mascio, P., Murphy, M. E., & Sies, H. (1991). Antioxidant defense system: The role of carotenoids, tocopherols and thiols. *The American Journal of Clinical Nutrition, 53*(1) (Suppl.), 194S–200S. https://doi.org/10.1093/ajcn/53.1.194S, PubMed: 1985387

Dikeman, M. E. (2007). Effects of metabolic modifiers on carcass traits and meat quality. *Meat Science, 77*(1), 121–135. https://doi.org/10.1016/j.meatsci.2007.04.011

Dinarello, C. A. (1996). Biological basis for interleukin-1 in disease. *Blood, 87*(6), 2095–2147. https://doi.org/10.1182/blood.V87.6.2095.bloodjournal8762095, PubMed: 8630372

Distl, O., & Schmid, D. (1994). Influence of biotin supplementation on the formation, hardness and health of claws in dairy cows. *Tierarztl. Umsch., 49*, 581–584.

Dittmer, K. E., & Thompson, K. G. (2011). Vitamin D metabolism and rickets in domestic animals: A review. *Veterinary Pathology, 48*(2), 389–407. https://doi.org/10.1177/0300985810375240

Dittmer, K. E., Thompson, K. G., & Blair, H. T. (2009). Pathology of inherited rickets in Corriedale sheep. *Journal of Comparative Pathology, 141*(2–3), 147–155. https://doi.org/10.1016/j.jcpa.2009.04.005

Dobsinska, E., Sova, Z., Kopak, V., & Trhon, M. (1981). Relations among glycemia, ascorbemia and weight gains in calves in a large capacity calf house. *Veterinary Medicine Praha, 26*, 203–212. PubMed: 6791354

Doğan, E. (2023). Effect of vitamin C on the immune system in cattle immunized with blackleg vaccine. *Veterinary Journal of Mehmet Akif Ersoy University.* J. Mehmet Akif Ersoy University, 8(2), 83–88. https://doi.org/10.24880/maeuvfd.1228850

Doğan, E., Merhan, O., Erdağ, D., Karamanci, E., Bozukluhan, K., & Doğan, A. N. C. (2021). The effect of vitamin C on oxidant and antioxidant parameters in anthrax vaccine administered cattle. *Van Veterinary Journal, 32*(3), 109–113. https://doi.org/10.36483/vanvetj.958358

Domingos, I. D., Xavier, A. A., Jorge, R. A., Mercadante, A. Z., Petenate, A. J., & Viotto, W. H. (2011). Riboflavin photodegradation in yogurt with added lutein. *Journal of Animal Science, 89*(1), 540 [Abstr.].

Dong, F. M., & Oace, S. M. (1975). Folate concentration and pattern in ovine milk. *Journal of Agricultural and Food Chemistry, 23*(3), 534–538. https://doi.org/10.1021/jf60199a014

Donoghue, S., Donawick, W. J., & Kronfeld, D. S. (1983). Transfer of vitamin A from intestine to plasma in lambs fed low and high intakes of vitamin A. *The Journal of Nutrition, 113*(11), 2197–2204. https://doi.org/10.1093/jn/113.11.2197

Dougherty, C. T., Lauriault, L. M., Bradley, N. W., Gay, N., & Cornelius, P. L. (1991). Induction of tall fescue toxicosis in heat-stressed cattle and its alleviation with thiamin. *Journal of Animal Science, 69*(3), 1008–1018. https://doi.org/10.2527/1991.6931008x

Drackley, J. K. (1992). Niacin and carnitine in the nutrition of dairy cows. *Proceedings of the Pacific Northwest Nutr. Conf. Tech.* symposium, October 20, Lonza Inc. & Spokane, WA, 8.

Drackley, J. K., Donkin, S. S., & Reynolds, C. K. (2006). Major advances in fundamental dairy cattle nutrition. *Journal of Dairy Science, 89*(4), 1324–1336. https://doi.org/10.3168/jds.S0022-0302(06)72200-7

Draper, H. H., & Johnson, B. C. (1952). Folic acid deficiency in the lamb. *The Journal of Nutrition, 46*(1), 123–131. https://doi.org/10.1093/jn/46.1.123

Driskell, J. A. (1984). Vitamin B$_6$. In L. J. Machlin (Ed.), *Handbook of vitamins*. Marcel Dekker, Inc.

Driver, L. S., Grummer, R. R., & Schultz, L. H. (1990). Effects of feeding heat-treated soybeans and niacin to high producing cows in early lactation. *Journal of Dairy Science, 73*(2), 463–469. https://doi.org/10.3168/jds.S0022-0302(90)78692-4

Droke, E. A., & Loerch, S. C. (1989). Effect of parenteral selenium and vitamin E on performance, health, and humoral immune response of steers new to the feedlot environment. *Journal of Animal Science, 67*(5), 1350–1359. https://doi.org/10.2527/jas1989.6751350x

Drouillard, J. S., Flake, A. S., & Kuhl, G. L. (1998). Effects of added fat, degradable intake protein, and ruminally protected choline in diets of finishing steers. Cattlemen's day, prog. Rep. 804. *Kansas Agric. Exp. Stn, Manhattan* (pp. 71–75).

Dryden, L. P., & Hartman, A. M. (1971). Variations in the amount and relative distribution of vitamin B$_{12}$ and its analogs in the bovine rumen. *Journal of Dairy Science, 54*(2), 235–246. https://doi.org/10.3168/jds.S0022-0302(71)85818-6

DSM Nutritional Products (2016) OVN Optimum Vitamin Nutrition® Guidelines.

dsm-firmenich. (2022a). *DSM Product Forms*. https://www.dsm.com/anh/news/downloads/infographics-checklists-and-guides/quality-feed-additives-for-more-sustainable-farming.html

dsm-firmenich. (2022b). *Vitamin supplementation guidelines 2022 for animal nutrition*. http://www.dsm.com/anh/en_NA/products-and-services/tools/ovn.html#ruminants

Duarte, T. L., & Almeida, I. F. (2012). Vitamin C, gene expression and skin health. In V. R. Preedy (Ed.), *Handbook of diet, nutrition and the skin. Human Health Handbooks no. 1, 2*, 114–127. Wageningen Academic Publishers. https://doi.org/10.3920/978-90-8686-729-5_7

Dubbs, M. D., & Gupta, R. B. (1998). Solubility of vitamin E (α-tocopherol) and vitamin K$_3$ (menadione) in ethanol–water mixture. *Journal of Chemical and Engineering Data, 43*(4), 590–591. https://doi.org/10.1021/je980017l

DuCoa, L. P. (1994). *Choline functions and requirements. DuCoa L.P., a DuPont/ConAgra Co, Higland*. IL.

Duello, T. J., & Matschiner, J. T. (1971). Characterization of vitamin K from pig liver and dog liver. *Archives of Biochemistry and Biophysics, 144*(1), 330–338. https://doi.org/10.1016/0003-9861(71)90485-1

Duffy, S. K., O'Doherty, J. V., Rajauria, G., Clarke, L. C., Cashman, K. D., Hayes, A., O'Grady, M. N., Kerry, J. P., & Kelly, A. K. (2017). Cholecalciferol supplementation of heifer diets increases beef vitamin D concentration and improves beef tenderness. *Meat Science, 134*, 103–110. https://doi.org/10.1016/j.meatsci.2017.07.024

Duffy, S. K., O'Doherty, J. V., Rajauria, G., Clarke, L. C., Hayes, A., Dowling, K. G., O'Grady, M. N., Kerry, J. P., Jakobsen, J., Cashman, K. D., & Kelly, A. K. (2018a). Vitamin D-biofortified beef: A comparison of cholecalciferol with synthetic versus UVB-mushroom-derived ergosterol as feed source. *Food Chemistry, 256*, 18–24. https://doi.org/10.1016/j.foodchem.2018.02.099

Duffy, S. K., Kelly, A. K., Rajauria, G., & O'Doherty, J. V. (2018b). Biofortification of meat with vitamin D. *CABI Reviews, 13*(045), 1–11. https://doi.org/10.1079/PAVSNNR201813045

Dumoulin, P. G., Girard, C. L., Matte, J. J., St-Laurent, G. J. (1991) Effects of a parenteral supplement of folic acid and its interaction with level of feed intake on hepatic tissues and growth performance of young dairy heifers. *Journal of Animal Science, 69*(4), 1657–1666. https://doi.org/10.2527/1991.6941657x

Duncan, C. W. (1944). Studies on the influence of ascorbic acid in calves with scurvy. *Journal of Dairy Science, 27*, 636.

Dunnett, C. E. (2003). Antioxidants in physiology and nutrition of exercising horses. In T. P. InLyons & K. P. Jacques (Eds.), *Nutritional biotechnology in the feed and food industries* (pp. 439–448) Nottingham University Press, G.B

Duplessis, M., & Girard, C. L. (2019). Effect of maternal biotin, folic acid, and vitamin B$_{12}$ supplementation before parturition on colostral and Holstein calf plasma concentrations in those vitamins. *Animal Feed Science and Technology*, 256, 114241. https://doi.org/10.1016/j.anifeedsci.2019.114241

Duplessis, M., Girard, C. L., Santschi, D. E., Laforest, J. P., Durocher, J., & Pellerin, D. (2014a). Effects of folic acid and vitamin B$_{12}$ supplementation on culling rate, diseases, and reproduction in commercial dairy herds. *Journal of Dairy Science*, 97(4), 2346–2354. https://doi.org/10.3168/jds.2013-7369

Duplessis, M., Girard, C. L., Santschi, D. E., Lefebvre, D. M., & Pellerin, D. (2014b). Milk production and composition, and body measurements of dairy cows receiving intramuscular injections of folic acid and vitamin B$_{12}$ in commercial dairy herds. *Livestock Science*, 167, 186–194. https://doi.org/10.1016/j.livsci.2014.06.022

Duplessis, M., Mann, S., Nydam, D. V., Girard, C. L., Pellerin, D., & Overton, T. R. (2015). Folates and vitamin B$_{12}$ in colostrum and milk from dairy cows fed different energy levels during the dry period. *Journal of Dairy Science*, 98(8), 5454–5459. https://doi.org/10.3168/jds.2015-9507

Duplessis, M., Lapierre, H., Ouattara, B., Bissonnette, N., Pellerin, D., Laforest, J. P., & Girard, C. L. (2017). Whole-body propionate and glucose metabolism of multiparous dairy cows receiving folic acid and vitamin B$_{12}$ supplements. *Journal of Dairy Science*, 100(10), 8578–8589. https://doi.org/10.3168/jds.2017-13056

Duplessis, M., Cue, R. I., Santschi, D. E., Lefebvre, D. M., & Girard, C. L. (2018). Relationships among plasma and milk vitamin B$_{12}$, plasma free fatty acids, and blood β-hydroxybutyrate concentrations in early lactation dairy cows. *Journal of Dairy Science*, 101(9), 8559–8565. https://doi.org/10.3168/jds.2018-14477

Duplessis, M., Pellerin, D., Robichaud, R., Fadul-Pacheco, L., & Girard, C. L. (2019). Impact of diet management and composition on vitamin B$_{12}$ concentration in milk of Holstein cows. *Animal*, 13(9), 2101–2109. https://doi.org/10.1017/S1751731119000211

Duplessis, M., Pellerin, D., Girard, C. L., Santschi, D. E., & Soyeurt, H. (2020a). Potential prediction of vitamin B$_{12}$ concentration based on mid-infrared spectral data using Holstein Dairy Herd Improvement milk samples. *Journal of Dairy Science*, 103(8), 7540–7546. https://doi.org/10.3168/jds.2019-17758

Duplessis, M., Ritz, K. E., Socha, M. T., & Girard, C. L. (2020b). Cross-sectional study of the effect of diet composition on plasma folate and vitamin B$_{12}$ concentrations in Holstein cows in the United States and Canada. *Journal of Dairy Science*, 103(3), 2883–2895. https://doi.org/10.3168/jds.2019-17657

Duplessis, M., Fréchette, A., Poisson, W., Blais, L., & Ronholm, J. (2021). Refining knowledge of factors affecting vitamin B$_{12}$ concentration in bovine milk. *Animals: An Open Access Journal from MDPI*, 11(2), 532. https://doi.org/10.3390/ani11020532

Duplessis, M., Lapierre, H., Sauerwein, H., & Girard, C. L. (2022). Combined biotin, folic acid, and vitamin B$_{12}$ supplementation given during the transition period to dairy cows: Part I. Effects on lactation performance, energy and protein metabolism, and hormones. *Journal of Dairy Science*, 105(8), 7079–7096. https://doi.org/10.3168/jds.2021-21677

Duplessis, M., Chorfi, Y., & Girard, C. L. (2023). Longitudinal data to assess relationships among plasma folate, vitamin B$_{12}$, non-esterified fatty acid, and β-hydroxybutyrate concentrations of Holstein cows during the transition period. *Metabolites*, 13(4), 547. https://doi.org/10.3390/metabo13040547

Duthie, G. G., Arthur, J. R., Mills, C. F., Morrice, P., & Nicol, F. (1987). Anomalous tissue vitamin E distribution in stress susceptible pigs after dietary vitamin E supplementation and effects on plasma pyruvate kinase and creatine kinase activities. *Livestock Production Science*, 17, 169–178. https://doi.org/10.1016/0301-6226(87)90062-5

Dutta-Roy, A. K., Gordon, M. J., Campbell, F. M., Duthie, G. G., & James, W. P. T. (1994). Vitamin E requirements, transport, and metabolism: Role of a-tocopherol-binding proteins. *The Journal of Nutritional Biochemistry*, 5(12), 562–570. https://doi.org/10.1016/0955-2863(94)90010-8

Dwenger, A., Pape, H. C., Bantel, C., Schweitzer, G., Krumm, K., Grotz, M., Lueken, B., Funck, M., & Regel, G. (1994). Ascorbic acid reduces the endotoxin-induced lung injury in awake sheep. *European Journal of Clinical Investigation*, 24(4), 229–235. https://doi.org/10.1111/j.1365-2362.1994.tb01079.x

Eastridge, M. L. (2006). Major advances in applied dairy cattle nutrition. *Journal of Dairy Science*, 89(4), 1311–1323. https://doi.org/10.3168/jds.S0022-0302(06)72199-3

Eaton, H. D., Rousseau, J. E., Hall, R. C., Jr., Frier, H. I., & Lucas, J. J. (1972). Revaluation of the minimum vitamin A requirements of Holstein male calves based upon elevated cerebrospinal fluid pressure. *Journal of Dairy Science*, 55(2), 232–237. https://doi.org/10.3168/jds.S0022-0302(72)85465-1

Eder, K., & Grundmann, S. M. (2022). Vitamin D in dairy cows: Metabolism, status and functions in the immune system. *Archives of Animal Nutrition*, 76(1), 1–33. https://doi.org/10.1080/1745039X.2021.2017747

Eder, K., Flader, D., Hirche, F., & Brandsch, C. (2002). Excess dietary vitamin E lowers the activities of anti-oxidative enzymes in erythrocytes of rats fed salmon oil. *The Journal of Nutrition*, 132(11), 3400–3404. https://doi.org/10.1093/jn/132.11.3400

Edwin, E. E., & Lewis, G. (1971). The implication of ruminal thiaminase in cerebrocortical necrosis. *The Proceedings of the Nutrition Society*, 30(1), 7A.

Edwin, E. E., Markson, L. M., Shreeve, J., Jackman, R., & Carroll, P. J. (1979). Diagnostic aspects of cerebrocortical necrosis. *The Veterinary Record*, 104(1), 4–8. https://doi.org/10.1136/vr.104.1.4

EFSA Panel on Additives and Products or Substances used in Animal Feed (FEEDAP)(2014)Scientific Opinion on the safety and efficacy of vitamin K3 (menadione sodium bisulphite and menadione nicotinamide bisulphite) as a feed additive for all animal species. *EFSA Journal*, 12(1), 3532. https://doi.org/10.2903/j.efsa.2014.3532

EFSA Panel on Dietetic Products, Nutrition and Allergies (NDA). (2010). Scientific Opinion on the substantiation of a health claim related to thiamine and carbohydrate and energy-yielding metabolism pursuant to Article 14 of Regulation (EC) No 1924/2006. *EFSA Journal*, 8(7)(1924/2006), 1690, article 14. https://doi.org/10.2903/j.efsa.2010.1690

Eggersdorfer, M., Laudert, D., Létinois, U., McClymont, T., Medlock, J., Netscher, T. and Bonrath, W. (2012) One hundred years of vitamins a success story of the natural sciences. *Angew. Chem. Int. Ed. Engl.* 51(52):12960–12990. https://doi.org/10.1002/anie.201205886. Eicher, S. D., Morrill, J. L., & Blecha, F. (1994). Vitamin concentration and function of leukocytes from dairy calves supplemented with vitamin A, vitamin E and beta-carotene. *Journal of Dairy Science*, 77(2), 560–565. https://doi.org/10.3168/jds.S0022-0302(94)76984-8

Eicher, S. D., Morrill, J. L., & Velazco, J. (1997). Bioavailability of α-tocopherol fed with retinol and relative bioavailability of d-α-tocopherol or dl-α-tocopherol acetate. *Journal of Dairy Science*, 80(2), 393–399. https://doi.org/10.3168/jds.S0022-0302(97)75949-6

Eicher-Pruiett, S. D., Morrill, J. L., Blecha, F., Higgins, J. J., Anderson, N. V., & Reddy, P. G. (1992). Neutrophil and lymphocyte response to supplementation with vitamins C and E in young calves. *Journal of Dairy Science*, 75(6), 1635–1642. https://doi.org/10.3168/jds.S0022-0302(92)77920-X

Ekanayake, A., & Nelson, P. E. (1990). Effect of thermal processing on lima bean vitamin B_6 availability. *Journal of Food Science*, 55(1), 154–157. https://doi.org/10.1111/j.1365-2621.1990.tb06040.x

Elam, N. A. (2006). Impact of vitamin E supplementation on newly received calves. *Proceedings of the Colorado Nutr. Round Table*. Colorado State University.

Elek, P., Newbold, J. R., Gaal, T., Wagner, L., & Husveth, F. (2008). Effects of rumen-protected choline supplementation on milk production and choline supply of periparturient dairy cows. *Animal*, 2(11), 1595–1601. https://doi.org/10.1017/S1751731108002917

Ellenbogen, L., & Cooper, B. A. (1991). Vitamin B_{12}. In J. Machlin (Ed.), *Handbook of Vitamins, 2nd ed.* L. Marcel Dekker, Inc.

Elliot, W., Wood, T. B., Elliot, W., & Crichton, A. (1926). Investigation on the mineral content of pasture grass and its effect on herbivora: II. Report on the effect of the addition of mineral salts to the ration of sheep. *Journal of Agricultural Science*, 16(1), 65–77. https://doi.org/10.1017/S0021859600088298.

El-Masry, K. A., Emara, S. S., & Eid, S. Y. (2020). Effect of β-carotene as antioxidant on immune response and blood biochemical changes in relation to growth performance of heat-stressed calves. *The Agriculturists Extension* J, 4(4), 166–175. https://www.academia.edu/download/87544635/06_AEXTJ_233_20.pdf

Elvehjem, C. A., Madden, R.J., Strong, F.M. and Wolley, D.W. (1974) The isolation and identification of the anti-black tongue factor. *Nutr. Rev.* 32(2):48–50. https://doi.org/10.1111/j.1753-4887.1974.tb06263.x.

Emanuele, S., Hickley, T., & Bicalho, R. C. (2007). Effect of rumen protected choline (Reashure®) and rumen protected methionine on milk yield, and composition in lactating dairy cows. *Journal of Dairy Science*, 90(1), 352–359 [Abstr.].

Emmanuel, B., & Kennelly, J. J. (1984). Kinetics of methionine and choline and their incorporation into plasma lipids and milk components in lactating goats. *Journal of Dairy Science, 67*(9), 1912–1918. https://doi.org/10.3168/jds.S0022-0302(84)81524-6

Emmert, J. L., & Baker, D. H. (1997). A chick bioassay approach for determining the bioavailable choline concentration in normal and overheated soybean meal, canola meal and peanut meal. *The Journal of Nutrition, 127*(5), 745–752. https://doi.org/10.1093/jn/127.5.745

Emmert, J. L., Garrow, T. A., & Baker, D. H. (1996). Development of an experimental diet for determining bio-available choline concentration and its application in studies with soybean lecithin. *Journal of Animal Science, 74*(11), 2738–2744. https://doi.org/10.2527/1996.74112738x

Ender, F., Dishington, I. W., & Helgebostad, A. (1971). Calcium balance studies in dairy cows under experimental induction and prevention of hypocalcemic *paresis puerperalis*. *Zeitschrift Fur Tierphysiologie, Tierernahrung und Futtermittelkunde, 28*(5), 233–256. https://doi.org/10.1111/j.1439-0396.1971.tb01573.x

Enevoldsen, C. (1993). Nutritional risk factors for milk fever in dairy cows: Meta-analysis revisited. *Acta Veterinaria Scandinavica, 89*, 131–134. PubMed: 8237649

Enjalbert, F., Nicot, M. C., & Packington, A. J. (2008). Effects of peripartum biotin supplementation of dairy cows on milk production and milk composition with emphasis on fatty acids profile. *Livestock Science, 114*(2–3), 287–295. https://doi.org/10.1016/j.livsci.2007.05.013

Ensminger, A. H., Ensminger, M. E., Konlande, J. E., & Robson, J. R. K. (1983). Foods and nutrition encyclopedia. In A. H. Ensminger (Ed.), *Ensminger pub*. CO.

Erdman, R. A. (1992). Vitamins. In H. H. Van Horn & C. J. Wilcox (Eds.), *Large Dairy herd management* (pp. 297–308). American Dairy Science Association.

Erdman, R. A., & Sharma, B. K. (1991). Effect of dietary rumen-protected choline in lactating dairy cows. *Journal of Dairy Science, 74*(5), 1641–1647. https://doi.org/10.3168/jds.S0022-0302(91)78326-4

Erdman, R. A., Shaver, R. D., & Vandersall, J. H. (1984). Dietary choline for the lactating cow: Possible effects on milk fat synthesis. *Journal of Dairy Science, 67*(2), 410–415. https://doi.org/10.3168/jds.S0022-0302(84)81317-X

Erickson, P. S., Trusk, A. M., & Murphy, M. R. (1990). Effects of niacin source on epinephrine stimulation of plasma nonesterified fatty acid and glucose concentrations, on diet digestibility and on rumen protozoal numbers in lactating dairy cows. *The Journal of Nutrition, 120*(12), 1648–1653. https://doi.org/10.1093/jn/120.12.1648

Erickson, P. S., Murphy, M. R., McSweeney, C. S., & Trusk, A. M. (1991). Niacin absorption from the rumen. *Journal of Dairy Science, 74*(10), 3492–3495. https://doi.org/10.3168/jds.S0022-0302(91)78540-8

Erickson, P. S., Murphy, M. R., & Clark, J. H. (1992). Supplementation of dairy cow diets with calcium salts of long-chain fatty acid in early lactation. *Journal of Dairy Science, 75*(4), 1078–1089. https://doi.org/10.3168/jds.S0022-0302(92)77852-7

Erskine, R. J., Bartlett, P. C., Herdt, T., & Gaston, P. (1997). Effects of parenteral administration of vitamin E on health of periparturient dairy cows. *Journal of the American Veterinary Medical Association, 211*(4), 466–469. https://doi.org/10.2460/javma.1997.211.04.466, PubMed: 9267510

Erskine, R. J., Eberhart, R. J., Grasso, P. J., & Scholz, R. W. (1989). Introduction of *Escherichia coli* mastitis in cows fed selenium-deficient or selenium-supplemented diets. *American Journal of Veterinary Research, 50*(12), 2093–2100. PubMed: 2558602

Eshaghian, M., Amini Pour, H., Hamedani, M. A., Jannat Abadi, A. A., & Ramshini, M. (2013). Effect of vitamin D on performance of ruminant animal: A review. *Journal of American Science, 3*, 130–138. https://www.cabdirect.org/cabdirect/abstract/20133161313

Esmon, C. T., Sadowski, J. A., & Suttie, J. W. (1975). A new carboxylation reaction. The vitamin K-dependent incorporation of H-14-CO3- into prothrombin. *The Journal of Biological Chemistry, 250*(12), 4744–4748. https://doi.org/10.1016/S0021-9258(19)41365-3, PubMed: 1141226

Esslemont, R. J. (1990). The cost of lameness in dairy herds: Update in cattle lameness. In *Proceedings of the "International Symposium on Diseases of the Ruminant Digest"*. Liverpool p. 237.

Esteban-Pretel, G., Marín, M. P., Renau-Piqueras, J., Barber, T., & Timoneda, J. (2010). Vitamin A deficiency alters rat lung alveolar basement membrane reversibility by retinoic acid. *The Journal of Nutritional Biochemistry, 21*(3), 227–236. https://doi.org/10.1016/j.jnutbio.2008.12.007

Eyles, D., Anderson, C., Ko, P., Jones, A., Thomas, A., Burne, T., Mortensen, P. B., Nørgaard-Pedersen, B., Hougaard, D. M., & McGrath, J. (2009). A sensitive LC/MS/MS assay of 25OH vitamin D_3 and 25OH vitamin D_2 in dried blood spots. *Clinica Chimica Acta; International Journal of Clinical Chemistry, 403*(1–2), 145–151. https://doi.org/10.1016/j.cca.2009.02.005

Fallah, R., Kiani, A., & Khaldari, M. (2021). Supplementing lycopene combined with corn improves circulating IgG concentration in pregnant ewes and their lambs. *Tropical Animal Health and Production, 53*(3), 360. https://doi.org/10.1007/s11250-021-02802-3

Farooq, U., Samad, H. A., Shehzad, F., & Qayyum, A. (2010). Physiological responses of cattle to heat stress. *World Applied Sciences Journal, 8*, 38–43.

Farrugia, W., Fortune, C. L., Heath, J., Caple, I. W., & Wark, J. D. (1989). Osteocalcin as an index of osteoblast function during and after ovine pregnancy. *Endocrinology, 125*(3), 1705–1710. https://doi.org/10.1210/endo-125-3-1705

Faulkner, H., O'Callaghan, T. F., McAuliffe, S., Hennessy, D., Stanton, C., O'Sullivan, M. G., Kerry, J. P., & Kilcawley, K. N. (2018). Effect of different forage types on the volatile and sensory properties of bovine milk. *Journal of Dairy Science, 101*(2), 1034–1047. https://doi.org/10.3168/jds.2017-13141

Faustman, C., & Cassens, R. G. (1990). The biochemical basis for discoloration in fresh meat: A review. *Journal of Muscle Foods, 1*(3), 217–243. https://doi.org/10.1111/j.1745-4573.1990.tb00366.x

Faustman, C., Cassens, R. G., Schaefer, D. M., Buege, D. R., Williams, S. N., & Scheller, K. K. (1989). Improvement of pigment and lipid stability in Holstein steer beef by dietary supplementation with vitamin E. *Journal of Food Science, 54*(4), 858–862. https://doi.org/10.1111/j.1365-2621.1989.tb07899.x

FEDNA (Federacion Española para el Desarrollo Nutricion Animal). (2018). Necesidades nutricionales en avicultura: Normas para la formulación de piensos. http://www.fundacionfedna.org/node/75

Fedosov, S. N., Nexo, E., & Heegaard, C. W. (2019). Vitamin B_{12} and its binding proteins in milk from cow and buffalo in relation to bioavailability of B_{12}. *Journal of Dairy Science, 102*(6), 4891–4905. https://doi.org/10.3168/jds.2018-15016

Feldman, D., Pike, J. W., & Glorieux, F. H. (2003). *Vitamin D*. Elsevier.

Fernandez, S. C., Budowski, P., Ascarelli, I., Neumark, H., & Bondi, A. (1976). Low utilization of carotene by sheep. *International Journal for Vitamin and Nutrition Research. Internationale Zeitschrift Fur Vitamin- und Ernahrungsforschung. Journal International de Vitaminologie et de Nutrition, 46*(4), 446–453. PubMed: 1010681

Fenstermacher, D. K., & Rose, R. C. (1986). Absorption of pantothenic acid in rat and chick intestine. *The American Journal of Physiology, 250*(2 Pt 1), G155–G160. https://doi.org/10.1152/ajpgi.1986.250.2.G155

Ferguson, E. G. W., Mitchell, G. B., & MacPherson, A. (1989). Cobalt deficiency and *Ostertagia circumcincta* infection in lambs. *The Veterinary Record, 124*(1), 20. https://doi.org/10.1136/vr.124.1.20

Ferland, G. (2006). Vitamin K. In B. A. Bowman & R. M. Russell (Eds.), *Present knowledge in nutrition* (9th ed.) (pp. 220–230). International Life Sciences Institute.

Ferreira, G., & Weiss, W. P. (2007). Effect of biotin on activity and gene expression of biotin- dependent carboxylases in the liver of dairy cows. *Journal of Dairy Science, 90*(3), 1460–1466. https://doi.org/10.3168/jds.S0022-0302(07)71631-4

Ferreira, G., Brown, A. N., & Teets, C. L. (2015). Effect of biotin and pantothenic acid on performance and concentrations of avidin-binding substances in blood and milk of lactating dairy cows. *Journal of Dairy Science, 98*(9), 6449–6454. https://doi.org/10.3168/jds.2015-9620

Ferreira, G., Weiss, W. P., & Willett, L. B. (2007). Changes in measures of biotin status do not reflect milk yield responses when dairy cows are fed supplemental biotin. *Journal of Dairy Science, 90*(3), 1452–1459. https://doi.org/10.3168/jds.S0022-0302(07)71630-2

Fichter, S. A., & Mitchell, G. E. (1997). Sheep blood response to orally supplemented vitamin K dissolved in coconut oil. *Journal of Animal Science, 72*(1), 266 [Abstr.].

Filmer, J. F. (1933). Enzootic marasmus of cattle and sheep. Preliminary report having special reference to iron and liver therapy. *Australian Veterinary Journal, 9*(5), 163–179. https://doi.org/10.1111/j.1751-0813.1933.tb03645.x

Finch, J. M., & Turner, R. J. (1989). Enhancement of ovine lymphocyte responses: A comparison of selenium and vitamin E supplementation. *Veterinary Immunology and Immunopathology, 23*(3–4), 245–256. https://doi.org/10.1016/0165-2427(89)90138-4

Finkelstein, J. D., Martin, J. J., Harris, B. J., & Kyle, W. E. (1982). Regulation of the betaine content of rat liver. *Archives of Biochemistry and Biophysics, 218*(1), 169–173. https://doi.org/10.1016/0003-9861(82)90332-0

Fisher, G. E. (1991). Effect of cobalt deficiency in the pregnant ewe on reproductive performance and lamb viability. *Research in Veterinary Science, 50*(3), 319–327. https://doi.org/10.1016/0034-5288(91)90132-8

Fitzgerald, T., Norton, B. W., Elliott, R., Podlich, H., & Svendsen, O. L. (2000). The influence of long-term supplementation with biotin on the prevention of lameness in pasture fed dairy cows. *Journal of Dairy Science, 83*(2), 338–344. https://doi.org/10.3168/jds.S0022-0302(00)74884-3

Flachowsky, G., Lober, U., Ast, H., Wolfram, D., & Mathey, M. (1988). *Influence of niacin on rumen fermentation variables in sheep and metabolic characteristics and performance in dairy cows*. Wiss, Z. Karl-marx-Univ. Leipzig math. Naturwiss R, 37, 55.

Flavin, M., & Ochoa, S. (1957). Metabolism of propionic acid in animal tissues. I. Enzymatic conversion of propionate to succinate. *The Journal of Biological Chemistry, 229*(2), 965–979. https://doi.org/10.1016/S0021-9258(19)63700-2, PubMed: 13502357

Flipse, R. J., Huffman, C. F., Duncan, C. W., & Thorp, Jr., F. (1948). Potassium vs. biotin in the treatment of experimentally induced paralysis in calves. *Animal Science Journal, 7*.

Flores-Villalva, S., O'Brien, M. B., Reid, C., Lacey, S., Gordon, S. V., Nelson, C., & Meade, K. G. (2021). Low serum vitamin D concentrations in Spring-born dairy calves are associated with elevated peripheral leukocytes. *Scientific Reports, 11*(1), 18969. https://doi.org/10.1038/s41598-021-98343-8

Flores-Villalva, S. (2022). *The effects of vitamin D on the cellular responses, molecular immunity, and mycobacterial killing in cattle*. https://researchrepository.ucd.ie/entities/publication/d79bb5b9-a8d8-4f32-a83a-b1a36e07be00/details. Retrieved Jan 2024 [Unpublished doctoral dissertation]. University College Dublin Press. School of Agriculture and Food Science.

Focant, M., Mignolet, E., Marique, M., Clabots, F., Breyne, T., Dalemans, D., & Larondelle, Y. (1998). The effect of vitamin E supplementation of cow diets containing rapeseed and linseed on the prevention of milk fat oxidation. *Journal of Dairy Science, 81*(4), 1095–1101. https://doi.org/10.3168/jds.S0022-0302(98)75671-1

Foley, J. A., & Otterby, D. E. (1978). Availability, storage, treatment, composition, and feeding value of surplus colostrum: A review. *Journal of Dairy Science, 61*(8), 1033–1060. https://doi.org/10.3168/jds.S0022-0302(78)83686-8

Folman, Y., Ascarelli, I., Herz, Z., Rosenberg, M., Davidson, M., & Halevi, A. (1979). Fertility of dairy heifers given a commercial diet free of beta-carotene. *The British Journal of Nutrition, 41*(2), 353–359. https://doi.org/10.1079/bjn19790044

Folman, Y., Ascarelli, I., Kraus, D., & Barash, H. (1987). Adverse effect of β-carotene in diet on fertility of dairy cows. *Journal of Dairy Science, 70*(2), 357–366. https://doi.org/10.3168/jds.S0022-0302(87)80017-6

Food and Agriculture Organization of the United Nations (FAO). (2004). *Vitamin and mineral requirements in human nutrition* (2nd ed.). https://www.who.int/publications/i/item/9241546123 Consulted: 1/15/2024.

Food Standards Australia/New Zealand Food Composition Database https://afcd.foodstandards.gov.au/fooddetails.aspx?PFKID=F005634

Foote, M. R., Horst, R. L., Huff-Lonergan, E. J., Trenkle, A. H., Parrish, Jr., F. C., & Beitz, D. C. (2004). The use of vitamin D_3 and its metabolites to improve beef tenderness. *Journal of Animal Science, 82*(1), 242–249. https://doi.org/10.2527/2004.821242x

Fox, H. M. (1991). Pantothenic Acid. In J. Machlin (Ed.), *Handbook of Vitamins, 2nd edition* L. Marcel Dekker, Inc.

Franceschi, R. T. (1992). The role of ascorbic acid in mesenchymal differentiation. *Nutrition Reviews, 50*(3), 65–70. https://doi.org/10.1111/j.1753-4887.1992.tb01271.x

Franco da Silva, L. A., Franco, L. G., Atayde, I. B., da Cunha, P. H., de Moura, M. I., & Goulart, D. S. (2010). Effect of biotin supplementation on claw horn growth in young, clinically healthy cattle. *Canadian Veterinary Journal, 51*(6), 607–610. PubMed: 20808571

Franco-Lopez, J., Duplessis, M., Bui, A., Reymond, C., Poisson, W., Blais, L., Chong, J., Gervais, R., Rico, D. E., Cue, R. I., Girard, C. L., & Ronholm, J. (2020). Correlations between the composition of the bovine microbiota and vitamin B$_{12}$ abundance. *mSystems, 5*(2):2, e00107-20. https://doi.org/10.1128/mSys tems.00107-20

Frank, A. A., Hedstrom, O. R., Braselton, W. E., Huckfeldt, R. E., & Snyder, S. P. (1992). Multifocal polio-encephalomyelomalacia in Simmental calves with elevated tissue aluminum and decreased tissue copper and manganese. *Journal of Veterinary Diagnostic Investigation, 4*(3), 353–355. https://doi. org/10.1177/104063879200400326

Franklin, S. T., Sorenson, C. E., & Hammell, D. C. (1998). Influence of vitamin A supplementation in milk on growth, health, concentration of vitamins in plasma, and immune parameters of calves. *Journal of Dairy Science, 81*(10), 2623–2632. https://doi.org/10.3168/jds.S0022-0302(98)75820-5

Fraser, D. R. (2021). Vitamin D toxicity related to its physiological and unphysiological supply. *Trends in Endocrinology and Metabolism, 32*(11), 929–940. https://doi.org/10.1016/j.tem.2021.08.006

Fredeen, A. H., DePeters, E. J., & Baldwin, R. L. (1988). Characterization of acid–base disturbances and effects on calcium and phosphorus balances of dietary fixed ions in pregnant or lactating does. *Journal of Animal Science, 66*(1), 159–173. https://doi.org/10.2527/jas1988.661159x

Freiser, H., & Jiang, Q. (2009). Optimization of the enzymatic hydrolysis and analysis of plasma conjugated gamma-CEHC and sulfated long-chain carboxychromanols, metabolites of vitamin E. *Analytical Biochemistry, 388*(2), 260–265. https://doi.org/10.1016/j.ab.2009.02.027

French, P. D. (2004). Nicotinic acid supplemented at a therapeutic level minimizes prepartum feed intake depression in dairy cows. *Journal of Dairy Science, 87*, 345 [Abstract].

FRIDA. *National Food Institute, Technical University of Denmark.* Foodata.dk. https://frida.fooddata.dk/food/1265?lang=en

Frieden, E. H., Mitchell, H. K., & Williams, R. J. (1944). Folic acid. II. Studies on adsorption. *Journal of the American Chemical Society, 66*(2), 269–271. https://doi.org/10.1021/ja01230a033

Friesecke, H. (1980). *Vitamin B$_{12}$, 1728.* F. Hoffmann-La Roche, and Co. Ltd.

Frigg, M. (1976). Bioavailability of biotin in cereals. *Poultry Science, 55*(6), 2310–2318. https://doi.org/10.3382/ps.0552310

Frigg, M. (1984). Available biotin content of various feed ingredients. *Poultry Science, 63*(4), 750–753. https://doi.org/10.3382/ps.0630750

Frigg, M., & Volker, L. (1994). Biotin inclusion helps optimize animal performance. *Feedstuffs, 66*(1), 12–13. ISSN: 0014-9624.

Frigg, M., Straub, O. C., & Hartmann, D. (1993). The bioavailability of supplemental biotin in cattle. *International Journal for Vitamin and Nutrition Research. Internationale Zeitschrift Fur Vitamin- und Ernahrungsforschung. Journal International de Vitaminologie et de Nutrition, 63*(2), 122–128. PubMed: 8407161

Fronk, T. J., & Schultz, L. H. (1979). Oral nicotinic acid as a treatment for ketosis. *Journal of Dairy Science, 62*(11), 1804–1807. https://doi.org/10.3168/jds.S0022-0302(79)83501-8

Frye, T. M. (1994). The performance of vitamins in multicomponent premixes. In *Proceedings of the Roche.*

Frye, T. M., Williams, S. N., & Graham, T. W. (1991). Vitamin deficiencies in cattle. *The Veterinary Clinics of North America. Food Animal Practice, 7*(1), 217–275. https://doi.org/10.1016/S0749-0720(15)30817-3

Funada, U., Wada, M., Kawata, T., Mori, K., Tamai, H., Isshiki, T., Onoda, J., Tanaka, N., Tadokoro, T., & Maekawa, A. (2001). Vitamin B$_{12}$ deficiency affects immunoglobulin production and cytokine levels in mice. *International Journal for Vitamin and Nutrition Research. Internationale Zeitschrift Fur Vitamin- und Ernahrungsforschung. Journal International de Vitaminologie et de Nutrition, 71*(1), 60–65. https://doi.org/10.1024/0300-9831.71.1.60

Funk, C. and Dubin, H.E. (1922) *The vitamins.* Williams & Wilkins, Co., Baltimore, MD.

Gadient, M. (1986). Effect of pelleting on nutritional quality of feed. In "Proc Maryland Nutrition Conference Feed Manufacturers, College Park, MD, *1986.*

Gagnon, A., Khan, D. R., Sirard, M. A., Girard, C. L., Laforest, J. P., & Richard, F. J. (2015). Effects of intramuscular administration of folic acid and vitamin B$_{12}$ on granulosa cells gene expression in postpartum dairy cows. *Journal of Dairy Science, 98*(11), 7797–7809. https://doi.org/10.3168/jds.2015-9623

Gallop, P. M., Lian, J. B., & Hauschka, P. V. (1980). Carboxylated calcium-binding proteins and vitamin K. *The New England Journal of Medicine, 302*(26), 1460–1466. https://doi.org/10.1056/NEJM198006263022608

Gallo-Torres, H. E. (1980a). *Absorption. In vitamin E: A comprehensive treatise* J. M. Lawrence (Ed.) (pp. 170–193). Marcel Dekker.

Gallo-Torres, H. E. (1970). Obligatory role of bile for the intestinal absorption of vitamin E. *Lipids, 5*(4), 379–384. https://doi.org/10.1007/BF02532102

Gálvez, I., Navarro, M. C., Martín-Cordero, L., Otero, E., Hinchado, M. D., & Ortega, E. (2022). The influence of obesity and weight loss on the bioregulation of innate/inflammatory responses: Macrophages and immunometabolism. *Nutrients, 14*(3), 612. https://doi.org/10.3390/nu14030612

Galyean, M. L., Perino, L. J., & Duff, G. C. (1999). Interaction of cattle health/immunity and nutrition. *Journal of Animal Science, 77*(5), 1120–1134. https://doi.org/10.2527/1999.7751120x

Gannon, B. M., Jones, C., & Mehta, S. (2020). Vitamin A requirements in pregnancy and lactation. *Current Developments in Nutrition, 4*(10), nzaa142. https://doi.org/10.1093/cdn/nzaa142

Garber, M. J., Roeder, R. A., Pumfrey, W. M., Schelling, G. T., & Davidson, P. M. (1996). Dose–response effects of vitamin E supplementation on growth performance and meat characteristics in beef and dairy steers. *Canadian Journal of Animal Science, 76*(1), 63–72. https://doi.org/10.4141/cjas96-009

Garcia, R., & Municio, A. M. (1990). Effect of *Escherichia coli* endotoxin on ascorbic acid transport in isolated adrenocortical cells. *Proceedings of the Society for Experimental Biology and Medicine. Society for Experimental Biology and Medicine, 193*(4), 280–284. https://doi.org/10.3181/00379727-193-43036

Gardner, H. W. (1989). Oxygen radical chemistry of polyunsaturated fatty acids. *Free Radical Biology and Medicine, 7*(1), 65–86. https://doi.org/10.1016/0891-5849(89)90102-0

Garrett, J. E., Oenga, G., Tayal, A., & Webster, T. M. (2007). Influence of encapsulation of ascorbic acid to fermentation by rumen bacteria, *in vitro*. *Journal of Dairy Science, 90*(1), 339 [Abstr.].

Garrow, T. A. (2007). Choline. In J. Zempleni, R. B. Rucker, D. B. McCormick, & J. W. Suttie (Eds.), *Handbook of vitamins* (4th ed.) (pp. 459–487). CRC Press.

Gasperi, V., Sibilano, M., Savini, I., & Catani, M. V. (2019). Niacin in the central nervous system: An update of biological aspects and clinical applications. *International Journal of Molecular Sciences, 20*(4), 974. https://doi.org/10.3390/ijms20040974

Gaynor, P. J., Mueller, F. J., Miller, J. K., Ramsey, N., Goff, J. P., & Horst, R. L. (1989). Parturient hypocalcemia in Jersey cows fed alfalfa haylage-based diets with different cation to anion ratios. *Journal of Dairy Science, 72*(10), 2525–2531. https://doi.org/10.3168/jds.S0022-0302(89)79392-9

Gentry, P. A., & Cooper, M. L. (1981). Effect of T-2 mycotoxin on the coagulation mechanism. *Thrombosis and Haemostasis, 46*(05), 1094. https://doi.org/10.1055/s-0038-1653046

Gershoff, S. N. (1993). Vitamin C (ascorbic acid) new roles, new requirements. *Nutrition Reviews, 51*(11), 313–326. https://doi.org/10.1111/j.1753-4887.1993.tb03757.x

Ghaffari, M. H., Bernhöft, K., Etheve, S., Immig, I., Hölker, M., Sauerwein, H., & Schweigert, F. J. (2019). Technical note: Rapid field test for the quantification of vitamin E, β-carotene, and vitamin A in whole blood and plasma of dairy cattle. *Journal of Dairy Science, 102*(12), 11744–11750. https://doi.org/10.3168/jds.2019-16755

Ghosh, H. P., Sarkar, P. K., & Guha, B. C. (1963). Distribution of the bound form of nicotinic acid in natural materials. *The Journal of Nutrition, 79*, 451–453. https://doi.org/10.1093/jn/79.4.451

Giguère, A., Matte, J. J., & Girard, C. L. (1998). Characterization of high-affinity folate-binding protein in serum of cow, pig and sheep. *Journal of Animal Science, 76*(1), 184.

Gilbert, R. O., Gröhn, Y. T., Miller, P. M., & Hoffman, D. J. (1993a). Effect of parity on periparturient neutrophil function in dairy cows. *Veterinary Immunology and Immunopathology, 36*(1), 75–82. https://doi.org/10.1016/0165-2427(93)90007-Q

Gilbert, R. O., Gröhn, Y. T., Guard, C. L., Surman, V., Neilsen, N., & Slauson, D. O. (1993b). Impaired postpartum neutrophil function in cows which retain fetal membranes. *Research in Veterinary Science, 55*(1), 15–19. https://doi.org/10.1016/0034-5288(93)90027-D

Girard, C. L. (1998). B-complex vitamins for dairy cows: A new approach. *Canadian Journal of Animal Science, 78*(Suppl.), 71.

Girard, C. L., & Duplessis, M. (2022). The importance of B vitamins in enhanced precision nutrition of dairy cows: The case of folates and vitamin B_{12}. *Canadian Journal of Animal Science, 102*(2), 201–210. https://doi.org/10.1139/cjas-2021-0065

Girard, C. L., & Duplessis, M. (2023). Review–State of knowledge on the importance of folates and cobalamin for dairy cow metabolism. *Animal*, 17(Suppl. 3), 100834. https://doi.org/10.1016/j.animal.2023.100834

Girard, C. L., & Graulet, B. (2021). Methods and approaches to estimate B vitamin status in dairy cows: Knowledge, gaps and advances. *Methods*, 186, 52–58. https://doi.org/10.1016/j.ymeth.2020.05.021

Girard, C. L., & Matte, J. J. (1998). Dietary supplements of folic acid during lactation: Effects on the performance of dairy cows. *Journal of Dairy Science*, 81(5), 1412–1419. https://doi.org/10.3168/jds.S0022-0302(98)75705-4

Girard, C. L., & Matte, J. J. (2005a). Folic acid and vitamin B_{12} requirements of dairy cows: A concept to be revised. *Livestock Production Science*, 98(1–2), 123–133. https://doi.org/10.1016/j.livprodsci.2005.10.009

Girard, C. L., & Matte, J. J. (2005b). Effects of intramuscular injections of vitamin B_{12} on lactation performance of dairy cow fed dietary supplements of folic acid and rumen-protected methionine. *Journal of Dairy Science*, 88(2), 671–676. https://doi.org/10.3168/jds.S0022-0302(05)72731-4

Girard, C. L., Chiquette, J., & Matte, J. J. (1994). Concentrations of folates in ruminal content of steers: Responses to a dietary supplement of folic acid in relation with the nature of the diet. *Journal of Animal Science*, 72(4), 1023–1028. https://doi.org/10.2527/1994.7241023x

Girard, C. L., Matte, J. J., & Tremblay, G. F. (1995). Gestation and lactation of dairy cows: A role for folic acid? *Journal of Dairy Science*, 78(2), 404–411. https://doi.org/10.3168/jds.S0022-0302(95)76649-8

Girard, C. L., Castonguay, F., Fahmy, M. H., & Matte, J. J. (1996). Serum and milk folates during the first two gestations and lactations in Romanov, Finnsheep and Suffolk ewes. *Journal of Animal Science*, 74(7), 1711–1715. https://doi.org/10.2527/1996.7471711x

Girard, C. L., Lapierre, H., Matte, J. J., & Lobley, G. E. (2005). Effects of dietary supplements of folic acid and rumen- protected methionine on lactational performance and folate metabolism of dairy cows. *Journal of Dairy Science*, 88(2), 660–670. https://doi.org/10.3168/jds.S0022-0302(05)72730-2

Girard, C. L., Santschi, D. E., Stabler, S. P., & Allen, R. H. (2009). Apparent ruminal synthesis and intestinal disappearance of vitamin B_{12} and its analogs in dairy cows. *Journal of Dairy Science*, 92(9), 4524–4529. https://doi.org/10.3168/jds.2009-2049

Girard, C. L., Vanacker, N., Beaudet, V., Duplessis, M., & Lacasse, P. (2019). Glucose and insulin responses to an intravenous glucose tolerance test administered to feed-restricted dairy cows receiving folic acid and vitamin B_{12} supplements. *Journal of Dairy Science*, 102(7), 6226–6234. https://doi.org/10.3168/jds.2019-16298

Gitter, M., Bradley, R., & Pepper, R. (1978). Nutritional myodegeneration in dairy cows. *The Veterinary Record*, 103(2), 24–26. https://doi.org/10.1136/vr.103.2.24

Godoy-Parejo, C., Deng, C., Zhang, Y., Liu, W., & Chen, G. (2020). Roles of vitamins in stem cells. *Cellular and Molecular Life Sciences*, 77(9), 1771–1791. https://doi.org/10.1007/s00018-019-03352-6

Godwin, K. O. (1975). The role and the metabolism of selenium in the animal. *Trace Elements in Soil-Plant-Animal Systems*, 259–270.

Goetsch, A. L., & Owens, F. N. (1987). Effects of supplement sulfate (Dynamate®) and thiamine-HCl on passage of thiamine to the duodenum and site of digestion in steers. *Archives of Animal Nutrition*, 37(12), 1075–1083. https://doi.org/10.1080/17450398709428275

Goff, J. P., Horst, R. L., Beitz, D. C., & Littledike, E. T. (1988). Use of 24-F-1,25-dihydroxyvitamin D_3 to prevent parturient paresis in dairy cows. *Journal of Dairy Science*, 71(5), 1211–1219. https://doi.org/10.3168/jds.S0022-0302(88)79676-9

Goff, J. P., Reinhardt, T. A., & Horst, R. L. (1989). Recurring hypocalcemia of bovine parturient paresis is associated with failure to produce 1, 25-dihydroxyvitamin D. *Endocrinology*, 125(1), 49–53. https://doi.org/10.1210/endo-125-1-49

Goff, J. P., & Horst, R. L. (1997). Physiological changes at parturition and their relationship to metabolic disorders. *Journal of Dairy Science*, 80(7), 1260–1268. https://doi.org/10.3168/jds.S0022-0302(97)76055-7

Goff, J. P., Horst, R. L., Mueller, F. J., Miller, J. K., Kiess, G. A., & Dowlen, H. H. (1991a). Addition of chloride to a prepartal diet high in cations increases 1,25-$(OH)_2$D response to hypocalcemia preventing milk fever. *Journal of Dairy Science*, 74(11), 3863–3871. https://doi.org/10.3168/jds.S0022-0302(91)78579-2

Goff, J. P., Reinhardt, T. A., & Horst, R. L. (1991b). Enzymes and factors controlling vitamin D metabolism and action in normal and milk fever cows. *Journal of Dairy Science*, 74(11), 4022–4032. https://doi.org/10.3168/jds.S0022-0302(91)78597-4

Goff, J. P., Kimura, K., & Horst, R. L. (2002). Effect of mastectomy on milk fever, energy, and vitamins A, E, and β-carotene at parturition. *Journal of Dairy Science*, *85*(6), 1427–1436. https://doi.org/10.3168/jds. S0022-0302(02)74210-0

Golder, H. M., McGrath, J., & Lean, I. J. (2021). Effect of 25-hydroxyvitamin D3 during prepartum transition and lactation on production, reproduction, and health of lactating dairy cows. *Journal of Dairy Science*, *104*(5), 5345–5374. https://doi.org/10.3168/jds.2020-18901

Goldschmidt, M. C. (1991). Reduced bactericidal activity in neutrophils from scorbutic animals and the effect of ascorbic acid on these target bacteria *in vivo* and *in vitro*. *The American Journal of Clinical Nutrition*, *54*(6)(Suppl.), 1214S–1220S. https://doi.org/10.1093/ajcn/54.6.1214s

Golub, M. S., & Gershwin, M. E. (1985). Stress-induced immunomodulation: What is it, if it is? In G. P. Moberg (Ed.), *Animal stress*. Springer. https://doi.org/10.1007/978-1-4614-7544-6_11

Goncalves, A., Roi, S., Nowicki, M., Dhaussy, A., Huertas, A., Amiot, M. J., & Reboul, E. (2015). Fat-soluble vitamin intestinal absorption: Absorption sites in the intestine and interactions for absorption. *Food Chemistry*, *172*, 155–160. https://doi.org/10.1016/j.foodchem.2014.09.021

González-Maldonado, J., Rangel-Santos, R., Rodríguez-de Lara, R., Ramírez-Valverde, G., Ramírez-Bribiesca, J. E., & Monreal-Díaz, J. C. (2019a). Supplementation of ascorbic acid to improve fertility in dairy cattle. Review [Review]. *Revista Mexicana de Ciencias Pecuarias*, *10*(4), 1000–1012. https://doi.org/10.22319/rmcp.v10i4.4703

González-Maldonado, J., Rangel-Santos, R., Rodríguez-de Lara, R., Rodríguez de Lara, R., Ramírez-Valverde, G., Ramírez Bribiesca, J. E., Vigil-Vigil, J. M., & García-Espinosa, M. F. (2019b). Effects of injecting increased doses of vitamins C and E on reproductive parameters of Holstein dairy cattle [Review]. *Revista Mexicana de Ciencias Pecuarias*, *10*(3), 571–582. https://doi.org/10.22319/rmcp.v10i3.4481

González-Montaña, J. R., Escalera-Valente, F., Alonso, A. J., Lomillos, J. M., Robles, R., & Alonso, M. E. (2020). Relationship between vitamin B$_{12}$ and cobalt metabolism in domestic ruminant: An update. *Animals: An Open Access Journal from MDPI*, *10*(10), 1855. https://doi.org/10.3390/ani10101855

Goodman, D. S. (1980). Vitamin A metabolism. *Federation Proceedings*, *39*(10), 2716–2722. https://doi.org/10.1097/00001433-199410000-00010, PubMed: 7190933

Goodman, D. S. (1984). Vitamin A and retinoids in health and disease. *The New England Journal of Medicine*, *310*(16), 1023–1031. https://doi.org/10.1056/NEJM198404193101605

Goodwin, T. W. (1984). The biochemistry of carotenoids. *Animals*. Chapman & Hall, *II*, (1–21). https://doi.org/10.1007/978-94-009-5542-4_1

Gorocica-Buenfil, M. A., Fluharty, F. L., Bohn, T., Schwartz, S. J., & Loerch, S. C. (2007a). Effect of low vitamin A diets with high-moisture or dry corn on marbling and adipose tissue fatty acid composition of beef steers. *Journal of Animal Science*, *85*(12), 3355–3366. https://doi.org/10.2527/jas.2007-0172

Gorocica-Buenfil, M. A., Fluharty, F. L., Reynolds, C. K., & Loerch, S. C. (2007b). Effect of dietary vitamin A concentration and roasted soybean inclusion on marbling, adipose cellularity, and fatty acid composition of beef. *Journal of Animal Science*, *85*(9), 2230–2242. https://doi.org/10.2527/jas.2006-780

Gorocica-Buenfil, M. A., Fluharty, F. L., Reynolds, C. K., & Loerch, S. C. (2007c). Effect of dietary vitamin A restriction on marbling and conjugated linoleic acid content in Holstein steers. *Journal of Animal Science*, *85*(9), 2243–2255. https://doi.org/10.2527/jas.2006-781

Gorocica-Buenfil, M. A., Fluharty, F. L., & Loerch, S. C. (2008). Effect of vitamin A restriction on carcass characteristics and immune status of beef steers. *Journal of Animal Science*, *86*(7), 1609–1616. https://doi.org/10.2527/jas.2007-0241

Gould, D. H. (1998). Polioencephalomalacia. *Journal of Animal Science*, *76*(1), 309–314. https://doi.org/10.2527/1998.761309x

Gould, D. H., McAllister, M. M., Savage, J. C., & Hamar, D. W. (1991). High sulfide concentrations in rumen fluid associated with nutritionally induced polioencephalomalacia in calves. *American Journal of Veterinary Research*, *52*(7), 1164–1169. https://doi.org/10.2460/ajvr.1991.52.07.1164, PubMed: 1892274

Gozalez-maldonado, J., Rangel-santos, R., Rodriguez-de Lara, R., & Ramirez-valverde, G. (2017). Impacts of vitamin C and E injections on ovarian structures and fertility in Holstein cows under heat stress conditions. *Turkish Journal of Veterinary and Animal Sciences*, *41*(3), 345–350. https://doi.org/10.3906/vet-1609-42

Grasso, P. J., Scholz, R. W., Erskine, R. J., & Eberhart, R. J. (1990). Phagocytosis, bactericidal activity, and oxidative metabolism of milk neutrophils from dairy cows fed selenium- supplemented and selenium-deficient diets. *American Journal of Veterinary Research, 51*(2), 269–274. https://doi.org/10.2460/ajvr.1990.51.02.269, PubMed: 2405755

Graulet, B., & Girard, C. L. (2017). B vitamins in cow milk: Their relevance to human health. In R. R. Watson, R. J. Collier, & V. R. Preedy (Eds.), *Dairy in human health and disease across the lifespan* (pp. 211–224). Elsevier. https://doi.org/10.1016/B978-0-12-809868-4.00015-7

Graulet, B., Matte, J. J., Desrochers, A., Doepel, L., Palin, M. F., & Girard, C. L. (2007). Effects of dietary supplements of folic acid and vitamin B_{12} on metabolism of dairy cows in early lactation. *Journal of Dairy Science, 90*(7), 3442–3455. https://doi.org/10.3168/jds.2006-718

Graulet, B., Martin, B., Agabriel, C., & Girard, C. L. (2013). Vitamins in milks. milk and dairy products in human nutrition: production. *Composition and health* (1st ed.). ISBN: 978-1-118-53422-9.

Graves-Hoagland, R. L., Hoagland, T. A., & Woody, C. O. (1988). Effect of beta-carotene and vitamin A on progesterone production by bovine luteal cells. *Journal of Dairy Science, 71*(4), 1058–1062. https://doi.org/10.3168/jds.S0022-0302(88)79652-6

Graves-Hoagland, R. L., Hoagland, T. A., & Woody, C. O. (1989). Relationship of plasma β-carotene and vitamin A to luteal function in postpartum cattle. *Journal of Dairy Science, 72*(7), 1854–1858. https://doi.org/10.3168/jds.S0022-0302(89)79303-6

Green, H. B., Horst, R. L., Beitz, D. C., & Littledike, E. T. (1981). Vitamin D metabolites in plasma of cows fed a prepartum low calcium diet for prevention of parturient hypocalcemia. *Journal of Dairy Science, 64*(2), 217–226. https://doi.org/10.3168/jds.S0022-0302(81)82557-X

Green, R., & Miller, J. W. (2013). Vitamin B_{12}. In J. Zempleni, J. Suttie, J. Gregory, & P. J. Stover (Eds.), *Handbook of vitamins* (5th ed.) (pp. 447–490). CRC Press, Taylor & Francis Group, LLC ISBN 9781466515567.

Greenberg, L. G., Bristol, F., Murphy, B. D., & Laarveld, B. (1986). Beta-carotene does not influence fertility in beef heifers. *Theriogenology, 26*(4), 491–508. https://doi.org/10.1016/0093-691X(86)90041-5

Gregoire, F. M., Smas, C. M., & Sul, H. S. (1998). Understanding adipocyte differentiation. *Physiological Reviews, 78*(3), 783–809. https://doi.org/10.1152/physrev.1998.78.3.783

Gregory III, J. F., & Ink, S. L. (1987). Identification and quantification of pyridoxine. Beta-glucoside as a major form of vitamin B_6 in plant-derived foods. *Journal of Agricultural and Food Chemistry, 35*(1), 76–82. https://doi.org/10.1021/jf00073a018

Gregory, J. F. (1989). Chemical and nutritional aspects of folate research: Analytical procedures, methods of folate synthesis, stability and bioavailability of dietary folates. *Advances in Food and Nutrition Research, 33*, 1–101. https://doi.org/10.1016/S1043-4526(08)60126-6

Gregory, J. F. (2001). Case study: Folate bioavailability. *The Journal of Nutrition, 131*(4)(Suppl.), 1376S–1382S. https://doi.org/10.1093/jn/131.4.1376S

Gregory, J. F., Trumbo, P. R., Bailey, L. B., Toth, J. P., Baumgartner, T. G., & Cerda, J. J. (1991a). Bioavailability of pyridoxine-5'-beta-D-glucoside determined in humans by stable-isotopic methods. *The Journal of Nutrition, 121*(2), 177–186. https://doi.org/10.1093/jn/121.2.177

Gregory, J. F., Bhandari, S. D., Bailey, L. B., Toth, J. P., Baumgartner, T. G., & Cerda, J. J. (1991b). Relative bioavailability of deuterium-labeled monoglutamyl and hexaglutamyl folates in human subjects. *The American Journal of Clinical Nutrition, 53*(3), 736–740. https://doi.org/10.1093/ajcn/53.3.736

Gregory, M. E. (1975). Reviews of the progress of Dairy Science. Water-soluble vitamins in milk and milk products. *The Journal of Dairy Research, 42*(1), 197–216. https://doi.org/10.1017/S0022029900015223

Griminger, P. (1984). Vitamin K in animal nutrition: Deficiency can be fatal. Part 1. *Feedstuffs, 56*(38), 24–25.

Griminger, P., & Donis, O. (1960). Potency of vitamin K_1 and two analogues in counteracting the effects of dicumarol and sulfaquinoxaline in the chick. *The Journal of Nutrition, 70*(3), 361–368. https://doi.org/10.1093/jn/70.3.361

Groziak, S. M., & Kirksey, A. (1987). Effects of maternal dietary restriction in vitamin B_6 on neocortex development in rats: B_6 vitamer concentrations, volume and cell estimates. *The Journal of Nutrition, 117*(6), 1045–1052. https://doi.org/10.1093/jn/117.6.1045

Groziak, S. M., & Kirksey, A. (1990). Effects of maternal dietary restriction in vitamin B$_6$ on neocortex development in rats: Neuron differentiation and synaptogenesis. *The Journal of Nutrition, 120*(5), 485–492. https://doi.org/10.1093/jn/120.5.485

Grummer, R. R., Armentano, L. E., & Marcus, M. S. (1987). Lactation response to short- term abomasal infusion of choline, inositol, and lecithin. *Journal of Dairy Science, 70*(12), 2518–2524. https://doi.org/10.3168/jds.S0022-0302(87)80320-X

Grummer, R. R., Mashek, D. G., & Hayırlı, A. (2004). Dry matter intake and energy balance in the transition period. *The Veterinary Clinics of North America. Food Animal Practice, 20*(3), 447–470. https://doi.org/10.1016/j.cvfa.2004.06.013

Guggenheim, K.Y. (1995) *Basic issues of the history of nutrition.* Magnes Press, Hebrew University.

Guidry, A. J., Paape, M. J., & Pearson, R. E. (1976). Effects of parturition and lactation on blood and milk cell concentrations, corticosteroids, and neutrophil phagocytosis in the cow. *American Journal of Veterinary Research, 37*(10), 1195–1200. PubMed: 984546

Guirgis, R. A., Ashmawy, G., & El-Ezz, S. S. A. (1982). Postnatal changes in some skin and wool characteristics associated with vitamin A blood concentration. *The Journal of Agricultural Science, 98*(1), 215–219. https://doi.org/10.1017/S0021859600041319

Gullickson, T. W. (1949). The relation of vitamin E to reproduction in dairy cattle. *Annals of the New York Academy of Sciences, 52*(3), 256–259. https://doi.org/10.1111/j.1749-6632.1949.tb55278.x

Guo, J., Jones, A. K., Givens, D. I., Lovegrove, J. A., & Kliem, K. E. (2018). Effect of dietary vitamin D3 and 25-hydroxyvitamin D3 supplementation on plasma and milk 25-hydroxyvitamin D3 concentration in dairy cows. *Journal of Dairy Science, 101*(4), 3545–3553. http://doi.org/10.3168/jds.2017-13824

Guss, S. B. (1977). Management and diseases of dairy goats. *Dairy goat* Journal Publishing Corporation. Scottsdale, AZ.

Gwazdauskas, F. C., Bibb, T. L., McGilliard, M. L., & Lineweaver, J. A. (1979) Effect of prepartum selenium-vitamin E injection on time for placenta to pass and on productive functions. *Journal of Dairy Science, 62*(6), 978–981. https://doi.org/10.3168/jds.S0022-0302(79)83357-3

Gyang, E. O., Stevens, J. B., Olson, W. G., Tsitsamis, S. D., & Usenik, E. A. (1984). Effects of selenium-vitamin E injection on bovine polymorphonucleated leukocytes phagocytosis and killing of *Staphylococcus aureus. American Journal of Veterinary Research, 45*(1), 175–177. PubMed: 6703453

Ha, T. Y., Otsuka, M., & Arakawa, N. (1994). Ascorbate indirectly stimulates fatty acid utilization in primary cultured guinea pig hepatocytes by enhancing carnitine synthesis. *The Journal of Nutrition, 124*(5), 732–737. https://doi.org/10.1093/jn/124.5.732

Hackbart, K. S., Ferreira, R. M., Dietsche, A. A., Socha, M. T., Shaver, R. D., Wiltbank, M. C., & Fricke, P. M. (2010). Effect of dietary organic zinc, manganese, copper, and cobalt supplementation on milk production, follicular growth, embryo quality, and tissue mineral concentrations in dairy cows. *Journal of Animal Science, 88*(12), 3856–3870. https://doi.org/10.2527/jas.2010-3055

Hadden, J. W. (1987). Neuroendocrine modulation of the thymus-dependent immune system. Agonists and mechanisms. *Annals of the New York Academy of Sciences, 496*(1), 39–48. https://doi.org/10.1111/j.1749-6632.1987.tb35744.x

Haga, S., Ishizaki, H., & Roh, S. (2021). The physiological roles of vitamin E and hypovitaminosis e in the transition period of high-yielding dairy cows. *Animals: An Open Access Journal from MDPI, 11*(4), 1088. https://doi.org/10.3390/ani11041088

Hale, W. H., Hubbert, F., & Taylor, R. E. (1961). The effect of feeding high levels of vitamin A to beef cattle upon performance and tissue vitamin A levels. *Journal of Animal Science, 20,* 668.

Halik, G., Lozicki, A., Dymnicka, M., Arkuszewska, E., Zielinska, M., & Rutkowska, H. (2016). The effect of feeding ration, enriched in synthetic and natural beta-carotene on the selected indicators of health condition of the cows and on reproduction parameters. *Animal Science.* Annals of Warsaw University of Life Sciences-SGGW, *55*(2), 167–175.

Haliloglu, S., Baspinar, N., Serpek, B., Erdem, H., & Bulut, Z. (2002). Vitamin A and beta carotene levels in plasma, *corpus luteum* and follicular fluid of cyclic and pregnant cattle. *Reproduction in Domestic Animals, 37*(2), 96–99. https://doi.org/10.1046/j.1439-0531.2002.00338.x

Halpin, C. G., Harris, D. J., Caple, I. W., & Petterson, D. S. (1984). Contribution of cobalamin analogues to plasma vitamin B_{12} concentrations in cattle. *Research in Veterinary Science, 37*(2), 249–251. https://doi.org/10.1016/S0034-5288(18)31915-5

Han, H. (1998). *Vitamin E in ruminant: The impact of form and dosing site on metabolism by steers.* PhD [Unpublished dissertation]. Oklahoma State University.

Hankes, L. V. (1984). Nicotinic acid and nicotinamide. In L. J. Machlin (Ed.), *Handbook of vitamins.* Marcel Dekker, Inc.

Hannah, S. M., & Stern, M. D. (1985). Effect of supplemental niacin or niacinamide and soybean source on ruminal bacterial fermentation in continuous culture. *Journal of Animal Science, 61*(5), 1253–1263. https://doi.org/10.2527/jas1985.6151253x

Hannah, S. S., & Norman, A. W. (1994). 1α,25(OH)2 vitamin D_3-regulated expression of the eukaryotic genome. *Nutrition Reviews, 52*(11), 376–382. https://doi.org/10.1111/j.1753-4887.1994.tb01368.x

Hardy, B., & Frape, D. L. (1983). Micronutrients and reproduction. Hoffmann-La Roche, Information Service, Anim. Nutr. Department.

Harmeyer, J., & Kollenkirchen, U. (1989). Thiamin and niacin in ruminant nutrition. *Nutrition Research Reviews, 2*(1), 201–225. https://doi.org/10.1079/NRR19890015

Harmon, B. G., Becker, D. E., Jensen, A. H., & Baker, D. H. (1969). Nicotinic acid-tryptophan relationship in the nutrition of the weanling pig. *Journal of Animal Science, 28*(6), 848–852. https://doi.org/10.2527/jas1969.286848x

Harper, H. A., Rodwell, V. W., & Mayes, P. A. (1977). *Review of physiological chemistry* (16th ed.). Lange Medical Publishers.

Harper, A. F., Knight, J. W., Kokue, E., & Usry, J. L. (2003). Plasma reduced folates, reproductive performance, and conceptus development in sows in response to supplementation with oxidized and reduced sources of folic acid. *Journal of Animal Science, 81*(3), 735–744. https://doi.org/10.2527/2003.813735x

Harris, C. L., Wang, B., Deavila, J. M., Busboom, J. R., Maquivar, M., Parish, S. M., McCann, B., Nelson, M. L., & Du, M. (2018). Vitamin A administration at birth promotes calf growth and intramuscular fat development in Angus beef cattle. *Journal of Animal Science and Biotechnology, 9*, 55. https://doi.org/10.1186/s40104-018-0268-7

Harris, H.F. (1919). *Pellagra.* Macmillan Co. New York, New York.

Harris, R. R., Yeates, H. F., & Barrett, Jr., J. E. (1966). Choline in a high roughage steer fattening ration. *Journal of Animal Science, 25*, 248 [Abstr.].

Harrison, E. H. (2012). Mechanisms involved in the intestinal absorption of dietary vitamin A and pro-vitamin A carotenoids Cell. Biol. Lipids BBA-Mol. *Cell Biology, 1821*(1), 70–77. https://doi.org/10.1016/j.bbalip.2011.06.002

Harrison, H. E., & Harrison, H. C. (1963). Sodium, potassium, and intestinal transport of glucose, l-tyrosine, phosphate, and calcium. *American Journal of Physiology-Legacy Content, 205*(1), 107–111. https://doi.org/10.1152/ajplegacy.1963.205.1.107

Harrison, J. H., Hancock, D. D., & Conrad, H. R. (1984). Vitamin E and selenium for reproduction of the dairy cow. *Journal of Dairy Science, 67*(1), 123–132. https://doi.org/10.3168/jds.S0022-0302(84)81275-8

Harrison, J. H., Hancock, D. D., St Pierre, N. S., Conrad, H. R., & Harvey, W. R. (1986). Effect of prepartum selenium treatment on uterine involution in the dairy cow. *Journal of Dairy Science, 69*(5), 1421–1425. https://doi.org/10.3168/jds.S0022-0302(86)80550-1

Hartley, W. J., & Grant, A. B. (1961). A review of selenium responsive diseases of New Zealand livestock. In *Federation Proceedings, 20*, 679–688.

Hartman, D., & Dryden, L. (1974). The vitamins in milk and milk products. In B. H. Webb, A. H. Johnson, & J. A. Alford (Eds.), *Fundamentals of dairy chemistry* (2nd ed.) AVI Publishing Co. Wesport. CT.

Hartwell, J. H., Cecava, M. J., Miller, B., & Donkin, S. S. (1999). Rumen protected choline and dietary protein for transition cows. *Journal of Dairy Science, 82*(Suppl. 1), 125.

Hartwell, J. R., Cecava, M. J., & Donkin, S. S. (2001). Rumen undegradable protein, rumen-protected choline and mRNA expression for enzymes in gluconeogenesis and ureagenesis in periparturient dairy cows. *Journal of Dairy Science, 84*(2), 490–497. https://doi.org/10.3168/jds.S0022-0302(01)74499-2

Hatfield, P. G., Daniels, J. T., Kott, R. W., Burgess, D. E., & Evans, T. J. (2000). Role of supplemental vitamin E in lamb survival and production: A review. *Journal of Animal Science, 77*(E–Suppl), 1–9. http://doi.org/10.2527/jas2000.77E-Suppl1a

Haug, A., Høstmark, A. T., & Harstad, O. M. (2007). Bovine milk in human nutrition – A review. *Lipids in Health and Disease, 6*, 25. https://doi.org/10.1186/1476-511X-6-25

Huang, H. Y., & Appel, L. J. (2003). Supplementation of diets with α-tocopherol reduces serum concentrations of γ- and δ-tocopherol in humans. *The Journal of Nutrition, 133*(10), 3137–3140. https://doi.org/10.1093/jn/133.10.3137

Hauschka, P. V., Lian, J. B., Cole, D. E., & Gundberg, C. M. (1989). Osteocalcin and matrix gla protein: Vitamin K-dependent proteins in bone. *Physiological Reviews, 69*(3), 990–1047. https://doi.org/10.1152/physrev.1989.69.3.990

Havemose, M. S., Weisbjerg, M. R., Bredie, W. L. P., & Nielsen, J. H. (2004). Influence of feeding different types of roughage on the oxidative stability of milk. *International Dairy Journal, 14*(7), 563–570. https://doi.org/10.1016/j.idairyj.2003.11.005

Haven, T. R. (1982). *Studies of thiamine destruction by ruminal bacteria in normal cattle and in cattle suffering from polioencephalomalacia.* University of Wyoming.

Haven, T. R., Caldwell, D. R., & Jensen, R. (1983). Role of predominant rumen bacteria in the cause of polio-encephalomalacia (cerebrocortical necrosis) in cattle. *American Journal of Veterinary Research, 44*(8), 1451–1455. PubMed: 6625295

Hayes, B. W., Mitchell, G. E., Little, C. O., & Bradley, N. W. (1966). Concentrations of B-vitamins in ruminal fluid of steers fed different levels and physical forms of hay and grain. *Journal of Animal Science, 25*(2), 539–542. https://doi.org/10.2527/jas1966.252539x

Hazzard, D. G., Woelfel, C. G., Calhoun, M. C., Rousseau, J. E., Eaton, H. D., Nielsen, S. W., Grey, R. M., & Lucas, J. J. (1964). Chronic hypervitaminosis A in Holstein male calves. *Journal of Dairy Science, 47*(4), 391–401. https://doi.org/10.3168/jds.S0022-0302(64)88673-2

He, C., Deng, J., Hu, X., Zhou, S., Wu, J., Xiao, D., Darko, K. O., Huang, Y., Tao, T., Peng, M., Wang, Z., & Yang, X. (2019). Vitamin A inhibits the action of LPS on the intestinal epithelial barrier function and tight junction proteins. *Food and Function, 10*(2), 1235–1242. https://doi.org/10.1039/c8fo01123k

Heaney, R. P., & Holick, M. F. (2011). Why the IOM Recommendations for vitamin D are deficient. *Journal of Bone and Mineral Research, 26*(3), 455–457. https://doi.org/10.1002/jbmr.328

Hedges, V., Blowey, R. W., Packington, A. J., O'Callaghan, C. J., & Green, L. E. (2001). A longitudinal field trial of the effect of biotin supplementation on lameness in dairy cows. *Journal of Dairy Science, 84*, 1969–1975. https://doi.org/10.3168/jds.S0022-0302(01)74639-5

Hegazy, E., & Schwenk, M. (1984). Choline uptake by isolated enterocytes of guinea pig. *The Journal of Nutrition, 114*(12), 2217–2220. https://doi.org/10.1093/jn/114.12.2217

Heirman, L. R. et al. (1990). Effects of dietary beta-carotene on lymphocyte function in peripartum dairy cows. *Journal of Dairy Science, 73*(Suppl. 1), 166.

Hemilä, H., & Douglas, R. M. (1999). Vitamin C and acute respiratory infections. *The International Journal of Tuberculosis and Lung Disease, 3*(9), 756–761. PubMed: 10488881

Hemingway, D. C. (1991). Vitamin C in the prevention of neonatal calf diarrhea. *Canadian Veterinary Journal, 32*(3), 184. http://www.ncbi.nlm.nih.gov/pmc/articles/pmc1480979/

Hemingway, R. G. (2003). The influences of dietary intakes and supplementation with selenium and vitamin E on reproduction diseases and reproduction efficiency in cattle and sheep. A review. *Veterinary Research Communications, 27*(2), 159–174. https://doi.org/10.1023/A:1022871406335

Henderson, L. M. (1984). Vitamin B$_6$. In R. E. Olson, H. P. Broquist, O. Chichester, W. J. Darby, A. C. Kolbye, & R. M. Stalvey (Eds.), *Nutrition reviews, present knowledge in nutrition* (5th ed.) The Nutrition Foundation, Inc.

Henderson, L. M., & Gross, C. J. (1979). Metabolism of niacin and niacinamide in perfused rat intestine. *The Journal of Nutrition, 109*(4), 654–662. https://doi.org/10.1093/jn/109.4.654

Hesselink, J. W., & Vellema, P. (1990). Cobalt deficiency and pholosensitization in a flock of Texel lambs. *Tijdschrift voor Diergeneeskunde, 115*(17), 789–794. PubMed: 2219077

Hibbs, J. W., & Conrad, H. R. (1976). Milk fever in dairy cows. VII. Effect of continuous vitamin D feeding on incidence of milk fever. *Journal of Dairy Science, 59*(11), 1944–1946. https://doi.org/10.3168/jds.S0022-0302(76)84465-7

Hibbs, J. W., & Conrad, H. R. (1983). *The relation of calcium and phosphorus intake on digestion and the effects of vitamin D feeding on the utilization of calcium and phosphorus by lactating dairy cows*. Rep. no. 1150. Ohio State University.

Hibbs, J. W., & Pounden, W. D. (1955). Studies on milk fever in dairy cows. IV. Prevention by short time prepartum feeding of massive doses of vitamin D. *Journal of Dairy Science, 38*(1), 65–72. https://doi.org/10.3168/jds.S0022-0302(55)94939-0

Hidiroglou, M. (1999). Technical note: Forms and route of vitamin C supplementation for cows. *Journal of Dairy Science, 82*(8), 1831–1833. https://doi.org/10.3168/jds.S0022-0302(99)75414-7

Hidiroglou, M., & Karpinski, K. (1987). Vitamin E kinetics in sheep. *The British Journal of Nutrition, 58*(1), 113–125. https://doi.org/10.1079/BJN19870075

Hidiroglou, N., & McDowell, L. R. (1987). Plasma and tissue levels of vitamin E in sheep following intramuscular administration in an oil carrier. *International Journal for Vitamin and Nutrition Research. Internationale Zeitschrift Fur Vitamin- und Ernahrungsforschung. Journal International de Vitaminologie et de Nutrition, 57*(3), 261–266. PubMed: 3679697

Hidiroglou, M., & Singh, K. (1991). Plasma α-tocopherol profiles in sheep after oral administration of dl-α-tocopheryl acetate and d-α-tocopheryl succinate. *Journal of Dairy Science, 74*(8), 2718–2723. https://doi.org/10.3168/jds.S0022-0302(91)78450-6

Hidiroglou, M., Hoffman, I., & Jenkins, K. J. (1969). Selenium distribution and radio tocopherol metabolism in the pregnant ewe and fetal lamb. *Canadian Journal of Physiology and Pharmacology, 47*(11), 953–962. https://doi.org/10.1139/y69-156

Hidiroglou, M., Batra, T. R., & Zhoa, X. (1977). Comparison of vitamin C bioavailability after multiple or single oral dosing of different formulations in sheep. *Reproduction Nutrition Developpement, 37*, 443–448. https://doi.org/10.1051/rnd:19970405

Hidiroglou, M., Ho, S. K., & Williams, C. J. (1978). Fate of tritiated cholecalciferol in healthy sheep and in those affected by osteodystrophy. *Canadian Journal of Animal Science, 58*(4), 621–630. https://doi.org/10.4141/cjas78-082

Hidiroglou, M., Proulx, J. G., & Roubos, D. (1979). 25-hydroxyvitamin D in plasma of cattle. *Journal of Dairy Science, 62*(7), 1076–1080. https://doi.org/10.3168/jds.S0022-0302(79)83377-9

Hidiroglou, N., Laflamme, L. F., & McDowell, L. R. (1988a). Blood plasma and tissue concentrations of vitamin E in beef cattle as influenced by supplementation of various tocopherol compounds. *Journal of Animal Science, 66*(12), 3227–3234. https://doi.org/10.2527/jas1988.66123227x

Hidiroglou, N., McDowell, L. R., & Pastrana, R. (1988b). Bioavailability of various vitamin E compounds in sheep. *International Journal for Vitamin and Nutrition Research. Internationale Zeitschrift Fur Vitamin- und Ernahrungsforschung. Journal International de Vitaminologie et de Nutrition, 58*(2), 189–197. PubMed: 3170092

Hidiroglou, N., McDowell, L. R., & Balbuena, O. (1989). Plasma tocopherol in sheep and cattle after ingesting free or acetylated tocopherol. *Journal of Dairy Science, 72*(7), 1793–1799. https://doi.org/10.3168/jds.S0022-0302(89)79296-1

Hidiroglou, N., McDowell, L. R., Papas, A. M., Antapli, M., & Wilkinson, N. S. (1992). Bioavailability of vitamin E compounds in lambs. *Journal of Animal Science, 70*(8), 2556–2561. https://doi.org/10.2527/1992.7082556x

Hidiroglou, M., Batra, T. R., Ivan, M., & Markham, F. (1995). Effects of supplemental vitamins E and C on the immune responses of calves. *Journal of Dairy Science, 78*(7), 1578–1583. https://doi.org/10.3168/jds.S0022-0302(95)76781-9

Hidiroglou, M., Batra, M. T., & Zhao, X. (1997a). Comparison of vitamin C bioavailability after multiple or single oral dosing of different formulations in sheep. *Reproduction Nutrition Developpement, 37*(4), 443–448. https://doi.org/10.1051/rnd:19970405

Hidiroglou, M., Batra, T. R., & Zhao, X. (1997b). Bioavailability of vitamin E compounds and the effect of supplementation on release of superoxide and hydrogen peroxide by bovine neutrophils. *Journal of Dairy Science, 80*(1), 187–193. https://doi.org/10.3168/jds.S0022-0302(97)75926-5

Hidiroglou, N., Madere, R., McDowell, L. R., & Toutain, P. L. (2003). Influence of sources of dietary vitamin E on the maternal transfer of alpha-tocopherol to fetal and neonatal guinea pigs as determined by a stable isotopic technique. *The British Journal of Nutrition, 89*(4), 455–466. https://doi.org/10.1079/BJN2002788

Hill, G. M., & Williams, S. E. (1993). Vitamin E in beef nutrition and meat quality. In *Proceedings of the 1993 Minnesota Nutr. Conf.*, Bloomington (pp. 197–211).

Hill, G. M., & Williams, S. E. (1995). *Vitamin E effects on performance of growing- finishing beef cattle and meat quality* p. 11. University of Georgia (UGA) Animal and Dairy Science [Annual report].

Hill, G. M., Williams, S. E., Williams, S. N., McDowell, L. R., Wilkinson, N., & Mullinix, B. E. (1995) *Vitamin A and vitamin E fed at high levels in steer feedlot diets: Tissue alpha- tocopherol and performance.* University of Georgia (UGA) Animal and Dairy Science Annual Report. 7.

Hines, E. A., Coffey, J. D., Starkey, C. W., Chung, T. K., & Starkey, J. D. (2013). Improvement of maternal vitamin D status with 25-hydroxycholecalciferol positively impacts porcine fetal skeletal muscle development and myoblast activity. *Journal of Animal Science, 91*(9), 4116–4122. https://doi.org/10.2527/jas.2013-6565

Hirsch, A. (1982). Vitamin D history, manufacture, analysis and metabolism: An overview. In *"Vitamins the life essentials"* National Feed Ingredients Association.

Hjarde, W., Hellstrum, V., & Akerberg, E. (1963). The contents of tocopherol and carotene in red clover as dependent on variety, conditions of cultivation and stage of development. *Acta Agriculturae Scandinavica, 13*, 1–16. https://doi.org/10.1080/00015126309434151

Hodges, R. E., Ohlson, M. A., & Bean, W. B. (1958). Pantothenic Acid deficiency in man. *The Journal of Clinical Investigation, 37*(11), 1642–1657. https://doi.org/10.1172/JCI103756

Hodges, S. J., Pitsillides, A. A., Ytrebø, L. M., & Soper, R. (2017). *Anti-inflammatory actions of vitamin K. Vitamin K_2: Vital for health and wellbeing, 153.* https://doi.org/10.5772/63891

Hodnik, J. J., Ježek, J., & Starič, J. (2020). A review of vitamin D and its importance to the health of dairy cattle. *The Journal of Dairy Research, 87*(S1)(Suppl. 1), 84–87. https://doi.org/10.1017/S0022029920000424

Hoekstra, W. G. (1975). Biochemical function of selenium and its relation to vitamin E. *Federation Proceedings, 34*(11), 2083–2089. PubMed: 1100437

Hoffbrand, A. V. (1978). Effects of folate deficiency in man. In CRC Press, Inc. (Ed.), *Handbook series in nutrition and food, section E: Nutritional disorders, 2m.* Rechcigl Jr. West.

Hoffmann-La Roche. (1984). Roche technical bulletin – Vitamin B_{12}. *RCD, 6723.*

Hogan, J. S., Smith, K. L., Weiss, W. P., Todhunter, D. A., & Schockey, W. L. (1990). Relationships among vitamin E, selenium, and bovine blood neutrophils. *Journal of Dairy Science, 73*(9), 2372–2378. https://doi.org/10.3168/jds.S0022-0302(90)78920-5

Hogan, J. S., Weiss, W. P., Todhunter, D. A., Smith, K. L., & Schoenberger, P. S. (1992). Bovine neutrophil response to parenteral vitamin E. *Journal of Dairy Science, 75*(2), 399–405. https://doi.org/10.3168/jds.S0022-0302(92)77775-3

Hogan, J. S., Weiss, W. P., & Smith, K. L. (1993). Role of vitamin E and selenium in host defense against mastitis. *Journal of Dairy Science, 76*(9), 2795–2803. https://doi.org/10.3168/jds.S0022-0302(93)77618-3

Holcombe, S. J., Wisnieski, L., Gandy, J., Norby, B., & Sordillo, L. M. (2018). Reduced serum vitamin D concentrations in healthy early-lactation dairy cattle. *Journal of Dairy Science, 101*(2), 1488–1494. https://doi.org/10.3168/jds.2017-13547

Holick, M. F. (2007). Vitamin D deficiency. *The New England Journal of Medicine, 357*(3), 266–281. https://doi.org/10.1056/NEJMra070553

Holland, R. E., Boyle, S. M., Herdt, T. H., Grimes, S. D., & Walker, R. D. (1992). Malabsorption of vitamin A in preruminating calves infected with *Cryptosporidium parvum. American Journal of Veterinary Research, 53*(10), 1947–1952. https://doi.org/10.2460/ajvr.1992.53.10.1947, PubMed: 1456546

Hollander, D. (1973). Vitamin K_1 absorption by everted intestinal sacs of the rat. *The American Journal of Physiology, 225*(2), 360–364. https://doi.org/10.1152/ajplegacy.1973.225.2.360

Höller, U., Bakker, S. J., Düsterloh, L., Frei, A., Körrle, B., Konz, J., Lietz, T., McCann, G., & Michels, A. (2018). Micronutrient status assessment in humans: Current methods of analysis and future trends. *Trends in Analytical Chemistry, 102*, 110–122. https://doi.org/10.1016/j.trac.2018.02.001

Hollis, L., Chappel, C. F., MacVicar, R., & Whitehair, C. K. (1954). Effect of ration on vitamin synthesis in rumen of sheep. *Journal of Animal Science, 13*(4), 732–738. https://doi.org/10.2527/jas1954.134732x

Hongtrakul, K., Kim, I. H., Loughmiller, J. A., Smith, J. W., Cao, H., Goodband, R. D., Tokach, M. D., & Nelssen, J. L. (1997). Effects of added choline on performance of weanling pigs. *Kansas Agricultural Experiment Station Research Reports*, (10), 70–71. https://doi.org/10.4148/2378-5977.6528

Hoppe, P. P., Chew, B. P., Safer, A., Stegemann, I., & Biesalski, H. K. (1996). Dietary beta-carotene elevates plasma steady-state and tissue concentrations of beta-carotene and enhances vitamin A balance in preruminant calves. *The Journal of Nutrition*, *126*(1), 202–208. https://doi.org/10.1093/jn/126.1.202

Hopper, J. H., & Johnson, B. C. (1955). The production and study of an acute nicotinic acid deficiency in the calf. *The Journal of Nutrition*, *56*(2), 303–310. https://doi.org/10.1093/jn/56.2.303

Horner, J. L., Coppock, C. E., Schelling, G. T., Labore, J. M., & Nave, D. H. (1986). Influence of niacin and whole cottonseed on intake, milk yield and composition, and systemic responses of dairy cows. *Journal of Dairy Science*, *69*(12), 3087–3093. https://doi.org/10.3168/jds.S0022-0302(86)80771-8

Horner, J. L., Windle, L. M., Coppock, C. E., Labore, J. M., Lanham, J. K., & Nave, D. H. (1988). Effects of whole cottonseed, niacin, and niacinamide on *in vitro* rumen fermentation and on lactating Holstein cows. *Journal of Dairy Science*, *71*(12), 3334–3344. https://doi.org/10.3168/jds.S0022-0302(88)79938-5

Hornig, B., Glatthar, B., & Mosw, U. (1984). General aspects of ascorbic acid and metabolism. In I. Wegger, F. J. Tagwerker, & J. Moustgaard (Eds.). *Proceedings of the Workshop Ascorbic Acid in Domest. Anim. the Royal Danish Agriculture Society*. Copenhagen, Denmark. ISBN: 8770262454.

Horst, R. L., & Littledike, E. T. (1982). Comparison of plasma concentration of vitamin D and its metabolites in young and aged domestic animals. Comp. *Biochemistry and Physiology*, *73*, 485. https://doi.org/10.1016/0305-0491(82)90064-5

Horst, R. L., Napoli, J. L., & Littledike, E. T. (1982). Discrimination in the metabolism of orally dosed ergocalciferol and cholecalciferol by the pig, rat and chick. *The Biochemical Journal*, *204*(1), 185–189. https://doi.org/10.1042/bj2040185

Horst, R. L., Goff, J. P., & Reinhardt, T. A. (1994). Calcium and vitamin D metabolism in the dairy cow. *Journal of Dairy Science*, *77*(7), 1936–1951. https://doi.org/10.3168/jds.S0022-0302(94)77140-X

Horst, R. L., Goff, J. P., Reinhardt, T. A., & Buxton, D. R. (1997). Strategies for preventing milk fever in dairy cattle. *Journal of Dairy Science*, *80*(7), 1269–1280. https://doi.org/10.3168/jds.S0022-0302(97)76056-9

Horst, R. L., Goff, J. P., & Reinhardt, T. A. (2005). Adapting to the transition between gestation and lactation: Differences between rat, human and dairy cow. *Journal of Mammary Gland Biology and Neoplasia*, *10*(2), 141–156. https://doi.org/10.1007/s10911-005-5397-x

Hove, K., Horst, R. L., & Littledike, E. T. (1983). Effects of 1α-hydroxyvitamin D_3, 1, 25-dihydroxyvitamin D_3, 1, 24, 25-trihydroxyvitamin D_3, and 1, 25, 26-trihydroxyvitamin D_3 on mineral metabolism and 1, 25-dihydroxyvitamin D concentrations in dairy cows. *Journal of Dairy Science*, *66*(1), 59–66. https://doi.org/10.3168/jds.S0022-0302(83)81753-6

Howe, A. M., & Webster, W. S. (1994). Vitamin K—Its essential role in craniofacial development: A review of the literature regarding vitamin K and craniofacial development. *Australian Dental Journal*, *39*(2), 88–92. https://doi.org/10.1111/j.1834-7819.1994.tb01379.x

Huang, S. W., Frankel, E. N., & German, J. B. (1995). Effects of individual tocopherols and tocopherol mixtures on the oxidative stability of corn oil triglycerides. *Journal of Agricultural and Food Chemistry*, *43*(9), 2345–2350. https://doi.org/10.1021/jf00057a006

Humer, E., Bruggeman, G., & Zebeli, Q. (2019). A meta-analysis on the impact of the supplementation of rumen-protected choline on the metabolic health and performance of dairy cattle. *Animals: An Open Access Journal from MDPI*, *9*(8), 566. https://doi.org/10.3390/ani9080566

Hungate, R. E. (1966). *The rumen and its microbes*. Academic Press, Inc.

Hurley, W. L., & Doane, R. M. (1989). Recent developments in the role of vitamins and minerals in reproduction. *Journal of Dairy Science*, *72*(3), 784–804. https://doi.org/10.3168/jds.S0022-0302(89)79170-0

Hustmyer, F. G., Beitz, D. C., Goff, J. P., Nonnecke, B. J., Horst, R. L., & Reinhardt, T. A. (1994). Effects of *in vivo* administration of 1,25-dihydroxyvitamin D_3 on *in vitro* proliferation of bovine lymphocytes. *Journal of Dairy Science*, *77*(11), 3324–3330. https://doi.org/10.3168/jds.S0022-0302(94)77273-8

Hutcheson, D. P. (1990). Rations for receiving and starting new cattle. Scott County Beef Cattle Conference.

Hutcheson, D. P., & Cole, N. A. (1985). Vitamin E and selenium for yearling feedlot cattle. *Federation Proceedings*, *44*, 549.

Hutchinson, L. J., Scholz, R. W., & Drake, T. R. (1982). Nutritional myodegeneration in a group of Chianina heifers. *Journal of the American Veterinary Medical Association, 181*(6), 581–584. PubMed: 7141951

Huyghebaert, A. (1991). Stability of vitamin K in a mineral premix. *World Poult., 7*, 71.

Hymøller, L., & Jensen, S. K. (2010a). Vitamin D_3 synthesis in the entire skin surface of dairy cows despite hair coverage. *Journal of Dairy Science, 93*(5), 2025–2029. https://doi.org/10.3168/jds.2009-2991

Hymøller, L., & Jensen, S. K. (2010b). Stability in the rumen and effect on plasma status of single oral doses of vitamin D and vitamin E in high-yielding dairy cows. *Journal of Dairy Science, 93*(12), 5748–5757. https://doi.org/10.3168/jds.2010-3338

Hymøller, L., & Jensen, S. K. (2011). Vitamin D_2 impairs utilization of vitamin D_3 in high-yielding dairy cows in a cross-over supplementation regimen. *Journal of Dairy Science, 94*(7), 3462–3466. https://doi.org/10.3168/jds.2010-4111

Ikeda, S., Takasu, M., Matsuda, T., Kakinuma, A., & Horio, F. (1997). Ascorbic acid deficiency decreases the renal level of kidney fatty acid-binding protein by lowering the alpha2u-globulin gene expression in liver in scurvy-prone ods rats. *The Journal of Nutrition, 127*(11), 2173–2178. https://doi.org/10.1093/jn/127.11.2173

Ikeda, S., Kitagawa, M., Imai, H., & Yamada, M. (2005). The roles of vitamin A for cytoplasmic maturation of bovine oocytes. *The Journal of Reproduction and Development, 51*(1), 23–35. https://doi.org/10.1262/jrd.51.23

Imawari, M. I. C. M. O., Kida, K., & Goodman, D. S. (1976). The transport of vitamin D and its 25-hydroxy metabolite in human plasma. Isolation and partial characterization of vitamin D and 25-hydroxyvitamin D binding protein. *The Journal of Clinical Investigation, 58*(2), 514–523. https://doi.org/10.1172/JCI108495

Inaba, T., Inoue, A., Shimizu, R., Nakano, Y., & Mori, J. (1986). Plasma concentrations of progesterone, estrogens, vitamin A and beta-carotene in cows retaining fetal membranes. *Nihon Juigaku Zasshi. the Japanese Journal of Veterinary Science, 48*(3), 505–508. https://doi.org/10.1292/jvms1939.48.505

Ingram, R. T., Park, Y. K., Clarke, B. L., & Fitzpatrick, L. A. (1994). Age- and gender-related changes in the distribution of osteocalcin in the extracellular matrix of normal male and female bone. Possible involvement of osteocalcin in bone remodeling. *The Journal of Clinical Investigation, 93*(3), 989–997. https://doi.org/10.1172/JCI117106

INRA. (1988). *Alimentation des bovins, ovins et caprins* p. 471. Institut National de la Recherche Agronomique.

INRA. (2018). Feeding system for ruminants. *Wageningen Academic Publishers* https://dx.doi.org/10.3920/978-90-8686-292-4 P. Nozière, D. Sauvant, & L. Delaby (Eds.), 640-p.

Iskakova, M., Karbyshev, M., Piskunov, A., & Rochette-Egly, C. R. (2015). Nuclear and extranuclear effects of vitamin A. *Canadian Journal of Physiology and Pharmacology, 93*(12), 1065–1075. https://doi.org/10.1139/cjpp-2014-0522

Itabisashi, T., Horino, R., Hirano, K., & Maeda, M. (1990). Electroencephalographic observation on sheep and cattle with experimental cerebrocortical necrosis. *Nihon Juigaku Zasshi. the Japanese Journal of Veterinary Science, 52*(3), 551–558. https://doi.org/10.1292/jvms1939.52.551

Itze, L. (1984). Ascorbic acid metabolism in ruminants. In I. Wegger, F. J. Tagwerker, & J. Moustgaard (Eds.). *Proceedings of the Workshop on Ascorbic Acid in Domestic Animals*. Royal Danish Agricultural Society, p. 126.

IUPAC. (1973). IUB. *The Biochemical Journal, 135*(1), 9–10. https://doi.org/10.1042/bj1350009

Iwańska, S., Lewicki, C., & Rybicka, M. (1985). The Effect of β-carotene supplementation on the β-carotene and vitamin A levels of blood plasma and some fertility indices of dairy cows. *Archiv für Tierernährung, 35*(8), 563–570. https://doi.org/10.1080/17450398509425220

Jackson, P. S., Furr, B. J. A., & Johnson, C. T. (1981). Endocrine and ovarian changes in dairy cattle fed a low beta-carotene diet during an estrus synchronization regime. *Research in Veterinary Science, 31*(3), 377–383. https://doi.org/10.1016/S0034-5288(18)32475-5

Jacob, R. A. (1995). The integrated antioxidant system. *Nutrition Research, 15*(5), 755–766. https://doi.org/10.1016/0271-5317(95)00041-G

Jacob, R. A. (2006). Niacin. In B. A. Bowman & R. M. Russell (Eds.), *Present knowledge in nutrition* (9th ed.) (pp. 261–268). International Life Sciences Institute.

Jacob, R. A., Wu, M. M., Henning, S. M., & Swendseid, M. E. (1994). Homocysteine increases as folate decreases in plasma of healthy men during short-term dietary folate and methyl group restriction. *The Journal of Nutrition, 124*(7), 1072–1080. https://doi.org/10.1093/jn/124.7.1072

Jagos, P., Bouda, J., & Dvorak, R. (1977). The ascorbic acid level in case of bronchopneumonia of calves. *Veterinary Medicine Praha, 22*, 133–136. PubMed: 407694

Jaster, E. H., & Ward, N. E. (1990). Supplemental nicotinic acid or nicotinamide for lactating dairy cows. *Journal of Dairy Science, 73*(10), 2880–2887. https://doi.org/10.3168/jds.S0022-0302(90)78975-8

Jaster, E. H., Hartnell, G. F., & Hutjens, M. F. (1983). Feeding supplemental niacin for milk production in six dairy herds. *Journal of Dairy Science, 66*(5), 1046–1051. https://doi.org/10.3168/jds.S0022-0302(83)81900-6

Jee, J., Hoet, A. E., Azevedo, M. P., Vlasova, A. N., Loerch, S. C., Pickworth, C. L., Hanson, J., & Saif, L. J. (2013). Effects of dietary vitamin A content on antibody responses of feedlot calves inoculated intramuscularly with an inactivated bovine coronavirus vaccine. *American Journal of Veterinary Research, 74*(10), 1353–1362. https://doi.org/10.2460/ajvr.74.10.1353

Jeng, K. C., Yang, C. S., Siu, W. Y., Tsai, Y. S., Liao, W. J., & Kuo, J. S. (1996). Supplementation with vitamins C and E enhances cytokine production by peripheral blood mononuclear cells in healthy adults. *The American Journal of Clinical Nutrition, 64*(6), 960–965. https://doi.org/10.1093/ajcn/64.6.960

Jensen, M., Fossum, C., Ederoth, M., & Hakkarainen, R. V. J. (1988). The effect of vitamin E on the cell-mediated immune response in pigs. *Zentralblatt Fur Veterinarmedizin. Reihe B. Journal of Veterinary Medicine. Series B, 35*(7), 549–555. https://doi.org/10.1111/j.1439-0450.1988.tb00528.x

Jensen, M. S., Gabert, V. M., Jorgensen, H., & Jensen, S. K. (1997). Dietary fat as a natural source of vitamin E and the influence of fatty acid composition on the apparent ileal and overall digestibility of protein, starch, fat and energy. *EAAP, 88*, 75–79.

Jensen, S. K., Nørgaard, J. V., & Lauridsen, C. (2006). Bioavailability of α-tocopherol stereoisomers in rats depends on dietary doses of all-rac- or RRR-α-tocopheryl acetate. *The British Journal of Nutrition, 95*(3), 477–487. https://doi.org/10.1079/BJN20051667

Ježek, J., Klinkon, M., Nemec, M., Hodnik, J. J., & Starič, J. (2020). β-carotene concentration in blood serum of cows from herds with impaired fertility. *Acta Fytotechnica et Zootechnica, 23*(Monothematic Issue), 162–166. https://doi.org/10.15414/afz.2020.23.mi-fpap.162-166

Jhoo, J. W., Lin, M. C., Sang, S., Cheng, X., Zhu, N., Stark, R. E., & Ho, C. T. (2002). Characterization of 2 methyl 4 amino 5 (2 methyl 3 furyl thiomethyl) pyrimidine from thermal degradation of thiamine. *Journal of Agricultural and Food Chemistry, 50*(14), 4055–4058. https://doi.org/10.1021/jf011591v

Jiang, Q., Christen, S., Shigenaga, M. K., & Ames, B. N. (2001). γ-Tocopherol, the major form of vitamin E in the US diet, deserves more attention. *The American Journal of Clinical Nutrition, 74*(6), 714–722. https://doi.org/10.1093/ajcn/74.6.714

Jiang, Q., Lin, L., Xie, F., Jin, W., Zhu, W., Wang, M., Qiu, Q., Li, Z., Liu, J., & Mao, S. (2022). Metagenomic insights into the microbe-mediated B and K_2 vitamin biosynthesis in the gastrointestinal microbiome of ruminants. *Microbiome, 10*(1), 109. https://doi.org/10.1186/s40168-022-01298-9

Jiang, X., Yan, J., & Caudill, M. A. (2013). Choline. In J. Zempleni, J. Suttie, J. Gregory, & P. J. Stover (Eds.), *Handbook of vitamins* (5th ed.) (pp. 491–514). CRC Press, Taylor & Francis Group.

Jin, L., Yan, S., Shi, B., Bao, H., Gong, J., Guo, X., & Li, J. (2014). Effects of vitamin A on the milk performance, antioxidant functions and immune functions of dairy cows. *Animal Feed Science and Technology, 192*, 15–23. https://doi.org/10.1016/j.anifeedsci.2014.03.003

Jin, Q., Cheng, H., Wan, F., Bi, Y., Liu, G., Liu, X., Zhao, H., You, W., Liu, Y., & Tan, X. (2015). Effects of feeding β-carotene on levels of β-carotene and vitamin A in blood and tissues of beef cattle and the effects on beef quality. *Meat Science, 110*, 293–301. https://doi.org/10.1016/j.meatsci.2015.07.019

Johansson, B., Persson Waller, K. P., Jensen, S. K., Lindqvist, H., & Nadeau, E. (2014). Status of vitamins E and A and β-carotene and health in organic dairy cows fed a diet without synthetic vitamins. *Journal of Dairy Science, 97*(3), 1682–1692. https://doi.org/10.3168/jds.2013-7388

Johnson, B. C., Mitchell, H. H., Hamilton, T. S., & Nevens, W. G. (1947). Vitamin deficiencies in the calf. *Federation Proceedings, 6*(1), 410.

Johnson, B. C., Hamilton, T. S., Nevens, W. B., Boley, L. E., Burke, K. A., & Pinkos, J. A. (1948). Thiamine deficiency in the calf. *The Journal of Nutrition, 35*(2), 137–145. https://doi.org/10.1093/jn/35.2.137

Johnson, B. C., Pinkos, J. A., & Burke, K. A. (1950). Pyridoxine deficiency in the calf. *The Journal of Nutrition*, *40*(2), 309–322. https://doi.org/10.1093/jn/40.2.309

Johnson, B. C., Mitchell, H. H., & Pinkos, J. A. (1951). Choline deficiency in the calf. *The Journal of Nutrition*, *43*(1), 37–48. https://doi.org/10.1093/jn/43.1.37

Johnson, E. J., Qin, J., Krinsky, N. I., & Russell, R. M. (1997). Ingestion by men of a combined dose of beta-carotene and lycopene does not affect the absorption of beta-carotene but improves that of lycopene. *The Journal of Nutrition*, *127*(9), 1833–1837. https://doi.org/10.1093/jn/127.9.1833

Johnson, M. A., & Kimlin, M. G. (2006). Vitamin D, aging, and the 2005 dietary guidelines for Americans. *Nutrition Reviews*, *64*(9), 410–421. https://doi.org/10.1111/j.1753-4887.2006.tb00226.x

Johnston, C. S. (2006). Vitamin C. In B. A. Bowman & R. M. Russell (Eds.), *Present knowledge in nutrition* (9th ed.) (pp. 233–241). International Life Sciences Institute.

Johnston, C. S., & Huang, S. N. (1991). Effect of ascorbic acid nutriture on blood histamine and neutrophil chemotaxis in guinea pigs. *The Journal of Nutrition*, *121*(1), 126–130. https://doi.org/10.1093/jn/121.1.126

Johnston, C. S., Martin, L. J., & Cai, X. (1992). Antihistamine effect of supplemental ascorbic acid and neutrophil chemotaxis. *Journal of the American College of Nutrition*, *11*(2), 172–176. https://doi.org/10.1080/07315724.1992.12098241

Johnston, C. S., Steinberg, F. M., & Rucker, R. B. (2013). Ascorbic acid. In J. Zempleni, J. Suttie, J. Gregory, & P. J. Stover (Eds.), *Handbook of vitamins* (5th ed.) (pp. 515–550). CRC Press, Taylor & Francis Group.

Johnston, L. A., & Chew, B. P. (1984). Peripartum changes of plasma and milk vitamin A and beta-carotene among dairy cows with or without mastitis. *Journal of Dairy Science*, *67*(8), 1832–1840. https://doi.org/10.3168/jds.S0022-0302(84)81511-8

Jolly, D. W., Craig, C., & Nelson, T. E. (1977). Estrogen and prothrombin synthesis: Effect of estrogen on absorption of vitamin K1. *The American Journal of Physiology*, *232*(1), H12–H17. https://doi.org/10.1152/ajpheart.1977.232.1.H12

Joyce, P. W., Sanchez, W. K., & Goff, J. P. (1997). Effect of anionic salts in prepartum diets based on alfalfa. *Journal of Dairy Science*, *80*(11), 2866–2875. https://doi.org/10.3168/jds.S0022-0302(97)76251-9

Juárez, M., Dugan, M. E., Aalhus, J. L., Aldai, N., Basarab, J. A., Baron, V. S., & McAllister, T. A. (2011). Effects of vitamin E and flaxseed on rumen-derived fatty acid intermediates in beef intramuscular fat. *Meat Science*, *88*(3), 434–440. https://doi.org/10.1016/j.meatsci.2011.01.023

Jukola, E., Hakkarainen, J., Saloniemi, H., & Sankari, S. (1996). Blood selenium, vitamin E, vitamin A and carotene concentrations and udder health, fertility treatments, and fertility. *Journal of Dairy Science*, *79*(5), 838–845. https://doi.org/10.3168/jds.S0022-0302(96)76432-9

Julien, W. E., Conrad, H. R., Jones, J. E., & Moxon, A. L. (1976a). Selenium and vitamin E and incidence of retained placenta in parturient dairy cows. *Journal of Dairy Science*, *59*(11), 1954–1959. https://doi.org/10.3168/jds.S0022-0302(76)84467-0

Julien, W. E., Conrad, H. R., & Moxon, A. L. (1976b). Selenium and vitamin E and incidence of retained placenta in parturient dairy cows. II. Prevention in commercial herds with prepartum treatment. *Journal of Dairy Science*, *59*(11), 1960–1962. https://doi.org/10.3168/jds.S0022-0302(76)84468-2

Jung, D. J. S., Kim, D. H., Beak, S. H., Cho, I. G., Hong, S. J., Lee, J., Lee, J. O., Kim, H. J., Malekkhahi, M., & Baik, M. (2023). Effects of vitamin E and selenium administration on transportation stress in pregnant dairy heifers. *Journal of Dairy Science*, *106*(12), 9576–9586. https://doi.org/10.3168/jds.2023-23463

Jurlin, K. E. (1965). On the effect of choline chloride and cyanocobalamin on the livers of cows with parturient paresis. *Nord. Veterinarmed.*, *17*, 169.

Kadek, R., Mikulková, K., Filípek, J., & Illek, J. (2021). The effect of parenteral application of vitamin A, vitamin E, and β-carotene to pregnant cows on selected indices in their calves. *Acta Veterinaria Brno*, *90*(2), 135–143. https://doi.org/10.2754/avb202190020135

Kaempf-Rotzoll, D. E., Traber, M. G., & Arai, H. (2003). Vitamin E and transfer proteins. *Current Opinion in Lipidology*, *14*(3), 249–254. https://doi.org/10.1097/00041433-200306000-00004

Kaewlamun, W., Okouyi, M., Humblot, P., Techakumphu, M., & Ponter, A. A. (2011). Does supplementing dairy cows with β-carotene during the dry period affect postpartum ovarian activity, progesterone, and cervical and uterine involution? *Theriogenology*, *75*(6), 1029–1038. https://doi.org/10.1016/j.theriogenology.2010.11.010

Kailasapathy, K. (2016). *Chemical composition, physical, and functional properties of milk and milk ingredients. Dairy processing and quality assurance* (2nd ed.). https://doi.org/10.1002/9781118810279.ch04

Kallner, A., Hartmann, D., & Hornig, D. (1977). On the absorption of ascorbic acid in man. *International Journal for Vitamin and Nutrition Research. Internationale Zeitschrift Fur Vitamin- und Ernahrungsforschung. Journal International de Vitaminologie et de Nutrition, 47*(4), 383–388. PubMed: 591210

Kamal-Eldin, A., & Appelqvist, L. A. (1996). The chemistry and antioxidant properties of tocopherols and tocotrienols. *Lipids, 31*(7), 671–701. https://doi.org/10.1007/BF02522884

Kandylis, K. (1984). Toxicology of sulfur in ruminants: Review. *Journal of Dairy Science, 67*(10), 2179–2187. https://doi.org/10.3168/jds.S0022-0302(84)81564-7

Kaneko, K., Kiyose, C., Ueda, T., Ichikawa, H., & Igarashi, O. (2000). Studies of the metabolism of a-tocopherol stereoisomers in rats using [5-methyl-14C] SRR- and RRR-a-tocopherol. *Journal of Lipid Research, 41*(3), 357–367. https://doi.org/10.1016/S0022-2275(20)34474-6

Kao, C., & Robinson, R. J. (1972). *Aspergillus flavus* deterioration of grain: Its effect on amino acids and vitamins in whole wheat. *Journal of Food Science, 37*(2), 261–263. https://doi.org/10.1111/j.1365-2621.1972.tb05831.x

Kappel, L. C., Ingraham, R. H., Morgan, E. B., Dixon, J. M., Zeringue, L., Wilson, D., & Babcock, D. K. (1984). Selenium concentrations in feeds and effects of treating pregnant Holstein cows with selenium and vitamin E on blood selenium values and reproductive performance. *American Journal of Veterinary Research, 45*(4), 691–694. PubMed: 6731980

Karapinar, T., Dabak, M., & Kizil, O. (2010). Thiamine status of feedlot cattle fed a high-concentrate diet. *The Canadian Veterinary Journal, 51*(11), 1251–1253. https://pubmed.ncbi.nlm.nih.gov/21286325

Kastner, P., Chambon, P., & Leid, M. (1994). *The role of nuclear retinoic acid receptors in the regulation of gene expression in "vitamin A in health and disease"* R. Blomhoff (Ed.) (pp. 189–238). Marcel Dekker. ISBN: 0-8247-9120-7.

Kaur, M., Hartling, I., Burnett, T. A., Polsky, L. B., Donnan, C. R., Leclerc, H., Veira, D., & Cerri, R. L. A. (2019). Rumen-protected B vitamin complex supplementation during the transition period and early lactation alters endometrium mRNA expression on day 14 of gestation in lactating dairy cows. *Journal of Dairy Science, 102*(2), 1642–1657. https://doi.org/10.3168/jds.2018-14622

Kawachi, H. (2006). Micronutrients affecting adipogenesis in beef cattle. *Animal Science Journal, 77*(5), 463–471. https://doi.org/10.1111/j.1740-0929.2006.00373.x

Kawas, J. R., Garcia-Mazcorro, J. F., Fimbres-Durazo, H., & Ortega-Cerrilla, M. E. (2020). Effects of rumen-protected choline on growth performance, carcass characteristics and blood lipid metabolites of feedlot lambs. *Animals: An Open Access Journal from MDPI, 10*(9), 1580. https://doi.org/10.3390/ani10091580

Kawashima, C., Kaneko, E., Amaya Montoya, C., Matsui, M., Yamagishi, N., Matsunaga, N., Ishii, M., Kida, K., Miyake, Y. I., & Miyamoto, A. (2006). Relationship between the first ovulation within three weeks postpartum and subsequent ovarian cycles and fertility in high producing dairy cows. *The Journal of Reproduction and Development, 52*(4), 479–486. https://doi.org/10.1262/jrd.18003

Kawashima, C., Kida, K., Schweigert, F. J., & Miyamoto, A. (2009a). Relationship between plasma β-carotene concentrations during the peripartum period and ovulation in the first follicular wave postpartum in dairy cows. *Animal Reproduction Science, 111*(1), 105–111. https://doi.org/10.1016/j.anireprosci.2008.02.008

Kawashima, C., Nagashima, S., Fujihara, Y., Schweigert, F. J., Sawada, K., Miyamoto, A., & Kida, K. (2009b). Effect of beta-carotene supply during the close-up dry period on ovulation at the first follicular wave postpartum in dairy cows. *Journal of Dairy Science, 92* E-Suppl.1:106.

Kay, J. K., Roche, J. R., Kolver, E. S., Thomson, N. A., & Baumgard, L. H. (2005). A comparison between feeding systems (pasture and TMR) and the effect of vitamin E supplementation on plasma and milk fatty acid profiles in dairy cows. *The Journal of Dairy Research, 72*(3), 322–332. https://doi.org/10.1017/S0022029905000944

Keener, H. A. (1954). The effect of various factors on the vitamin D content of several common forages. *Journal of Dairy Science, 37*(11), 1337–1345. https://doi.org/10.3168/jds.S0022-0302(54)91411-3

Kehrli, Jr., M. E., & Goff, J. P. (1989). Periparturient hypocalcemia in cows: Effects on peripheral blood neutrophil and lymphocyte function. *Journal of Dairy Science, 72*(5), 1188–1196. https://doi.org/10.3168/jds.S0022-0302(89)79223-7

Kennedy, D. G., Blanchflower, W. J., Scott, J. M., Weir, D. G., Molloy, A. M., Kennedy, S., & Young, P. B. (1992). Cobalt-vitamin B_{12} deficiency decreases methionine synthase activity and phospholipid methylation in sheep. *The Journal of Nutrition, 122*(7), 1384–1390. https://doi.org/10.1093/jn/122.7.1384

Kennedy, D. G., Kennedy, S., Blanchflower, W. J., Scott, J. M., Weir, D. G., Molloy, A. M., & Young, P. B. (1994). Cobalt-vitamin B_{12} deficiency causes accumulation of odd-numbered, branched chain fatty acids in the tissues of sheep. *The British Journal of Nutrition, 71*(1), 67–76. https://doi.org/10.1079/bjn19940111

Kennedy, D. G., Young, P. B., Kennedy, S., Scott, J. M., Molloy, A. M., Weir, D. G., & Price, J. (1995). Cobalt-vitamin B_{12} deficiency and the activity of methylmalonyl CoA mutase and methionine synthase in cattle. *International Journal for Vitamin and Nutrition Research. Internationale Zeitschrift Fur Vitamin- und Ernahrungsforschung. Journal International de Vitaminologie et de Nutrition, 65*(4), 241–247. PubMed: 8789620

Kennedy, D. G., Kennedy, S., & Young, P. B. (1996). Effects of low concentrations of dietary cobalt on rumen succinate concentration in sheep. *International Journal for Vitamin and Nutrition Research. Internationale Zeitschrift Fur Vitamin- und Ernahrungsforschung. Journal International de Vitaminologie et de Nutrition, 66*(1), 86–92. PubMed: 8698552

Kennedy, S., McConnell, S., Anderson, H., Kennedy, D. G., Young, P. B., & Blanchflower, W. J. (1997). Histopathologic and ultrastructural alterations of white liver disease in sheep experimentally depleted of cobalt. *Veterinary Pathology, 34*(6), 575–584. https://doi.org/10.1177/030098589703400605

Kesavan, V., & Noronha, J. M. (1983). Folate malabsorption in aged rats related to low levels of pancreatic folyl conjugase. *The American Journal of Clinical Nutrition, 37*(2), 262–267. https://doi.org/10.1093/ajcn/37.2.262

Khan, H. M., Bhakat, M., Mohanty, T. K., & Pathbanda, T. K. (2014). Influence of vitamin E, macro and micro minerals on reproductive performance of cattle and buffalo- a review. *Agricultural Reviews, 35*(2), 113–121. https://doi.org/10.5958/0976-0741.2014.00088.9

Khan, M. Z., Khan, A., Xiao, J., Dou, J., Liu, L., & Yu, Y. (2020a). Overview of folic acid supplementation alone or in combination with vitamin B_{12} in dairy cattle during periparturient period. *Metabolites, 10*(6), 263. https://doi.org/10.3390/metabo10060263

Khan, M. Z., Liu, L., Zhang, Z., Khan, A., Wang, D., Mi, S., Usman, T., Liu, G., Li, X., Wang, Y., & Yu, Y. (2020b). Folic acid supplementation regulates milk production variables, metabolic associated genes and pathways in perinatal Holsteins. *Journal of Animal Physiology and Animal Nutrition, 104*, 438–492. https://doi.org/10.1111/jpn.13313

Khan, M. Z., Zhang, Z., Liu, L., Wang, D., Mi, S., Liu, X., Liu, G., Guo, G., Li, X., Wang, Y., & Yu, Y. (2020c). Folic acid supplementation regulates key immunity-associated genes and pathways during the periparturient period in dairy cows. *Asian-Australasian Journal of Animal Sciences, 33*(9), 1507–1519. https://doi.org/10.5713/ajas.18.0852

Khan, M. Z., Ma, Y., Xiao, J., Chen, T., Ma, J., Liu, S., Wang, Y., Khan, A., Alugongo, G. M., & Cao, Z. (2022). Role of selenium and vitamins E and B9 in the alleviation of bovine mastitis during the periparturient period. *Antioxidants, 11*(4), 657. https://doi.org/10.3390/antiox11040657

Khan, N., Kewalramani, N., Mahajan, V., Haq, Z., & Kumar, B. (2018). Effect of supplementation of niacin on physiological and blood biochemical parameters in crossbred cows during heat stress. *The Indian Journal of Animal Sciences, 88*(1), 58–65. https://doi.org/10.56093/ijans.v88i1.79498

Kiani, A. (2017). Effect of lycopene and energy supplementation on serum and colostrum IgG concentrations in pregnant ewes. *Animal Production, 19*(3), 557–567. https://doi.org/10.22059/jap.2018.223175.623146

Kichura, T. S., Horst, R. L., Beitz, D. C., & Littledike, E. T. (1982). Relationships between prepartal dietary calcium and phosphorus, vitamin D metabolism and parturient paresis in dairy cows. *The Journal of Nutrition, 112*(3), 480–487. https://doi.org/10.1093/jn/112.3.480

Kim, H. S., Lee, J. M., Park, S. B., Jeong, S. G., Jung, J. K., & Im, K. S. (1997). Effect of vitamin E and selenium administration on the reproductive performance of dairy cows. *Asian-Australian Journal of Animal Science, 10*, 308–312. https://doi.org/10.5713/ajas.1997.308

Kim, Y. I., Miller, J. W., Da Costa, K. A., Nadeau, M., Smith, D., Selhub, J., Zeisel, S. H., & Mason, J. B. (1994). Severe folate deficiency causes secondary depletion of choline and phosphocholine in rat liver. *The Journal of Nutrition, 124*(11), 2197–2203. https://doi.org/10.1093/jn/124.11.2197

Kam, K. T., R., Deng, Y., Chen, Y., & Zhao, H. (2012). Retinoic acid synthesis and functions in early embryonic development. *Cell and Bioscience, 2*, 1–14. https://doi.org/10.1186/2045-3701-2-11

Kincaid, R. L., & Socha, M. T. (2007). Effect of cobalt supplementation during late gestation and early lactation on milk and serum measures. *Journal of Dairy Science, 90*(4), 1880–1886. https://doi.org/10.3168/jds.2006-296

Kirdeci, A., Çetin, H., & Raza, S. (2021). Effect of vitamin C on pregnancy rate and 8-OHdG levels during heat stress in post-partum dairy cattle. *Journal of Animal Reproduction and Biotechnology, 36*(4), 194–202. https://doi.org/10.12750/JARB.36.4.194

Kirkland, J. B. (2013). Niacin. In J. Zempleni, J. Suttie, J. Gregory, & P. J. Stover (Eds.), *Handbook of vitamins* (5th ed.) (pp. 149–190). Taylor & Francis Group.

Kiyose, C., Muramatsu, R., Ueda, T., & Igarashi, O. (1995). Change in the distribution of a-tocopherol stereoisomers in rats after intravenous administration. *Bioscience, Biotechnology, and Biochemistry, 59*(5), 791–795. https://doi.org/10.1271/bbb.59.791

Kleczkowski, M., Kluciński, W., Shaktur, A., & Sikora, J. (2005). Concentration of ascorbic acid in the blood of cows with subclinical mastitis. *Polish Journal of Veterinary Sciences, 8*(2), 121–125. PubMed: 15989131

Kliewer, S. A., Umesono, K., Mangelsdorf, D. J., & Evans, R. M. (1992). Retinoid X receptor interacts with nuclear receptors in retinoic acid, thyroid hormone and vitamin D_3 signaling. *Nature, 355*(6359), 446–449. https://doi.org/10.1038/355446a0

Kliewer, S. A., Umesono, K., Evans, R. M., & Mangelsdorf, D. (1994). Retinoid X receptor interacts with nuclear receptors in retinoic acid, thyroid hormone and vitamin D_3 signaling. In R. Blomhoff (Ed.), *Vitamin A in health and disease* p. 239. Marcel Dekker. ISBN: 0-8247-9120-7.

Kluenter, A. M., & Steinberg, W. (1993). Influence of biotin supplementation on the concentration of biotin in the blood plasma and milk of dairy cows. Proc. Soc. Nutr. Physiol., 1, 67.

Kobeisy, M. A., Salem, I. A., Zenhom, M., & Hayder, M. (1997). The effect of giving ascorbic acid on some physiological and hematological parameters of suckling lambs exposed to solar radiation and exercise. Assiut. Vet. *Medical Journal, 37*, 120–132. https://doi.org/10.21608/AVMJ.1997.183420

Kodentsova, V. M., Iakushina, L. M., Vrzhesinskaia, O. A., Beketova, N. A., & Spirichev, V. B. (1993). Effect of riboflavin administration on vitamin B_6 metabolism. *Voprosy Pitaniia, 5*(5), 32–36. PubMed: 8042309

Kodicek, E., Ashby, D. R., Muller, M., & Carpenter, K. J. (1974). The conversion of bound nicotinic acid to free nicotinamide on roasting sweet corn. *The Proceedings of the Nutrition Society, 33*(3), 105A–106A. PubMed: 4282141

Kohler, M., Leiber, F., Willems, H., Merbold, L., & Liesegang, A. (2013). Influence of altitude on vitamin D and bone metabolism of lactating sheep and goats. *Journal of Animal Science, 91*(11), 5259–5268. https://doi.org/10.2527/jas.2013-6702

Kolb, E. (1984). Metabolism of ascorbic acid in livestock under pathological conditions. In I. Wegger, F. J. Tagwerker, & J. Moustgaard (Eds.) [Workshop]. Danish, R. Agr. Soc. *Ascorbic acid in domestic animals* (pp. 162–175). Copenhagen.

Kolb, E., & Seehawer, J. (1997). The significance of carotenes and of vitamin A for the reproduction of cattle, of horses, and of pigs – A review. Det. *Der Praktische Tierarzt, 78*(9), 783–789.

Kominato, T. (1971). Speed of vitamin B_{12} turnover and its relation to the intestine in the rat. *Vitamins, 44*, 76–83.

Kontoghiorghes, G. J., Kolnagou, A., Kontoghiorghe, C. N., Mourouzidis, L., Timoshnikov, V. A., & Polyakov, N. E. (2020). Trying to solve the puzzle of the interaction of ascorbic acid and iron: Redox, chelation and therapeutic implications. *Medicines, 7*(8), 45. https://doi.org/10.3390/medicines7080045

Kornegay, E. T. (1986). Biotin in swine production: A review. *Livestock Production Science, 14*(1), 65–89. https://doi.org/10.1016/0301-6226(86)90097-7

Koutsoumpas, A. T., Giadinis, N. D., Petridou, E. J., Konstantinou, E., Brozos, C., Lafi, S. Q., Fthenakis, G. C., & Karatzias, H. (2013). Consequences of reduced vitamin A administration on mammary health of dairy ewes. *Small Ruminant Research, 110*(2–3), 120–123. https://doi.org/10.1016/j.smallrumres.2012.11.018

Kozicki, L., Silva, R. G., & Barnabe, R. C. (1981). Effects of vitamins A, D$_3$, E, and C on the characteristics of bull semen. *Zentralblatt für Veterinärmedizin. Reihe A, 28*(7), 538–546. https://doi.org/10.1111/j.1439-0442.1981.tb01224.x

Krinke, G. J., & Fitzgerald, R. E. (1988). The pattern of pyridoxine-induced lesion: Difference between the high and the low toxic level. *Toxicology, 49*(1), 171–178. https://doi.org/10.1016/0300-483X(88)90190-4

Król, J., Wawryniuk, A., Brodziak, A., Barłowska, J., & Kuczyńska, B. (2020). The effect of selected factors on the content of fat-soluble vitamins and macro-elements in raw milk from Holstein-Friesian and Simmental cows and acid curd cheese (tvarog). *Animals: An Open Access Journal from MDPI, 10*(10). https://doi.org/10.3390/ani10101800

Krone, K. G., Ward, A. K., Madder, K. M., Hendrick, S., McKinnon, J. J., & Buchanan, F. C. (2015). Interaction of vitamin A supplementation level with ADH1C genotype on intramuscular fat in beef steers. *Animal, 10*, 3. https://doi.org/10.1017/S1751731115002153

Krüger, K. A., Blum, J. W., & Greger, D. L. (2005). Expression of nuclear receptor and target genes in liver and intestine of neonatal calves fed colostrum and vitamin A. *Journal of Dairy Science, 88*(11), 3971–3981. https://doi.org/10.3168/jds.S0022-0302(05)73083-6

Krueger, L. A., Beitz, D. C., Onda, K., Osman, M., O'Neil, M. R., Lei, S., Wattoo, F. H., Stuart, R. L., Tyler, H. D., & Nonnecke, B. (2014). Effects of d-α-tocopherol and dietary energy on growth and health of preruminant dairy calves. *Journal of Dairy Science, 97*(6), 3715–3727. https://doi.org/10.3168/jds.2013-7315

Krueger, L. A., Reinhardt, T. A., Beitz, D. C., Stuart, R. L., & Stabel, J. R. (2016). Effects of fractionated colostrum replacer and vitamins A, D, and E on haptoglobin and clinical health in neonatal Holstein calves challenged with Mycobacterium avium ssp. paratuberculosis. *Journal of Dairy Science, 99*(4), 2884–2895. https://doi.org/10.3168/jds.2015-10395

Kruk, Z. A., Bottema, C. D. K., Davis, J. J., Siebert, B. D., Harper, G. S., Di, J., & Pitchford, W. S. (2008). Effects of vitamin A on growth performance and carcass quality in steers. *Livestock Science, 119*(1–3), 12–21. https://doi.org/10.1016/j.livsci.2008.02.008

Krumdieck, C. L. (1990). Folic acid. In M. L. Brown (Ed.) Int., *Present knowledge in nutrition* (6th ed.) (pp. 179–188) Life Sci. Institute/Nutrition Foundation.

Kucmyj, A. (1955). Vitamin C in cow's milk and colostrum and some questions of increasing its content. *Voprosy Pitanija, 14*, 3.

Kuhn, M. J., & Sordillo, L. M. (2021). Vitamin E analogs limit in vitro oxidant damage to bovine mammary endothelial cells. *Journal of Dairy Science, 104*(6), 7154–7167. https://doi.org/10.3168/jds.2020-19675

Kumar, S., Pandey, A. K., Rao, M. M., & Razzaque, W. A. A. (2010). Role of β carotene/vitamin A in animal reproduction. *Veterinary World, 3*(5), 236–237. https://citeseerx.ist.psu.edu/document?repid=rep1&type=pdf&doi=cf5ec43107d11ffa6e92de8f1811485ab0e73813

Kung, L., Gubert, K., & Huber, J. T. (1980). Supplemental niacin for lactating cows fed diets of natural protein or nonprotein nitrogen. *Journal of Dairy Science, 63*(12), 2020–2025. https://doi.org/10.3168/jds.S0022-0302(80)83178-X

Kurnick, A. A., Hanold, F. J., & Stangeland, V. A. (1972) Problems in the use of feed ingredient vitamin values in formulating feeds. *Proceedings of the 1972 Georgia Nutr. Conf. Feed Industry.*

Kuroiwa, T., Ohtani, Y., Obara, Y., Terada, F., Watanabe, K., Shirakawa, H., Komai, M., Satoh, H., Sato, S., & Ichijo, T. (2022). Effect of vitamin K3 supplementation on immunoglobulin G concentration in colostrum of periparturient Holstein dairy cows. *Journal of Animal Science, 93*, 1. https://doi.org/10.1111/asj.13706

Lacetera, N., Bernabucci, U., Ronchi, B., & Nardone, A. (1996). Effects of selenium and vitamin E administration during a late stage of pregnancy on colostrum and milk production in dairy cows, and on passive immunity and growth of their offspring. *American Journal of Veterinary Research, 57*(12), 1776–1780. https://doi.org/10.2460/ajvr.1996.57.12.1776, PubMed: 8950434

LaCount, D. W., Drackley, J. K., & Weigel, D. J. (1995). Responses of dairy cows during early lactation to ruminal or abomasal administration of L-carnitine. *Journal of Dairy Science, 78*(8), 1824–1836. https://doi.org/10.3168/jds.S0022-0302(95)76807-2

LaCount, D. W., Emmert, L. S., & Drackley, J. K. (1996b). Dose response of dairy cows to abomasal administration of four amounts of L-carnitine. *Journal of Dairy Science, 79*(4), 591–602. https://doi.org/10.3168/jds.S0022-0302(96)76404-4

LaCount, D. W., Ruppert, L. D., & Drackley, J. K. (1996a). Ruminal degradation and dose response of dairy cows to dietary L-carnitine. *Journal of Dairy Science*, *79*(2), 260–269. https://doi.org/10.3168/jds.S0022-0302(96)76359-2

Ladeira, M. M., de Oliveira, D. M., Schoonmaker, J. P., Chizzotti, M. L., Barreto, H. G., Paiva, L. V., Coelho, T. C., Machado Neto, O. R. M., Gionbelli, M. P., & Chalfun-Junior, A. (2020). Expression of lipogenic genes in the muscle of beef cattle fed oilseeds and vitamin E. *Agri Gene*, *15*, 100097. https://doi.org/10.1016/j.aggene.2019.100097

Laflamme, L. F., & Hidiroglou, M. (1991). Effects of selenium and vitamin E administration on breeding of replacement beef heifers. In *Annales de Recherches Veterinaires. Annals of Veterinary Research*, *22*(1), 65–69. PubMed: 2042908

Lakshmi, A. V., Prasad, R. K., & Bamji, M. S. (1990). Effect of riboflavin deficiency on collagen content of cornea and bone. *Journal of Clinical Biochemistry and Nutrition*, *9*(2), 115–118. https://doi.org/10.3164/jcbn.9.115

Lakshmi, R., Lakshmi, A. V., & Bamji, M. S. (1989). Skin wound healing in riboflavin deficiency. *Biochemical Medicine and Metabolic Biology*, *42*(3), 185–191. https://doi.org/10.1016/0885-4505(89)90054-6

Lanari, M. C., Cassens, R. G., Schaefer, D. M., & Scheller, K. K. (1994). Effect of dietary vitamin E on pigment and lipid stability of frozen beef: A kinetic analysis. *Meat Science*, *38*(1), 3–15. https://doi.org/10.1016/0309-1740(94)90091-4

Lane, M. D., Young, D. L., & Lynen, F. (1964). The enzymatic synthesis of holotranscarboxylase from apo-transcarboxylase and (+)-biotin: I. Purification of the apoenzyme and synthetase; characteristics of the reaction. *The Journal of Biological Chemistry*, *239*(9), 2858–2864. https://doi.org/10.1016/S0021-9258(18)93825-1

Lanham, J. K., Coppock, C. E., Brooks, K. N., Wilks, D. L., & Horner, J. L. (1992). Effects of whole cottonseed or niacin or both on casein synthesis by lactating Holstein cows. *Journal of Dairy Science*, *75*(1), 184–192. https://doi.org/10.3168/jds.S0022-0302(92)77752-2

Lardinois, C. C., Mills, R. C., Elvehjem, C. A., & Hart, E. B. (1944). Rumen synthesis of the vitamin B complex as influenced by ration composition. *Journal of Dairy Science*, *27*(7), 579–583. https://doi.org/10.3168/jds.S0022-0302(44)92635-4

Larkin, P. J., & Yates, R. J. (1964). Vitamin deficiencies in farm animals in the tropics. *East African Agricultural and Forestry Journal*, *30*(1), 11–20. https://doi.org/10.1080/00128325.1964.11661951

Larson, L. L., Wang, J. Y., Owen, F. G., & Meader, J. E. (1983). Effect of beta-carotene supplementation during early lactation on reproduction. *Journal of Dairy Science*, *66*(1), 240.

Lashkari, S., Jensen, S. K., Hansen, C. B., Krogh, K., Theilgaard, P., Raun, B. M. L., & Vestergaard, M. (2021). Feeding concentrate pellets enriched by natural vitamin E keeps the plasma vitamin E above the critical level in calves post-weaning. *Livestock Science*, *253*, 104672. https://doi.org/10.1016/j.livsci.2021.104672

Lassiter, C. A., Ward, G. M., Huffman, C. F., Duncan, C. W., & Webster, H. D. (1953). Crystalline vitamin B_{12} requirement of the young dairy calf. Journal of Dairy Science, 36(9), 997–1005. https://doi.org/10.3168/jds.S0022-0302(53)91587-2

Latteur, J. P. (1962). Cobalt Deficiencies and Sub deficiencies in Ruminants *Center information du cobalt, Brussels, Belgium.*

Lauriault, L. M., Dougherty, C. T., Bradley, N. W., & Cornelius, P. L. (1990). Thiamin supplementation and the ingestive behavior of beef cattle grazing endophyte-infected tall fescue. *Journal of Animal Science*, *68*(5), 1245–1253. https://doi.org/10.2527/1990.6851245x

Le Grusse, J., & Watier, B. (1993). Les vitamins. *Données biochimiques, nutritionnelles et cliniques. Centre d'étude et d'information sur les vitamins, Produits Roche.* Neuilly-sur-Seine, France.

Lean, I. J., & Rabiee, A. R. (2011). Effect of feeding biotin on milk production and hoof health in lactating dairy cows: A quantitative assessment. *Journal of Dairy Science*, *94*(3), 1465–1476. https://doi.org/10.3168/jds.2010-3682

LeBlanc, S. J., Duffield, T. F., Leslie, K. E., Bateman, K. G., Tenhag, J., Walton, J. S., & Johnson, W. H. (2002). The effect of prepartum injection of vitamin E on health in transition dairy cows. *Journal of Dairy Science*, *85*(6), 1416–1426. https://doi.org/10.3168/jds.S0022-0302(02)74209-4

LeBlanc, S. J., Herdt, T. H., Seymour, W. M., Duffield, T. F., & Leslie, K. E. (2004). Peripartum serum vitamin E, retinol, and beta-carotene in dairy cattle and their association with disease. *Journal of Dairy Science, 87*(3), 609–619. https://doi.10.3168/jds.S0022-0302(04)73203-8. https://doi.org/10.3168/jds.S0022-0302(04)73203-8

Lee, H. J. (1963). *Cobalt deficiency. Animal health, production and pasture* A. N. Worden, K. C. Sellers, & D. E. Tribe (Eds.) (pp. 662–680). Longmans, Green.

Lee, H. J. (1963). Animal health, production and pasture. In A. H. Worden, K. O. Seller, & D. E. Tribe (Eds.). 662. Longmans.

Lee, L. C., Carlson, R. W., Judge, D. L., & Ogawa, M. (1973). The absorption cross sections of N_2, O_2, CO, NO, CO_2, N_2O, CH_4, C_2H_4, C_2H_6 and C_4H_{10} from 180 to 700A. *Journal of Quantitative Spectroscopy and Radiative Transfer, 13*(10), 1023–1031. https://doi.org/10.1016/0022-4073(73)90075-7

Lee, R. W., Stuart, R. L., Perryman, K. R., & Ridenour, K. W. (1985). Effect of vitamin supplementation on the performance of stressed beef calves. *Journal of Animal Science, 61*(Suppl. 1), 425.

Leedle, R. A., Leedle, J. A. Z., & Butine, M. D. (1993). Vitamin E is not degraded by ruminal microorganisms: Assessment with ruminal contents from a steer fed a high-concentrate diet. *Journal of Animal Science, 71*(12), 3442–3450. https://doi.org/10.2527/1993.71123442x

Lehninger, A. L. (1982). *Principles of biochemistry*. Worth Publishers, Inc.

Lehr, H. A., Vajkoczy, P., & Menger, M. D. (1998). Vitamin E: Focus on microcirculation. *Microcirculation, 5*(2–3), 117–128. https://doi.org/10.1080/mic.5.2-3.117.128

Lemire, J. M. (1992). Immunomodulatory role of 1,25 dihydroxy. *Journal of Cellular Biochemistry, 49*(1), 26–31. https://doi.org/10.1002/jcb.240490106

Leonard, S. W., Terasawa, Y., Farese, R. V., & Traber, M. G. (2002). Incorporation of deuterated RRR- or all-rac-a-tocopherol in plasma and tissues of a-tocopherol transfer protein-null mice. *The American Journal of Clinical Nutrition, 75*(3), 555–560. https://doi.org/10.1093/ajcn/75.3.555

Lester, G. E. (1986). Cholecalciferol and placental calcium transport. *Federation Proceedings, 45*(10), 2524–2527. PubMed: 3017769

Lewis, L. L., Stark, C. R., Fahrenholz, A. C., Bergstrom, J. R., & Jones, C. K. (2015). Evaluation of conditioning time and temperature on gelatinized starch and vitamin retention in a pelleted swine diet. *Journal of Animal Science, 93*(2), 615–619. https://doi.org/10.2527/jas.2014-8074

Li, H. Q., Liu, Q., Wang, C., Yang, Z. M., Guo, G., Huo, W. J., Pei, C. X., Zhang, Y. L., Zhang, S. L., Wang, H., Liu, J. X., & Huang, Y. X. (2016). Effects of dietary supplements of rumen-protected folic acid on lactation performance, energy balance, blood parameters and reproductive performance in dairy cows. *Animal Feed Science and Technology, 213*, 55–63. https://doi.org/10.1016/j.anifeedsci.2016.01.005

Li, Z., Wang, B., Li, H., Jian, L., Luo, H., Wang, B., Zhang, C., Zhao, X., Xue, Y., Peng, S., & Zuo, S. (2020). Maternal folic acid supplementation differently affects the small intestinal phenotype and gene expression of newborn lambs from differing litter sizes. *Animals: An Open Access Journal from MDPI, 10*(11), 2183. https://doi.org/10.3390/ani10112183

Li, Q., Wang, Y. S., Wang, L. J., Zhang, H., Li, R. Z., Cui, C. C., Li, W. Z., Zhang, Y., & Jin, Y. P. (2014). Vitamin C supplementation enhances compact morulae formation but reduces the hatching blastocyst rate of bovine somatic cell nuclear transfer embryos. *Cellular Reprogramming, 16*(4), 290–297. https://doi.org/10.1089/cell.2013.0088

Liesegang, A., Sassi, M.-L., Risteli, J., Eicher, R., Wanner, M., & Riond, J.-L. (1998). Physiology of bone resorption during hypocalcemia in dairy cows. *Journal of Animal Physiology and Animal Nutrition, 80*(1–5), 82–85. https://doi.org/10.1111/j.1439-0396.1998.tb00507.x

Liesegang, A., Eicher, R., Sassi, M. L., Risteli, J., Kraenzlin, M., Riond, J. L., & Wanner, M. (2000). Biochemical markers of bone formation and resorption around parturition and during lactation in dairy cows with high and low standard milk yields. *Journal of Dairy Science, 83*(8), 1773–1781. https://doi.org/10.3168/jds.S0022-0302(00)75048-X

Lindemann, M. D. (1988). Further research supports value of folic acid in sow diets. *Feedstuffs, 60*(46), 15.

Lindley, C. E., Brugman, H. H., Cunha, T. J., & Warwick, E. J. (1949). The effect of vitamin A deficiency on semen quality and the effect of testosterone and pregnant mare serum on vitamin A deficient rams. *Journal of Animal Science, 8*(4), 590–602. https://doi.org/10.2527/jas1949.84590x

Lindmark-Månsson, H., Fondén, R., & Pettersson, H. E. (2003). Composition of Swedish milk. *International Dairy Journal, 13*(6), 409–425. https://doi.org/10.1016/S0958-6946(03)00032-3

Lindshield, B. L., & Erdman, J. W. (2006). Carotenoids. In B. A. Bowman & R. M. Russell (Eds.), *Present knowledge in nutrition* (9th ed.) (pp. 184–197). International Life Sciences Institute.

Lischer, Ch. J., Koller, U., Geyer, H., Mülling, Ch., Schulze, J., & Ossent, P. (2002). Effect of therapeutic dietary biotin on the healing of uncomplicated sole ulcers in dairy cattle–a double blinded controlled study. *Veterinary Journal, 163*(1), 51–60. https://doi.org/10.1053/tvjl.2001.0627

Littledike, E. T., & Horst, R. L. (1982). Vitamin D$_3$ toxicity in dairy cows. *Journal of Dairy Science, 65*(5), 749–759. https://doi.org/10.3168/jds.S0022-0302(82)82263-7

Liu, Y., Zhang, J., Wang, C., Liu, Q., Guo, G., Huo, W., Chen, L., Zhang, Y., Pei, C., & Zhang, S. (2022). Effects of folic acid and cobalt sulphate supplementation on growth performance, nutrient digestion, rumen fermentation and blood metabolites in holstein calves. *The British Journal of Nutrition, 127*(9), 1313–1319. https://doi.org/10.1017/S000711452100221X

Loew, F. M., & Dunlop, R. H. (1972). Induction of thiamine inadequacy and polioencephalomalacia in adult sheep with amprolium. *American Journal of Veterinary Research, 33*(11), 2195–2205. PubMed: 5081481

Loew, F. M., Bettany, J. M., & Halifax, C. E. (1975). Apparent thiamin status of cattle and its relationship to polioencephalomalacia. *Canadian Journal of Comparative Medicine: Revue Canadienne de Medecine Comparee, 39*(3), 291–295. http://www.ncbi.nlm.nih.gov/pmc/articles/pmc1277459/

Lomba, F. G., Chauvaux, G., Teller, E., Lengele, L., & Bienfet, V. (1978). Calcium digestibility in cows as influenced by excess of alkaline ions over stable acid ions in their diets. *The British Journal of Nutrition, 39*(3), 425–429. https://doi.org/10.1079/bjn19780058

Loneragan, G. H., Gould, D. H., Callan, R. J., Sigurdson, C. J., & Hamar, D. W. (1998). Association of excess sulfur intake and an increase in hydrogen sulfide concentrations in the ruminal cap of recently weaned beef calves with polioencephalomalacia. *Journal of the American Veterinary Medical Association, 213*(11), 1599–1604. https://doi.org/10.2460/javma.1998.213.11.1599, PubMed: 9838961

Lopes, M. M., Brito, T. R., Lage, J. F., Costa, T. C., Fontes, M. M. D. S., Serão, N. V. L., Mendes, T. A. O., Reis, R. A., Veroneze, R., E Silva, F. F., & Duarte, M. S. (2021). Proteomic analysis of liver from finishing beef cattle supplemented with a rumen-protected b-vitamin blend and hydroxy trace minerals. *Animals: An Open Access Journal from MDPI, 11*(7), 1934. https://doi.org/10.3390/ani11071934

López-Constantino, S., Barragan, E. A., & Alfonseca-Silva, E. (2022). Reduced levels of serum 25 (OH) D3 are associated with tuberculosis positive cattle under conditions of high natural exposure to *Mycobacterium bovis. Comparative Immunology, Microbiology and Infectious Diseases, 81*, 101746. https://doi.org/10.1016/j.cimid.2022.101746

Lopez-Diaz, M. C., & Bosu, W. T. K. (1992). A review and an update of cystic ovarian degeneration in ruminants. *Theriogenology, 37*(6), 1163–1183. https://doi.org/10.1016/0093-691X(92)90173-O

Losada, H., Dixon, F., & Preston, T. R. (1971). Thiamine and molasses toxicity. 1. Effects with roughage free diets. *Rev. Cubana Cienc. Agríc, 5*(3), 369–378.

Lotthammer, K. H. (1979). Importance of beta-carotene for the fertility of dairy cattle. *Feedstuffs, 51*(43), 16.

Lotthammer, K. H., Ahlswede, L., & Meyer, H. (1976). Studies on a specific vitamin A unrelated effect of beta-carotene on the fertility of cattle. 2. Further clinical findings and fertilization results (experiment III). *DTW. Deutsche Tierarztliche Wochenschrift, 83*(8), 353–358. PubMed: 791616

Lotthammer, K. H., Ahlswede, L., & Meyer, H. (1979). Untersuchungen über eine spezifische, vitamin-A-unabhängige Wirkung des b-carotins auf die Fertilität des Rindes. 2. *Mitt.: Weitere Klinische Befunde und Befruchtungsergebnisse. Dtsch. Tierärztl. Wochenschr., 83*, 353.

Lucas, A., Agabriel, C., Martin, B., Ferlay, A., Verdier-Metz, I., Coulon, J. B., & Rock, E. (2006). Relationships between the conditions of cow's milk production and the contents of components of nutritional interest in raw milk farmhouse cheese. *Le Lait, 86*(3), 177–202. http://doi.org/10.1051/lait:2005049

Luce, W. G., Peo, E. R., & Hudman, D. B. (1966). Availability of niacin in wheat for swine. *The Journal of Nutrition, 88*(1), 39–44. https://doi.org/10.1093/jn/88.1.39

Luce, W. G., Peo, E. R., & Hudman, D. B. (1967). Availability of niacin in corn and milo for swine. *Journal of Animal Science, 26*(1), 76–84. https://doi.org/10.2527/jas1967.26176x

Luciano, G., Moloney, A. P., Priolo, A., Röhrle, F. T., Vasta, V., Biondi, L., López-Andrés, P., Grasso, S., & Monahan, F. J. (2011). Vitamin E and polyunsaturated fatty acids in bovine muscle and the oxidative stability of beef from cattle receiving grass or concentrate-based rations. *Journal of Animal Science*, *89*(11), 3759–3768. https://doi.org/10.2527/jas.2010-3795

Luck, M. R., Jeyaseelan, I., & Scholes, R. A. (1995). Ascorbic-acid and fertility. *Biology of Reproduction*, *52*(2), 262–266. https://doi.org/10.1095/biolreprod52.2.262

Lynch, G. P. (1983). Changes of tocopherols in blood serum of cows fed hay or silage. *Journal of Dairy Science*, *66*(7), 1461–1465. https://doi.org/10.3168/jds.S0022-0302(83)81960-2

Ma, Y., Zhang, Y., Zhang, H., Wang, H., & Elmhadi, M. (2021). Thiamine alleviates high-concentrate-diet-induced oxidative stress, apoptosis, and protects the rumen epithelial barrier function in goats. *Frontiers in Veterinary Science*, *8*, 663698. https://doi.org/10.3389/fvets.2021.663698

Maas, J., Bulgin, M. S., Anderson, B. C., & Frye, T. M. (1984). Nutritional myodegeneration associated with vitamin E deficiency and normal selenium status in lambs. *Journal of the American Veterinary Medical Association*, *184*(2), 201–204. PubMed: 6698855

Machado, M., Castro, M. B., Gimeno, E. J., Barros, S. S., & Riet-Correa, F. (2020). Enzootic calcinosis in ruminants: A review. *Toxicon*, *187*, 1–9. https://doi.org/10.1016/j.toxicon.2020.08.009

Machlin, L. J. (1988). *Free radical tissue damage and the protective role of antioxidant nutrients*. Special Report 414. https://mospace.umsystem.edu/xmlui/bitstream/handle/10355/56845/AESSpecialReport.pdf?sequence=1 Retrieved Jan 2024. Agricultural Experiment Station. University of Missouri – Columbia.

Machlin, L. J. (1991). Vitamin E. In L. J. Machlin (Ed.), *Handbook of vitamins* (2nd ed.). Marcel Dekker.

Machlin, L. J. (1994). New views on the function and health effects of vitamins. Nutrition, 10(6), 562. https://doi.org/10.1097/00017285-199401000-00006

Maciel, F. C., Machado Neto, O. R., Duarte, M. S., Du, M., Lage, J. F., Teixeira, P. D., Martins, C. L., Domingues, E. H. R., Fogaça, L. A., & Ladeira, M. M. (2022). Effect of vitamin A injection at birth on intramuscular fat development and meat quality in beef cattle. *Meat Science*, *184*, 108676. https://doi.org/10.1016/j.meatsci.2021.108676

Mackenzie, A. M., Drennan, M., Rowan, T. G., Dixon, J. B., & Carter, S. D. (1997). Effect of transportation and weaning on humoral immune responses of calves. *Research in Veterinary Science*, *63*(3), 227–230. https://doi.org/10.1016/s0034-5288(97)90025-4

MacLeod, D., Ozimek, L., & Kennelly, J. J. (1996). Supplemental vitamin C may enhance immune function in dairy cows. Adv. dairy tech, *8*, 227–235. https://wcds.ualberta.ca/wcds/wp-content/uploads/sites/57/wcds_archive/Archive/1996/wcd96227.htm

MacPherson, A. (1982). Dietary vitamin B_{12} and cobalt for ruminants. Roche Vitamin Symposium: Recent Research on the Vitamin Requirements of Ruminants. Hoffmann–La Roche.

MacRae, J., O'Reilly, L., & Morgan, P. (2005). Desirable characteristics of animal products from a human health perspective. *livestock Production Science*, *94*(1–2), 95–103. https://doi.org/10.1016/j.livprodsci.2004.11.030

Madureira, A. M. L., Pohler, K. G., Guida, T. G., Wagner, S. E., Cerri, R. L. A., & Vasconcelos, J. L. M. (2020). Association of concentrations of beta-carotene in plasma on pregnancy per artificial insemination and pregnancy loss in lactating Holstein cows. *Theriogenology*, *142*, 216–221. https://doi.org/10.1016/j.theriogenology.2019.10.006

Maeda, Y., Kawata, S., Inui, Y., Fukuda, K., Igura, T., & Matsuzawa, Y. (1996). Biotin deficiency decreases ornithine transcarbamylase activity and mRNA in rat liver. *The Journal of Nutrition*, *126*(1), 61–66. https://doi.org/10.1093/jn/126.1.61

Maggini, S., & Walter, P. (1997). Effects of vitamin C on phosphoenolpyruvate carboxykinase from rat liver. *International Journal for Vitamin and Nutrition Research. Internationale Zeitschrift Fur Vitamin- und Ernahrungsforschung. Journal International de Vitaminologie et de Nutrition*, *67*(6), 437–443. PubMed: 9433678

Mahalle, N., Bhide, V., Greibe, E., Heegaard, C. W., Nexo, E., Fedosov, S. N., & Naik, S. (2019). Comparative bio-availability of synthetic B_{12} and dietary vitamin B_{12} present in cow and buffalo milk: A prospective study in lactovegetarian Indians. *Nutrients*, *11*(2), 304. https://doi.org/10.3390/nu11020304

Majee, D. N., Schwab, E. C., Bertics, S. J., Seymour, W. M., & Shaver, R. D. (2003). Lactation performance by dairy cows fed supplemental biotin and a B-vitamin blend. *Journal of Dairy Science*, *86*(6), 2106–2112. https://doi.org/10.3168/jds.S0022-0302(03)73800-4

Majumdar, B. N., & Gupta, B. N. (1960). Studies on carotene metabolism in goats. *Indian Journal of Medical Research*, *48*, 388.

Mallard, B. A., Dekkers, J. C., Ireland, M. J., Leslie, K. E., Sharif, S., Vankampen, C. L., Wagter, L., & Wilkie, B. N. (1998). Alteration in immune responsiveness during the peripartum period and its ramification on dairy cow and calf health. *Journal of Dairy Science*, *81*(2), 585–595. https://doi.org/10.3168/jds.S0022-0302(98)75612-7

Malone, J. I. (1975). Vitamin passage across the placenta. *Clinics in Perinatology*, *2*(2), 295–307. PubMed: 1102224

Mancinelli, R., Ceccanti, M., Guiducci, M. S., Sasso, G. F., Sebastiani, G., Attilia, M. L., & Allen, J. P. (2003). Simultaneous liquid chromatographic assessment of thiamine, thiamine monophosphate and thiamine diphosphate in human erythrocytes: A study on alcoholics. *Journal of Chromatography B*, *789*(2), 355–363. https://doi.org/10.1016/S1570-0232(03)00139-9

Manthey, K. C., Griffin, J. B., & Zempleni, J. (2002). Biotin supply affects expression of biotin transporters, biotinylation of carboxylases and metabolism of interleukin-2 in Jurkat cells. *The Journal of Nutrition*, *132*(5), 887–892. https://doi.org/10.1093/jn/132.5.887

Marca, M. C., Ramos, J. J., Sáez, T., Sanz, M. C., Verde, M. T., & Fernández, A. (1996). Vitamin B_{12} supplementation of lambs. *Small Ruminant Research*, *20*(1), 9–14. https://doi.org/10.1016/0921-4488(95)00772-5

Marcek, J. M., Appell, L. H., Hoffman, C. C., Moredick, P. T., & Swanson, L. V. (1985). Effect of supplemental beta-carotene on incidence and responsiveness of ovarian cysts to hormone treatment. *Journal of Dairy Science*, *68*(1), 71–77. https://doi.org/10.3168/jds.S0022-0302(85)80799-2

Margerison, J. K., Winkler, B., Penny, G., & Packington, A. (2003). The effect of biotin supplementation on milk yield, reproduction and lameness in dairy cattle. *Journal of Dairy Science*, *86*, 250. https://doi.org/10.3168/jds.S0022-0302(00)74884-3

Marks, J. (1975). In *A Guide to the vitamins. Their role in health and disease*. Springer.

Martin, F. H., Ullrey, D. E., Miller, E. R., Kemp, K. E., Geasler, M. R., & Henderson, H. E. (1971). Vitamin A status of steers as influenced by corn silage harvest date and supplemental vitamin A. *Journal of Animal Science*, *32*(6), 1233–1238. https://doi.org/10.2527/jas1971.3261233x

Martinez, N., Rodney, R. M., Block, E., Hernandez, L. L., Nelson, C. D., Lean, I. J., & Santos, J. E. P. (2018a). Effects of prepartum dietary cation–anion difference and source of vitamin D in dairy cows: Health and reproductive responses. *Journal of Dairy Science*, *101*(3), 2563–2578. https://doi.org/10.3168/jds.2017-13740

Martinez, N., Rodney, R. M., Block, E., Hernandez, L. L., Nelson, C. D., Lean, I. J., & Santos, J. E. P. (2018b). Effects of prepartum dietary cation–anion difference and source of vitamin D in dairy cows: Lactation performance and energy metabolism. *Journal of Dairy Science*, *101*(3), 2544–2562. https://doi.org/10.3168/jds.2017-13739

Martins, T. E., Acedo, T. S., Gouvea, V. N., Vasconcellos, G. S., Arrigoni, M. B., Martins, C. L., Millen, D. D., Pai, M. D., Perdigão, A., Melo, G. F., Rizzieri, R. A., Rosolen, L. M., Costa, C., & Sartor, A. B. (2020). PSVII-6 Effects of 25-hydroxycholecalciferol supplementation on gene expression of feedlot cattle. *Journal of Animal Science*, *98*(4)(Suppl. 4), 302–303. https://doi.org/10.1093/jas/skaa278.542

Mary, A. E. P., Artavia Mora, J. I., Ronda Borzone, P. A., Richards, S. E., & Kies, A. K. (2021). Vitamin E and beta-carotene status of dairy cows: A survey of plasma levels and supplementation practices. *Animal*, *15*(8), 100303. https://doi.org/10.1016/j.animal.2021.100303

Mason, J. B. (2003). Biomarkers of nutrient exposure and status in one-carbon (methyl) metabolism. *The Journal of Nutrition*, *133*(3)(Suppl. 3), 941S–947S. https://doi.org/10.1093/jn/133.3.941S

Mathison, G. W. (1986). B-vitamins, choline, inositol and para aminobenzoic acid for ruminants. In 21st Annual Pacific Northwest Animal Nutrition Conference. Vancouver (pp. 107–157).

Mathison, G. W. (1989). B vitamins for ruminants. In *Proceedings of the 3rd Western Nutrition Conference* p. 125. Winnipeg, Manitoba, Canada.

Matsui, T. (2012). Vitamin C nutrition in cattle. *Asian-Australasian Journal of Animal Sciences*, *25*(5), 597–605. https://doi.org/10.5713/ajas.2012.r.01

Maurya, V. K., & Aggarwal, M. (2017). Factors influencing the absorption of vitamin D in GIT: An overview. *Journal of Food Science and Technology*, *54*(12), 3753–3765. https://doi.org/10.1007/s13197-017-2840-0

Maynard, L. A., Loosli, J. K., Hintz, H. F., & Warner, R. G. (1979). *Animal nutrition* (7th ed.). McGraw-Hill Book, Co.

Mburu, J. N., Kamau, J. M., & Badamana, M. S. (1993). Changes in serum levels of vitamin B$_{12}$, feed intake, live-weight and hematological parameters in cobalt deficient small east African goats. *International Journal for Vitamin and Nutrition Research. Internationale Zeitschrift Fur Vitamin- und Ernahrungsforschung. Journal International de Vitaminologie et de Nutrition, 63*(2), 135–139. PubMed: 8407163

McAllister, M. M., Gould, D. H., Raisbeck, M. F., Cummings, B. A., & Loneragan, G. H. (1997). Evaluation of ruminal sulfide concentrations and seasonal outbreaks of polioencephalomalacia in beef cattle in the feedlot. *Journal of the American Veterinary Medical Association, 211*(10), 1275–1279. https://doi.org/10.2460/javma.1997.211.10.1275, PubMed: 9373365

McCandless, D. W. (2010). *Thiamine deficiency and associated clinical disorders* (pp. 1–192). Humana Press.

McCay, P. B. (1985). Vitamin E: Interactions with free radicals and ascorbate. *Annual Review of Nutrition, 5*(1), 323–340. https://doi.org/10.1146/annurev.nu.05.070185.001543

McCay, P. B., Gibson, D. D., & Hornbrook, K. R. (1981). Glutathione dependent inhibition of lipid peroxidation by a soluble heat-labile factor not glutathione peroxidase. *Federation Proceedings, 40*(2), 199–205. PubMed: 7461144

McCollum, E.V. (1957) *A history of nutrition*. Houghton Mifflin Co., Boston, MA.

McCormick, C. C., & Parker, R. S. (2004). The cytotoxicity of vitamin E is both vitamer- and cell-specific and involves a selectable trait. *The Journal of Nutrition, 134*(12), 3335–3342. https://doi.org/10.1093/jn/134.12.3335

McCormick, D. B. (1990). Riboflavin. In M. L. Brown (Ed.), *Nutrition reviews, present knowledge in nutrition* (6th ed.). Washington, DC, p. 146. International Life Sci. Inst.

McCormick, D. B. (2006). Vitamin B$_6$. In B. A. Bowman & R. M. Russell (Eds.), *Present knowledge in nutrition* (9th ed.) (pp. 269–277). International Life Sciences Institute.

McDowell, L. R. (1985). *Nutrition of grazing ruminants in warm climates*. Academic Press.

McDowell, L. R. (1992). *Minerals in animal and human nutrition*. Academic Press.

McDowell, L. R. (2000a). *Vitamins in animal and human nutrition*. Iowa State University Press.

McDowell, L. R. (2000b). Reevaluation of the metabolic essentiality of the vitamins – Review -. *Asian-Australasian Journal of Animal Sciences, 13*(1), 115–125. https://doi.org/10.5713/ajas.2000.115

McDowell, L. R. (2004). Re-evaluation of the essentiality of the vitamins. In California Animal Nutrition Conference, Fresno, CA (pp. 37–67).

McDowell, L. R. (2006). Vitamin nutrition of livestock animals: Overview from vitamin discovery to today. *Canadian Journal of Animal Science, 86*(2), 171–179. https://doi.org/10.4141/A05-057

McDowell, L.R. (2013) *Vitamin history, the early years*. Design Publishing Inc. Sarasora, FL, USA.

McDowell, L. R., & Arthington, J. D. (2005). *Minerals for grazing ruminants in tropical regions* (4th ed), *2005* (pp. 1–86) [Bulletin]. University of Florida, Institute of Food and Agricultural Sciences, Department of Animal Sciences.

McDowell, L. R., Conrad, J. H., & Ellis, G. L. (1984). Mineral deficiencies and imbalances and their diagnosis. In "Symposium on Herbivore Nutrition in Sub-Tropics and Tropics-Problems and Prospects" (F.M.C. Gilchrist and R.I. Mackie, eds.). Pretoria, South Africa. p. 67.

McDowell, L. R., Williams, S. N., Hidiroglou, N., Njeru, C. A., Hill, G. M., Ochoa, L., & Wilkinson, N. S. (1996). Vitamin E supplementation for the ruminant. *Animal Feed Science and Technology, 60*(3–4), 273–296. https://doi.org/10.1016/0377-8401(96)00982-0

McDowell, L. R., Wilkinson, N., Madison, R., & Felix, T. (2007). Vitamins and minerals functioning as antioxidants with supplementation considerations. In Florida Ruminant Nutrition Symposium; Best Western Gateway Grand: Gainesville, FL, USA, 3(30–31).

McElroy, L. W., & Goss, H. (1939). Report on four members of the vitamin B complex synthesized in the rumen of the sheep. *Journal of Biological Chemistry, 130*(1), 437–438. https://doi.org/10.1016/S0021-9258(18)73603-X

McElroy, L. W., & Goss, H. (1940). A quantitative study of vitamins in the rumen contents of sheep and cows fed vitamin-low diets: I. *The Journal of Nutrition, 20*(6), 527–540. https://doi.org/10.1093/jn/22.6.527

McFadden, J. W., Girard, C. L., Tao, S., Zhou, Z., Bernard, J. K., Duplessis, M., & White, H. M. (2020). Symposium review: One-carbon metabolism and methyl donor nutrition in the dairy cow. *Journal of Dairy Science, 103*(6), 5668–5683. https://doi.org/10.3168/jds.2019-17319

McGill, J. L., Kelly, S. M., Guerra-Maupome, M., Winkley, E., Henningson, J., Narasimhan, B., & Sacco, R. E. (2019). Vitamin A deficiency impairs the immune response to intranasal vaccination and RSV infection in neonatal calves. *Scientific Reports*, 9(1), 15157. https://doi.org/10.1038/s41598-019-51684-x

McGinnis, C. H. (1986a). *Bioavailability of nutrients in feed ingredients*. National Feed Ingredient Association.

McGinnis, C. H. (1986b). Vitamin stability and activity of water-soluble vitamins as influenced by manufacturing processes and recommendations for the water-soluble vitamin. In *Bioavailability of nutrients in feed. Proceedings of the NFIA Nutrition Institute* (pp. 1–44).

McGinnis, C. H. (1988). New concepts in vitamin nutrition. In *Proceedings of the 1988 Georgia Nutrition Conference of the Feed Industry*.

McGrath, J. J., Savage, D. B., Nolan, J. V., & Elliott, R. (2012). Phosphorus and calcium retention in steers fed a roughage diet is influenced by dietary 25OH-vitamin D. *Animal Production Science*, 52(7), 636–640. https://doi.org/10.1071/AN11293

McGrath, J. J., Savage, D. B., & Godwin, I. R. (2013). The potential for pharmacological supply of 25-hydroxyvitamin D to increase phosphorus utilisation in cattle. *Animal Production Science*, 53(11), 1238–1245. https://doi.org/10.1071/AN13193

McGrath, J., Duval, S. M., Tamassia, L. F. M., Kindermann, M., Stemmler, R. T., de Gouvea, V. N., Acedo, T. S., Immig, I., Williams, S. N., & Celi, P. (2018). Nutritional strategies in ruminants: A lifetime approach. *Research in Veterinary Science*, 116, 28–39. https://doi.org/10.1016/j.rvsc.2017.09.011

McKenzie, R. A., Carmichael, A. M., Schibrowski, M. L., Duigan, S. A., Gibson, J. A., & Taylor, J. D. (2009). Sulfur-associated polioencephalomalacia in cattle grazing plants in the Family Brassicaceae. *Australian Veterinary Journal*, 87(1), 27–32. https://doi.org/10.1111/j.1751-0813.2008.00387.x

McMurray, C. H., & Rice, D. A. (1982). Vitamin E and selenium deficiency diseases. *Irish Veterinary Journal*, 36, 57–67.

McMurray, C. H., Rice, D. A., & Blanchflower, W. J. (1980). Changes in plasma levels on linoleic and linolenic acids in calves recently introduced to spring pasture. *Proceedings of the Nutrition Society*, 39, 65 [Abstr.].

McMurray, C. H., Rice, D. A., & Kennedy, S. (1983). January. Experimental models for nutritional myopathy. In *Ciba Foundation Symposium*. John Wiley & Sons, Ltd, 101-Biology of Vitamin E (201-223).

McNeil, C. J., Hay, S. M., Rucklidge, G. J., Reid, M. D., Duncan, G. J., & Rees, W. D. (2009). Maternal diets deficient in folic acid and related methyl donors modify mechanisms associated with lipid metabolism in the fetal liver of the rat. *The British Journal of Nutrition*, 102(10), 1445–1452. https://doi.org/10.1017/S0007114509990389

Meglia, G. E., Jensen, S. K., Lauridsen, C., & Persson Waller, K. P. (2006). α-Tocopherol concentration and stereoisomer composition in plasma and milk from dairy cows fed natural or synthetic vitamin E around calving. *The Journal of Dairy Research*, 73(2), 227–234. https://doi.org/10.1017/S0022029906001701

Mehansho, H., & Henderson, L. M. (1980). Transport and accumulation of pyridoxine and pyridoxal by erythrocytes. *The Journal of Biological Chemistry*, 255(24), 11901–11907. https://doi.org/10.1016/S0021-9258(19)70220-8, PubMed: 7440576

Melendez, P., Riquelme, P., & Reyes, C. (2021). Effect of rumen protected thiamine on blood concentration of beta-hydroxyl butyrate in postpartum Holstein cows: A pilot study. *Ciencia Veterinaria*, 24, 1. https://doi.org/10.19137/cienvet202224106

Mella, C. M., Perez-Oliva, O., & Loew, F. M. (1976). Induction of bovine polioencephalomalacia with a feeding system based on molasses and urea. *Canadian Journal of Comparative Medicine: Revue Canadienne de Medecine Comparee*, 40(1), 104–110. https://pubmed.ncbi.nlm.nih.gov/1000370

Mendiratta, S., Qu, Z. C., & May, J. M. (1998). Erythrocyte ascorbate recycling: Antioxidant effects in blood. *Free Radical Biology and Medicine*, 24(5), 789–797. https://doi.org/10.1016/S0891-5849(97)00351-1

Mengal, M. A., Galbraith, H., & Scaife, J. R. (1998). Effect of biotin supplementation on hoof growth of Angora and Cashmere goats. *Proceedings of the British Society of Animal Science* [Abstr.], 1998, 212–212. https://doi.org/10.1017/S1752756200598640

Merrill, Jr., A. H., & McCormick, D. B. (2020). Riboflavin. In *Present knowledge in nutrition* (pp. 189–207). Academic Press. https://doi.org/10.1016/B978-0-323-66162-1.00011-1

Merriman, K. E., Kweh, M. F., Powell, J. L., Lippolis, J. D., & Nelson, C. D. (2015). Multiple β-defensin genes are upregulated by the vitamin D pathway in cattle. *The Journal of Steroid Biochemistry and Molecular Biology*, 154, 120–129. https://doi.org/10.1016/j.jsbmb.2015.08.002

Meydani, N., & Han, S. N. (2006). Nutrient regulation of the immune response: The case of vitamin E. In B. A. Bowman & R. M. Russell (Eds.), *Present knowledge in nutrition* (9th ed.) (pp. 585–603). International Life Sciences Institute.

Meydani, S. N., & Blumberg, J. B. (2020). Vitamin E and the immune response. In *Nutrient modulation of the immune response* (pp. 223–238). CRC Press.

Meydani, S. N., Ribaya-Mercado, J. D., Russell, R. M., Sahyoun, N., Morrow, F. D., & Gershoff, S. N. (1991). Vitamin B_6 deficiency impairs interleukin 2 production and lymphocyte proliferation in elderly adults. *The American Journal of Clinical Nutrition*, 53(5), 1275–1280. https://doi.org/10.1093/ajcn/53.5.1275

Meyer, E., Lamote, I., & Burvenich, C. (2005). Retinoids and steroids in bovine mammary gland immunobiology. *Livestock Production Science*, 98(1–2), 33–46. https://doi.org/10.1016/j.livprodsci.2005.10.011

Mgongo, F. O., Gombe, S., & Ogaa, J. S. (1984). The influence of cobalt/vitamin B_{12} deficiency as a stressor affecting adrenal cortex and ovarian activities in goats. *Reproduction, Nutrition, Developpement*, 24(6), 845–854. https://doi.org/10.1051/rnd:19840703

Michal, J. J., Heirman, L. R., Wong, T. S., Chew, B. P., Frigg, M., & Volker, L. (1994). Modulatory effects of dietary carotene on blood and mammary leukocyte function in periparturient dairy cows. *Journal of Dairy Science*, 77(5), 1408–1421. https://doi.org/10.3168/jds.S0022-0302(94)77079-X

Midla, L. T., Hoblet, K. H., Weiss, W. P., & Moeschberger, M. L. (1998). Supplemental dietary biotin for prevention of lesions associated with aseptic clinical laminitis (*pododermatitis aseptica diffusa*) in primiparous Holsteins. *American Journal of Veterinary Research*, 59, 33. PubMed: 9622743

Miquel Becker, E. M., Christensen, J., Frederiksen, C. S., & Haugaard, V. K. (2003). Front-face fluorescence spectroscopy and chemometrics in analysis of yogurt: Rapid analysis of riboflavin. Journal of Dairy Science, 86(8), 2508–2515. https://doi.org/10.3168/jds.S0022-0302(03)73845-4

Miles, W. H., & McDowell, L. R. (1983). *Mineral deficiencies in the llanos rangelands of Colombia [cattle feed]. World animal review.* Food and Agriculture Organization.

Millar, K. R., Craig, J., & Dawe, L. (1973). α-Tocopherol and selenium levels in pasteurised cows' milk from different areas of New Zealand. *New Zealand Journal of Agricultural Research*, 16(2), 301–303. https://doi.org/10.1080/00288233.1973.10421149

Miller, B. L., Meiske, J. C., & Goodrich, R. D. (1986). Effects of grain source and concentrate level on B-vitamin production and absorption in steers. *Journal of Animal Science*, 62(2), 473–483. https://doi.org/10.2527/jas1986.622473x

Miller, E. R., Schmidt, D. A., Hoefer, J. A., & Luecke, R. W. (1957). The pyridoxine requirement of the baby pig. *The Journal of Nutrition*, 62(3), 406–419. https://doi.org/10.1093/jn/62.3.407

Miller, G. Y., Bartlett, P. C., Erskine, R. J., & Smith, K. L. (1995). Factors affecting serum selenium and vitamin E concentrations in dairy cows. *Journal of the American Veterinary Medical Association*, 206(9), 1369–1373. https://doi.org/10.2460/javma.1995.206.09.1369, PubMed: 7775251

Miller, J. K., Brzezinska-Slebodzinska, E., & Madsen, F. C. (1993). Oxidative stress, antioxidants and animal function. *Journal of Dairy Science*, 76(9), 2812–2823. https://doi.org/10.3168/jds.S0022-0302(93)77620-1

Miller, J. K., Campbell, M. H., Motjope, L., Cunningham, P. F., & Madsen, F. C. (1997). September. Antioxidant nutrients and reproduction in dairy cattle. In *Proceedings of the Minn. Nutr. Conf* (p. 1).

Miller, J. W., Rogerf, L. M., & Rucker, R. B. (2006). Pantothenic acid. In B. A. Bowman & R. M. Russell (Eds.), *Present knowledge in nutrition* (9th ed.) (pp. 327–339). International Life Sciences Institute, D.C.

Miller, R. H., Ffrench-Constant, C., & Raff, M. C. (1989). The macroglial cells of the rat optic nerve. *Annual Review of Neuroscience*, 12(1), 517–534. https://doi.org/10.1146/annurev.ne.12.030189.002505

Miller, R. W., Hemken, R. W., Waldo, D. R., & Moore, L. A. (1969). Effect of ethyl alcohol on the vitamin A status of Holstein heifers. *Journal of Dairy Science*, 52(12), 1998–2000. https://doi.org/10.3168/jds.S0022-0302(69)86885-2

Milligan, L. P., Asplund, J. M., & Robblee, A. R. (1967). *In vitro* studies on the role of biotin in the metabolism of rumen microorganisms. *Canadian Journal of Animal Science*, 47(1), 57–64. https://doi.org/10.4141/cjas67-008

Mirvish, S. S. (1986). Effects of vitamins C and E on N-nitroso compound formation, carcinogenesis, and cancer. *Cancer, 58*(8), 1842–1850. https://doi.org/10.1002/1097-0142(19861015)58:8+<1842::AID-CNCR282 0581410>3.0.CO;2-%23

Mishra, A., Aderao, G. N., Chaudhary, S. K., Raje, K., Singh, A., & Bisht, P. (2018). Effect of niacin supplementation on milk yield and composition during heat stress in dairy cows: A review. *Int. J. Curr. Microbiol., 6*(3), 1719–1724. E-ISSN: 2320-7078

Misir, R., & Blair, R. (1984). Effect of biotin supplementation on performance of biotin-deficient sows. *J. Ani. Sci., 59*(Suppl. 1), 254.

Mittal, P. K., Anand, M., Madan, A. K., Yadav, S., & Kumar, J. (2014). Antioxidative capacity of vitamin E, vitamin C and their combination in cryopreserved Bhadavari bull semen. *Veterinary World, 7*(12), 1127–1131. http://doi.org/10.14202/vetworld.2014.1127-1131

Miyake, N., Kim, M., & Kurata, T. (1999). Stabilization of L-ascorbic acid by superoxide dismutase and catalase. *Bioscience, Biotechnology, and Biochemistry, 63*(1), 54–57. https://doi.org/10.1271/bbb.63.54

Mizutani, A., Maki, H., Torii, Y., Hitomi, K., & Tsukagoshi, N. (1998). Ascorbate-dependent enhancement of nitric oxide formation in activated macrophages. *Nitric Oxide: Biology and Chemistry, 2*(4), 235–241. https://doi.org/10.1006/niox.1998.0182

Mizwicki, K. L. (1976). *Niacin and nitrogen metabolism in sheep* [Unpublished MSc thesis]. University of Illinois.

Mizwicki, K. L., Owens, F. N., Isaacson, H. R., & Shockey, B. (1975). Supplemental niacin for lambs. *Journal of Animal Science, 41*, 411 [Abstr.].

Mladěnka, P., Macáková, K., Kujovská Krčmová, L., Javorská, L., Mrštná, K., Carazo, A., Protti, M., Remião, F., Nováková, L. and OEMONOM Researchers and Collaborators (2022) Vitamin K–sources, physiological role, kinetics, deficiency, detection, therapeutic use, and toxicity. Nutr. Rev. 80(4):677-698. https://doi.org/10.1093/nutrit/nuab061

Mock, D. M. (1990). Biotin. In R. E. Olson (Ed.) Nutritional Foundation, *Nutrition reviews, present knowledge in nutrition*.

Mock, D. M. (1991). Skin manifestations of biotin deficiency. *Seminars in Dermatology, 10*(4), 296–302. PubMed: 1764357

Mock, D. M. (1996). In E. E. Ziegler & L. J. Filer, Jr. (Eds.). *Present knowledge in nutrition* (7th ed.) (pp. 220–235). International Life Sciences Institute Research Foundation Press, DC1996

Mock, D. M. (2013). Biotin. In J. Zempleni, J. Suttie, J. Gregory, & P. J. Stover (Eds.), *Handbook of vitamins* (5th ed.) (pp. 397–420). CRC Press, Taylor & Francis Group.

Mock, D. M., & Malik, M. I. (1992). Distribution of biotin in human plasma: Most of the biotin is not bound to protein. *The American Journal of Clinical Nutrition, 56*(2), 427–432. https://doi.org/10.1093/ajcn/56.2.427

Mock, N. I., & Mock, D. M. (1992). Biotin deficiency in rats: Disturbances of leucine metabolism are detectable early. *The Journal of Nutrition, 122*(7), 1493–1499. https://doi.org/10.1093/jn/122.7.1493

Moghimi-Kandelousi, M., Alamouti, A. A., Imani, M., & Zebeli, Q. (2020). A meta-analysis and meta-regression of the effects of vitamin E supplementation on serum enrichment, udder health, milk yield, and reproductive performance of transition cows. *Journal of Dairy Science, 103*(7), 6157–6166. https://doi.org/10.3168/jds.2019-17556

Mohammed, R., & Lamand, M. (1986). Cardiovascular lesions in cobalt-vitamin B_{12} deficient sheep. *Annales de Recherches Veterinaires. Annals of Veterinary Research, 17*(4), 447–450. https://hal.science/hal-00901681

Mohri, M., Seifi, H. A., & Khodadadi, J. (2005). Effects of preweaning parenteral supplementation of vitamin E and selenium on hematology, serum proteins, and weight gain in dairy calves. *Comparative Clinical Pathology, 14*(3), 149–154. https://doi.org/10.1007/s00580-005-0581-3

Molina, P. E., Myers, N., Smith, R. M., Lang, C. H., Yousef, K. A., Tepper, P. G., & Abumrad, N. N. (1994). Nutritional and metabolic characterization of a thiamine-deficient rat model. *JPEN. Journal of Parenteral and Enteral Nutrition, 18*(2), 104–111. https://doi.org/10.1177/0148607194018002104

Monegue, J. S. (2013). *Evaluation of the effects of vitamin K on growth performance and bone health in swine*. https://uknowledge.uky.edu/animalsci_etds/26/ [Unpublished Doctorate dissertation].

Montgomery, J. L., Parrish, Jr., F. C., Beitz, D. C., Horst, R. L., Huff-Lonergan, E. J., & Trenkle, A. H. (2000). The use of vitamin D₃ to improve beef tenderness. *Journal of Animal Science, 78*(10), 2615–2621. https://doi.org/10.2527/2000.78102615x

Montgomery, J. L., Carr, M. A., Kerth, C. R., Hilton, G. G., Price, B. P., Galyean, M. L., Horst, R. L., & Miller, M. F. (2002). Effect of vitamin D₃ supplementation level on the postmortem tenderization of beef from steers. *Journal of Animal Science, 80*(4), 971–981. https://doi.org/10.2527/2002.804971x

Montgomery, J. L., Blanton, Jr., J. R., Horst, R. L., Galyean, M. L., Morrow, Jr., K. J., Wester, D. B., & Miller, M. F. (2004). Effects of biological type of beef steers on vitamin D, calcium, and phosphorus status. *Journal of Animal Science, 82*(7), 2043–2049. https://doi.org/10.2527/2004.8272043x

Mora, O., Romano, J. L., González, E., Ruiz, F. J., & Shimada, A. (1999). *In vitro* and *in situ* disappearance of beta-carotene and lutein from lucerne (*Medicago sativa*) hay in bovine and caprine ruminal fluids. *Journal of the Science of Food and Agriculture, 79*(2), 273–276. https://doi.org/10.1002/(SICI)1097-0010(199902)79:2<273::AID-JSFA191>3.0.CO;2-V

Mora, O., Romano, J. L., Gonzalez, E., Ruiz, F., & Shimada, A. (2000). Low cleavage activity of 15,15' dioxygenase to convert β-carotene to retinal in cattle compared with goats, is associated with the yellow pigmentation of adipose tissue. *International Journal for Vitamin and Nutrition Research. Internationale Zeitschrift Fur Vitamin- und Ernahrungsforschung. Journal International de Vitaminologie et de Nutrition, 70*(5), 199–205. https://doi.org/10.1024/0300-9831.70.5.199

Moreiras, o., Carbajal, A., Cabrera, L., & Cuadrado, C. (2013). Tablas de composición de alimentos. Editorial pirámide (16th ed.).

Morgante, M., Beghelli, D., Pauselli, M., Dall'Ara, P., Capuccella, M., & Ranucci, S. (1999). Effect of administration of vitamin E and selenium during the dry period on mammary health and milk cell counts in dairy ewes. *Journal of Dairy Science, 82*(3), 623–631. https://doi.org/10.3168/jds.S0022-0302(99)75276-8

Mori, M., Padilla, L., Matsui, T., Yano, H., Matsui, Y., & Yamada, H. (2006). *Effects of vitamin C supplementation on plasma vitamin C level and fattening traits in Japanese Black cattle on a fattening farm.* Bull. Beef cattle sci, 81, 15–19.

Moriguchi, S., & Kaneyasu, M. (2004). Role of vitamin E in immune system. *Journal of Clinical Biochemistry and Nutrition, 34*(3), 97–109. https://doi.org/10.3164/jcbn.34.97

Moriguchi, S., & Muraga, M. (2000). Vitamin E and immunity. *Vitamins and Hormones, 59*, 305–336. https://doi.org/10.1016/S0083-6729(00)59011-6

Morrill, J. L., & Reddy, P. G. (1987). Evaluation of a calf starter supplement. *Kansas Agricultural Experiment Station Research Reports, 0*(2), 50–52. https://doi.org/10.4148/2378-5977.3035

Morris, K. M. L. (1982). Plant induced calcinosis: A review. *Veterinary and Human Toxicology, 24*(1), 34–48. PubMed: 6277082

Morris, M. S., Sakakeeny, L., Jacques, P. F., Picciano, M. F., & Selhub, J. (2010). Vitamin B₆ intake is inversely related to, and the requirement is affected by, inflammation status. *The Journal of Nutrition, 140*(1), 103–110. https://doi.org/10.3945/jn.109.114397

Morrison, E. I., Reinhardt, H., Leclerc, H., DeVries, T. J., & LeBlanc, S. J. (2018). Effect of rumen-protected B vitamins and choline supplementation on health, production, and reproduction in transition dairy cows. *Journal of Dairy Science, 101*(10), 9016–9027. https://doi.org/10.3168/jds.2018-14663

Morrissey, P. A., & Sheehy, P. J. A. (1999). Optimal nutrition: Vitamin E. *The Proceedings of the Nutrition Society, 58*(2), 459–468. https://doi.org/10.1017/S0029665199000609

Moser, U., & Bendich, A. (1991). Vitamin C. In L. J. Machlin (Ed.), *Handbook of vitamins* (2nd ed.) (p. 195). Marcel Dekker.

Muggli, R. (1994). Physiological requirements of vitamin E as a function of the amount and type of polyunsaturated fatty acid. *World Review of Nutrition and Dietetics, 75*, 166–168. https://doi.org/10.1159/000423574

Mujica-Álvarez, J., Gil-Castell, O., Barra, P. A., Ribes-Greus, A., Bustos, R., Faccini, M., & Matiacevich, S. (2020). Encapsulation of vitamins A and E as spray-dried additives for the feed industry. *Molecules, 25*(6), 1357. https://doi.org/10.3390/molecules25061357

Mullenax, C. H., Baumann, L. E., McDowell, L. R., & Norman, B. B. (1992). Secadera. *American Association of Bovine Practitioners Conference Proceedings. Am. Ass. Bovine Pract. Conference Proceedings, 2*, 57–62. https://doi.org/10.21423/aabppro19926488

Muller, L. D., Heinrichs, A. J., Cooper, J. B., & Atkin, Y. H. (1986). Supplemental niacin for lactating cows during summer feeding. *Journal of Dairy Science, 69*(5), 1416–1420. https://doi.org/10.3168/jds.S0022-0302(86)80549-5

Mülling, C. K., Bragulla, H. H., Reese, S., Budras, K. D., & Steinberg, W. (1999). How structures in bovine hoof epidermis are influenced by nutritional factors. *Anatomia, Histologia, Embryologia, 28*(2), 103–108. https://doi.org/10.1046/j.1439-0264.1999.00180.x

von Muralt, A. (1962). The role of thiamine in neurophysiology. *Annals of the New York Academy of Sciences, 98*(2), 499–507. https://doi.org/10.1111/j.1749-6632.1962.tb30571.x

Muri, C., Schottstedt, T., Hammon, H. M., Meyer, E., & Blum, J. W. (2005). Hematological, metabolic, and endocrine effects of feeding vitamin A and lactoferrin in neonatal calves. *Journal of Dairy Science, 88*(3), 1062–1077. https://doi.org/10.3168/jds.S0022-0302(05)72774-0

Muth, O. H. (1955). White muscle disease (myopathy) in lambs and calves. I. Occurrence and nature of the disease under Oregon conditions. *Journal of the American Veterinary Medical Association, 126*(938), 355–361.

Nabokina, S. M., Kashyap, M. L., & Said, H. M. (2005). Mechanism and regulation of human intestinal niacin uptake. *American Journal of Physiology. Cell Physiology, 289*(1), C97–C103. https://doi.org/10.1152/ajpcell.00009.2005

Nagaraj, R. Y., Wu, W. D., & Vesonder, R. F. (1994). Toxicity of corn culture material of Fusarium proliferatum M-7176 and nutritional intervention in chicks. *Poultry Science, 73*(5), 617–626. https://doi.org/10.3382/ps.0730617

Naito, Y., Shindo, N., Sato, R., & Murakami, D. (1990). Plasma osteocalcin in preparturient and postparturient cows: Correlation with plasma 1,25-dihydroxyvitamin D, calcium and inorganic phosphorus. *Journal of Dairy Science, 73*(12), 3481–3484. https://doi.org/10.3168/jds.S0022-0302(90)79047-9

Nakagawa, K., Shibata, A., Yamashita, S., Tsuzuki, T., Kariya, J., Oikawa, S., & Miyazawa, T. (2007). *In vivo* angiogenesis is suppressed by unsaturated vitamin E, tocotrienol. *The Journal of Nutrition, 137*(8), 1938–1943. https://doi.org/10.1093/jn/137.8.1938

Nakano, H., & Gregory, J. F. (1995). Pyridoxine and pyridoxine-5'-β-D-glucoside exert different effects on tissue B$_6$ vitamers but similar effects on β-glucosidase activity in rats. *The Journal of Nutrition, 125*(11), 2751–2762. https://doi.org/10.1093/jn/125.11.2751

Nakano, H., McMahon, L. G., & Gregory, J. F. (1997). Pyridoxine-5'-beta-glucoside exhibits incomplete bioavailability as a source of vitamin B$_6$ and partially inhibits the utilization of co-ingested pyridoxine in humans. *The Journal of Nutrition, 127*(8), 1508–1513. https://doi.org/10.1093/jn/127.8.1508

Nam, K. C., & Ahn, D. U. (2003). Effects of ascorbic acid and antioxidants on the color of irradiated ground beef. *Journal of Food Science, 68*(5), 1686–1690. https://doi.org/10.1111/j.1365-2621.2003.tb12314.x

Naresh, R., Dwivedi, S. K., Swarup, D., & Patra, R. C. (2002). Evaluation of ascorbic acid treatment in clinical and subclinical mastitis of Indian dairy cows. *Asian-Australasian Journal of Animal Sciences, 15*(6), 905–911. https://doi.org/10.5713/ajas.2002.905

Narkewicz, M. R., Jones, G., Thompson, H., Kolhouse, F., & Fennessey, P. V. (2002). Folate cofactors regulate serine metabolism in fetal ovine hepatocytes. *Pediatric Research, 52*(4), 589–594. https://doi.org/10.1203/00006450-200210000-00020

NASEM (National Academy of Sciences Engineering and Medicine). (2021). *Nutrient requirements of dairy cattle eighth* (rev. ed.). The National Academies Press. https://doi.org/10.17226/25806

National Health and Medical Research Council of Autralia and New Zealand (NHMRC). (2006). *Nutrient reference values for Australia and New Zealand including recommended dietary intakes.* http://www.nrv.gov.au/_resources/n35-vitamine.pdf. (*Referenced.* 04/12/2008).

Ndiweni, N., & Finch, J. M. (1995). Effects of *in vitro* supplementation of bovine mammary gland macrophages and peripheral blood lymphocytes with α-tocopherol and sodium selenite: Implications for udder defences. *Veterinary Immunology and Immunopathology, 47*(1–2), 111–121. https://doi.org/10.1016/0165-2427(94)05382-3

Ndiweni, N., & Finch, J. M. (1996). Effects of *in vitro* supplementation with tocopherol and selenium on bovine neutrophil functions: Implications for resistance to mastitis. *Veterinary Immunology and Immunopathology, 51*(1–2), 67–78. https://doi.org/10.1016/0165-2427(95)05515-0

Neill, A. R., Grime, D. W., Snoswell, A. M., Northrop, A. J., Lindsay, D. B., & Dawson, R. M. C. (1979). The low availability of dietary choline for the nutrition of the sheep. *The Biochemical Journal, 180*(3), 559–565. https://doi.org/10.1042/bj1800559

Nelsestuen, G. L., Zytkovicz, T. H., & Howard, J. B. (1974). The mode of action of vitamin K. Identification of gamma-carboxyglutamic acid as a component of prothrombin. *The Journal of Biological Chemistry, 249*(19), 6347–6350. https://doi.org/10.1016/S0021-9258(19)42259-X

Nelson, C. D., & Merriman, K. E. (2014). *Vitamin D metabolism in dairy cattle and implications for dietary requirements.*

Nelson, C. D., Reinhardt, T. A., Thacker, T. C., Beitz, D. C., & Lippolis, J. D. (2010). Modulation of the bovine innate immune response by production of 1α, 25-dihydroxyvitamin D_3 in bovine monocytes. *Journal of Dairy Science, 93*(3), 1041–1049. https://doi.org/10.3168/jds.2009-2663

Nelson, C. D., Reinhardt, T. A., Lippolis, J. D., Sacco, R. E., & Nonnecke, B. J. (2012). Vitamin D signaling in the bovine immune system: A model for understanding human vitamin D requirements. *Nutrients, 4*(3), 181–196. https://doi.org/10.3390/nu4030181

Nelson, C. D., Powell, J. L., Price, D. M., Hersom, M. J., Yelich, J. V., Drewnoski, M. E., Bird, S. L., & Bridges, G. A. (2016a). Assessment of serum 25-hydroxyvitamin D concentrations of beef cows and calves across seasons and geographical locations. *Journal of Animal Science, 94*(9), 3958–3965. https://doi.org/10.2527/jas.2016-0611

Nelson, C. D., Lippolis, J. D., Reinhardt, T. A., Sacco, R. E., Powell, J. L., Drewnoski, M. E., O'Neil, M., Beitz, D. C., & Weiss, W. P. (2016b). Vitamin D status of dairy cattle: Outcomes of current practices in the dairy industry. *Journal of Dairy Science, 99*(12), 10150–10160. https://doi.org/10.3168/jds.2016-11727

Nelson, C. D., Merriman, K. E., Poindexter, M. B., Kweh, M. F., & Blakely, L. P. (2018). Symposium review: Targeting antimicrobial defenses of the udder through an intrinsic cellular pathway. *Journal of Dairy Science, 101*(3), 2753–2761. https://doi.org/10.3168/jds.2017-13426

Nesheim, R. O., & Johnson, B. C. (1950). Effect of a high level of methionine on the dietary choline requirement of the baby pig. *The Journal of Nutrition, 41*(1), 149–152. https://doi.org/10.1093/jn/41.1.149

Nestor, K. E., & Conrad, H. R. (1990). Metabolism of vitamin K and influence on prothrombin time in milk-fed preruminant calves. *Journal of Dairy Science, 73*(11), 3291–3296. https://doi.org/10.3168/jds.S0022-0302(90)79022-4

New Zealand legislation. (2019). *Climate change response (zero carbon) amendment act.* https://www.legislation.govt.nz/act/public/2019/0061/latest/LMS183848.html#LMS183790

Nguyen, D. V., Nguyen, O. C., & Malau-Aduli, A. E. O. (2021). Main regulatory factors of marbling level in beef cattle. *Veterinary and Animal Science, 14*, 100219. https://doi.org/10.1016/j.vas.2021.100219

Niehues, M. B., Perdigão, A., de Carvalho, V. V., Acedo, T., Vasconcellos, G. S. F. M., Tamassia, L. F., Martins, C., Millen, D., & Arrigoni, M. (2020). *Feeding essential oils and α-amylase or its association with25-hydroxyvitamin-D3 improves productive performance by feedlot cattle.* ASAS-CSAS-WSASAS virtual annual meeting [Abstract].

Niki, E. (2016). Oxidative stress and antioxidants: Distress or estress? *Archives of Biochemistry and Biophysics, 595*, 19–24. https://doi.org/10.1016/j.abb.2015.11.017

Nisar, M., Beigh, S. A., Mir, A. Q., Hussain, S. A., Dar, A. A., Yatoo, I., & Khan, A. M. (2024). Association of vitamin D status with redox balance and insulin resistance and its predicting ability for subclinical pregnancy toxemia in pregnant sheep. *Domestic Animal Endocrinology, 86*, 106823. https://doi.org/10.1016/j.domaniend.2023.106823

Njeru, C. A., McDowell, L. R., Wilkinson, N. S., Linda, S. B., & Williams, S. N. (1994a). Pre-and postpartum supplemental DL-α-tocopheryl acetate effects on placental and mammary vitamin E transfer in sheep. *Journal of Animal Science, 72*(6), 1636–1640. https://doi.org/10.2527/1994.7261636x

Njeru, C. A., McDowell, L. R., Wilkinson, N. S., & Williams, S. N. (1994b). Assessment of vitamin E nutritional status in sheep. *Journal of Animal Science, 72*(12), 3207–3212. https://doi.org/10.2527/1994.721 23207x

Njeru, C. A., McDowell, L. R., Shireman, R. M., Wilkinson, N. S., Rojas, L. X., & Williams, S. N. (1995). Assessment of vitamin E nutritional status in yearling beef heifers. *Journal of Animal Science, 73*(5), 1440–1448. https://doi.org/10.2527/1995.7351440x

Noble, R. C., Moore, J. H., & Harfoot, C. G. (1974). Observations on the pattern on biohydrogenation of ester-ified and unesterified linoleic acid in the rumen. *The British Journal of Nutrition*, *31*(1), 99–108. https://doi.org/10.1079/BJN19740012

Nockels, C. F. (1988). The role of vitamins in modulating disease resistance. *The Veterinary Clinics of North America. Food Animal Practice*, 4(3), 531–542. https://doi.org/10.1016/S0749-0720(15)31030-6

Nockels, C. F. (1990). Mineral alterations associated with stress, trauma and infection and the effect on immunity. Cont. Educ. *Practicing Veterinarian*, *12*(8), 1133–1139. ISSN: 0193-1903.

Nonnecke, B. J., Horst, R. L., Waters, W. R., Dubeski, P., & Harp, J. A. (1999). Modulation of fat-soluble vitamin concentrations and blood mononuclear leukocyte populations in milk replacer-fed calves by dietary vitamin A and beta-carotene. *Journal of Dairy Science*, *82*(12), 2632–2641. https://doi.org/10.3168/jds.S0022-0302(99)75520-7

Nonnecke, B. J., Roberts, M. P., Godkin, J. D., Horst, R. L., Hammell, D. C., & Franklin, S. T. (2001). Influence of supplemental, dietary vitamin A on retinol-binding protein concentrations in the plasma of preruminant calves. *Journal of Dairy Science*, *84*(3), 641–648. https://doi.org/10.3168/jds.S0022-0302(01)74519-5

Nonnecke, B. J., Foote, M. R., Miller, B. L., Beitz, D. C., & Horst, R. L. (2010). Short communication: Fat-soluble vitamin and mineral status of milk replacer-fed dairy calves: Effect of growth rate during the prerumi-nant period. *Journal of Dairy Science*, *93*(6), 2684–2690. https://doi.org/10.3168/jds.2009-2892

Nonnecke, B. J., McGill, J. L., Ridpath, J. F., Sacco, R. E., Lippolis, J. D., & Reinhardt, T. A. (2014). Acute phase response elicited by experimental bovine diarrhea virus (BVDV) infection is associated with decreased vitamin D and E status of vitamin-replete preruminant calves. *Journal of Dairy Science*, *97*(9), 5566–5579. https://doi.org/10.3168/jds.2014-8293

Norman, A. W. (2006). Minireview: Vitamin D receptor: New assignments for an already busy receptor. *Endocrinology*, *147*(12), 5542–5548. https://doi.org/10.1210/en.2006-0946

Norman, A. W., & Henry, H. C. (2007). Vitamin D. In J. Zempleni, R. B. Rucker, D. B. McCormick, & J. W. Suttle (Eds.), *Handbook of vitamins* (4th ed.) (pp. 47–99). CRC Press.

Norrman, J., David, C. W., Sauter, S. N., Hammon, H. M., & Blum, J. W. (2003). Effects of dexamethasone on lymphoid tissue in the gut and thymus of neonatal calves fed with colostrum and milk replacer. *Journal of Animal Science*, *81*(9), 2322–2332. https://doi.org/10.2527/2003.8192322x

Nozière, P., Graulet, B., Lucas, A., Martin, B., Grolier, P., & Doreau, M. (2006). Carotenoids for ruminants: From forages to dairy products. *Animal Feed Science and Technology*, *131*(3–4), 418–450. https://doi.org/10.1016/j.anifeedsci.2006.06.018

NRC. (1979). *Nutrient requirements of domestic animals: Nutrient requirements of swine 9th* (rev. ed.). National Academies.

NRC. (1980). Mineral tolerance of domestic animals. *National Academy of Sciences-National Research Council, Washington DC*. https://doi.org/10.17226/25

NRC. (1981). Nutrient requirements of domestic animals: Nutrient requirements of goats. *National Academy of Sciences-National Research Council, Washington DC*. https://doi.org/10.17226/30

NRC. (1982). United States-Canadian tables of feed composition. *Third* (rev. ed.) National Academy of Sciences- National Research Council. *Washington, D.C.*. https://doi.org/10.17226/1713

NRC. (1983). *Selenium in nutrition* (rev. ed.). National Academies Press. https://doi.org/10.17226/40

NRC. (1985). Nutrient requirements of sheep (Sixth Rev. Ed.). *National Academy of Sciences-National Research Council, Washington, DC*.

NRC. (1987). Vitamin tolerance of domestic animals. Natl. Academ. Press. Washington DC. https://doi.org/10.17226/949

NRC. (1989). Nutrient requirements of dairy cattle. 6th (rev. ed.) Natl. Academ. Press. Washington DC.

NRC. (1996). *Nutrient requirements of beef cattle*. 7th (rev. ed.) Natl. Academ. Press. Washington DC. https://doi.org/10.17226/9791

NRC. (1998). *Nutrient requirements of domestic animals: Nutrient requirements of swine 10th* (rev. ed.) Natl. Academ. Press. Washington DC. https://doi.org/10.17226/6016

NRC. (2000). *Nutrient requirements of beef cattle*. 7th (rev. ed.): update. Natl. Academ. Press. Washington DC. https://doi.org/10.17226/9791

NRC. (2001). *Nutrient requirements of dairy cattle*. 7th (rev. ed.) Natl. Academ. Press. Washington DC. https://doi.org/10.17226/9825

NRC. (2016). *Nutrient Requirements of Beef Cattle: 8th* (rev. ed.). Natl. Academ. Press. Washington DC. https://doi.org/10.17226/19014

NRC. (2007). *Committee on Nutrient Requirements of Small Ruminants Nutrient requirements of small ruminants: Sheep, goats, cervids, and new world camelids*. Natl. Academ. Press. Washington DC. https://doi.org/10.17226/11654

Nunnery, G. A., Galyean, M. L., Harris, S. C., Sayler, G. B., & Defoor, P. J. (1999). Effects of source and level of ruminally protected choline on performance and carcass characteristics of finishing beef steers. *Journal of Animal Science, 77*(Suppl. 1), 273–282.

O'Byrne, S. M., & Blaner, W. S. (2013). Retinol and retinyl esters: Biochemistry and physiology. *Journal of Lipid Research, 54*(7), 1731–1743. https://doi.org/10.1194/jlr.R037648

Oetzel, G. R., Olson, J. D., Curtis, C. R., & Fettman, M. J. (1988). Ammonium chloride and ammonium sulfate for prevention of parturient paresis in dairy cows. *Journal of Dairy Science, 71*(12), 3302–3309. https://doi.org/10.3168/jds.S0022-0302(88)79935-X

Oka, A., Dohgo, T., Juen, M., & Saito, T. (1997). Effects of vitamin A on beef quality, weight gain, and serum concentrations of thyroid hormones, insulin-like growth factor-I, and insulin in Japanese Black steers. *Animal Science and Technology (Jpn), 69*(2), 90–99.

Oka, A., Maruo, Y., Miki, T., Yamasaki, T., & Saito, T. (2018). Influence of vitamin A on the quality of beef from the Tajima strain of Japanese Black cattle. *Meat Science, 48*(1–2), 159–167. https://doi.org/10.1016/S0309-1740(97)00086-7

Okada, K. A., Carrillo, B. J., & Tilley, M. (1977). *Solanum malacoxylon* Sendtner: A toxic plant in Argentina. *Economic Botany, 31*(2), 225–236. https://doi.org/10.1007/BF02866593

Oldfield, J. E. (1987). History of nutrition: Development of the concept of antimetabolites. Introduction [Introduction]. *The Journal of Nutrition, 117*(7), 1322–1323. https://doi.org/10.1093/jn/117.7.1322

Oldham, E. R., Eberhart, R. J., & Muller, L. D. (1991). Effects of supplemental vitamin A or carotene during the dry period and early lactation on udder health. *Journal of Dairy Science, 74*(11), 3775–3781. https://doi.org/10.3168/jds.S0022-0302(91)78569-X

Olivares, M., Pizarro, F., Pineda, O., Name, J. J., Hertrampf, E., & Walter, T. (1997). Milk inhibits and ascorbic acid favors ferrous bis-glycine chelate bioavailability in humans. *The Journal of Nutrition, 127*(7), 1407–1411. https://doi.org/10.1093/jn/127.7.1407

Olkowski, A. A., Gooneratne, S. R., & Christensen, D. A. (1990). Effects of diets of high sulphur content and varied concentrations of copper, molybdenum and thiamine on *in vitro* phagocytic and candidacidal activity of neutrophils in sheep. *Research in Veterinary Science, 48*(1), 82–86. https://doi.org/10.1016/S0034-5288(18)31514-5

Olkowski, A. A., Christensen, D. A., & Gooneratne, S. R. (1991). The effects of copper status on thiamine metabolism in sheep fed a high sulfur diet. *Canadian Journal of Animal Science, 71*(3), 813–824. https://doi.org/10.4141/cjas91-096

Ollilainen, V.-M. (1999). HPLC analysis of vitamin B_6 in foods. *Agricultural and Food Science, 8*(6), 515–619. https://doi.org/10.23986/afsci.5632

Olson, J. A. (1984). Vitamin A. In L. J. Machlin (Ed.), *Handbook of vitamins*. Marcel Dekker, Inc.

Olson, R. E. (1973). Vitamin E and its relation to heart disease. *Circulation, 48*(1), 179–184. https://doi.org/10.1161/01.cir.48.1.179

Olson, R. E. (1990). Pantothenic acid. In R. E. Olson (Ed.), *Nutrition reviews, present knowledge in nutrition*. Nutrition Foundation, p. 208.

Oltjen, R. R., Sirny, R. J., & Tillman, A. D. (1962). Effects of B vitamins and mineral mixtures upon growth and rumen function of ruminants fed purified diets. *The Journal of Nutrition, 77*(3), 269–277. https://doi.org/10.1093/jn/77.3.269

Omur, A., Kirbas, A., Aksu, E., Kandemir, F., Dorman, E., Kaynar, O., & Ucar, O. (2016). Effects of antioxidant vitamins (A, D, E) and trace elements (Cu, Mn, Se, Zn) on some metabolic and reproductive profiles in dairy cows during transition period. *Polish Journal of Veterinary Sciences, 19*(4), 697–706. https://doi.org/10.1515/pjvs-2016-0088

Oohashi, H., Takizawa, H., & Matsui, M. (2000). Effect of vitamin C administration on the improvement of the meat quality in Japanese Black steers. *Research Bulletin of the Aichi-Ken Agricultural Research Center*, *32*, 207–214.

Overfield, J. R., & Hatfield, E. E. (1976). Dietary niacin for steers fed corn silage diets. *Journal of Animal Science*, *43*, 329.

Padh, H. (1991). Vitamin C: Newer insights into its biochemical functions. *Nutrition Reviews*, *49*(3), 65–70. https://doi.org/10.1111/j.1753-4887.1991.tb07407.x

Padilla, L., Matsui, T., Kamiya, Y., Kamiya, M., Tanaka, M., & Yano, H. (2006). Heat stress decreases plasma vitamin C concentration in lactating cows. *Livestock Science*, *101*(1–3), 300–304. https://doi.org/10.1016/j.livprodsci.2005.12.002

Padilla, L., Matsui, T., Ikeda, S., Kitagawa, M., & Yano, H. (2007). The effect of vitamin C supplementation on plasma concentration and urinary excretion of vitamin C in cattle. *Journal of Animal Science*, *85*(12), 3367–3370. https://doi.org/10.2527/jas.2007-0060

Palagina, N. K., Meledina, T. V., & Karpisheva, I. A. (1990). Simplified method for determining pantothenic acid in molasses. *Applied Biochemistry and Microbiology*, *26*, 688.

Palludan, B., & Wegger, I. (1984). Plasma ascorbic acid in calves. In I. Wegger, F. Tagwerker, & J. Moustgaard (Eds.), *Ascorbic acid in domestic animals* (pp. 131–138). Royal Danish Agricultural Society.

Pan, X. H., Yang, L., Xue, F. G., Xin, H. R., Jiang, L. S., Xiong, B. H., & Beckers, Y. (2016). Relationship between thiamine and subacute ruminal acidosis induced by a high-grain diet in dairy cows. *Journal of Dairy Science*, *99*(11), 8790–8801. https://doi.org/10.3168/jds.2016-10865

Pan, X. H., Yang, L., Beckers, Y., Xue, F. G., Tang, Z. W., Jiang, L. S., & Xiong, B. H. (2017). Thiamine supplementation facilitates thiamine transporter expression in the rumen epithelium and attenuates high-grain-induced inflammation in low-yielding dairy cows. *Journal of Dairy Science*, *100*(7), 5329–5342. https://doi.org/10.3168/jds.2016-11966

Pan, X. H., Nan, X., Yang, L., Jiang, L., & Xiong, B. (2018). Thiamine status, metabolism and application in dairy cows: A review. *The British Journal of Nutrition*, *120*(5), 491–499. https://doi.org/10.1017/S0007114518001666

Panagabko, C., Morley, S., Neely, S., Lei, H., Manor, D., & Atkinson, J. (2002). Expression and refolding of recombinant human alpha-tocopherol transfer protein capable of specific alpha-tocopherol binding. *Protein Expression and Purification*, *24*(3), 395–403. https://doi.org/10.1006/prep.2001.1576

Panda, D. K., Miao, D., Tremblay, M. L., Sirois, J., Farookhi, R., Hendy, G. N., & Goltzman, D. (2001). Targeted ablation of the 25-hydroxyvitamin D 1alpha-hydroxylase enzyme: Evidence for skeletal, reproductive, and immune dysfunction. *Proceedings of the National Academy of Sciences of the United States of America*, *98*(13), 7498–7503. https://doi.org/10.1073/pnas.131029498

Panda, S., Panda, N., Panigrahy, K. K., Gupta, S. K., Mishra, S. P., & Laishram, M. (2017). Role of niacin supplementation in dairy cattle: A review. *Asian Journal of Dairy and Food Research*, *36*(2), 93–99. https://doi.org/10.18805/ajdfr.v36i02.7949

Panganamala, R. V., & Cornwell, D. G. (1982). The effects of vitamin E on arachidonic acid metabolism. *Annals of the New York Academy of Sciences*, *393*, 376–391. https://doi.org/10.1111/j.1749-6632.1982.tb31277.x

Pappu, A. S., Fatterpaker, P., & Sreenivasan, A. (1978). Possible interrelationships between vitamins E and B$_{12}$ in the disturbance in methylmalonate metabolism in vitamin E deficiency. *The Biochemical Journal*, *172*(1), 115–121. https://doi.org/10.1042/bj1720115

Park, S. J., Beak, S. H., Jung, D. J. S., Kim, S. Y., Jeong, I. H., Piao, M. Y., Kang, H. J., Fassah, D. M., Na, S. W., Yoo, S. P., & Baik, M. (2018). Genetic, management, and nutritional factors affecting intramuscular fat deposition in beef cattle—A review. *Asian-Australasian Journal of Animal Sciences*, *31*(7), 1043–1061. https://doi.org/10.5713/ajas.18.0310

Parker, R. S. (1989). Dietary and biochemical aspects of vitamin E. *Advances in Food and Nutrition Research*, *33*, 157–232. https://doi.org/10.1016/S1043-4526(08)60128-X

Parsons, J. L., & Klostermann, H. J. (1967). Dakota scientists report new antibiotic found in flaxseed. *Feedstuffs*, *39*(45), 74.

Pascoe, G. A., & Reed, D. J. (1989). Cell calcium, vitamin E, and the thiol redox system in cytotoxicity. *Free Radical Biology and Medicine*, *6*(2), 209–224. https://doi.org/10.1016/0891-5849(89)90118-4

Patel, B. M., Patel, C. A., & Shukla, P. C. (1966). Effect of drying and storage on the carotene content and other constituents in lucerne. *Indian J. Vet. Sci. Anim. Husb, 36*, 124–129.

Paterson, J. E., & MacPherson, A. (1990). The influence of a low cobalt intake on the neutrophil function and severity of *Ostertagia* infection in cattle. *The British Veterinary Journal, 146*(6), 519–530. https://doi.org/10.1016/0007-1935(90)90055-8

Patterson, H.H., Johnson, P.S. and Epperson, W.B. (2003) Effect of total dissolved solids and sulfates in drinking water for growing steers. Proceedings Wester section, American Society of Animal Science. 54

Patterson, K. Y., Duvall, M. L., Howe, J. C., & Holden, J. M. (2011). USDA nutrient data set for retail beef cuts. http://www.researchgate.net/publication/237518570_USDA_Nutrient_Data_Set_for_Retail_Beef_Cuts

Paul, S. S., & Dey, A. (2015). Nutrition in health and immune function of ruminants. *The Indian Journal of Animal Sciences, 85*(2), 103–112. http://doi.org/10.56093/ijans.v85i2.46557

Paulson, S. K., & Langman, C. B. (1990). Plasma vitamin D metabolite levels in pregnant and nonpregnant ewes. *Comparative Biochemistry and Physiology. A, Comparative Physiology, 96*(2), 347–349. https://doi.org/10.1016/0300-9629(90)90703-u

Pearson, P. B., Struglia, L., & Lindahl, I. L. (1953). The fecal and urinary excretion of certain B vitamins by sheep fed hay and semi-synthetic rations. *Journal of Animal Science, 12*(1), 213–218. https://doi.org/10.2527/jas1953.121213x

Peng, D. Q., Lee, J. S., Kim, W. S., Kim, Y. S., Bae, M. H., Jo, Y. H., Oh, Y. K., Baek, Y. C., Hwang, S. G., & Lee, H. G. (2019). Effect of vitamin A restriction on carcass traits and blood metabolites in Korean native steers. *Animal Production Science, 59*(12), 2138–2146. https://doi.org/10.1071/AN17733

Perry, T. W. (1980). *Beef cattle feeding and nutrition*. Academic Press.

Pethes, G., Rudas, P., & Huszenicza, G. (1985). Conversion of thyroxine to triiodothyronine in liver biopsy samples of beta-carotene and vitamin A supplemented dairy cows. Zbl. *Veterinary Medicine A, 32*, 512–517. https://doi.org/10.1111/j.1439-0442.1985.tb01971.x

Petroff, B. K., Ciereszko, R. E., Dabrowski, K., Ottobre, A. C., Pope, W. F., & Ottobre, J. S. (1996). Prostaglandin F2a depletes the porcine *corpus luteum* of vitamin C by inducing secretion of the vitamin into the bloodstream. *The Ohio State Res. and Rev.*, (321–327).

Petrović, K., Stojanovic, D., Cincovic, M. R., Belic, B., Lakic, I., & Dokovic, R. (2020). Influence of niacin application on inflammatory parameters, nonesterified fatty acids and functional status of liver in cows during early lactation. *Large Animal Review*. http://www.largeanimalreview.com/index.php/lar/article/view/223.

Phillippo, M., Reid, G. W., & Nevison, I. M. (1994). Parturient hypocalcemia in dairy cows: Effects of dietary acidity on plasma minerals and calciotrophic hormones. *Research in Veterinary Science, 56*(3), 303–309. https://doi.org/10.1016/0034-5288(94)90146-5

Pickworth, C. L., Loerch, S. C., & Fluharty, F. L. (2012a). Restriction of vitamin A and D in beef cattle finishing diets on feedlot performance and adipose accretion. *Journal of Animal Science, 90*(6), 1866–1878. https://doi.org/10.2527/jas.2010-3590

Pickworth, C. L., Loerch, S. C., Kopec, R. E., Schwartz, S. J., & Fluharty, F. L. (2012b). Concentration of provitamin A carotenoids in common beef cattle feedstuffs. *Journal of Animal Science, 90*(5), 1553–1561. https://doi.org/10.2527/jas.2011-4217

Piepenbrink, M. S., & Overton, T. R. (2003). Liver metabolism and production of cows fed increasing amounts of rumen-protected choline during the periparturient period. *Journal of Dairy Science, 86*(5), 1722–1733. https://doi.org/10.3168/jds.S0022-0302(03)73758-8

Pinotti, L., Baldi, A., & Dell'orto, V. (2002). Comparative mammalian choline metabolism with emphasis on the high- yielding dairy cow. *Nutrition Research Reviews, 15*(2), 315–332. https://doi.org/10.1079/NRR200247

Pinotti, L., Baldi, A., Politis, I., Rebucci, R., Sangalli, L., & Dell'orto, V. (2003). Rumen- protected choline administration to transition cows: Effects on milk production and vitamin E status. *Journal of Veterinary Medicine. A, Physiology, Pathology, Clinical Medicine, 50*(1), 18–21. https://doi.org/10.1046/j.1439-0442.2003.00502.x

Pinotti, L., Campagnoli, A., Dell'orto, V., & Baldi, A. (2005). Choline: Is there a need in the lactating dairy cow? *Livestock Production Science, 98*(1–2), 149–152. https://doi.org/10.1016/j.livprodsci.2005.10.013

Pinotti, L., Manoni, M., Fumagalli, F., Rovere, N., Tretola, M., & Baldi, A. (2020). The role of micronutrients in high-yielding dairy ruminants: Choline and vitamin E. *Ankara Üniversitesi Veteriner Fakültesi Dergisi*, *67*(2), 209–214. https://doi.org/10.33988/auvfd.695432

Pinto, J. T., & Rivlin, R. S. (2013). Riboflavin (vitamin B_2). In J. Zempleni, J. Suttie, J. Gregory, & P. J. Stover (Eds.), *Handbook of vitamins* (5th ed.) (pp. 191–266). CRC Press, Taylor & Francis Group.

Pires, J. A. A., & Grummer, R. R. (2007). The use of nicotinic acid to induce sustained low plasma nonesterified fatty acids in feed-restricted Holstein cows. *Journal of Dairy Science*, *90*(8), 3725–3732. https://doi.org/10.3168/jds.2006-904

Playford, R. J., & Weiser, M. J. (2021). Bovine colostrum: Its constituents and uses. *Nutrients*, *13*(1), 265. https://doi.org/10.3390/nu13010265

Podda, M., & Grundmann-Kollmann, M. (2001). Low molecular weight antioxidants and their role in skin ageing. *Clinical and Experimental Dermatology*, *26*(7), 578–582. https://doi.org/10.1046/j.1365-2230.2001.00902.x

Pogge, D. J., & Hansen, S. L. (2013). Supplemental vitamin C improves marbling in feedlot cattle consuming high sulfur diets. *Journal of Animal Science*, *91*(9), 4303–4314. https://doi.org/10.2527/jas.2012-5638

Poindexter, M. B., Kweh, M. F., Zimpel, R., Zuniga, J., Lopera, C., Zenobi, M. G., Jiang, Y., Engstrom, M., Celi, P., Santos, J. E. P., & Nelson, C. D. (2020). Feeding supplemental 25-hydroxyvitamin D_3 increases serum mineral concentrations and alters mammary immunity of lactating dairy cows. *Journal of Dairy Science*, *103*(1), 805–822. https://doi.org/10.3168/jds.2019-16999

Poindexter, M. B., Zimpel, R., Vieira-Neto, A., Husnain, A., Silva, A. C. M., Faccenda, A., Sanches de Avila, A., Celi, P., Cortinhas, C., Santos, J. E. P., & Nelson, C. D. (2023a). Effect of prepartum source and amount of vitamin D supplementation on lactation performance of dairy cows. *Journal of Dairy Science*, *106*(2), 974–989. https://doi.org/10.3168/jds.2022-22388

Poindexter, M. B., Zimpel, R., Vieira-Neto, A., Husnain, A., Silva, A. C. M., Faccenda, A., Sanches de Avila, A., Celi, P., Cortinhas, C., Santos, J. E. P., & Nelson, C. D. (2023b). Effect of source and amount of vitamin D on serum concentrations and retention of calcium, magnesium, and phosphorus in dairy cows. *Journal of Dairy Science*, *106*(2), 954–973. https://doi.org/10.3168/jds.2022-22386

Polak, D. M., Elliot, J. M., & Haluska, M. (1979). Vitamin B_{12} binding proteins in bovine serum. *Journal of Dairy Science*, *62*(5), 697–701. https://doi.org/10.3168/jds.S0022-0302(79)83312-3

Polcz, M. E., & Barbul, A. (2019). The role of vitamin A in wound healing. *Nutrition in Clinical Practice*, *34*(5), 695–700. https://doi.org/10.1002/ncp.10376

Polegato, B. F., Pereira, A. G., Azevedo, P. S., Costa, N. A., Zornoff, L. A. M., Paiva, S. A. R., & Minicucci, M. F. (2019). Role of thiamin in health and disease. *Nutrition in Clinical Practice*, *34*(4), 558–564. https://doi.org/10.1002/ncp.10234

Politis, I., Bizelis, I., Tsiaras, A., & Baldi, A. (2004). Effect of vitamin E supplementation on neutrophil function, milk composition and plasmin activity in dairy cows in a commercial herd. *The Journal of Dairy Research*, *71*(3), 273–278. https://doi.org/10.1017/S002202990400010X

Politis, I., Hidiroglou, M., Batra, T. R., Gilmore, J. A., Gorewit, R. C., & Scherf, H. (1995). Effects of vitamin E on immune function of dairy cows. *American Journal of Veterinary Research*, *56*(2), 179–184. https://doi.org/10.2460/ajvr.1995.56.02.179, PubMed: 7717582

Politis, I., Hidiroglou, N., White, J. H., Gilmore, J. A., Williams, S. N., Scherf, H., & Frigg, M. (1996). Effects of vitamin E on mammary and blood leukocyte function, with emphasis on chemotaxis, in periparturient dairy cows. *American Journal of Veterinary Research*, *57*(4), 468–471. https://doi.org/10.2460/ajvr.1996.57.04.468, PubMed: 8712508

Politis, I. (2012). Reevaluation of vitamin E supplementation of dairy cows: Bioavailability, animal health and milk quality. *Animal*, *6*(9), 1427–1434. https://doi.org/10.1017/S1751731112000225

Pollock, J. M., McNair, J., Kennedy, S., Kennedy, D. G., Walsh, D. M., Goodall, E. A., Mackie, D. P., & Crockard, A. D. (1994). Effects of dietary vitamin E and selenium on *in vitro* cellular immune responses in cattle. *Research in Veterinary Science*, *56*(1), 100–107. https://doi.org/10.1016/0034-5288(94)90203-8

Półtorak, A., Moczkowska, M., Wyrwisz, J., & Wierzbicka, A. (2017). Beef tenderness improvement by dietary vitamin D supplementation in the last stage of fattening of cattle. *Journal of Veterinary Research*, *61*(1), 59–67. https://doi.org/10.1515/jvetres-2017-0008

Poor, C. L., Bierer, T. L., Merchen, N. R., Fahey, G. C., & Erdman, J. W. (1993). The accumulation of alpha- and beta-carotene in serum and tissues of preruminant calves fed raw and steamed carrot slurries. *The Journal of Nutrition, 123*(7), 1296–1304. https://doi.org/10.1093/jn/123.7.1296

Porter, J. W. G. (1961). Vitamin synthesis in the rumen. In D. Lewis (Ed.), *Digestive physiology and nutrition of the ruminants*. Butterworths p. 226.

Porter, S. B., Ong, D. E., & Chytil, F. (1986). Vitamin A status affects chromatin structure. *International Journal for Vitamin and Nutrition Research. Internationale Zeitschrift Fur Vitamin- und Ernahrungsforschung. Journal International de Vitaminologie et de Nutrition, 56*(1), 11–20. PubMed: 2423469

Potkanski, A. A., Tucker, R. E., Mitchell, G. E., & Schelling, G. T. (1974). Pre-intestinal losses of carotene in sheep fed high-starch or high-cellulose diets. International Journal for Vitamin and Nutrition Research. Internationale Zeitschrift Fur Vitamin- und Ernahrungsforschung. Journal International de Vitaminologie et de Nutrition, 44(2), 147–150

Potter, M. J., & Broom, D. M. (1990). Behavior and welfare aspects of cattle lameness in relation to building design. Update in cattle lameness. In *Proceedings*: "International symposium on diseases of the ruminant digest" Liverpool, 80–84.

Pottier, J., Focant, M., Debier, C., De Buysser, G., Goffe, C., Mignolet, E., Froidmont, E., & Larondelle, Y. (2006). Effect of dietary vitamin E on rumen biohydrogenation pathways and milk fat depression in dairy cows fed high-fat diets. *Journal of Dairy Science, 89*(2), 685–692. https://doi.org/10.3168/jds.S0022-0302(06)72131-2

Potts, S. B., Scholte, C. M., Moyes, K. M., & Erdman, R. A. (2020). Production responses to rumen-protected choline and methionine supplemented during the periparturient period differ for primi- and multiparous cows. *Journal of Dairy Science, 103*(7), 6070–6086. https://doi.org/10.3168/jds.2019-17591

Pötzsch, C. J., Hedges, V. J., Blowey, R. W., Packington, A. J., & Green, L. E. (2003). The impact of parity and duration of biotin supplementation on white line disease lameness in dairy cattle. *Journal of Dairy Science, 86*(8), 2577–2582. https://doi.org/10.3168/jds.S0022-0302(03)73852-1

Poulsen, N. A., Rybicka, I., Larsen, L. B., Buitenhuis, A. J., & Larsen, M. K. (2015). Short communication: Genetic variation of riboflavin content in bovine milk. *Journal of Dairy Science, 98*(5), 3496–3501. https://doi.org/10.3168/jds.2014-8829

Pour, H. A., Branch, S., & Sarab, I. (2017). *Vitamin H and their role in ruminants: A review*. https://doi.org/10.7537/marscbj070417.08

Powers, H. J., Weaver, L. T., Austin, S., Wright, A. J., & Fairweather-Tait, S. J. (1991) Riboflavin deficiency in the rat: Effects on iron utilization and loss. *The British Journal of Nutrition, 65*(3), 487–496. https://doi.org/10.1079/BJN19910107

Powers, H. J., Weaver, L. T., Austin, S., & Beresford, J. K. (1993). A proposed intestinal mechanism for the effect of riboflavin deficiency on iron loss in the rat. *The British Journal of Nutrition, 69*(2), 553–561. https://doi.org/10.1079/bjn19930055

Prasad, P. D., Ramamoorthy, S., Leibach, F. H., & Ganapathy, V. (1997). Characterization of a sodium-dependent vitamin transporter mediating the uptake of pantothenate, biotin and lipoate in human placental choriocarcinoma cells. *Placenta, 18*(7), 527–533. https://doi.org/10.1016/0143-4004(77)90006-6

Premkumar, V. G., Yuvaraj, S., Shanthi, P., & Sachdanandam, P. (2008). Co-enzyme Q10, riboflavin and niacin supplementation on alteration of DNA repair enzyme and DNA methylation in breast cancer patients undergoing tamoxifen therapy. *The British Journal of Nutrition, 100*(6), 1179–1182. https://doi.org/10.1017/S0007114508968276

Preś, J., Fuchs, B., & Schleicher, A. (1993). The efect of carotene and vitamins A and E supplementation on reproduction of sows. *Archivum Veterinarium Polonicum, 33*(1–2), 55–64. PubMed: 8055056

Preynat, A., Lapierre, H., Thivierge, M. C., Palin, M. F., Matte, J. J., Desrochers, A., & Girard, C. L. (2009). Effects of supplements of folic acid, vitamin B_{12}, and rumen-protected methionine on whole body metabolism of methionine and glucose in lactating dairy cows. *Journal of Dairy Science, 92*(2), 677–689. https://doi.org/10.3168/jds.2008-1525

Preynat, A., Lapierre, H., Thivierge, M. C., Palin, M. F., Cardinault, N., Matte, J. J., Desrochers, A., & Girard, C. L. (2010). Effects of supplementary folic acid and vitamin B_{12} on hepatic metabolism of dairy cows according to methionine supply. *Journal of Dairy Science, 93*(5), 2130–2142. https://doi.org/10.3168/jds.2009-2796

Pribyl, E. (1963). *Diseases of young cattle, 230*. Praha.

Price, M. Y., & Preedy, V. R. (2020). Reference dietary requirements of vitamins in different stages of life. *Molecular Nutrition*, 3–32. https://doi.org/10.1016/B978-0-12-811907-5.00002-6

Priolo, A., Micol, D., Agabriel, J., Prache, S., & Dransfield, E. (2002). Effect of grass or concentrate feeding systems on lamb carcass and meat quality. *Meat Science, 62*(2), 179–185. https://doi.org/10.1016/S0309-1740(01)00244-3

Pritchard, D. G., Markson, L. M., Brush, P. J., Sawtell, J. A., & Bloxham, P. A. (1983). Haemorrhagic syndrome of cattle associated with the feeding of sweet vernal (*Anthoxanthum odoratum*) hay containing dicoumarol. *The Veterinary Record, 113*(4), 78–84. https://doi.org/10.1136/vr.113.4.78

Pritchard, R. H. (2007). Corn by-products: Considerations involving sulfur. In *Proceedings of the Plains Nutrition Council Spring Conference* p. 6500 Amarillo Blvd. Plains Nutrition Council. West.

Prom, C. M., Engstrom, M. A., & Drackley, J. K. (2022). Effects of prepartum supplementation of β-carotene in Holstein cows. *Journal of Dairy Science, 105*(5), 4116–4127. https://doi.org/10.3168/jds.2021-21482

Puchala, R., Banskalieva, V., Goetsch, A. L., Prieto, I., & Sahlu, T. (1999). Effects of dietary protein and ruminally protected betaine or choline on productivity of Angora doelings. *Journal of Animal Science, 77*(Suppl. 1), 261.

Pullar, J. M., Carr, A. C., & Vissers, M. C. M. (2017). The roles of vitamin C in skin health. *Nutrients, 9*(8), 866–892. https://doi.org/10.3390/nu9080866

Puschner, B., Galey, F. D., Holstege, D. M., & Palazoglu, M. (1998). Sweet clover poisoning in dairy cattle in California. *Journal of the American Veterinary Medical Association, 212*(6), 857–859. https://doi.org/10.2460/javma.1998.212.06.857, PubMed: 9530428

Putman, A. K. (2023). *Novel insights into biomarker potential and physiological roles of isoprostanes in dairy cattle*. https://doi.org/10.3390/antiox10020145 ([Unpublished doctoral dissertation]. Michigan State University).

Puvogel, G., Baumrucker, C. R., Sauerwein, H., Rühl, R., Ontsouka, E., Hammon, H. M., & Blum, J. W. (2005). Effects of an enhanced vitamin A intake during the dry period on retinoids, lactoferrin, IGF-system, mammary gland epithelial cell apoptosis and subsequent lactation in dairy cows. *Journal of Dairy Science, 88*(5), 1785–1800. https://doi.org/10.3168/jds.S0022-0302(05)72853-8

Puvogel, G., Baumrucker, C., & Blum, J. W. (2008). Plasma vitamin A status in calves fed colostrum from cows that were fed vitamin A during late pregnancy. *Journal of Animal Physiology and Animal Nutrition, 92*(5), 614–620. https://doi.org/10.1111/j.1439-0396.2007.00757.x

Pyatt, N. A., & Berger, L. L. (2005). Review: Potential effects of vitamins A and D on marbling deposition in beef cattle. *The Professional Animal Scientist, 21*(3), 174–181. https://doi.org/10.15232/S1080-7446(15)31199-2

Pyatt, N. A., Berger, L. L., & Nash, T. G. (2005). Effects of vitamin A and restricted intake on performance, carcass characteristics, and serum retinol status in Angus× Simmental feedlot cattle. *The Professional Animal Scientist, 21*(4), 318–331. https://doi.org/10.15232/S1080-7446(15)31223-7

Qu, Y., Lytle, K., Traber, M. G., & Bobe, G. (2013). Depleted serum vitamin E concentrations precede left displaced abomasum in early-lactation dairy cows. *Journal of Dairy Science, 96*(5), 3012–3022. http://doi.org/10.3168/jds.2012-6357

Quackenbush, F. W. (1963). Corn carotenoids: Effect of temperature and moisture on losses during storage. *Cereal Chemistry, 40*, 266.

Quigley, J. D., III, & Bernard, J. K. (1995). Effects of addition of vitamin E to colostrum on serum α-tocopherol and immunoglobulin concentrations in neonatal calves. *Food and Agricultural Immunology, 7*(3), 295–298. https://doi.org/10.1080/09540109509354887

Quigley, J. D., III, & Drewry, J. J. (1998). Nutrient and immunity transfer from cow to calf pre- and postcalving. *Journal of Dairy Science, 81*(10), 2779–2790. https://doi.org/10.3168/jds.S0022-0302(98)75836-9

Qureshi, A. A., Salser, W. A., Parmar, R., & Emeson, E. E. (2001). Novel tocotrienols of rice bran inhibit atherosclerotic lesions in C57BL/6 apoE-deficient mice. *The Journal of Nutrition, 131*(10), 2606–2618. https://doi.org/10.1093/jn/131.10.2606

Rabia, S. A., Ali, I., & Muhammad, B. H. (2018). Nutritional composition of meat. *Meat Sci. and Nutr.*. https://doi.org/10.5772/intechopen.77045

Radostits, O. M., & Bell, J. M. (1970). Nutrition of the preruminant dairy calf with special reference to the digestion and absorption of nutrients: A review. *Canadian Journal of Animal Science*, 50(3), 405–452. https://doi.org/10.4141/cjas70-063

Ragaller, V., Hüther, L., & Lebzien, P. (2008). Folic acid in ruminant nutrition: A review. *British Journal of Nutrition*, 1–12. https://doi.org/10.1017/S0007114508051556

Ragaller, V., Lebzien, P., Bigalke, W., Südekum, K. H., Hüther, L., & Flachowsky, G. (2011). Effects of a pantothenic acid supplementation to different rations on ruminal fermentation, nutrient flow at the duodenum, and on blood and milk variables of dairy cows. *Journal of Animal Physiology and Animal Nutrition*, 95(6), 730–743. https://doi.org/10.1111/j.1439-0396.2010.01103.x

Rajaraman, V., Nonnecke, B. J., & Horst, R. L. (1997). Effects of replacement of native fat in colostrum and milk with coconut oil on fat-soluble vitamins in serum and immune function in calves. *Journal of Dairy Science*, 80(10), 2380–2390. https://doi.org/10.3168/jds.S0022-0302(97)76189-7

Rakes, A. H., Owens, M. P., Britt, J. H., & Whitlow, L. W. (1985). Effects of adding beta-carotene to rations of lactating cows consuming different forages. *Journal of Dairy Science*, 68(7), 1732–1737. https://doi.org/10.3168/jds.S0022-0302(85)81019-5

Rammell, C. G., & Hill, J. H. (1986). A review of thiamine deficiency and its diagnosis, especially in ruminants. *New Zealand Veterinary Journal*, 34(12), 202–204. https://doi.org/10.1080/00480169.1986.35350

Rammell, C. G., Thompson, K. G., Bentley, G. R., & Gibbons, M. W. (1989). Selenium, vitamin E and polyunsaturated fatty acid concentrations in goat kids with and without nutritional myodegeneration. *New Zealand Veterinary Journal*, 37(1), 4–6. https://doi.org/10.1080/00480169.1989.35536

Ramos, J. J., Ferrer, L. M., García, L., Fernández, A., & Loste, A. (2005). Polioencephalomalacia in adult sheep grazing pastures with prostrate pigweed. *The Canadian Veterinary Journal*, 46(1), 59–61. http://www.ncbi.nlm.nih.gov/pmc/articles/pmc1082858/

Ranjan, R., Swarup, D., Naresh, R., & Patra, D. (2005). Ameliorative potential of L-ascorbic acid in bovine clinical mastitis. *Indian Journal of Animal Sciences*, 75, 174–177.

Ranjan, R., Ranjan, A., Dhaliwal, G. S., & Patra, R. C. (2012). L-ascorbic acid (vitamin C) supplementation to optimize health and reproduction in cattle. *The Veterinary Quarterly*, 32(3–4), 145–150. https://doi.org/10.1080/01652176.2012.734640

Rapoport, R., Sklan, D., Wolfenson, D., Shaham-Albalancy, A., & Hanukoglu, I. (1998). Antioxidant capacity is correlated with steroidogenic status of the *corpus luteum* during the bovine estrous cycle. *Biochimica et Biophysica Acta*, 1380(1), 133–140. https://doi.org/10.1016/S0304-4165(97)00136-0

Rather, S. A., Masoodi, F. A., Akhter, R., Rather, J. A., & Shiekh, K. A. (2016). Advances in use of natural antioxidants as food additives for improving the oxidative stability of meat products. *MJFT*, 1(1), 10–17. http://doi.org/10.18689/mjft.2016-102

Rathman, S. C., Eisenschenk, S., & McMahon, R. J. (2002). The abundance and function of biotin-dependent enzymes are reduced in rats chronically administered carbamazepine. *The Journal of Nutrition*, 132(11), 3405–3410. https://doi.org/10.1093/jn/132.11.3405

Rawling, J. M., Jackson, T. M., Driscoll, E. R., & Kirkland, J. B. (1994). Dietary niacin deficiency lowers tissue poly(ADP-ribose) and NAD+ concentrations in Fischer-344 rats. *The Journal of Nutrition*, 124(9), 1597–1603. https://doi.org/10.1093/jn/124.9.1597

Reboul, E., & Borel, P. (2011). Proteins involved in uptake, intracellular transport and basolateral secretion of fat-soluble vitamins and carotenoids by mammalian enterocytes. *Progress in Lipid Research*, 50(4), 388–402. https://doi.org/10.1016/j.plipres.2011.07.001

Reddy, M. U., & Pushpamma, P. (1986). Effect of storage and insect infestation on thiamine and niacin content in different varieties of rice, sorghum, and legumes. *Nutrition Reports International*, 34, 393–401.

Reddy, P. G., Morrill, J. L., Frey, R. A., Morrill, M. B., Minocha, H. C., Galitzer, S. J., & Dayton, A. D. (1985). Effects of supplemental vitamin E on the performance and metabolic profiles of dairy calves. *Journal of Dairy Science*, 68(9), 2259–2266. https://doi.org/10.3168/jds.S0022-0302(85)81098-5

Reddy, P. G., Morrill, J. L., Minocha, H. C., Morrill, M. B., Dayton, A. D., & Frey, R. A. (1986). Effect of supplemental vitamin E on the immune system of calves. *Journal of Dairy Science*, 69(1), 164–171. https://doi.org/10.3168/jds.S0022-0302(86)80382-4

Reddy, P. G., Morrill, J. L., Minocha, H. C., & Stevenson, J. S. (1987). Vitamin E is Immunostimulatory in Calves. Journal of Dairy Science, 70(5), 993–999. https://doi.org/10.3168/jds.S0022-0302(87)80104-2

Reffett, J. K., Spears, J. W., & Brown, T. T. (1988). Effect of dietary selenium and vitamin E on the primary and secondary immune response in lambs challenged with parainfluenza3 virus. *Journal of Animal Science*, 66(6), 1520–1528. https://doi.org/10.2527/jas1988.6661520x

Reinhardt, T. A., & Hustmyer, F. G. (1987). Role of vitamin D in the immune system. *Journal of Dairy Science*, 70(5), 952–962. https://doi.org/10.3168/jds.S0022-0302(87)80099-1

Ren, N., Zhang, X., Hao, X., Dong, Y., Wang, X., & Zhang, J. (2023). Effect of dietary inclusion of riboflavin on growth, nutrient digestibility and ruminal fermentation in Hu lambs. *Animals: An Open Access Journal from MDPI*, 13(1), 26. https://doi.org/10.3390/ani13010026

Rérat, A., Champigny, O., & Jacquot, R. (1959). Methods of vitamin absorption in ruminants: Form and availability of the B vitamins of the alimentary bolus at different digestive levels. *Comptes Rendus Hebdomadaires des Seances de l'Académie des Sciences*, 249, 1274–1276. PubMed: 14437424

Reynolds, C. K. (2006). Production and metabolic effects of site of starch digestion in dairy cattle. *Animal Feed Science and Technology*, 130(1–2), 78–94. https://doi.org/10.1016/j.anifeedsci.2006.01.019

Reynolds, C. K., Beever, D. E., Steinberg, W., & Packington, A. J. (2007). Net nutrient absorption and liver metabolism in lactating dairy cows fed supplemental dietary biotin. *Animal*, 1(3), 375–380. https://doi.org/10.1017/S1751731107666105

Rezamand, P., Hoagland, T. A., Moyes, K. M., Silbart, L. K., & Andrew, S. M. (2007). Energy status, lipid-soluble vitamins, and acute phase proteins in periparturient Holstein and Jersey dairy cows with or without subclinical mastitis. *Journal of Dairy Science*, 90(11), 5097–5107. https://doi.org/10.3168/jds.2007-0035

Rhodes, S. G., Terry, L. A., Hope, J., Hewinson, R. G., & Vordermeier, H. M. (2003). 1,25-dihydroxyvitamin D3 and development of tuberculosis in cattle. *Clinical and Diagnostic Laboratory Immunology*, 10(6), 1129–1135. https://doi.org/10.1128/cdli.10.6.1129-1135.2003

Ribeiro, A. M., Estevinho, B. N., & Rocha, F. (2021). The progress and application of vitamin E encapsulation–A review. *Food Hydrocolloids*, 121, 106998. https://doi.org/10.1016/j.foodhyd.2021.106998

Rice, D. A., Blanchflower, W. J., & McMurray, C. H. (1981). Reproduction of nutritional degenerative myopathy in the post ruminant calf. *The Veterinary Record*, 109(8), 161–162. https://doi.org/10.1136/vr.109.8.161

Richter, V. G. H., Flachowsky, F., Matthey, F., Ochrimenko, W. I., Wolfram, W. I., & Schade, T. (1990). Influence of stall resp. Outdoor husbandry on the 25(OH)vitamin D$_3$ blood plasma concentration in fattening bulls. Mh. Vet. El Medico, 45, 227.

Riddell, D. O., Bartley, E. E., & Dayton, A. D. (1981). Effect of nicotinic acid on microbial protein synthesis *in vitro* and on dairy cattle growth and milk production. *Journal of Dairy Science*, 64(5), 782–791. https://doi.org/10.3168/jds.S0022-0302(81)82648-3

Riddell, D. O., Bartley, E. E., & Dayton, A. D. (1980). Effect of nicotinic acid on rumen fermentation *in vitro* and *in vivo*. *Journal of Dairy Science*, 63(9), 1429–1436. https://doi.org/10.3168/jds.S0022-0302(80)83100-6

Rigotti, A. (2007). Absorption, transport, and tissue delivery of vitamin E. *Molecular Aspects of Medicine*, 28(5–6), 423–436. https://doi.org/10.1016/j.mam.2007.01.002

Riley, W. W., Nickerson, J. G., Mogg, T. J., & Burton, G. W. (2023). Oxidized β-carotene is a novel phytochemical immune modulator that supports animal health and performance for antibiotic-free production. *Animals: An Open Access Journal from MDPI*, 13(2), 289. https://doi.org/10.3390/ani13020289

Rivera, J. D., Duff, G. C., Galyean, M. L., Walker, D. A., & Nunnery, G. A. (2002). Effects of supplemental vitamin E on performance, health, and humoral immune response of beef cattle. *Journal of Animal Science*, 80(4), 933–941. https://doi.org/10.2527/2002.804933x

Rivera, J. D., Duff, G. C., Galyean, M. L., Hallford, D. M., & Ross, T. T. (2003). Effects of graded levels of vitamin E on inflammatory response and evaluation of methods of supplementing vitamin E on performance and health of beef steers11This research was supported by funds from the New Mexico Agric. Exp. Stn., Las Cruces, NM 88005. *The Professional Animal Scientist*, 19(2), 171–177. https://doi.org/10.15232/S1080-7446(15)31396-6

Riveron-Negrete, L., & Fernandez-Mejia, C. (2017). Pharmacological effects of biotin in animals. *Mini Reviews in Medicinal Chemistry, 17*(6), 529–540. https://doi.org/10.2174/1389557516666160923132611

Rivlin, R. S. (2006). Riboflavin. In B. A. Bowman & R. M. Russell (Eds.), *Present knowledge in nutrition* (9th ed.) (pp. 250–259). International Life Sciences Institute.

Robbins, K., Jensen, J., Ryan, K. J., Homco-Ryan, C., McKeith, F. K., & Brewer, M. S. (2003). Effect of dietary vitamin E supplementation on textural and aroma attributes of enhanced beef clod roasts in a cook/ hot-hold situation. *Meat Science, 64*(3), 317–322. https://doi.org/10.1016/S0309-1740(02)00203-6

Roberson, J. R., Swecker, W. S., & Hullender, L. L. (2000). Hypercalcemia and hypervitaminosis D in two lambs. *Journal of the American Veterinary Medical Association, 216*(7), 1115–1118. https://doi.org/10.2460/javma.2000.216.1115

Robinson, P. H. (2019). Vitamin B requirements and duodenal deliveries in lactating dairy cows: Organization of a limited literature. *Livestock Science, 226*, 48–60. https://doi.org/10.1016/j.livsci.2019.06.004

Rode, L. M., McAllister, T. A., & Cheng, K.-J. (1990). Microbial degradation of vitamin A in rumen fluid from steers fed concentrate, hay or straw diets. *Canadian Journal of Animal Science, 70*(1), 227–233. https://doi.org/10.4141/cjas90-026

Rodney, R. M., Martinez, N., Block, E., Hernandez, L. L., Celi, P., Nelson, C. D., Santos, J. E. P., & Lean, I. J. (2018). Effects of prepartum dietary cation–anion difference and source of vitamin D in dairy cows: Vitamin D, mineral, and bone metabolism. *Journal of Dairy Science, 101*(3), 2519–2543. https://doi.org/10.3168/jds.2017-13737

Rodrigues, I. (2014). A review on the effects of mycotoxins in dairy ruminants. *Animal Production Science, 54*(9), 1155–1165. http://doi.org/10.1071/AN13492

Rodriguez, M., Enger, B. D., Weiss, W. P., Lee, K., & Lee, C. (2023). Effects of different vitamin A supplies on performance and the risk of ketosis in transition cows. *Journal of Dairy Science, 106*(4), 2361–2373. https://doi.org/10.3168/jds.2022-22491

Rodríguez-Meléndez, R., & Zempleni, J. (2003). Regulation of gene expression by biotin (review) [Review]. *The Journal of Nutritional Biochemistry, 14*(12), 680–690. https://doi.org/10.1016/j.jnutbio.2003.07.001

Rodríguez-Meléndez, R., Cano, S., Méndez, S. T., & Velázquez, A. (2001). Biotin regulates the genetic expression of holocarboxylase synthetase and mitochondrial carboxylases in rats. *The Journal of Nutrition, 131*(7), 1909–1913. https://doi.org/10.1093/jn/131.7.1909

Roest, J. (1993). Foot care. *Veepro Holland Magazine, 17*, 22–23.

Röhrle, F. T., Moloney, A. P., Black, A., Osorio, M. T., Sweeney, T., Schmidt, O., & Monahan, F. J. (2011). α-Tocopherol stereoisomers in beef as an indicator of vitamin E supplementation in cattle diets. *Food Chemistry, 124*(3), 935–940. https://doi.org/10.1016/j.foodchem.2010.07.023

Rohlfs, E. M., Garner, S. C., Mar, M. H., & Zeisel, S. H. (1993). Glycerophosphocholine and phosphocholine are the major choline metabolites in rat milk. *The Journal of Nutrition, 123*(10), 1762–1768. https://doi.org/10.1093/jn/123.10.1762

Rojas, C., Cadenas, S., Herrero, A., Méndez, J., & Barja, G. (1996). Endotoxin depletes ascorbate in the guinea pig heart. Protective effects of vitamins C and E against oxidative stress. *Life Sciences, 59*(8), 649–657. https://doi.org/10.1016/0024-3205(96)00346-3

Romagnoli, E., Caravella, P., Scarnecchia, L., Martinez, P., & Minisola, S. (1999). Hypovitaminosis D in an Italian population of healthy subjects and hospitalized patients. *The British Journal of Nutrition, 81*(2), 133–137. https://doi.org/10.1017/S0007114599000264

Rose, R. (1990). Vitamin absorption. In *Developments in vitamin nutrition and health applications. Proceedings of the National Feed Ingr. Ass., Nutr. Inst. Kansas City.* National Feed Ingredients Association.

Rose, R. C., & Bode, A. M. (1993). Biology of free radical scavengers: An evaluation of ascorbate. *FASEB Journal, 7*(12), 1135–1142. https://doi.org/10.1096/fasebj.7.12.8375611, PubMed: 8375611

Rose, R. C., McCorrmick, D. B., Li, T. K., Lumeng, L., Haddad, J. G., & Spector, R. (1986). Transport and metabolism of vitamins. *Federation Proceedings, 45*(1), 30–39. PubMed: 3000833

Rosenberg, I. H. (2012). A history of the isolation and identification of vitamin B_6. *Annals of Nutrition and Metabolism, 61*(3), 236–238. https://doi.org/10.1159/000343113

Rosendo, O., Bates, D. B., McDowell, L. R., Staples, C. R., McMahon, R., & Wilkinson, N. S. (2003). Availability and ability of biotin for promoting forage fiber *in vitro* ruminal digestibility. *Journal of Animal and Veterinary Advances*, 2, 350–357. https://medwelljournals.com/abstract/?doi=javaa.2003.350.357

Rosendo, O., Staples, C. R., McDowell, L. R., McMahon, R., Badinga, L., Martin, F. G., Shearer, J. F., Seymour, W. M., & Wilkinson, N. S. (2004). Effects of biotin supplementation on peripartum performance and metabolites of Holstein cows. *Journal of Dairy Science*, 87(8), 2535–2545. https://doi.org/10.3168/jds.S0022-0302(04)73378-0

Rosendo, O., McDowell, L. R., Staples, C., Shearer, J. K., Wilkinson, N. S., & Seymour, W. M. (2010). Relationship of mild fatty liver, β-carotene, vitamin A and E status of periparturient Holstein cows. *Revista Científica*, 20(4), 399–408.

Ross, A. C. (1993). Overview of retinoid metabolism. *The Journal of Nutrition*, 123(2)(Suppl.), 346–350. https://doi.org/10.1093/jn/123.suppl_2.346

Ross, A. C. (2003). Retinoid production and catabolism: Role of diet in regulating retinol esterification and retinoic acid oxidation. *The Journal of Nutrition*, 133(1), 291S–296S. https://doi.org/10.1093/jn/133.1.291S

Ross, A. C., & Harrison, E. H. (2013). Vitamin A: Nutritional aspects of retinoids and carotenoids. In J. Zempleni, J. Suttie, J. Gregory, & P. J. Stover (Eds.), *Handbook of vitamins* (5th ed.) (pp. 1–50). CRC Press, Taylor & Francis Group, LLC.

Ross, S. A., McCaffery, P. J., Drager, U. C., & De Luca, L. M. (2000). Retinoids in embryonal development. *Physiological Reviews*, 80(3), 1021–1054. https://doi.org/10.1152/physrev.2000.80.3.1021

Roth, J. A., & Kaeberle, M. L. (1985). *In vivo* effect of ascorbic acid on neutrophil function in healthy and dexamethasone- treated cattle. *American Journal of Veterinary Research*, 46(12), 2434–2436. PubMed: 4083574

Roudbari, Z., Coort, S. L., Kutmon, M., Eijssen, L., Melius, J., Sadkowski, T., & Evelo, C. T. (2020). Identification of biological pathways contributing to marbling in skeletal muscle to improve beef cattle breeding. *Frontiers in Genetics*, 10, 1370. https://doi.org/10.3389/fgene.2019.01370

Rousseau, J. E., Eaton, H. D., Helmboldt, C. F., Jungherr, E. L., Robrish, S. A., Beal, G., & Moore, L. A. (1954). Relative Value of Carotene from Alfalfa and Vitamin A from a Dry Carrier Fed at Minimum Levels to Holstein Calves. Journal of Dairy Science, 37(7), 889–899. https://doi.org/10.3168/jds.S0022-0302(54)91341-7

Rowe, L. J., Maddock, K. R., Lonergan, S. M., & Huff-Lonergan, E. (2004). Influence of early postmortem protein oxidation on beef quality. *Journal of Animal Science*, 82(3), 785–793. https://doi.org/10.2527/2004.823785x

Roy, J. H. B. (1980). Symposium: Disease prevention in calves. Factors affecting susceptibility of calves to disease. *Journal of Dairy Science*, 63(4), 650–664. https://doi.org/10.3168/jds.S0022-0302(80)82987-0

Rucker, R. B., & Bauerly, K. (2013). Pantothenic acid. In J. Zempleni, J. Suttie, J. Gregory, & P. J. Stover (Eds.), *Handbook of vitamins* (5th ed.) (pp. 289–313). CRC Press, Taylor & Francis Group, LLC ISBN 9781466515567.

Rumsey, T. S. (1975). Vitamin requirements for ruminants. *Feedstuffs*, 47(7), 30.

Rumsey, T. S. (1989). Effect of choline in all concentrate diets of feedlot steers and on rumen acidosis. *Canadian Journal of Animal Science*, 65, 135–146. https://doi.org/10.4141/cjas85-014

Rungruang, S., Collier, J. L., Rhoads, R. P., Baumgard, L. H., De Veth, M. J., & Collier, R. J. (2014). A dose–response evaluation of rumen-protected niacin in thermoneutral or heat-stressed lactating Holstein cows. *Journal of Dairy Science*, 97(8), 5023–5034. https://doi.org/10.3168/jds.2013-6970

Rupel, I. W., Bohstedt, G., & Hart, E. B. (1933). Vitamin D in the nutrition of the dairy calf. Wis. Agric. exp. Stn. *Research Bulletin*, 115.

Russell, W. C. (1929). The effect of the curing process upon the vitamin A and D content of alfalfa. *Journal of Biological Chemistry*, 85(1), 289–297. https://doi.org/10.1016/S0021-9258(18)76998-6

Ryu, K. S., Roberson, K. D., Pesti, G. M., & Eitenmiller, R. R. (1995). The folic acid requirements of starting broiler chicks fed diets based on practical ingredients: 1. Interrelationships with dietary choline. *Poultry Science*, 74(9), 1447–1455. https://doi.org/10.3382/ps.0741447

Sacadura, F. C., Robinson, P. H., Evans, E., & Lordelo, M. (2008). Effects of a ruminally protected B-vitamin supplement on milk yield and composition of lactating dairy cows. *Animal Feed Science and Technology*, 144(1–2), 111–124. https://doi.org/10.1016/j.anifeedsci.2007.10.005

Sadler, W. C., Mahoney, J. H., Puch, H. C., Williams, D. L., & Hodge, D. E. (1983). Relationship between sulfate and polioencephalomalacia in cattle. *Journal of Animal Science*, *57*(Suppl. 1), 467.

Saeed, A., Dullaart, R. P. F., Schreuder, T. C. M. A., Blokzijl, H., & Faber, K. N. (2017). Disturbed vitamin A metabolism in non-alcoholic fatty liver disease (NAFLD). *Nutrients*, *10*(1). http://doi.org/10.3390/nu10010029

Safford, J. W., Swingle, K. F., & Marsh, H. (1954). Vitamin deficiency in calves. *American Journal of Veterinary Research*, *15*(56), 373–384.

Safonova, I., Darimont, C., Amri, E. Z., Grimaldi, P., Ailhaud, G., Reichert, U., & Shroot, B. (1994). Retinoids are positive effectors of adipose cell differentiation. *Molecular and Cellular Endocrinology*, *104*(2), 201–211. https://doi.org/10.1016/0303-7207(94)90123-6

Said, H. M. (2011). Intestinal absorption of water-soluble vitamins in health and disease. *The Biochemical Journal*, *437*(3), 357–372. https://doi.org/10.1042/BJ20110326

Said, H. M. (2012). Biotin: Biochemical, physiological and clinical aspects. In *Water soluble vitamins* (pp. 1–19). https://doi.org/10.1007/978-94-007-2199-9_1

Said, H. M., & Derweesh, I. (1991). Carrier-mediated mechanism for biotin transport in rabbit intestine: Studies with brush–border membrane vesicles. *The American Journal of Physiology*, *261*(1 Pt 2), R94–R97. https://doi.org/10.1152/ajpregu.1991.261.1.R94

Said, H. M., Redha, R., & Nylander, W. (1988). Biotin transport in the human intestine: Site of maximum transport and effect of pH. *Gastroenterology*, *95*(5), 1312–1317. https://doi.org/10.1016/0016-5085(88)90366-6

Said, H. M., Hoefs, J., Mohammadkhani, R., & Horne, D. W. (1992). Biotin transport in human liver basolateral membrane vesicles: A carrier-mediated, Na+ gradient-dependent process. *Gastroenterology*, *102*(6), 2120–2125. https://doi.org/10.1016/0016-5085(92)90341-u

Sakurai, T., Asakura, T., Mizuno, A., & Matsuda, M. (1992). Absorption and metabolism of pyridoxamine in mice II. Transformation of pyridoxamine to pyridoxal in intestinal tissues. *Journal of Nutritional Science and Vitaminology*, *38*(3), 227–233. https://doi.org/10.3177/jnsv.38.227

Salami, S. A., Guinguina, A., Agboola, J. O., Omede, A. A., Agbonlahor, E. M., & Tayyab, U. (2016). Review: *In vivo* and postmortem effects of feed antioxidants in livestock: A review of the implications on authorization of antioxidant feed additives. *Animal*, *10*(8), 1375–1390. https://doi.org/10.1017/S1751731115002967

Sales, J., & Koukolová, V. (2011). Dietary vitamin E and lipid and color stability of beef and pork: Modeling of relationships. *Journal of Animal Science*, *89*(9), 2836–2848. https://doi.org/10.2527/jas.2010-3335

Salinas-Chavira, J., Arrizon, A. A., Barreras, A., Chen, C. Z., Plascencia, A., & Zinn, R. A. (2014). Evaluation of supplemental vitamin A and E on 56-day growth performance, dietary net energy, and plasma retinol and tocopherol concentrations in Holstein steer calves. *The Professional Animal Scientist*, *30*(5), 510–514. https://doi.org/10.15232/pas.2014-01316

Salisbury, G. W. (1944). A controlled experiment in feeding wheat germ oil as a supplement to the normal ration of bulls used for artificial insemination. *Journal of Dairy Science*, *27*(7), 551–562. https://doi.org/10.3168/jds.S0022-0302(44)92632-9

Samuelson, K. L., Hubbert, M. E., Galyean, M. L., & Löest, C. A. (2016). Nutritional recommendations of feedlot consulting nutritionists: The 2015 New Mexico State and Texas Tech University survey. *Journal of Animal Science*, *94*(6), 2648–2663. https://doi.org/10.2527/jas.2016-0282

Santschi, D. E., Berthiaume, R., Matte, J. J., Mustafa, A. F., & Girard, C. L. (2005a). Fate of supplementary B-vitamins in the gastrointestinal tract of dairy cows. *Journal of Dairy Science*, *88*(6), 2043–2054. https://doi.org/10.3168/jds.S0022-0302(05)72881-2

Santschi, D. E., Chiquette, J., Berthiaume, R., Martineau, R., Matte, J. J., Mustafa, A. F., & Girard, C. L. (2005b). Effects of the forage to concentrate ratio on B-vitamin concentrations in different ruminal fractions of dairy cows. *Canadian Journal of Animal Science*, *85*(3), 389–399. https://doi.org/10.4141/A05-012

Sauberlich, H. E. (1985). Bioavailability of vitamins. *Progress in Food and Nutrition Science*, *9*(1–2), 1–33. PubMed: 3911266

Sauberlich, H. E. (1990). Ascorbic acid. In R. E. Olson (Ed.), 132, *Nutrition reviews, present knowledge in nutrition*. Nutrition Foundation.

Sauberlich, H. E. (1994). Pharmacology of vitamin C. *Annual Review of Nutrition*, *14*, 371–391. https://doi.org/10.1146/annurev.nu.14.070194.002103

Sauberlich, H. E. (1999). *Laboratory tests for the assessment of nutritional status* (2nd ed.). Routledge. https://doi.org/10.1201/9780203749647

Savage, D. G., & Lindenbaum, J. (1995). Folate-cobalamin interactions. In L. B. Bailey (Ed.), 237. Marcel Dekker, *Folate in health and disease.* New York.

Schaefer, D. M., Scheller, K. K., Arp, S. C., Buege, D. R., & Lane, S. F. (1989). Growth of Holstein steers and beef color as affected by dietary vitamin E supplementation. *Journal of Animal Science, 68*(Suppl. 1), 190.

Schaefer, D. M., Arnold, R. N., Scheller, K. K., Arp, S. C., & Williams, S. N. (1991). *Proceedings of the Holstein Beef Prod. Symp.* Northeast Regional Agricultural Engineering Service p.175.

Schaeffer, M. C. (1993). Excess dietary vitamin B$_6$ alters startle behavior of rats. *The Journal of Nutrition, 123*(8), 1444–1452. https://doi.org/10.1093/jn/123.8.1444

Schaffer, S., Müller, W. E., & Eckert, G. P. (2005). Tocotrienols: Constitutional effects in aging and disease. *The Journal of Nutrition, 135*(2), 151–154. https://doi.org/10.1093/jn/135.2.151

Schams, D., Hoffmann, B., Lotthammer, K. H., & Ahlswede, L. (1977). Researches on a specific effect of β-carotene, not dependent on vitamin A, on the fertility of cattle. 4. Importance of hormonal parameters during the cycle. *Dt. Tierdrzl. Wschr., 84,* 307–310.

Schelling, G. T., Roeder, R. A., Garber, M. J., & Pumfrey, W. M. (1995). Bioavailability and interaction of vitamin A and vitamin E in ruminants. *The Journal of Nutrition, 125*(6)(Suppl.), 1799S–1803S. https://doi.org/10.1093/jn/125.suppl_6.1799S

Scherf, H., Machlin, L. J., Frye, T. M., Krautmann, B. A., & Williams, S. N. (1996). Vitamin E biopotency: Comparison of various'natural-derived'and chemically synthesized α-tocopherols. *Animal Feed Science and Technology, 59*(1–3), 115–126. https://doi.org/10.1016/0377-8401(95)00892-6

Schingoethe, D. J., Kirkbride, C. A., Palmer, I. S., Owens, M. J., & Tucker, W. L. (1982). Response of cows consuming adequate selenium to vitamin E and selenium supplementation prepartum. *Journal of Dairy Science, 65*(12), 2338–2344. https://doi.org/10.3168/jds.S0022-0302(82)82506-X

Schmidt, H. (1941). Vitamin A deficiencies in ruminants. *American Journal of Veterinary Research, 2,* 373.

Schneider, J. (1986). Vitamin stability and activity of fat-soluble vitamins as influenced by manufacturing processes. In Proc, *National feed Ingred. assoc. nutr., 1986.* Institut "Bioavailability of vitamins in feed ingredients,". National Feed Ingredients Association.

Schönfeldt, H. C., Naudé, R. T., & Boshoff, E. (2010). Effect of age and cut on the nutritional content of South African beef. *Meat Science, 86*(3), 674–683. https://doi.org/10.1016/j.meatsci.2010.06.004

Schottstedt, T., Muri, C., Morel, C., Philipona, C., Hammon, H. M., & Blum, J. W. (2005). Effects of feeding vitamin A and lactoferrin on epithelium of lymphoid tissues of intestine of neonatal calves. *Journal of Dairy Science, 88*(3), 1050–1061. https://doi.org/10.3168/jds.S0022-0302(05)72773-9

Schröder, B., Breves, G., & Pfeffer, E. (1990). Binding properties of duodenal 1,25-dihydroxyvitamin D$_3$ receptors as affected by phosphorus depletion in lactating goats. *Comparative Biochemistry and Physiology. A, Comparative Physiology, 96*(4), 495–498. https://doi.org/10.1016/0300-9629(90)90668-i

Schultze, J., & Willy, V. (1997). Biological efficacy of Rovimix Stay-C 35 as a source of vitamin C for dogs, poultry, calves, growing pigs and horses. Roche Vitamins Research Report, *167,* 495.

Schurgers, L. J., & Vermeer, C. (2002). Differential lipoprotein transport pathways of K-vitamins in healthy subjects. *Biochimica et Biophysica Acta, 1570*(1), 27–32. https://doi.org/10.1016/S0304-4165(02)00147-2

Schwab, E. C., & Shaver, R. D. (2005). B-vitamin nutrition for dairy cattle. Penn State Dairy-Cattle Nutrition Workshop, *Grantville, PA.*

Schwab, E. C., Caraviello, D. Z., & Shaver, R. D. (2005). REVIEW: A meta-analysis of lactation responses to supplemental dietary niacin in dairy cows. *The Professional Animal Scientist, 21*(4), 239–247. https://doi.org/10.15232/S1080-7446(15)31214-6

Schwab, E. C., Schwab, C. G., Shaver, R. D., Girard, C. L., Putnam, D. E., & Whitehouse, N. L. (2006). Dietary forage and nonfiber carbohydrate contents influence B-vitamin intake, duodenal flow, and apparent ruminal synthesis in lactating dairy cows. *Journal of Dairy Science, 89*(1), 174–187. https://doi.org/10.3168/jds.S0022-0302(06)72082-3

Schwarz, K. (1962). Vitamin E, trace elements and sulfhydryl groups in respiratory decline: (an approach to the mode of action of tocopherol and related compounds). In *Vitamins and Hormones.* Academic Press, *20.* https://doi.org/10.1016/S0083-6729(08)60730-X

Schweigert, F. J., & Zucker, H. (1988). Concentrations of vitamin A, beta-carotene and vitamin E in individual bovine follicles of different quality. *Journal of Reproduction and Fertility*, *82*(2), 575–579. https://doi.org/10.1530/jrf.0.0820575

Schweigert, F. J., Wierich, M., Rambeck, W. A., & Zucker, H. (1988). Carotene cleavage activity in bovine ovarian follicles. *Theriogenology*, *30*(5), 923–930. https://doi.org/10.1016/S0093-691X(88)80054-2

Scott, J. M. (1999). Folate and vitamin B$_{12}$. *The Proceedings of the Nutrition Society*, *58*(2), 441–448. https://doi.org/10.1017/s0029665199000580

Scott, M. L. (1966). Factors modifying the practical vitamin requirements of poultry. In *Proceedings of the 1966 Cornell Nutrition Conference for the Feed Manufacturers* 35. Ithaca, NY.

Seck, M., Linton, J. A. V., Allen, M. S., Castagnino, D. S., Chouinard, P. Y., & Girard, C. L. (2017). Apparent ruminal synthesis of B vitamins in lactating dairy cows fed diets with different forage-to-concentrate ratios. *Journal of Dairy Science*, *100*(3), 1914–1922. https://doi.org/10.3168/jds.2016-12111

Segerson, E. C., Riviere, G. J., Dalton, H. L., & Whitacre, M. D. (1981). Retained placenta of Holstein cows treated with selenium and vitamin E. *Journal of Dairy Science*, *64*(9), 1833–1836. https://doi.org/10.3168/jds.S0022-0302(81)82772-5

Sehested, J., Jørgensen, C., Mortensen, S. B., Jensen, S. K., Vestergaard, M., Koch, P., Jungersen, G., & Eriksen, L. (2004). Effect of oral alpha-tocopherol and zinc on plasma status, IGF-I levels, weight gain and immune response in young calves. *Journal of Animal and Feed Sciences*, *13*(Suppl. 1), 609–612. https://doi.org/10.22358/jafs/74066/2004

Seifi, H. A., Mokhber, M., Dezfuly, R., & Bolurchi, M. (1996). The effectiveness of ascorbic acid in the prevention of calf neonatal diarrhoea. *Journal of Veterinary Medicine*, *43*, 189–191. https://doi.org/10.1111/j.1439-0450.1996.tb00304.x

Sergeev, I. N., Arkhapchev, Y. P., & Spirichev, V. B. (1990). The role of vitamin E in the metabolism and reception of vitamin E. Biokhimiya-Engl. Tr, *55*(11), 1483. PubMed: 1964807

Seymour, W. M. (2000). Biotin, hoof health and milk production in dairy cows. In 12th Annual Florida Ruminant Nutrition Symposium, FL, United States (pp. 70–78).

Seymour, W. M. (2004). Recent developments in vitamin nutrition of dairy cattle. http://www.dsm.com/enUS/downloads/dnpus/seymour_dairy1.pdf. In *Proceedings of the Intermountain Nutr. Conf. Available at* (pp. 43–64).

Seyoum, E., & Selhub, J. (1998). Properties of food folates determined by stability and susceptibility to intestinal pteroyl polyglutamate hydrolase action. *The Journal of Nutrition*, *128*(11), 1956–1960. https://doi.org/10.1093/jn/128.11.1956

Shanker, A. (2006). Nutritional modulation of immune function and infectious disease. In B. A. Bowman & R. M. Russell (Eds.), *Present knowledge in nutrition* (9th ed.) (pp. 604–624). International Life Sciences Institute.

Shappell, N. W., Herbein, J. H., Deftos, L. J., & Aiello, R. J. (1987). Effects of dietary calcium and age on parathyroid hormone, calcitonin and serum and milk minerals in the periparturient dairy cow. *The Journal of Nutrition*, *117*(1), 201–207. https://doi.org/10.1093/jn/117.1.201

Sharma, B. K., & Erdman, R. A. (1988). Effects of high amounts of dietary choline supplementation on duodenal choline flow and production responses of dairy cows. *Journal of Dairy Science*, *71*(10), 2670–2676. https://doi.org/10.3168/jds.S0022-0302(88)79860-4

Sharma, B. K., & Erdman, R. A. (1989a). *In vitro* degradation of choline from selected feedstuffs and choline supplements. *Journal of Dairy Science*, *72*(10), 2772–2776. https://doi.org/10.3168/jds.S0022-0302(89)79421-2

Sharma, B. K., & Erdman, R. A. (1989b). Effects of dietary and abomasally infused choline on milk production responses of lactating dairy cows. *The Journal of Nutrition*, *119*(2), 248–254. https://doi.org/10.1093/jn/119.2.248

Shaver, R. D., & Bal, M. A. (2000). Effect of dietary thiamin supplementation on milk production by dairy cows. *Journal of Dairy Science*, *83*(10), 2335–2340. https://doi.org/10.3168/jds.S0022-0302(00)75121-6

Shea, M. K., & Booth, S. L. (2008). Update on the role of vitamin K in skeletal health. *Nutrition Reviews*, *66*(10), 549–557. https://doi.org/10.1111/j.1753-4887.2008.00106.x

Shearer, J. K., & Van Amstel, S. R. (1997). Claw disorders: A primary cause of lameness in dairy cattle. In *Manual for the master hoof care technician program* (pp. 18–32). Gainesville, FL.

Shearer, M. J., Barkhan, P., & Webster, G. R. (1970). Absorption and excretion of an oral dose of tritiated vitamin K$_1$ in man. *British Journal of Haematology*, *18*(3), 297–308. https://doi.org/10.1111/j.1365-2141.1970.tb01444.x

Sheffy, B. E., & Schultz, R. D. (1979). Influence of vitamin E and selenium on immune response mechanisms. *Federation Proceedings*, *38*(7), 2139–2143. https://doi.org/10.1111/j.1365-2141.1970.tb01444.x, PubMed: 312742

Shenkoru, T., Owens, F. N., Puchala, R., & Sahlu, T. (1999). Effect of ruminally protected choline on productivity of Angora goats. *Journal of Animal Science*, *77*(Suppl. 1), 271.

Sheppard, A. J., & Johnson, B. C. (1957). Pantothenic acid deficiency in the growing calf. *The Journal of Nutrition*, *61*(2), 195–205. https://doi.org/10.1093/jn/61.2.195

Sheridan, P. A., & Beck, M. A. (2008). The immune response to herpes simplex virus encephalitis in mice is modulated by dietary vitamin E. *The Journal of Nutrition*, *138*(1), 130–137. https://doi.org/10.1093/jn/138.1.130

Shetty, S. A., Young, M. F., Taneja, S., & Rangiah, K. (2020). Quantification of B-vitamins from different fresh milk samples using ultra-high performance liquid chromatography mass spectrometry/selected reaction monitoring methods. *Journal of Chromatography. A*, *1609*, 460452. https://doi.org/10.1016/j.chroma.2019.460452

Shideler, C. E. (1983). Vitamin B$_6$: An overview. *The American Journal of Medical Technology*, *49*(1), 17–22. PubMed: 6342384

Shields, R. G., Campbell, D. R., Huges, D. M., & Dillingham, D. A. (1982). Researchers study vitamin A stability in feeds. *Feedstuffs*, *54*(47), 22.

Shin, D. J., & McGrane, M. M. (1997). Vitamin A regulates genes involved in hepatic gluconeogenesis in mice: Phosphoenolpyruvate carboxykinase, fructose-1,6-bisphosphatase and 6-phosphofructo-2-kinase/fructose-2,6-bisphosphatase. *The Journal of Nutrition*, *127*(7), 1274–1278. https://doi.org/10.1093/jn/127.7.1274

Siebert, B. D., Pitchford, W. S., Kruk, Z. A., Kuchel, H., Deland, M. P. B., & Bottema, C. D. K. (2003). Differences in Δ9 desaturase activity between Jersey and Limousin- sired cattle. *Lipids*, *38*(5), 539–543. https://doi.org/10.1007/s11745-003-1339-7

Siebert, B. D., Kruk, Z. A., Davis, J., Pitchford, W. S., Harper, G. S., & Bottema, C. D. K. (2006). Effect of low vitamin A status on fat deposition and fatty acid desaturation in beef cattle. *Lipids*, *41*(4), 365–370. https://doi.org/10.1007/s11745-006-5107-5

Silva, A. S., Cortinhas, C. S., Acedo, T. S., Morenz, M. J. F., Lopes, F. C. F., Arrigoni, M. B., Ferreira, M. H., Jaguaribe, T. L., Ferreira, L. D., Gouvêa, V. N., & Pereira, L. G. R. (2022). Effects of feeding 25-hydroxyvitamin D3 with an acidogenic diet during the prepartum period in dairy cows: Mineral metabolism, energy balance, and lactation performance of Holstein dairy cows. *Journal of Dairy Science*, *105*(7), 5796–5812. https://doi.org/10.3168/jds.2021-21727

Simon, J. (1999). Choline, betaine and methionine interactions in chickens, pigs and fish (including crustaceans). *World's Poultry Science Journal*, *55*(4), 353–374. https://doi.org/10.1079/WPS19990025

Singh, R. (1957). *B-vitamins and vitamin C levels in blood and milk of cattle under different environmental temperature conditions* [Unpublished PhD dissertation]. University Missouri.

Singh, U., Devaraj, S., & Jialal, I. (2005). Vitamin E, oxidative stress, and inflammation. *Annual Review of Nutrition*, *25*, 151–174. https://doi.org/10.1146/annurev.nutr.24.012003.132446

Sitara, D., Razzaque, M. S., St-Arnaud, R., Huang, W., Taguchi, T., Erben, R. G., & Lanske, B. (2006). Genetic ablation of vitamin D activation pathway reverses biochemical and skeletal anomalies in FGF23-null animals. *The American Journal of Pathology*, *169*(6), 2161–2170. https://doi.org/10.2353/ajpath.2006.060329

Sitrin, M. D., Lieberman, F., Jensen, W. E., Noronha, A., Milburn, C., & Addington, W. (1987). Vitamin E deficiency and neurologic disease in adults with cystic fibrosis. *Annals of Internal Medicine*, *107*(1), 51–54. https://doi.org/10.7326/0003-4819-107-1-51

Skaar, T. C., Grummer, R. R., Dentine, M. R., & Stauffacher, R. H. (1989). Seasonal effects of prepartum and postpartum fat and niacin feeding on lactation performance and lipid metabolism. *Journal of Dairy Science*, *72*(8), 2028–2038. https://doi.org/10.3168/jds.S0022-0302(89)79326-7

Sklan, D. (1983). Carotene cleavage activity in the *corpus luteum* of cattle. *International Journal for Vitamin and Nutrition Research. Internationale Zeitschrift Fur Vitamin- und Ernahrungsforschung. Journal International de Vitaminologie et de Nutrition*, 53(1), 23–26. PubMed: 6406383

Smit, J. J., Schonewille, J. T., & Beynen, A. C. (1999). Transient lowering of plasma vitamin B_{12} concentrations in Ouessant sheep fed on a potassium-rich ration. *International Journal for Vitamin and Nutrition Research. Internationale Zeitschrift Fur Vitamin- und Ernahrungsforschung. Journal International de Vitaminologie et de Nutrition*, 69(4), 273–276. https://doi.org/10.1024/0300-9831.69.4.273

Smith, C. M., & Song, W. O. (1996). Comparative nutrition of pantothenic acid. *The Journal of Nutritional Biochemistry*, 7(6), 312–321. https://doi.org/10.1016/0955-2863(96)00034-4

Smith, K. L., Conrad, H. R., Amiet, B. A., & Todhunter, D. A. (1984). Incidence of environmental mastitis as influenced by vitamin E and selenium. *Kiel. Milchwirstsch. Forschungsber*, 37, 482.

Smith, K. L., Conrad, H. R., Amiet, B. A., Schoenberger, P. S., & Todhunter, D. A. (1985). Effect of vitamin E and selenium dietary supplementation on mastitis in first lactation dairy cows. *Journal of Dairy Science*, 68(Suppl. 1), 190.

Smith, K. L., Hogan, J. S., & Weiss, W. P. (1997). Dietary vitamin E and selenium affect mastitis and milk quality. *Journal of Animal Science*, 75(6), 1659–1665. https://doi.org/10.2527/1997.7561659x

Smith, R. (1994). Assay for vitamin E represents a major step to longer, redder beef color. *Feedstuffs*, 66(16), 9.

Smith, R. M., & Marston, H. R. (1970). Production, absorption, distribution and excretion of vitamin B_{12} in sheep. *The British Journal of Nutrition*, 24(4), 857–877. https://doi.org/10.1079/BJN19700092

Sobel, B. E., & Shell, W. E. (1972). Serum enzyme determinations in the diagnosis and assessment of myocardial infarction. *Circulation*, 45(2), 471–482. https://doi.org/10.1161/01.CIR.45.2.471

Soldatenkov, P. F., & Suganova, N. M. (1966). On the vitamin C exchange in cattle. *Selskochoz Biol.*, 1, 446.

Solomons, N. W. (2006). Vitamin A. In B. Bowman & R. Russell (Eds.), *Present knowledge in nutrition* (9th ed.) (pp. 157–183). International Life Sciences Institute.

Sommerfeldt, J. L., Horst, R. L., Littledike, E. T., Beitz, D. C., & Napoli, J. L. (1981). Metabolism of orally administered 3H-vitamin D_2 and 3H-vitamin D_3 by dairy calves. *Journal of Dairy Science*, 64(1), 157–160 [Abstr.]. https://doi.org/10.3168/jds.S0022-0302(81)82543-X

Sommerfeldt, J. L., Napoli, J. L., Littledike, E. T., & Horst, R. L. (1983). Metabolism of orally administered [3H]cholecalciferol by dairy cows. *Journal of Nutrition*, 113, 2595–2600. https://doi.org/10.1093/jn/113.12.2595

Sone, H., Ito, M., Sugiyama, K., Ohneda, M., Maebashi, M., & Furukawa, Y. (1999). Biotin enhances glucose-stimulated insulin secretion in the isolated perfused pancreas of the rat. *The Journal of Nutritional Biochemistry*, 10(4), 237–243. https://doi.org/10.1016/S0955-2863(99)00003-0

Southern, L. L., & Baker, D. H. (1981). Bioavailable pantothenic acid in cereal grains and soybean meal. *Journal of Animal Science*, 53(2), 403–408. https://doi.org/10.2527/jas1981.532403x

Spasevski, N. J., Vukmirovic, D., Levic, J., & Kokic, B. (2015). Influence of pelleting process and material particle size on the stability of retinol acetate. *Arch. Zootech.*, 18(2), 67–72

Spears, J. W. (2000). Micronutrients and immune function in cattle. *The Proceedings of the Nutrition Society*, 59(4), 587–594. https://doi.org/10.1017/s0029665100000835

Spears, J. W., & Weiss, W. P. (2014). Invited review: Mineral and vitamin nutrition in ruminants. *The Professional Animal Scientist*, 30(2), 180–191. https://doi.org/10.15232/S1080-7446(15)30103-0

Spencer, R. P., Purdy, S., Hoeldtke, R., Bow, T. M., & Markulis, M. A. (1963). Studies on intestinal absorption of L-ascorbic acid-1-C14. *Gastroenterology*, 44(6), 768–773. https://doi.org/10.1016/S0016-5085(63)80086-4

Stabel, J. R., Reinhardt, T. A., Stevens, M. A., Kehrli, Jr., M. E., & Nonnecke, B. J. (1992). Vitamin E effects on *in vitro* immunoglobulin M and interleukin-Lβ production and transcription in dairy cattle. *Journal of Dairy Science*, 75(8), 2190–2198. https://doi.org/10.3168/jds.S0022-0302(92)77979-X

Stabler, S. P. (2006). Vitamin B_{12}. In B. A. Bowman & R. M. Russell (Eds.), *Present knowledge in nutrition* (9th ed.) (pp. 302–313). International Life Sciences Institute.

Stacchiotti, V., Rezzi, S., Eggersdorfer, M., & Galli, F. (2021). Metabolic and functional interplay between gut microbiota and fat-soluble vitamins. *Critical Reviews in Food Science and Nutrition*, 61(19), 3211–3232. https://doi.org/10.1080/10408398.2020.1793728

Stahl, W., Schwarz, W., Von Laar, J., & Sies, H. (1995). All-trans beta-carotene preferentially accumulates in human chylomicrons and very low-density lipoproteins compared with the 9-cis geometrical isomer. *The Journal of Nutrition*, *125*(8), 2128–2133. https://doi.org/10.1093/jn/125.8.2128

Stangl, G. I., Schwarz, F. J., & Kirchgessner, M. (1998). Amino acid changes in plasma and liver of cobalt-deficient cattle. *Journal of Animal Physiology and Animal Nutrition*, *80*(1–5), 40–48. https://doi.org/10.1111/j.1439-0396.1998.tb00498.x

Stangl, G. I., Schwarz, F. J., & Kirchgessner, M. (1999). Cobalt deficiency effects on trace elements, hormones and enzymes involved in energy metabolism of cattle. *International Journal for Vitamin and Nutrition Research. Internationale Zeitschrift Fur Vitamin- und Ernahrungsforschung. Journal International de Vitaminologie et de Nutrition*, *69*(2), 120–126. https://doi.org/10.1024/0300-9831.69.2.120

Stangl, G. I., Schwarz, F. J., Müller, H., & Kirchgessner, M. (2000). Evaluation of the cobalt requirement of beef cattle based on vitamin B_{12}, folate, homocysteine and methylmalonic acid. *The British Journal of Nutrition*, *84*(5), 645–653. https://doi.org/10.1017/S0007114500001987

Steenbock, H. (1924) The induction of growth promoting and calcifying properties in a ration by exposure to light. *Science* 60(1549):224–225. https://doi.org/10.1126/science.60.1549.224

Stein, J., Daniel, H., Whang, E., Wenzel, U., Hahn, A., & Rehner, G. (1994). Rapid postabsorptive metabolism of nicotinic acid in rat small intestine may affect transport by metabolic trapping. *The Journal of Nutrition*, *124*(1), 61–66. https://doi.org/10.1093/jn/124.1.61

Steinberg, W., Kluenter, A. M., & Shuep, W. (1994). Plasma kinetics and excretion of biotin in dairy cows after intravenous and intraruminal application. Proc. Soc. Nutr., *3*, 226.

Steinberg, W., Griggio, C., Bohn, N., Kluenter, A. M., & Schuep, W. (1996). Influence of graded biotin supplementation on biotin concentration in blood plasma and milk of dairy cows. Roche res. *Rep. B.* Basel, Switzerland, *166*, 726.

Steiner, M., & Anastasi, J. (1976). Vitamin E. An inhibitor of the platelet release reaction. *The Journal of Clinical Investigation*, *57*(3), 732–737. https://doi.org/10.1172/JCI108331

Stemme, K., Meyer, U., Flachowsky, G., & Scholz, H. (2006). The influence of an increased cobalt supply to dairy cows on the vitamin B_{12} status of their calves. *Journal of Animal Physiology and Animal Nutrition*, *90*(3–4), 173–176. https://doi.org/10.1111/j.1439-0396.2005.00584.x

Stemme, K., Lebzien, P., Flachowsky, G., & Scholz, H. (2008). The influence of an increased cobalt supply on ruminal parameters and microbial vitamin B_{12} synthesis in the rumen of dairy cows. *Archives of Animal Nutrition*, *62*(3), 207–218. https://doi.org/10.1080/17450390802027460

Stephens, L. C., McChesney, A. E., & Nockels, C. F. (1979). Improved recovery of vitamin E-treated lambs that have been experimentally infected with intratracheal chlamydia. *The British Veterinary Journal*, *135*(3), 291–293. https://doi.org/10.1016/S0007-1935(17)32890-7

Stephensen, C. B., Moldoveanu, Z., & Gangopadhyay, N. N. (1996). Vitamin A deficiency diminishes the salivary immunoglobulin A response and enhances the serum immunoglobulin G response to influenza A virus infection in BALB/c mice. *The Journal of Nutrition*, *126*(1), 94–102. https://doi.org/10.1093/jn/126.1.94

Stobo, I. J. F. (1983). Milk replacers for calves. In *Recent advances in animal nutrition*, 113. Butterworths.

Stowe, H. D., Thomas, J. W., Johnson, T., Marteniuk, J. V., Morrow, D. A., & Ullrey, D. E. (1988). Responses of dairy cattle to long term and short-term supplementation with oral selenium and vitamin E. *Journal of Dairy Science*, *71*(7), 1830–1839. https://doi.org/10.3168/jds.S0022-0302(88)79752-0

Strickland, J. M., Wisnieski, L., Herdt, T. H., & Sordillo, L. M. (2021). Serum retinol, β-carotene, and α-tocopherol as biomarkers for disease risk and milk production in periparturient dairy cows. *Journal of Dairy Science*, *104*(1), 915–927. https://doi.org/10.3168/jds.2020-18693

Strickland, J. M., Wisnieski, L., Mavangira, V., & Sordillo, L. M. (2021). Serum vitamin D is associated with antioxidant potential in peri-parturient cows. *Antioxidants*, *10*(9), 1420. https://doi.org/10.3390/antiox10091420

Stubbs, R. L., Morgan, J. B., Ray, F. K., & Dolezal, H. G. (2002). Effect of supplemental dietary vitamin E on the color and case-life of top loin steaks and ground chuck patties in various case- ready retail packaging systems. *Meat Science*, *61*(1), 1–5. https://doi.org/10.1016/s0309-1740(01)00148-6

Styskal, J., Van Remmen, H., Richardson, A., & Salmon, A. B. (2012). Oxidative stress and diabetes: What can we learn about insulin resistance from antioxidant mutant mouse models? *Free Radical Biology and Medicine*, *52*(1), 46–58. https://doi.org/10.1016/j.freeradbiomed.2011.10.441

Su, Y., Sun, Y., Ju, D., Chang, S., Shi, B., & Shan, A. (2018). The detoxification effect of vitamin C on zearalenone toxicity in piglets. *Ecotoxicology and Environmental Safety*, *158*, 284–292. https://doi.org/10.1016/j.ecoenv.2018.04.046

Sun, M. K., & Alkon, D. L. (2008). Synergistic effects of chronic bryostatin-1 and α-tocopherol on spatial learning and memory in rats. *European Journal of Pharmacology*, *584*(2–3), 328–337. https://doi.org/10.1016/j.ejphar.2008.02.014

Surai, P. F., & Dvorska, J. E. (2005). *Effects of mycotoxins on antioxidant status and immunity. The mycotoxin blue book*, 1. ISBN: 1904761194.

Suter, C. (1990). Vitamins at the molecular level. In *Proceedings of the 'National Feed Ingr. Ass. Nutr. Inst.'*: *"Developments in Vitamin Nutrition and Health Applications"* Kansas City, MO. National Feed Ingredients Association.

Suttie, J. W. (2007). Vitamin K. In J. Zempleni, R. B. Rucker, D. B. McCormick, & J. W. Suttie (Eds.), *Handbook of vitamins* (4th ed.) (pp. 111–139). CRC Press. https://doi.org/10.2527/1997.751112x

Suttie, J. W. (2013). Vitamin K. In J. Zempleni, J. W. Suttie, J. Gregory, & P. J. Stover (Eds.), *Handbook of vitamins* (5th ed.) (pp. 89–124). CRC Press, Taylor & Francis Group, LLC.

Suttie, J. W., & Jackson, C. M. (1977). Prothrombin structure, activation, and biosynthesis. *Physiological Reviews*, *57*(1), 1–70. https://doi.org/10.1152/physrev.1977.57.1.1

Suttie, J. W., & Olson, R. E. (1990). Vitamin K. In *"Nutrition reviews, present knowledge in nutrition"* Nutrition Foundation R. E. Olson (Ed.). (122).

Suttle, N. F., & Jones, D. G. (1989). Recent developments in trace element metabolism and function: Trace elements, disease resistance and immune responsiveness in ruminants. *The Journal of Nutrition*, *119*(7), 1055–1061. https://doi.org/10.1093/jn/119.7.1055

Sutton, A. L., & Elliot, J. M. (1972). Effect of ration of roughage to concentrate and level of feed intake on ovine ruminal vitamin B_{12} production. *The Journal of Nutrition*, *102*(10), 1341–1346. https://doi.org/10.1093/jn/102.10.1341

Sutton, R. A. L., & Dirks, J. H. (1978). Renal handling of calcium. *Federation Proceedings*, *37*(8), 2112–2119. PubMed: 658450

Swanek, S. S., Morgan, J. B., Owens, F. N., Gill, D. R., Strasia, C. A., Dolezal, H. G., & Ray, F. K. (1999). Vitamin D_3 supplementation of beef steers increases *longissimus* tenderness. *Journal of Animal Science*, *77*(4), 874–881. https://doi.org/10.2527/1999.774874x

Swanson, E. W., Martin, G. G., Pardue, F. E., & Gorman, G. M. (1968). Milk production of cows fed diets deficient in vitamin A. *Journal of Animal Science*, *27*(2), 541. https://doi.org/10.2527/jas1968.272541x

Swanson, K. S., Merchen, N. R., Erdman, Jr., J. W., Drackley, J. K., Orias, F., Morin, D. E., & Haddad, M. F. (2000). Influence of vitamin A concentrations and health in preruminant Holstein calves fed milk replacer. *Journal of Dairy Science*, *83*(9), 2027–2036. https://doi.org/10.3168/jds.S0022-0302(00)75083-1

Swensson, C., & Lindmark-Månsson, H. (2007). The prospect of obtaining beneficial mineral and vitamin contents in cow's milk through feed. *Journal of Animal and Feed Sciences*, *16*(Suppl. 1), 21–41. https://doi.org/10.22358/jafs/74110/2007

Swingle, R. S., & Dyer, I. A. (1970). Effects of choline on rumen microbial metabolism. *Journal of Animal Science*, *31*(2), 404–408. https://doi.org/10.2527/jas1970.312404x

Takahashi, E., Matsui, T., Wakamatsu, S., Yuri, N., Shiojiri, Y., Matsuyama, R., Murakami, H., Tanaka, S., Torii, S., & Yano, H. (1999). Serum vitamin C concentration in fattening and fattened beef cattle. *Nihon Chikusan Gakkaiho*, *70*(8), 119–122. https://doi.org/10.2508/chikusan.70.8_119

Taljaard, T. L. (1993). Cabbage poisoning in ruminants. *Journal of the South African Veterinary Association*, *64*(2), 96–100. PubMed: 8410951

Tanaka, K. A., Szlam, F., Dickneite, G., & Levy, J. H. (2008). Effects of prothrombin complex concentrate and recombinant activated factor VII on vitamin K antagonist induced anticoagulation. *Thrombosis Research*, *122*(1), 117–123. https://doi.org/10.1016/j.thromres.2007.09.002

Tang, F. I., & Wei, I. L. (2004). Vitamin B$_6$ deficiency prolongs the time course of evoked dopamine release from rat striatum. *The Journal of Nutrition*, *134*(12), 3350–3354. https://doi.org/10.1093/jn/134.12.3350

Tani, M., & Iwai, K. (1984). Some nutritional effects of folate-binding protein in bovine milk on the bioavailability of folate to rats. *The Journal of Nutrition*, *114*(4), 778–785. https://doi.org/10.1093/jn/114.4.778

Tanumihardjo, S. A. (2013). Vitamin A and bone health: The balancing act. *Journal of Clinical Densitometry*, *16*(4), 414–419. https://doi.org/10.1016/j.jocd.2013.08.016

Tanumihardjo, S. A., & Howe, J. A. (2005). Twice the amount of alpha-carotene isolated from carrots is as effective as beta-carotene in maintaining the vitamin A status of Mongolian gerbils. *The Journal of Nutrition*, *135*(11), 2622–2626. https://doi.org/10.1093/jn/135.11.2622

Taylor, M. S., Knowlton, K. F., McGilliard, M. L., Seymour, W. M., & Herbein, J. H. (2008). Blood mineral, hormone, and osteocalcin responses of multiparous jersey cows to an oral dose of 25–hydroxyvitamin D$_3$ or vitamin D$_3$ before parturition. *Journal of Dairy Science*, *91*(6), 2408–2416. https://doi.org/10.3168/jds.2007-0750

Taylor, T., Hawkins, D. R., Hathway, D. E., & Partington, H. (1972). A new urinary metabolite of pantothenate in dogs. *British Veterinary Journal*, *128*(10), 500–505. https://doi.org/10.1016/S0007-1935(17)36734-9

Tekpetey, F. R., Palmer, W. M., & Ingalls, J. R. (1987a). Reproductive performance of prepuberal dairy heifers on low or high beta-carotene diets. *Canadian Journal of Animal Science*, *67*(2), 477–489. https://doi.org/10.4141/cjas87-046

Tekpetey, F. R., Palmer, W. M., & Ingalls, J. R. (1987b). Seasonal variation in serum beta-carotene and vitamin A and their association with postpartum reproductive performance of Holstein cow. *Canadian Journal of Animal Science*, *67*(2), 491–500. https://doi.org/10.4141/cjas87-047

Tengerdy, R. P. (1980). Disease resistance: Immune response. In *Vitamin e a Comprehensive Treatise* (Basic & Clinical Nutrition Series) Marcel" Machlin, L. J. (Ed.). *Dekker Inc.*. https://doi.org/10.1007/978-1-4613-0553-8_9

Thafvelin, B., & Oksanen, H. E. (1966). Vitamin E and linolenic acid content of hays as related to different drying conditions. *Journal of Dairy Science*, *49*(3), 282–286. https://doi.org/10.3168/jds.S0022-0302(66)87850-5

Tharnish, T. A., & Larson, L. L. (1992). Vitamin A supplementation of Holsteins at high concentrations: Progesterone and reproductive responses. *Journal of Dairy Science*, *75*(9), 2375–2381. https://doi.org/10.3168/jds.S0022-0302(92)77998-3

Thierry, M. J., Hermodson, M. A., & Suttie, J. W. (1970). Vitamin K and warfarin distribution and metabolism in the warfarin-resistant rat. *The American Journal of Physiology*, *219*(4), 854–859. https://doi.org/10.1152/ajplegacy.1970.219.4.854

Thomas, J. W., Loosli, J. K., & William, J. P. (1947). Placental and mammary transfer of vitamin A in swine and goats as affected by the prepartum diet. *Journal of Animal Science*, *6*(2), 141–145. https://doi.org/10.2527/jas1947.62141x

Thornber, E. J. (1979). *Biochemical studies of thiamine deficiency in the lamb* ([Unpublished doctoral dissertation]. Murdoch University).

Tiffany, M. E., & Spears, J. W. (2005). Differential responses to dietary cobalt in finishing steers fed corn vs. barley-based diets. *Journal of Animal Science*, *83*(11), 2580–2589. https://doi.org/10.2527/2005.83112580x

Tiffany, M. E., Spears, J. W., Xi, L., & Horton, J. (2003). Influence of supplemental cobalt source and concentration on performance, vitamin B$_{12}$ status, and ruminal and plasma metabolites in growing and finishing steers. *Journal of Animal Science*, *81*(12), 3151–3159. https://doi.org/10.2527/2003.81123151x

Tjoelker, L. W., Chew, B. P., Tanaka, T. S., & Daniel, L. R. (1988). Bovine vitamin A and beta-carotene intake and lactational status. 2. Responsiveness of mitogen stimulated peripheral blood lymphocytes to vitamin A and beta-carotene challenge *in vitro*. *Journal of Dairy Science*, *71*(11), 3120–3127. https://doi.org/10.3168/jds.S0022-0302(88)79912-9

Tjoelker, L. W., Chew, B. P., Tanaka, T. S., & Daniel, L. R. (1990). Effect of vitamin A and beta carotene on polymorphonuclear leukocyte and lymphocyte function in dairy cows during the early dry period. *Journal of Dairy Science*, *73*(4), 1017–1022. https://doi.org/10.3168/jds.S0022-0302(90)78760-7

Tligui, N., & Ruth, G. R. (1994). *Ferula communis* variety *brevifolia* intoxication of sheep. *American Journal of Veterinary Research*, 55(11), 1558–1563. https://doi.org/10.2460/ajvr.1994.55.11.1558, PubMed: 7879979

Toghdory, A., Emanuele, S., Goorchi, T., & Nasorian, A. (2007). Effects of choline and rumen protected choline (Reashure®) on milk production, milk composition and blood metabolites of lactating dairy cows. *Journal of Dairy Science* 90 [Suppl., 1], *353*.

Tomkins, N. W., Elliott, R., McGrath, J. J., & Schatz, T. (2020). Managing plasma P concentrations in beef heifers with a slow-release vitamin D supplementation. *Animal Production Science*, 60(5), 610–617. https://doi.org/10.1071/AN17601

Tomlinson, D. J., Mülling, C. H., & Fakler, T. M. (2004). Invited review: Formation of keratins in the bovine claw: Roles of hormones, minerals, and vitamins in functional claw integrity. *Journal of Dairy Science*, 87(4), 797–809. https://doi.org/10.3168/jds.S0022-0302(04)73223-3

Tomkins, A., & Hussey, G. (1989). Vitamin A, immunity and infection. Nutrition Research Reviews, 2(1), 17–28. https://doi.org/10.1079/NRR19890005

Torquato, P., Bartolini, D., Giusepponi, D., Piroddi, M., Sebastiani, B., Saluti, G., Galarini, R., & Galli, F. (2019). Increased plasma levels of the lipoperoxyl radical-derived vitamin E metabolite α-tocopheryl quinone are an early indicator of lipotoxicity in fatty liver subjects. *Free Radical Biology and Medicine*, 131, 115–125. https://doi.org/10.1016/j.freeradbiomed.2018.11.036

Toutain, P. L., Béchu, D., & Hidiroglou, M. (1997). Ascorbic acid disposition kinetics in the plasma and tissues of calves. *The American Journal of Physiology*, 273(5), R1585–R1597. https://doi.org/10.1152/ajpregu.1997.273.5.R1585

Traber, M. G. (2006). Vitamin E. In B. A. Bowman & R. M. Russell (Eds.), *Present knowledge in nutrition* (9th ed.) (pp. 211–219). International Life Sciences Institute.

Traber, M. G. (2013). Vitamin E. In J. Zempleni, J. Suttie, J. Gregory, & P. J. Stover (Eds.), *Handbook of vitamins* (5th ed.) (pp. 125–148). CRC Press, Taylor & Francis Group, LLC.

Traber, M. G., & Head, B. (2021). Vitamin E: How much is enough, too much and why! *Free Radical Biology and Medicine*, 177, 212–225. https://doi.org/10.1016/j.freeradbiomed.2021.10.028

Traber, M. G., & Kamal-Eldin, A. (2022). Oxidative stress and vitamin E in anemia. In Nutritional Anemia. Springer International Publishing, (205–219)

Traber, M. G., & Sies, H. (1996). Vitamin E in humans: Demand and delivery. *Annual Review of Nutrition*, 16(1), 321–347. https://doi.org/10.1146/annurev.nu.16.070196.001541

Traber, M. G., Rader, D., Acuff, R. V., Ramakrishnan, R., Brewer, H. B., & Kayden, H. J. (1998). Vitamin E dose response studies in humans using deuterated RRR-a-tocopherol. *The American Journal of Clinical Nutrition*, 68(4), 847–853. https://doi.org/10.1093/ajcn/68.4.847

Tramontano, W. A., Ganci, D., Pennino, M., & Dierenfeld, E. S. (1993). Distribution of α-tocopherol in early foliage samples in several forage crops. *Phytochemistry*, 34(2), 389–390. https://doi.org/10.1016/0031-9422(93)80013-I

Tsuchiya, H., & Bates, C. J. (1997). Vitamin C and copper interactions in guinea pigs and a study of collagen cross-links. *The British Journal of Nutrition*, 77(2), 315–325. https://doi.org/10.1079/bjn19970032

Tsukaguchi, H., Tokui, T., Mackenzie, B., Berger, U. V., Chen, X. Z., Wang, Y., Brubaker, R. F., & Hediger, M. A. (1999). A family of mammalian Na+-dependent L-ascorbic acid transporters. *Nature*, 399(6731), 70–75. https://doi.org/10.1038/19986

Tunca, R., Erdoğan, H. M., Sözmen, M., Çitil, M., Devrim, A. K., Erginsoy, S., & Uzlu, E. (2009). Evaluation of cardiac troponin I and inducible nitric oxide synthase expressions in lambs with white muscle disease. *Turkish Journal of Veterinary and Animal Sciences*, 33(1), 53–59. https://doi.org/10.3906/vet-0710-6

Turley, C. P., & Brewster, M. A. (1993). α-tocopherol protects against a reduction in adenosylcobalamin in oxidatively stressed human cells. *The Journal of Nutrition*, 123(7), 1305–1312. https://doi.org/10.1093/jn/123.7.1305

Turner, R. J., & Finch, J. M. (1990). Immunological malfunctions associated with low selenium-vitamin E diets in lambs. *Journal of Comparative Pathology*, 102(1), 99–109. https://doi.org/10.1016/S0021-9975(08)80012-6

Twining, S. S., Schulte, D. P., Wilson, P. M., Fish, B. L., & Moulder, J. E. (1997). Vitamin A deficiency alters rat neutrophil function. *The Journal of Nutrition*, 127(4), 558–565. https://doi.org/10.1093/jn/127.4.558

Uhl, E. W. (2018). The pathology of vitamin D deficiency in domesticated animals: An evolutionary and comparative overview. *International Journal of Paleopathology*, *23*, 100–109. https://doi.org/10.1016/j.ijpp.2018.03.001

Ullrey, D. E. (1972). Biological availability of fat- soluble vitamins: Vitamin A and carotene. *Journal of Animal Science*, *35*(3), 648–657. https://doi.org/10.2527/jas1972.353648x

Ulvund, M. J., & Pestalozzi, M. (1990). Ovine white-liver disease (OWLD) in Norway: Clinical symptoms and preventative measures. *Acta Veterinaria Scandinavica*, *31*(1), 53–62. https://doi.org/10.1186/BF03547577

Underwood, E. J. (1977). *Trace elements in human and animal nutrition*. Academic Press

Underwood, E. J. (1979). The detection and correction of trace mineral deficiencies and toxicities. In *Proceedings of the of the Florida Nutrition Conference*. University of Florida p.203.

Underwood, E. J. (1981). *The mineral nutrition of livestock*. Commonwealth Agricultural Bureaux.

United States Pharmacopeia. (1980) (20th ed.) Mack Printing Comp., Easton, Pennsylvania.

United States Department of Agriculture. *Food Data Central https://fdc.nal.usda.gov/fdc-app.html#/food-details/746782/nutrients*.

USDA (United States Department of Agriculture). (2023). https://www.nass.usda.gov/Charts_and_Maps/Milk_Production_and_Milk_Cows/cowrates.php

Van de Braak, A. E., Van't Klooster, A. T., Goedegebuure, S. A., & Faber, J. A. J. (1987). Effects of calcium and magnesium intakes and feeding level during the dry period on bone resorption in dairy cows at parturition. *Research in Veterinary Science*, *43*(1), 7–12. https://doi.org/10.1016/S0034-5288(18)30732-X

Van den Ouweland, J. M. W. (2016). Analysis of vitamin D metabolites by liquid chromatography-tandem mass spectrometry, TrAC Trends Anal. Chem. MassSpectrom. *Clinical Laboratory*, *84*, 117.e130. https://doi.org/10.1016/j.tr.c.2016.02.005

Van der Lugt, J. J., & Prozesky, L. (1989). The pathology of blindness in new-born calves caused by hypovitaminosis A. http://hdl.handle.net/2263/42135. *The Onderstepoort Journal of Veterinary Research*, *56*(2), 99–109.

van Het Hof, K. H., West, C. E., Weststrate, J. A., & Hautvast, J. G. (2000). Dietary factors that affect the bioavailability of carotenoids. *The Journal of Nutrition*, *130*(3), 503–506. https://doi.org/10.1093/jn/130.3.503

Van Merris, V., Meyer, E., Duchateau, L., Blum, J., & Burvenich, C. (2004). All-trans retinoic acid is increased in the acute phase-related hyporetinemia during *Escherichia coli* mastitis. *Journal of Dairy Science*, *87*(4), 980–987. https://doi.org/10.3168/jds.S0022-0302(04)73243-9

Van Mosel, M., van 't Klooster, A. Th., & Wouterse, H. S. (1991). Effects of a deficient magnesium supply during the dry period on bone turnover of dairy cows at parturition. *The Veterinary Quarterly*, *13*(4), 199–208. https://doi.org/10.1080/01652176.1991.9694309

Van Saun, R. J., Herdt, T. H., & Stowe, H. D. (1989). Maternal and fetal vitamin E interrelationship in dairy cattle. *The Journal of Nutrition*, *119*(8), 1156–1164. https://doi.org/10.1093/jn/119.8.1156

Van Vleet, J. F., & Ferrans, V. J. (1992). Etiologic factors and pathologic alterations in selenium-vitamin E deficiency and excess in animals and humans. *Biological Trace Element Research*, *33*, 1–21. https://doi.org/10.1007/BF02783988

van Vliet, T., van Vlissingen, M. F., van Schaik, F., & van den Berg, H. (1996). β-carotene absorption and cleavage in rats is affected by the vitamin A concentration of the diet. *The Journal of Nutrition*, *126*(2), 499–508. https://doi.org/10.1093/jn/126.2.499

Vanderschueren, D., Gevers, G., Raymaekers, G., Devos, P., & Dequeker, J. (1990). Sex- and age-related changes in bone and serum osteocalcin. *Calcified Tissue International*, *46*(3), 179–182. https://doi.org/10.1007/BF02555041

Vasconcelos, J. T., & Galyean, M. L. (2007). Nutritional recommendations of feedlot consulting nutritionists: The 2007 Texas Tech University survey. *Journal of Animal Science*, *85*(10), 2772–2781. https://doi.org/10.2527/jas.2007-0261

Vasquez, F., Bunting, L. D., Gantt, D. T., Hoyt, P. G., Adkinson, R. W., & Fernandez, J. M. (1999). Metabolic responses and early lactation performance of primiparous heifers fed rumen-protected choline. *Journal of Dairy Science*, *82* (Suppl. 1), 125.

Vaxman, F., Olender, S., Lambert, A., Nisand, G., Aprahamian, M., Bruch, J. F., Didier, E., Volkmar, P., & Grenier, J. F. (1995). Effect of pantothenic acid and ascorbic acid supplementation on human skin wound healing process. A double-blind, prospective and randomized trial. *European Surgical Research. Europaische Chirurgische Forschung. Recherches Chirurgicales Europeennes, 27*(3), 158–166. https://doi.org/10.1159/000129395

Velásquez-Pereira, J., Chenoweth, P. J., McDowell, L. R., Risco, C. A., Staples, C. A., Prichard, D., Martin, F. G., Calhoun, M. C., Williams, S. N., & Wilkinson, N. S. (1998). Reproductive effects of feeding gossypol and vitamin E to bulls. *Journal of Animal Science, 76*(11), 2894–2904. https://doi.org/10.2527/1998.76112894x

Velásquez -Pereira, J., Risco. C.A., McDowell. *Law Review, Staples,* C.R., Prichard, D., Chenoweth, P.J., Martin, F.G., Williams, S.N., Rojas, L.X., Calhoun, M.C. and Wilkinson, N.S. (1999) Long-term effects of feeding gossypol and vitamin E to dairy calves. JDS 82(6):1240-1251. https://doi.org/10.3168/jds.S0022-0302(99)75347-6.

Vellema, P., Rutten, V. P., Hoek, A., Moll, L., & Wentink, G. H. (1996). The effect of cobalt supplementation on the immune response in vitamin B_{12} deficient Texel lambs. *Veterinary Immunology and Immunopathology, 55*(1–3), 151–161. https://doi.org/10.1016/S0165-2427(96)05560-2

Vellema, P., Van den Ingh, T. S., & Wouda, W. (1999). Pathological changes in cobalt-supplemented and non-supplemented twin lambs in relation to blood concentrations of methylmalonic acid and homo-cysteine. *The Veterinary Quarterly, 21*(3), 93–98. https://doi.org/10.1080/01652176.1999.9695001

Verbeeck, J. (1975). Vitamin behavior in premixes. *Feedstuffs, 47*(36), 4.

Vermeer, C. (1984). The vitamin K-dependent carboxylation reaction. *Molecular and Cellular Biochemistry, 61*(1), 17–35. https://doi.org/10.1007/BF00239604

Vermeer, C. (1986). Comparison between hepatic and nonhepatic vitamin K-dependent carboxylase. *Haemostasis, 16*(3–4), 239–245. https://doi.org/10.1159/000215296

Vermeer, C., Jie, K. S., & Knapen, M. H. J. (1995). Role of vitamin K in bone metabolism. *Annual Review of Nutrition, 15*(1), 1–22. https://doi.org/10.1146/annurev.nu.15.070195.000245

Vermunt, J. J., & Greenough, P. R. (1994). Predisposing factors of laminitis in cattle. *The British Veterinary Journal, 150*(2), 151–164. https://doi.org/10.1016/S0007-1935(05)80223-4

Vermunt, J. J., & Greenough, P. R. (1995). Structural characteristics of the bovine claw: Horn growth and wear, horn hardness and claw conformation. *The British Veterinary Journal, 151*(2), 157–180. https://doi.org/10.1016/s0007-1935(95)80007-7

Vieira-Neto, A., Negro, G., Zimpel, R., Poindexter, M., Lopes, Jr., F., Thatcher, W. W., Nelson, C. D., & Santos, J. E. P. (2021a). Effects of injectable calcitriol on mineral metabolism and postpartum health and perfor-mance in dairy cows. *Journal of Dairy Science, 104*(1), 683–701. https://doi.org/10.3168/jds.2020-18448

Vieira-Neto, A., Poindexter, M. B., Nehme Marinho, M. N., Zimpel, R., Husnain, A., Silva, A. C. M., Prim, J. G., Nelson, C. D., & Santos, J. E. P. (2021b). Effect of source and amount of vitamin D on function and mRNA expression in immune cells in dairy cows. *Journal of Dairy Science, 104*(10), 10796–10811. https://doi.org/10.3168/jds.2021-20284

Vinet, C., Conrad, H. R., Reinhardt, T. A., & Horst, R. L. (1985). Minimal requirements for vitamin D in lactating cows. *Federation Proceedings, 28*, 549 [Abstr.].

Vlasova, A. N., Chattha, K. S., Kandasamy, S., Siegismund, C. S., & Saif, L. J. (2013). Prenatally acquired vitamin A deficiency alters innate immune responses to human rotavirus in a gnotobiotic pig model. *Journal of Immunology, 190*(9), 4742–4753. https://doi.org/10.4049/jimmunol.1203575

Vlasova, A. N., & Saif, L. J. (2021). Bovine immunology: Implications for dairy cattle. *Frontiers in Immunology, 12*, 643206. http://doi.org/10.3389/fimmu.2021.643206

Wagner, C. (1995). Biochemical role of folate in cellular metabolism. *Clinical Research and Regulatory Affairs, 18*(3), 161–180. https://doi.org/10.1081/CRP-100108171

Wagner, C., Briggs, W. T., & Cook, R. J. (1984). Covalent binding of folic acid to dimethylglycine dehydrogenase. *Archives of Biochemistry and Biophysics, 233*(2), 457–461. https://doi.org/10.1016/0003-9861(84)90467-3

Waldner, C. L., & Uehlinger, F. D. (2016). Factors associated with serum vitamin A and vitamin E concen-trations in beef calves from Alberta and Saskatchewan and the relationship between vitamin con-centrations and calf health outcomes. *Canadian Journal of Animal Science, 97*(1), 65–82. https://doi.org/10.1139/CJAS-2016-0055

Walker, C. K., & Elliot, J. M. (1972). Lactational trends in vitamin B_{12} status on conventional and restricted-rough-age rations. *Journal of Dairy Science, 55*(4), 474–479. https://doi.org/10.3168/jds.S0022-0302(72)85518-8

Waller, K. P., Sandgren, C. H., Emanuelson, U., & Jensen, S. K. (2007). Supplementation of RRR-α-tocopheryl acetate to periparturient dairy cows in commercial herds with high mastitis incidence. *JDS*, *90*(8), 3640–3646. https://doi.org/10.3168/jds.2006-421

Wallis, G. C. (1946). *Vitamin D deficiency in dairy cows*. S.D. Agric. Exp. Stn. Bull. http://openprairie. sdstate.edu/agexperimentsta_bulletins/372?utm_source=openprairie.sdstate.edu%2Fagexperiment sta_bulletins%2F372&utm_medium=PDF&utm_campaign=PDFCoverPages, *372*. South Dakota State University.

Wallis, G. C., Kennedy, G. H., & Fishman, R. H. (1958). The vitamin D content of roughages. *Journal of Animal Science*, *17*(2), 410–415. https://doi.org/10.2527/jas1958.172410x

Walsh, D. M., Kennedy, S., Blanchflower, W. J., Goodall, E. A., & Kennedy, D. G. (1993). Vitamin E and selenium deficiencies increase indices of lipid peroxidation in muscle tissue of ruminant calves. *International Journal for Vitamin and Nutrition Research. Internationale Zeitschrift Fur Vitamin- und Ernahrungsforschung. Journal International de Vitaminologie et de Nutrition*, *63*(3), 188–194. PubMed: 8300329

Wang, B., Nie, W., Fu, X., De Avila, J. M., Ma, Y., Zhu, M. J., Maquivar, M., Parish, S. M., Busboom, J. R., Nelson, M. L., & Du, M. (2018). Neonatal vitamin A injection promotes cattle muscle growth and increases oxidative muscle fibers. *Journal of Animal Science and Biotechnology*, *9*, 82. https://doi.org/10.1186/s40104-018-0296-3

Wang, C., Zhang, J., Guo, G., Huo, W., Xia, C. Q., Chen, L., Zhang, Y., Pei, C., & Liu, Q. (2023). Effects of folic acid and riboflavin on growth performance, nutrient digestion and rumen fermentation in Angus bulls. *The British Journal of Nutrition*, *129*(1), 1–9. https://doi.org/10.1017/S0007114522000630

Wang, C., Zhang, J., Liu, Q., Guo, G., Huo, W. J., Pei, C. X., Xia, C. Q., Chen, L., & Zhang, Y. W. (2022). Rumen pro-tected riboflavin and rumen protected pantothenate improved growth performance, nutrient digestion and rumen fermentation in Angus bulls. *Animal Feed Science and Technology*, *291*, 115394. https://doi.org/10.1016/j.anifeedsci.2022.115394

Wang, H., Pan, X., Wang, C., Wang, M., & Yu, L. (2015). Effects of different dietary concentrate to forage ratio and thiamine supplementation on the rumen fermentation and ruminal bacterial community in dairy cows. *Animal Production Science*, *55*(2), 189–193. https://doi.org/10.1071/AN14523

Wang, J. Y., Larson, L. L., & Owen, F. G. (1982). Effect of beta-carotene supplementation on reproductive per-formance of dairy heifers. *Theriogenology*, *18*(4), 461–473. https://doi.org/10.1016/0093-691X(82)90168-6

Wang, J. Y., Hafi, C. B., & Larson, L. L. (1988a). Effect of supplemental β-carotene on luteinizing hormone released in response to gonadotropin-releasing hormone challenge in ovariectomized Holstein cows. *Journal of Dairy Science*, *71*(2), 498–504. https://doi.org/10.3168/jds.S0022-0302(88)79580-6

Wang, J. Y., Owen, F. G., & Larson, L. L. (1988b). Effect of beta-carotene supplementation on reproductive performance of lactating Holstein cows. *Journal of Dairy Science*, *71*(1), 181–186. https://doi.org/10.3168/jds.S0022-0302(88)79540-5

Wang, Y., Russo, T. A., Kwon, O., Chanock, S., Rumsey, S. C., & Levine, M. (1997). Ascorbate recycling in human neutrophils: Induction by bacteria. *Proceedings of the National Academy of Sciences of the United States of America*, *94*(25), 13816–13819. https://doi.org/10.1073/pnas.94.25.13816

Wang, L. H., Zhang, C. R., Zhang, Q. Y., Xu, H. J., Feng, G. Z., Zhang, G. N., & Zhang, Y. G. (2022). Effects of feed-ing different doses of 25-hydroxyvitamin D3 on the growth performance, blood minerals, antioxidant status and immunoglobulin of preweaning calves. *Animal Feed Science and Technology*, *285*, 115220. https://doi.org/10.1016/j.anifeedsci.2022.115220

Ward, A. K., McKinnon, J. J., Hendrick, S., & Buchanan, F. C. (2012). The impact of vitamin A restriction and ADH1C genotype on marbling in feedlot steers. *Journal of Animal Science*, *90*(8), 2476–2483. https://doi.org/10.2527/jas.2011-4404

Ward, E. H., & Patterson, H. H. (2004). Effects of thiamine supplementation on performance and health of growing steers consuming high sulfate water. *Proceedings of the West Sec. Am. Soc. Anim. Sci. 55*: 375–378. https://doi.org/10.2527/jas.2011-4404

Ward, G., Dobson, R. C., & Dunham, J. R. (1972). Influences of calcium and phosphorus intakes, vitamin D supplement, and lactation on calcium and phosphorus balances. *Journal of Dairy Science*, *55*(6), 768–776. https://doi.org/10.3168/jds.S0022-0302(72)85571-1

Warner, R. L. Mitchell Jr, G.E., *Little, C.O. and Alderson, N.E.* (1970) Pre-intestinal disappearance of vitamin A in steers fed different levels of corn. Int. Vit, J. Res, *40*, 585. PubMed: 5504691

Washburn, M. P., & Wells, W. W. (1999). Identification of the dehydroascorbic acid reductase and thioltransferase activities of bovine erythrocyte glutathione peroxidase. *Biochemical and Biophysical Research Communications*, *257*(2), 567–571. https://doi.org/10.1006/bbrc.1999.0508

Washko, P. W., Wang, Y., & Levine, M. (1993). Ascorbic acid recycling in human neutrophils. *The Journal of Biological Chemistry*, *268*(21), 15531–15535. https://doi.org/10.1016/S0021-9258(18)82289-X

Wasserman, R. H. (1975). Active vitamin D-like substances in *Solanum malacoxylon* and other calcinogenic plants. *Nutrition Reviews*, *33*(1), 1–5. https://doi.org/10.1111/j.1753-4887.1975.tb07074.x

Wasserman, R. H. (1981). Intestinal absorption of calcium and phosphorus. *Federation Proceedings*, *40*(1), 68–72. PubMed: 7192650

Watanabe, F., & Bito, T. (2018). Vitamin B_{12} sources and microbial interaction. *Experimental Biology and Medicine*, *243*(2), 148–158. https://doi.org/10.1177/1535370217746612

Waterman, R., Schwalm, J. W., & Schultz, L. H. (1972). Nicotinic acid treatment of bovine ketosis. I. Effects on circulatory metabolites and interrelationships. *Journal of Dairy Science*, *55*(10), 1447–1453. https://doi.org/10.3168/jds.S0022-0302(72)85692-3

Waterman, R. A. (1978). Nutrient toxicities in animals and man: Niacin. In M. Rechcigl, Jr. (Ed.), *Handbook series in nutrition and food, section E: Nutritional disorders*, 1 p. 29. CRC Press.

Watkins, B. A. (1989). Influence of biotin deficiency and dietary trans-fatty acids on tissue lipids in chickens. *The British Journal of Nutrition*, *61*(1), 99–111. https://doi.org/10.1079/BJN19890096

Watkins, B. A., & Kratzer, F. H. (1987). Effects of dietary biotin and linoleate on polyunsaturated fatty acids in tissue phospholipids. *Poultry Science*, *66*(12), 2024–2031. https://doi.org/10.3382/ps.0662024

Webb, Jr., K. E., Mitchell, G. E., Little, C. O., Schmitt, G. H., ... Schmitt, G. H.. (1968) Polyuria in vitamin A-deficient sheep. *Journal of Animal Science*, *27*(6), 1657–1662. https://doi.org/10.2527/jas1968.2761657x

Weber, F. (1983). Biochemical mechanisms of vitamin A action. *The Proceedings of the Nutrition Society*, *42*(1), 31–41. https://doi.org/10.1079/pns19830005

Weerathilake, W. A. D. V., Brassington, A. H., Williams, S. J., Kwong, W. Y., Sinclair, L. A., & Sinclair, K. D. (2019). Added dietary cobalt or vitamin B_{12}, or injecting vitamin B_{12} does not improve performance or indicators of ketosis in pre- and post-partum Holstein-Friesian dairy cows. *Animal*, *13*(4), 750–759. https://doi.org/10.1017/S175173111800232X

Wei, I. L., & Young, T. K. (1994). Vitamin B_6 metabolism is altered in chronic renal failure rats. *Nutrition Research*, *14*(2), 271–278. https://doi.org/10.1016/S0271-5317(05)80385-9

Wei, R. R., Wamer, W. G., Lambert, L. A., & Kornhauser, A. (1998). Beta-carotene uptake and effects on intracellular levels of retinol *in vitro*. *Nutrition and Cancer*, *30*(1), 53–58. https://doi.org/10.1080/01635589809514640

Weir, R. R., Johnston, M., Lowis, C., Fearon, A. M., Stewart, S., Strain, J. J., & Pourshahidi, L. K. (2021). Vitamin D3 content of cows' milk produced in Northern Ireland and its efficacy as a vehicle for vitamin D fortification: A UK model. *International Journal of Food Sciences and Nutrition*, *72*(4), 447–455. https://doi.org/10.1080/09637486.2020.1837743

Weiser, H., & Vecchi, M. (1982). Stereoisomers of alpha-tocopheryl acetate. II. Biopotencies of all eight stereoisomers, individually or in mixtures, as determined by rat resorption-gestation tests. *International Journal for Vitamin and Nutrition Research. Internationale Zeitschrift für Vitamin- und Ernahrungsforschung. Journal International de Vitaminologie et de Nutrition*, *52*(3), 351–370. PubMed: 7174231

Weiss, W. P. (1998). Requirements of fat-soluble vitamins for dairy cows: A review. *Journal of Dairy Science*, *81*(9), 2493–2501. https://doi.org/10.3168/jds.S0022-0302(98)70141-9

Weiss, W. P. (2005). *Antioxidant nutrients, cow health, and milk quality*. Penn State Dairy-Cattle Nutrition Workshop (pp. 11–18).

Weiss, J. P. (2007). An update on vitamins for dairy cattle. http://www.ads.uga.edu/extension/dairycattle/documents/MasterSEDHM2007. In *Proceedings of the Southeast Dairy HERD Management Conference*.

Weiss, W. P., & Ferreira, G. (2006a). Water soluble vitamins for dairy cattle. https://www.researchgate.net/profile/William-Weiss-4/publication/228344104_Water_soluble_vitamins_for_dairy_cattle/links/53ed f08c0cf23733e80b1aef/Water-soluble-vitamins-for-dairy-cattle.pdf?_tp=eyJjb250ZXh0Ijp7ImZpccнN0UG FnZSI6InB1YmxpY2F0aW9uIiwicGFnZSI6InB1YmxpY2F0aW9uIn19. Tri-State Dairy Nutrition Conference. Ohio, USA (pp. 51–63).

Weiss, W. P., & Fereira, G. (2006b). Are your cows getting the vitamins that they need WCDS Advances in Dairy Technology, *18*, 249–259. https://www.researchgate.net/profile/William-Weiss-4/publica tion/251640629_Are_Your_Cows_Getting_the_Vitamins_They_Need/links/53edf0860cf23733e80b1aeb/ Are-Your-Cows-Getting-the-Vitamins-They-Need.pdf?_tp=eyJjb250ZXh0Ijp7ImZpccнN0UGFnZSI6In B1YmxpY2F0aW9uIiwicGFnZSI6InB1YmxpY2F0aW9uIn19

Weiss, W. P., & Hogan, J. S. (2007). Effects of dietary vitamin C on neutrophil function and responses to intramammary infusion of lipopolysaccharide in periparturient dairy cows. *Journal of Dairy Science*, *90*(2), 731–739. https://doi.org/10.3168/jds.S0022-0302(07)71557-6

Weiss, W. P., & Wyatt, D. J. (2003). Effect of dietary fat and vitamin E on α-tocopherol in milk from dairy cows. *Journal of Dairy Science*, *86*(11), 3582–3591. https://doi.org/10.3168/jds.S0022-0302(03)73964-2

Weiss, W. P., Hogan, J. S., Smith, K. L., & Hoblet, K. H. (1990a). Relationships among selenium, vitamin E and mammary gland health in commercial dairy herds. *Journal of Dairy Science*, *73*(2), 381–390. https://doi.org/10.3168/jds.S0022-0302(90)78684-5

Weiss, W. P., Todhunter, D. A., Hogan, J. S., & Smith, K. L. (1990b). Effect of duration of supplementation of selenium and vitamin E on periparturient dairy cows. *Journal of Dairy Science*, *73*(11), 3187–3194. https://doi.org/10.3168/jds.S0022-0302(90)79009-1

Weiss, W. P., Hogan, J. S., Smith, K. L., Todhunter, D. A., & Williams, S. N. (1992). Effect of supplementing par-turient cows with vitamin E on distribution of α-tocopherol in blood. *Journal of Dairy Science*, *75*(12), 3479–3485. https://doi.org/10.3168/jds.S0022-0302(92)78124-7

Weiss, W. P., Hogan, J. S., Smith, K. L., & Williams, S. N. (1994). Effect of dietary fat and vitamin E on α-tocoph-erol and β-carotene in blood of peripartum cows. *Journal of Dairy Science*, *77*(5), 1422–1429. https://doi.org/10.3168/jds.S0022-0302(94)77080-6

Weiss, W. P., Smith, K. L., Hogan, J. S., & Steiner, T. E. (1995). Effect of forage to concentrate ratio on dis-appearance of vitamins A and E during *in vitro* ruminal fermentation. *Journal of Dairy Science*, *78*(8), 1837–1842. https://doi.org/10.3168/jds.S0022-0302(95)76808-4

Weiss, W. P., Hogan, J. S., Todhunter, D. A., & Smith, K. L. (1997). Effect of vitamin E supplementation in diets with a low concentration of selenium on mammary gland health of dairy cows. *Journal of Dairy Science*, *80*(8), 1728–1737. https://doi.org/10.3168/jds.S0022-0302(97)76105-8

Weiss, W. P., Hogan, J. S., & Smith, K. L. (2004). Changes in vitamin C concentrations in plasma and milk from dairy cows after an intramammary infusion of Escherichia coli. *Journal of Dairy Science*, *87*(1), 32–37. https://doi.org/10.3168/jds.S0022-0302(04)73138-0

Weiss, W. P., Hogan, J. S., & Wyatt, D. J. (2009). Relative bioavailability of all-rac and RRR vitamin E based on neutrophil function and total α-tocopherol and isomer concentrations in periparturient dairy cows and their calves. *Journal of Dairy Science*, *92*(2), 720–731. https://doi.org/10.3168/jds.2008-1635

Wellmann, K. B., Kim, J. K., Urso, P. M., Smith, Z. K., & Johnson, B. J. (2020). Evaluation of the dietary vitamin A requirement of finishing steers via systematic depletion and repletion, and its effects on performance and carcass characteristics. *Journal of Animal Science*, *98*(9). https://doi.org/10.1093/jas/skaa266

Wernery, U., Haydn-Evans, J., & Kinne, J. (1998). Amprolium-induced cerebrocortical necrosis (CCN) in dromedary racing camels. *Journal of Veterinary Medicine Series B*, *45*, (1–10):335-343. https://doi.org/10.1111/j.1439-0450.1998.tb00802.x

Wertz, A. E., Knight, T. J., Trenkle, A., Sonon, R., Horst, R. L., Huff-Lonergan, E. J., & Beitz, D. C. (2004). Feeding 25-hydroxyvitamin D$_3$ to improve beef tenderness. *Journal of Animal Science*, *82*(5), 1410–1418. https://doi.org/10.2527/2004.8251410x

Whanger, P. D. (1981). Selenium and heavy metal toxicity. In J. E. Spallholz, J. L. Martin, & H. E. Ganther (Eds.), *In "selenium in biology and medicine"*. AVI Publishing, Co.

Wherry, T. L., Dassanayake, R. P., Casas, E., Mooyottu, S., Bannantine, J. P., & Stabel, J. R. (2022). Exogenous vitamin D3 modulates response of bovine macrophages to Mycobacterium avium subsp. paratuber-culosis infection and is dependent upon stage of Johne's disease. *Frontiers in Cellular and Infection Microbiology*, *11*, 1446. https://doi.org/10.3389/fcimb.2021.773938

White, W. S., Peck, K. M., Ulman, E. A., & Erdman, Jr., J. W. (1993). The ferret as a model for evaluation of the bioavailabilities of all-trans-β-carotene and its isomers. *The Journal of Nutrition*, 123(6), 1129–1139. https://doi.org/10.1093/jn/123.6.1129

Whited, L. J., Hammond, B. H., Chapman, K. W., & Boor, K. J. (2002). Vitamin A degradation and light-oxidized flavor defects in milk. *Journal of Dairy Science*, 85(2), 351–354. https://doi.org/10.3168/jds.S0022-0302(02)74080-0

Whitfield, G. K., Hsieh, J. C., Jurutka, P. W., Selznick, S. H., Haussler, C. A., MacDonald, P. N., & Haussler, M. R. (1995). Genomic actions of 1,25-dihydroxyvitamin D3. *The Journal of Nutrition*, 125(6) (Suppl.), 1690S–1694S. https://doi.org/10.1093/jn/125.suppl_6.1690S

Whiting, F., & Loosli, J. K. (1948). The placental and mammary transfer of tocohperols [vitamin E] in sheep, goats and swine. *The Journal of Nutrition*, 36(6), 721–726. https://doi.org/10.1093/jn/36.6.721

Wiedermann, U., Hanson, L. A., Kahu, H., & Dahlgren, U. I. (1993). Aberrant T-cell function *in vitro* and impaired T-cell dependent antibody response *in vivo* in vitamin A-deficient rats. *Immunology*, 80(4), 581–586. PubMed: 8307607

Wiese, A. C., Johnson, B. C., & Nevens, W. B. (1946). Biotin deficiency in the dairy calf. *Proceedings of the Society for Experimental Biology and Medicine. Society for Experimental Biology and Medicine*, 63(3), 521. https://doi.org/10.3181/00379727-63-15657p

Williams, P. E. V., Ballet, N., & Robert, J. C. (1998) Provision of Vitamins and Amino Acids for Ruminants. A review of the provision of vitamins for ruminants. In *Proceedings of the Preconference Symposium of the Cornell Nutrition Conference* (pp. 7–37). Rhône Poulenc Animal Nutrition.

Williams, P. G. (2007). Nutritional composition of red meat. *Nutrition and Dietetics*, 64(s4), S113–S119. https://doi.org/10.1111/j.1747-0080.2007.00197.x

Wing, J. M. (1969). Effect of source and season on apparent digestibility of carotene in forage by cattle. *Journal of Dairy Science*, 52(4), 479–483. https://doi.org/10.3168/jds.S0022-0302(69)86591-4

Wise, M. B., Blumer, T. N., & Barrick, E. R. (1964) Effect of various levels of choline on performance and carcass characteristics of finishing steers fed on an all-concentrate ration. North Carolina Agri. Exp. Station. ANS Report 139.A.H, 10 p. 22.

Wisnieski, L., Brown, J. L., Holcombe, S. J., Gandy, J. C., & Sordillo, L. M. (2019). Serum vitamin D concentrations at dry-off and close-up predict increased postpartum urine ketone concentrations in dairy cattle. *Journal of Dairy Science*, 103(2), 1795–1806. https://doi.org/10.3168/jds.2019-16599

Witkowska, D., Sedrowicz, L., & Oledzka, R. (1992). Effect of a diet with an increased content of vitamin B$_6$ on the absorption of amino acids in the intestine of rats intoxicated with carbaryl propoxur and thiuram. Methionine. *Bromatologia Chemia Toksykoleziczna*, 25, 25.

Wolf, G. (1991). The intracellular vitamin A-binding proteins: An overview of their functions. *Nutrition Reviews*, 49(1), 1–12. https://doi.org/10.1111/j.1753-4887.1991.tb07349.x

Wolf, G. (1993). The newly discovered retinoic acid-X receptors (RXRs). *Nutrition Reviews*, 51(3), 81–84. https://doi.org/10.1111/j.1753-4887.1993.tb03075.x

Wolf, G. (1995). The enzymatic cleavage of beta-carotene: Still controversial. *Nutrition Reviews*, 53(5), 134–137. https://doi.org/10.1111/j.1753-4887.1995.tb01537.x

Wolf, G. (2006). How an increased intake of α-tocopherol can suppress the bioavailability of gamma-tocopherol. *Nutrition Reviews*, 64(6), 295–299. https://doi.org/10.1111/j.1753-4887.2006.tb00213.x

Wolf, G. (2007). Identification of a membrane receptor for retinol-binding protein functioning in the cellular uptake of retinol. *Nutrition Reviews*, 66(8), 385–388. https://doi.org/10.1111/j.1753-4887.2007.tb00316.x

Wolf, G. and Carpenter, K.J. (1997) Early Research into the vitamins: the work of Wilhelm Stepp. *J. Nutr.* 127(7):1255–1259. https://doi.org/10.1093/jn/127.7.1255

Won, J. H., Oishi, N., Kawamura, T., Sugiwaka, T., Fukuda, S., Sato, R., & Naito, Y. (1996). Mineral metabolism in plasma, urine and bone of periparturient cows fed anionic diets with different calcium and phosphorus contents. *The Journal of Veterinary Medical Science*, 58(12), 1187–1192. https://doi.org/10.1292/jvms.58.12_1187

Woolley, D. W. (2012). Antimetabolites of the water-soluble vitamins. "*Metabolic Inhibitors*". https://dtk.tankonyvtar.hu/xmlui/bitstream/handle/123456789/8939/B9780123956224500173.pdf?sequence=17&isAllowed=y. In.

Wu, H. M., Zhang, J., Wang, C., Liu, Q., Guo, G., Huo, W. J., Chen, L., Zhang, Y. L., Pei, C. X., & Zhang, S. L. (2021). Effects of riboflavin supplementation on performance, nutrient digestion, rumen microbiota composition and activities of Holstein bulls. *The British Journal of Nutrition*, *126*(9), 1288–1295. https://doi.org/10.1017/S0007114520005243

Xiao, J., Khan, M. Z., Ma, Y., Alugongo, G. M., Ma, J., Chen, T., Khan, A., & Cao, Z. (2021). The antioxidant properties of selenium and vitamin E; their role in periparturient dairy cattle health regulation. *Antioxidants*, *10*(10), 1555. https://doi.org/10.3390/antiox10101555

Xu, H. G., Zhang, Q. Y., Wang, L. H., Zhang, C., Li, Y., & Zhang, Y. G. (2021). Effects of 25-hydroxyvitamin D3 and oral calcium bolus on lactation performance, Ca homeostasis, and health of multiparous dairy cows. *Animals: An Open Access Journal from MDPI*, *11*(6), 1576. https://doi.org/10.3390/ani11061576

Xu, Y., Chen, J., Yu, X., Tao, W., Jiang, F., Yin, Z., & Liu, C. (2010). Protective effects of chlorogenic acid on acute hepatotoxicity induced by lipopolysaccharide in mice. *Inflammation Research*, *59*(10), 871–877. https://doi.org/10.1007/s00011-010-0199-z

Xu, Y., Sladky, J. T., & Brown, M. J. (1989). Dose-dependent expression of neuronopathy after experimental pyridoxine intoxication. *Neurology*, *39*(8), 1077–1083. https://doi.org/10.1212/wnl.39.8.1077

Xue, G. P., Snoswell, A. M., & Runciman, W. B. (1986). Perturbation of methionine metabolism in sheep with nitrous-oxide-induced inactivation of cobalamin. *Biochemistry International*, *12*(1), 61–69. PubMed: 2868723

Yamada, K., Shimodaira, M., Chida, S., Yamada, N., Matsushima, N., Fukuda, M., & Yamada, S. (2008). Degradation of vitamin B$_{12}$ in dietary supplements. *International Journal for Vitamin and Nutrition Research. Internationale Zeitschrift Fur Vitamin- und Ernahrungsforschung. Journal International de Vitaminologie et de Nutrition*, *78*(4–5), 195–203. https://doi.org/10.1024/0300-9831.78.45.195

Yang, A., Larsen, T. W., & Tume, R. K. (1992). Carotenoid and retinol concentrations in serum, adipose tissue and liver and carotenoid transport in sheep, goats and cattle. *Australian Journal of Agricultural Research*, *43*(8), 1809–1817. https://doi.org/10.1071/AR9921809

Yang, A., Brewster, M. J., Lanari, M. C., & Tume, R. K. (2002a). Effect of vitamin E supplementation on α-tocopherol and β-carotene concentrations in tissues from pasture- and grain-fed cattle. *Meat Science*, *60*(1), 35–40. https://doi.org/10.1016/S0309-1740(01)00102-4

Yang, A., Lanari, M. C., Brewster, M., & Tume, R. K. (2002b). Lipid stability and meat colour of beef from pasture- and grain-fed cattle with or without vitamin E supplement. *Meat Science*, *60*(1), 41–50. https://doi.org/10.1016/S0309-1740(01)00103-6

Yang, P., & Ma, Y. (2021). Recent advances of vitamin D in immune, reproduction, performance for pig: A review. *Animal Health Research Reviews*, *22*(1), 85–95. https://doi.org/10.1017/S1466252321000049

Yang, P., Wang, H., Li, L., Zhang, N., & Ma, Y. (2021a). The stability of vitamin A from different sources in vitamin premixes and vitamin-trace mineral premixes. *Applied Sciences*, *11*(8), 3657. https://doi.org/10.3390/app11083657

Yang, P., Wang, H., Li, L., Zhang, N., & Ma, Y. (2021b). Determination and evaluation of bioavailability of vitamins from different multivitamin supplements using a pig model. *Agriculture*, *11*(5), 418. https://doi.org/10.3390/agriculture11050418

Yang, P., Wang, H. K., Zhu, M., Li, L. X., & Ma, Y. X. (2021c). Degradation kinetics of vitamins in premixes for pig: Effects of choline, high concentrations of copper and zinc, and storage time. *Animal Bioscience*, *34*(4), 701–713. https://doi.org/10.5713/ajas.20.0026

Yao, X., Ei-Samahy, M. A., Yang, H., Feng, X., Li, F., Meng, F., Nie, H., & Wang, F. (2018). Age-associated expression of vitamin D receptor and vitamin D-metabolizing enzymes in the male reproductive tract and sperm of Hu sheep. *Animal Reproduction Science*, *190*, 27–38. https://doi.org/10.1016/j.anireprosci.2018.01.003

Yassen, H. A., Attia, K. A. A., Shamiah, S. M., El-Arian, M. N., & El-Harairy, M. A. (2020). Effect of addition vitamin C and zinc chloride in vitrification medium on viability, in vitro maturation and ultrastructure changes of vitrified immature bovine oocytes. *Journal of Animal and Poultry Production*, 441–447. https://doi.org/10.21608/jappmu.2020.130060

Yeum, K. J., dos Anjos Ferreira, A. L., Smith, D., Krinsky, N. I., & Russell, R. M. (2000). The effect of α-tocopherol on oxidative cleavage of beta carotene. *Free Radical Biology and Medicine*, *29*(2), 105–114. https://doi.org/10.1016/S0891-5849(00)00296-3

Yonekura, L., & Nagao, A. (2007). Intestinal absorption of dietary carotenoids. *Molecular Nutrition and Food Research*, *51*(1), 107–115. https://doi.org/10.1002/mnfr.200600145

Young, L. G., Lun, A., Pos, J., Forshaw, R. P., & Edmeades, D. (1975). Vitamin E stability in corn and mixed feed. *Journal of Animal Science*, *40*(3), 495–499. https://doi.org/10.2527/jas1975.403495x

Yue, Y., Hymøller, L., Jensen, S. K., & Lauridsen, C. (2018). Effect of vitamin D treatments on plasma metabolism and immune parameters of healthy dairy cows. *Archives of Animal Nutrition*, *72*(3), 205–220. https://doi.org/10.1080/1745039X.2018.1448564

Zahra, L. C., Duffield, T. F., Leslie, K. E., Overton, T. R., Putnam, D., & LeBlanc, S. J. (2006). Effects of rumen-protected choline and monensin on milk production and metabolism of periparturient dairy cows. *Journal of Dairy Science*, *89*(12), 4808–4818. https://doi.org/10.3168/jds.S0022-0302(06)72530-9

Zamora, R., Hidalgo, F. J., & Tappel, A. L. (1991). Comparative antioxidant effectiveness of dietary beta carotene, vitamin E, selenium and coenzyme Q10 in rat erythrocytes and plasma. *The Journal of Nutrition*, *121*(1), 50–56. https://doi.org/10.1093/jn/121.1.50

Zanker, I. A., Hammon, H. M., & Blum, J. W. (2000). Beta-carotene, retinol and alpha- tocopherol status in calves fed the first colostrum at 0–2, 6–7, 12–13 or 24–25 hours after birth. *International Journal for Vitamin and Nutrition Research. Internationale Zeitschrift Fur Vitamin- und Ernahrungsforschung. Journal International de Vitaminologie et de Nutrition*, *70*(6), 305–310. https://doi.org/10.1024/0300-9831.70.6.305

Zebeli, Q., & Ametaj, B. N. (2009). Relationships between rumen lipopolysaccharide and mediators of inflammatory response with milk fat production and efficiency in dairy cows. *Journal of Dairy Science*, *92*(8), 3800–3809. https://doi.org/10.3168/jds.2009-2178

Zee, J. A., Carmichael, L., Codère, D., Poirier, D., & Fournier, M. (1991). Effect of storage conditions on the stability of vitamin C in various fruits and vegetables produced and consumed in Quebec. *Journal of Food Composition and Analysis*, *4*(1), 77–86. https://doi.org/10.1016/0889-1575(91)90050-G. Zee, J. A., Carmichael, L., Codère, D., Poirier, D., & Fournier, M.. (1991) Effect of storage conditions on the stability of vitamin C in various fruits and vegetables produced and consumed in Quebec. *Journal of Food Composition and Analysis*, *4*(1), 77–86. https://doi.org/10.1016/0889-1575(91)90050-G

Zeisel, S. H. (1990). Choline deficiency. *The Journal of Nutritional Biochemistry*, *1*(7), 332–349. https://doi.org/10.1016/0955-2863(90)90001-2

Zeisel, S. H. (2006). Choline: Critical role during fetal development and dietary requirements in adults. *Annual Review of Nutrition*, *26*, 229–250. https://doi.org/10.1146/annurev.nutr.26.061505.111156

Zeisel, S. H., Klatt, K. C., & Caudill, M. A. (2018). Choline. *Advances in Nutrition*, *9*(1), 58–60. https://doi.org/10.1093/advances/nmx004

Zeisel, S. H., & Niculescu, M. D. (2006). Perinatal choline influences brain structure and function. *Nutrition Reviews*, *64*(4), 197–203. https://doi.org/10.1111/j.1753-4887.2006.tb00202.x

Zempleni, J., & Mock, D. M. (1999). Biotin biochemistry and human requirements. *The Journal of Nutritional Biochemistry*, *10*(3), 128–138. https://doi.org/10.1016/S0955-2863(98)00095-3

Zempleni, J., Rucker, R. B., McCormick, D. B., & Suttie, J. W. (2007). Handbook of vitamins" R. B. Rucker, J. W. Suttie, D. B. McCormick, & L. J. Machlin (Eds.) (4th ed.). CRC Press, Taylor & Francis Group, LLC Ratón Fl. USA. 593.

Zenobi, M. G., Gardinal, R., Zuniga, J. E., Mamedova, L. K., Driver, J. P., Barton, B. A., Santos, J. E. P., Staples, C. R., & Nelson, C. D. (2020). Effect of prepartum energy intake and supplementation with ruminally protected choline on innate and adaptive immunity of multiparous Holstein cows. *Journal of Dairy Science*, *103*(3), 2200–2216. https://doi.org/10.3168/jds.2019-17378

Zhang, J. Z., Henning, S. M., & Swendseid, M. E. (1993). Poly(ADP-ribose) polymerase activity and DNA strand breaks are affected in tissues of niacin-deficient rats. *The Journal of Nutrition*, *123*(8), 1349–1355. https://doi.org/10.1093/jn/123.8.1349

Zhang, Y., Gao, E., Guan, H., Wang, Q., Zhang, S., Liu, K., Yan, F., Tian, H., Shan, D., Xu, H., & Hou, J. (2020). Vitamin C treatment of embryos, but not donor cells, improves the cloned embryonic development in sheep. *Reproduction in Domestic Animals*, *55*(3), 255–265. https://doi.org/10.1111/rda.13606

Zhao, Z., & Ross, A. C. (1995). Retinoic acid repletion restores the number of leukocytes in vitamin A deficient rats. *The Journal of Nutrition*, *125*(8), 2064–2073. https://doi.org/10.1093/jn/125.8.2064

Zheng, W., & Teegarden, D. (2013). Vitamin D. In J. Zempleni, J. Suttie, J. Gregory, & P. J. Stover (Eds.), *Handbook of vitamins* (5th ed.) (pp. 51–88). CRC Press, Taylor & Francis Group, LLC. https://doi.org/10.1201/b15413

Zhou, P., McEvoy, T. G., Gill, A. C., Lambe, N. R., Morgan-Davies, C. R., Hurst, E., Sargison, N. D., & Mellanby, R. J. (2019). Investigation of relationship between vitamin D status and reproductive fitness in Scottish hill sheep. *Scientific Reports*, *9*(1), 1162. https://doi.org/10.1038/s41598-018-37843-6

Zimbelman, R. B., Baumgard, L. H., & Collier, R. J. (2010). Effects of encapsulated niacin on evaporative heat loss and body temperature in moderately heat-stressed lactating Holstein cows. *Journal of Dairy Science*, *93*(6), 2387–2394. https://doi.org/10.3168/jds.2009-2557

Zimmerly, C. A., & Weiss, W. P. (2001). Effects of supplemental biotin on performance of Holstein cows in early lactation. *Journal of Dairy Science*, *84*(2), 498–506. https://doi.org/10.3168/jds.S0022-0302(01)74500-6

Zimmerman, C. A., Rakes, A. H., Daniel, T. E., & Hopkins, B. A. (1992). Influence of dietary protein and supplemental niacin on lactational performance of cows fed normal and low fiber diets. *Journal of Dairy Science*, *75*(7), 1965–1978. https://doi.org/10.3168/jds.S0022-0302(92)77956-9

Zinn, R. A. (1992). B-vitamins in beef cattle nutrition. In Takeda Technical Symposium. 53rd Minnesota Nutrition Conference. September 21.

Zinn, R. A., Owens, F. N., Stuart, R. L., Dunbar, J. R., & Norman, B. B. (1987). B-vitamin supplementation of diets for feedlot calves. *Journal of Animal Science*, *65*(1), 267–277. https://doi.org/10.2527/jas1987.651267x

Zinn, R. A., Alvarez, E., & Stuart, R. L. (1996). Interaction of supplemental vitamin A and E on health and performance of crossbred and Holstein calves during the receiving period. *The Professional Animal Scientist*, *12*(1), 14–20. https://doi.org/10.15232/S1080-7446(15)32476-1

Zobell, D. R., Schaefer, A. L., LePage, P. L., Eddy, L., Briggs, G., & Stanley, R. (1995). Gestational vitamin E supplementation in beef cows: Effect on calf immunological competence, growth and morbidity. *Proceedings of the West Sect. Am. Soc. Animal Science*, *46*, 464.

Zom, R., Van Baal, J., De Veth, M. J., Goselink, R. M. A., Widjaja-Greefkes, H. C. A., Bakker, J. A., & Van Vuuren, A. M. (2010). Effects of rumen-protected choline on performance and hepatic fat metabolism in periparturient dairy cattle. *Journal of Dairy Science*, *93*(1), 781. https://doi.org/10.3168/jds.2011-4233

Index